Multiple Myeloma

Morie A. Gertz • S. Vincent Rajkumar
Editors

Multiple Myeloma

Diagnosis and Treatment

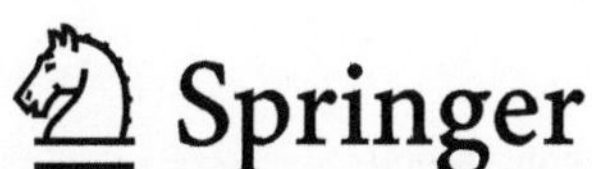

Springer

Editors
Morie A. Gertz, M.D., M.A.C.P.
Department of Internal Medicine
Division of Hematology
Mayo Clinic
Rochester, MN, USA

S. Vincent Rajkumar, M.D.
Myeloma Amyloidosis Dysproteinemia Group
Division of Hematology
Mayo Clinic
Rochester, MN, USA

ISBN 978-1-4614-8519-3 ISBN 978-1-4614-8520-9 (eBook)
DOI 10.1007/978-1-4614-8520-9
Springer New York Heidelberg Dordrecht London

Library of Congress Control Number: 2013949155

Printed on acid-free paper

Springer is part of Springer Science+Business Media (www.springer.com)

Preface

Advances in multiple myeloma and related plasma cell disorders are occurring at an unprecedented pace. These include dramatic changes not only in diagnosis and therapy but also in our understanding of the biological basis of these complex neoplastic disorders. We are thrilled with the advances, but at the same time recognize the challenges and confusion that occur. There are a plethora of guidelines and recommendations from expert panels that are often contradictory. Furthermore, availability and access to modern drugs are not uniform across the world, resulting in widely varied treatment approaches. In this book, we have assembled a multidisciplinary collection of experts from the Mayo Clinic to present the latest aspects of the biology and management of a wide spectrum of plasma cell disorders. Every chapter is written by a recognized authority in the field. As editors, we have ensured that the authors provide clear guidelines on diagnosis and therapy.

The book covers all aspects of multiple myeloma, including molecular classification, diagnosis, risk stratification, and therapy. In addition, we have also included and discussed in detail closely related plasma cell disorders such as solitary plasmacytoma, Waldenstrom macroglobulinemia, and light chain amyloidosis. Often neglected areas such as the role of radiation therapy, vertebral augmentation, and supportive care are also discussed in detail.

This work represents the collective view of a large group of physicians who are uniquely positioned to address the complexity of the issues not only based on the large patient volume we serve but also because of the close interactions that can only occur in an integrated and collaborative practice environment. We have very much enjoyed putting this book together, and we hope that it is of use and value to clinicians and researchers interested in this fascinating group of disorders.

Rochester, MN, USA Morie A. Gertz
Rochester, MN, USA S. Vincent Rajkumar

Contents

Contributors

Stephen M. Ansell M.D., Ph.D., Division of Hematology, Mayo Clinic, Rochester, MN, USA

Camilo Ayala-Breton Department of Molecular Medicine, Mayo Clinic, Rochester, MN, USA

P. Leif Bergsagel M.D., Division of Hematology Research and Division of Hematoloy/Oncology, Mayo Clinic, Scottsdale, AZ, USA

Francis Buadi M.B., Ch.B., Division of Hematology, Mayo Clinic, Rochester, MN, USA

Marta Chesi Ph.D., Division of Biochemistry and Molecular Biology, Mayo Clinic, Scottsdale, AZ, USA

David Dingli M.D., Ph.D., Division of Hematology, Department of Internal Medicine, Mayo Clinic, Rochester, MN, USA

Angela Dispenzieri M.D., Division of Hematology, Mayo Clinic, Rochester, MN, USA

Kathleen A. Donovan Ph.D., Division of Hematology, Mayo Clinic, Rochester, MN, USA

Matthew T. Drake M.D., Ph.D., Division of Endocrinology, Mayo Clinic, Rochester, MN, USA

Rafael Fonseca M.D., Center for Individualized Medicine, Mayo Clinic Cancer Center, Scottsdale, AZ, USA

Division of Hematology, Mayo Clinic, SW, Rochester, MN, USA

Morie A. Gertz M.D., M.A.C.P., Division of Hematology, Mayo Clinic, Rochester, MN, USA

Philip R. Greipp M.D., Division of Hematology, Mayo Clinic, Rochester, MN, USA

Suzanne R. Hayman Division of Hematology, Mayo Clinic, Rochester, MN, USA

Lucy S. Hodge Division of Hematology, Mayo Clinic, Rochester, MN, USA

Diane F. Jelinek Ph.D., Division of Hematology, Department of Immunology, Mayo Clinic, Rochester, MN, USA

Dragan Jevremovic M.D., Ph.D., Division of Hematopathology, Mayo Clinic, Rochester, MN, USA

David Kallmes M.D., Division of Radiology, Mayo Clinic, Rochester, MN, USA

Prashant Kapoor M.D., Division of Hematology, Department of Internal Medicine, Mayo Clinic, Rochester, MN, USA

Chafic Y. Karam M.D., Department of Neurology, Mayo Clinic, Rochester, MN, USA

Jerry A. Katzmann Ph.D., Division of Clinical Biochemistry & Immunology, Department of Laboratory Medicine & Pathology, Mayo Clinic, Rochester, MN, USA

Asher Chanan Khan M.D., Division of Hematology and Medical Oncology, Mayo Clinic Florida, Jacksonville, FL, USA

Omar Khan M.D., Division of Radiology, Mayo Clinic, Rochester, MN, USA

Shaji Kumar M.D., Division of Hematology, Mayo Clinic, Rochester, MN, USA

Robert A. Kyle M.D., Division of Hematology, Mayo Clinic, Rochester, MN, USA

Martha Q. Lacy M.D., Division of Hematology, Mayo Clinic, Rochester, MN, USA

Nelson Leung M.D., Division of Hematology, Mayo Clinic, Rochester, MN, USA

John A. Lust M.D., Ph.D., Division of Hematology, Mayo Clinic, Rochester, MN, USA

James A. Martenson M.D., Division of Radiation Oncology, Mayo Clinic, Rochester, MN, USA

Michelle L. Mauermann M.D., Department of Neurology, Mayo Clinic, Rochester, MN, USA

Arleigh McCurdy M.D., Division of Hematology, Mayo Clinic, Rochester, MN, USA

Joseph Mikhael M.D., Division of Hematology and Medical Oncology, Mayo Clinic Arizona, Scottsdale, AZ, USA

William Morice M.D., Ph.D., Division of Hematopathology, Mayo Clinic, Rochester, MN, USA

Kah-Whye Peng Department of Molecular Medicine, Mayo Clinic, Rochester, MN, USA

S. Vincent Rajkumar M.D., Myeloma Amyloidosis Dysproteinemia Group, Division of Hematology, Mayo Clinic, Rochester, MN, USA

Craig B. Reeder M.D., Division of Hematology/Oncology, Mayo Clinic, Scottsdale, AZ, USA

Vivek Roy M.D., Division of Hematology and Oncology, Mayo Clinic, Jacksonville, FL, USA

Stephen J. Russell M.D., Ph.D., Division of Hematology and Department of Molecular Medicine, Mayo Clinic, Rochester, MN, USA

Steven R. Schuster M.D., Division of Hematology and Medical Oncology, Mayo Clinic Arizona, Scottsdale, AZ, USA

Keith Stewart M.B., Ch.B., Division of Hematology, Mayo Clinic, SW, Rochester, MN, USA

Mayo Clinic in Arizona, Scottsdale, AZ, USA

Steven R. Zeldenrust M.D., Ph.D., Division of Hematology, Mayo Clinic, Rochester, MN, USA

1 Criteria for Diagnosis and Response

Robert A. Kyle and S. Vincent Rajkumar

Introduction

Multiple myeloma accounts for about 1 % of all types of malignancy and slightly more than 10 % of hematologic malignancies [1]. The incidence of multiple myeloma in the United States has increased from 0.8/100,000 persons in 1949 to 1.7/100,000 in 1963 and then to 3.5/100,000 for males in 1988. The incidence was 3.1/100,000 from 1945 to 1964 in Olmsted County, Minnesota, 2.7/100,000 from 1965 to 1977, 4.1/100,000 from 1978 to 1990, and 4.3/100,000 from 1991 to 2001 [2]. There was no change in incidence in Olmsted County over the 56-year period. The increased incidence reported during the past few decades in The United States is most likely due to the increased availability of medical facilities for elderly patients and improved diagnostic techniques rather than an actual increased incidence. The incidence of multiple myeloma is approximately twice as high in the African-American population as in the white population.

R.A. Kyle, M.D. (✉)
Division of Hematology, Mayo Clinic,
200 First Street, SW, Rochester, MN 55905, USA
e-mail: kyle.robert@mayo.edu

S.V. Rajkumar, M.D.
Division of Hematology, Myeloma Amyloidosis
Dysproteinemia Group, Mayo Clinic,
Rochester, MN, USA
e-mail: rajkumar.vincent@mayo.edu

Clinical Manifestations

Symptoms

The most important symptom of multiple myeloma is bone pain which is reported by more than 60 % of patients at the time of diagnosis [3]. The pain occurs most often in the back or ribs and less often in the extremities and is usually induced by movement. Sudden pain in the ribs accompanied by localized tenderness indicates a rib fracture even if the X-rays show no abnormalities. Sudden, severe back pain from a compression fracture may occur after a fall or even lifting a minor object. During the course of the disease a patient may lose 5 or 6 inches in height because of multiple vertebral collapses.

Weakness and fatigue may be a major complaint. This is often due to anemia which is present initially in more than 70 % of patients at diagnosis and occurs in almost all patients during the course of their disease. The anemia is normocytic and normochromic and often is due to bone marrow replacement by myeloma cells or renal insufficiency.

Symptoms may result from renal insufficiency, hypercalcemia, or neurologic features and will be discussed separately.

M.A. Gertz and S.V. Rajkumar (eds.), *Multiple Myeloma: Diagnosis and Treatment*,
DOI 10.1007/978-1-4614-8520-9_1,

Physical Findings

The most frequent physical finding is pallor. Skeletal deformities, pathologic fractures, localized bone tenderness, or purpura may also be present. Extramedullary plasmacytomas may present as purplish subcutaneous masses that range from less than 1 cm to more than 10 cm. They occur initially in approximately 5 % of patients and in an additional 5 % of patients during long-term follow-up.

The liver is palpable in less than 5 % of patients while splenomegaly is present in approximately 1 %. Lymphadenopathy is uncommon.

Multiple myeloma is a disease of older persons. The age ranges from the teens to the 90s [4]. The median age is about 70 years with 90 % of patients older than 50 years. Only 2 % of patients are less than 40 years of age while 0.3 % are less than 30 years of age. Very rarely myeloma can occur in children, but most of the reports in the older literature of children with myeloma are probably erroneous. Almost 60 % of patients in our practice are male.

Renal Involvement

Patients with multiple myeloma may present with acute or more often chronic renal failure. Almost one-half of patients have an elevated serum creatinine at diagnosis. The serum creatinine is >2 mg/dL in approximately 20 % of our patients at the time of diagnosis. The major causes of renal failure are "myeloma kidney" from cast nephropathy or hypercalcemia. Cast nephropathy is characterized by the presence of large, waxy, laminated casts consisting mostly of precipitated monoclonal light chains (Bence Jones protein) and are seen mainly in the distal and collecting tubules. The extent of cast formation correlates in general with the amount of free urinary light chain and the severity of renal insufficiency. Other causes of renal insufficiency include light chain (AL) amyloidosis, light chain deposition disease, or drug-induced renal damage.

Acute renal failure may be the initial manifestation of multiple myeloma. The diagnosis of multiple myeloma may not be apparent until the recognition of Bence Jones proteinuria or other features of myeloma. Dehydration or hypotension are major precipitating events. Intravenous urography rarely causes renal failure if dehydration is avoided.

An Acquired Fanconi Syndrome may develop. It is characterized by proximal tubular dysfunction that results in glycosuria, phosphaturia, and aminoaciduria. A common clue is a very low serum uric acid value without an apparent cause [5].

Hypercalcemia

Hypercalcemia (≥11 mg/dL) is found in 10–15 % of patients at diagnosis. It may develop at any time during the course of the disease. Symptoms include weakness, fatigue, polydipsia, polyuria, constipation, anorexia, nausea, vomiting, confusion, stupor, or coma. The patient or caregiver must be alert for this complication and notify his/her physician so that a serum calcium can be obtained. Lack of recognition may lead to chronic renal failure or even death. Rarely the patient's monoclonal protein may bind calcium producing a very high serum calcium level without symptoms of hypercalcemia because the ionized calcium level is normal. These patients must be recognized and not treated for hypercalcemia [6].

Neurological Involvement

Radiculopathy is the most frequently observed neurological complication. It is usually caused by compression of a nerve by a paravertebral plasma cell tumor or rarely by the collapsed bone itself.

Spinal cord compression results when a plasmacytoma arising in the marrow cavity of the vertebra extends into the extradural space compressing the spinal cord. It occurs in less than 5 % of patients with multiple myeloma. It should always be suspected in patients with back pain accompanied by paresthesias of the lower extremities, weakness of the legs or bladder or bowel dysfunction. Patients must contact their physician immediately and have magnetic resonance imaging (MRI) or computed tomographic myelography (CT) as an emergency. The entire spine must be examined because extramedullary plasmacytomas may occur at multiple levels. The thoracic spine is most often involved. Immediate therapy with dexamethasone and local radiation therapy often leads to recovery.

Peripheral neuropathy is uncommon in multiple myeloma and when present is usually due to AL amyloidosis or another unrelated cause. The possibility of POEMS syndrome (osteosclerotic myeloma) must be considered in any patient with a serum M-protein and bone marrow plasmacytosis. In addition to the peripheral neuropathy, osteosclerotic bone lesions occur in almost all patients with POEMS. Enlargement of the liver or spleen may be present as well as multiple endocrine abnormalities, a plasma cell proliferative process, and skin changes [7].

Leptomeningeal Myelomatosis

Leptomeningeal myelomatosis is uncommon but is being recognized more frequently in advanced stages of myeloma [8]. It is more likely to be found in patients with chromosome 17p 13.1 (p53) deletions [9]. Survival may have improved modestly with the use of novel agents, but it is a very serious complication [10]. The cerebrospinal fluid contains monoclonal plasma cells.

Intracranial plasmacytomas are rare and, when present, are usually from extensions of a myelomatous lesion of the skull expanding inward or involvement of the clivus or base of the skull. Encephalopathy from high blood levels of ammonia have been recognized [11].

Infection

Infections are common in patients with multiple myeloma. The cause of infections is multifactorial and due to an impaired antibody response, reduction in normal polyclonal (background) immunoglobulin levels, neutropenia, and corticosteroid therapy. Infection is often manifested by pneumonia, septicemia, or meningitis. Streptococcus pneumonia and gram negative organisms are the most frequent causes.

Organ Infiltration

Organ infiltration may occur. Occasionally plasma cells infiltrate the rugal folds of the stomach or a plasmacytoma develops in the stomach with bleeding and pain as the initial symptoms. Hepatomegaly, jaundice, ascites, and plasma cell infiltration are uncommon. Rarely the gallbladder, bile ducts, pancreas, and large and small bowel are involved by plasma cell infiltration. IgA myeloma is more common than IgG when the GI tract is involved.

The ribs and sternum are frequently involved and characterized by localized, painless swelling associated with the plasma cell tumors. Pain develops when a pathologic fracture occurs. Asymptomatic plasmacytomas may appear on a routine chest X-ray. Occasionally the radiographic changes are interpreted as a primary tumor of the lung and the rib involvement is overlooked. Occasionally extramedullary involvement of the mediastinum, mediastinal lymph nodes, or lung is an initial finding. Pleural effusion associated with plasma cell deposits in the pleura may occur late in the disease. Rarely myeloma involves the pericardium and produces effusion and tamponade. Myeloma may involve the orbit and produce diplopia or subsequently loss of vision.

Both bleeding and thrombotic events may occur. Bleeding is often aggravated by thrombocytopenia or qualitative platelet abnormalities presumably due to the presence of a large monoclonal protein. Abnormalities of clot retraction may contribute to bleeding along with hyperviscosity, intravascular coagulation, and the presence of amyloidosis. Deep vein thrombosis and pulmonary embolism may also be the precipitating event of multiple myeloma.

Laboratory Findings

Anemia

Normocytic normochromic anemia is present at the time of diagnosis in about 70 % of patients with symptomatic multiple myeloma. Leukocyte and neutrophil levels are usually normal, but thrombocytopenia is found in about 5 % of patients at diagnosis. Overt hemolytic anemia is rare in patients with myeloma.

Peripheral Blood Smear

The most frequent finding in the peripheral blood smear is rouleaux formation and should alert the examiner to the possibility of myeloma. A leukoerythroblastic condition (presence of immature leukocytes and nucleated red cells) may be present.

Only an occasional monoclonal plasma cell is found in the Wright stain smear in myeloma. However, circulating monoclonal plasma cells can be detected using a slide-based immunofluorescence assay or flow cytometry by gating on CD38 plus/CD45 negative cells. Approximately 10 % of patients have an absolute peripheral blood plasma cell count ≥100 cells/μL ($\geq 0.1 \times 10^9$/L). The presence of plasma cell leukemia occurs in approximately 1 % of patients with myeloma. It is characterized by the presence of more than 20 % circulating plasma cells and/or an absolute count $>2 \times 10^9$/L plasma cells in the peripheral blood [12, 13].

Serum and Urine M-Proteins

The serum protein electrophoretic pattern shows a single narrow peak or localized band in 80 % of patients. Hypogammaglobulinemia is present in 10 % while the remainder have an equivocal abnormality or a normal-appearing pattern. IgG accounts for approximately 50 % of cases while IgA is found in 20 % and light chain only in 15–20 %. IgD is present in 2 % while IgM is found in 0.5 % and a biclonal protein is found in 2 %. Immunofixation will identify a monoclonal protein in the serum in more than 90 % of patients. Kappa light chains are found twice as often as lambda.

Ninety percent of myeloma patients have a reduction of one of the uninvolved immunoglobulins. For example, reduction of IgM or IgG in the presence of an IgA myeloma occurs in 90 % of patients while both uninvolved immunoglobulins are reduced in almost three-fourths of patients. Normal values of the uninvolved immunoglobulins were present at diagnosis in 3 % of IgA patients, 8 % of nonsecretory patients, 12 % of IgG, and 13 % of patients with light chain myeloma.

Urinalysis

The dipstick examination of urine detects albumin but frequently does not recognize light chains. Consequently, sulfosalicylic acid is necessary for detecting light chain protein in the urine. A 24-h urine collection should be done and an aliquot concentrated and then electrophoresis and immunofixation is performed. The presence of light chains in the urine produces a spike or localized band. This allows the laboratory to quantitate the amount of light chain produced per 24 h.

Between 15 and 20 % of patients with multiple myeloma have only light chains in the serum or urine and these are classified as "light chain myeloma." Approximately one-third of patients with light chain myeloma have a serum creatinine ≥2 mg/dL, but the overall survival is not different when compared to all cases of myeloma.

Nonsecretory Myeloma

Nonsecretory myeloma is characterized by the absence of M-protein in the serum or urine on immunofixation. The free light chain (FLC) assay will be abnormal in two-thirds myeloma patients who have a negative serum and urine immunofixation [14, 15]. A normal FLC ratio is found in patients with polyclonal increases of immunoglobulins or in the presence of renal insufficiency [16].

Patients with a negative serum and urine immunofixation and a normal serum FLC assay are considered to have nonsecretory myeloma. Almost 90 % of these patients will have an M-protein in the cytoplasm of the monoclonal plasma cells when utilizing immunochemistry. In the majority of patients with nonsecretory myeloma, they remain nonsecretory throughout the course of the disease. These patients do not develop myeloma kidney. Patients with nonsecretory myeloma must be monitored on the basis of imaging tests of the bone and bone marrow studies unless the FLC value is abnormal.

Oligosecretory Myeloma

Oligosecretory myeloma occurs in 5–10 % of patients and is defined as a serum M-protein <1 g/dL and urine M-protein <200 mg/24 h. These patients do not have a measurable M-protein in the serum or urine. The serum FLC assay is helpful in monitoring these patients if the involved FLC level is ≥10 mg/dL [17].

Bone Marrow Examination

A bone marrow aspirate and biopsy are essential for making the diagnosis of multiple myeloma. Monoclonal plasma cells usually account for more than 10 % of the bone marrow cells. However, we found in our series of 1,027 patients with symptomatic MM that 4 % had fewer than 10 % plasma cells. The median number of plasma cells in the bone marrow was 50 %. The patients with <10 % plasma cells had typical MM with lytic bone lesions, M-protein in the serum and urine, often anemia and required therapy. Presumably the small number of plasma cells detected is due to patchy involvement of the bone marrow. Consequently if fewer than 10 % plasma cells are found, the marrow aspirate and biopsy should be repeated at another site. Biopsy of a lytic lesion or an extramedullary plasmacytoma may also provide the diagnosis. The morphology is considered plasmablastic when plasmablasts comprise 2 % or more of the plasma cells [18].

The cytosplasm of the plasma cells contains either kappa or lambda light chains but not both. The normal kappa/lambda ratio in the bone marrow is 2:1, but a ratio greater than 4:1 or less than 1:1 meets the definition of kappa or lambda monoclonal protein, respectively. This is a critical determination because patients with both kappa and lambda staining (polyclonal) have a reactive plasma cell process due to metastatic carcinoma, chronic liver disease, autoimmune diseases, or chronic infection. Staining with CD138 identifies a plasma cell and is helpful in determining the number involved. Myeloma cells express CD38 and CD138. About two-thirds will express CD56 while CD19 is expressed in 10–15 % of patients.

Cytogenetics

There is no single cytogenetic abnormality that is typical or diagnostic of MM. Almost all myeloma tumors have genetic abnormalities that can be detected with interphase fluorescence in situ hybridization (FISH). Patients with deletion of 17p, t(14;16), or t(14;20) are considered to have high-risk myeloma and constitute about 20 % of patients. The presence of t(4;14) is an intermediate risk level while patients with t(11;14) and t(6;14) as well as hyperdiploidy are considered to be in the standard risk group [19]. Patients with deletion of chromosome 13 with conventional cytogenetics or hyperdiploidy are in an intermediate risk group. Gene expression profiling (GEP) may also prove to be useful.

Skeletal Findings

Conventional radiographs reveal lytic lesions, osteoporosis, or pathologic fractures in almost 80 % of patients at the time of diagnosis. The vertebra, skull, thoracic cage, pelvis, and proximal humeri and femori are the most frequently involved. Osteosclerotic changes are rare in MM [20]. When present, osteosclerotic lesions are often associated with metastatic cancer from the prostate or breast. Technetium (Tc-99M) bone scanning should not be used because it is inferior to conventional radiography. In fact, large lytic lesions may be overlooked because there is an absence of bone formation. Computerized tomography (CT), MRI, and Positron Emission Tomography (PET-CT) are more sensitive for detecting skeletal involvement.

MRI can detect diffuse and focal bone marrow lesions in patients with MM without osteopenia or lytic lesions on standard metastatic bone surveys. In one study of 611 patients with MM who had both MRI studies as well as a standard metastatic bone survey, the MRI detected focal lesions in 52 % of those with negative bone surveys while bone surveys detected focal lesions in 20 % of those with a negative MRI [21]. Gadolinium has been associated with nephrogenic systemic fibrosis when given to patients with moderate to advanced renal failure.

PET/CT scanning with Fluorine-18-labeled FDG correlates with areas of active bone disease; however, both false positive as well as false negative results have been reported [22].

Diagnosis

The diagnosis of MM is usually not difficult because most patients present with typical symptoms or laboratory abnormalities. Patients should initially have a complete history and physical examination. The family history should focus on first-degree relatives with the diagnosis of hematologic malignancies, especially monoclonal gammopathy of undetermined significance (MGUS), multiple myeloma and related disorders, and all types of leukemia and lymphoma. The past medical history should address comorbid conditions that may affect treatment decisions such as coronary artery disease, congestive heart failure, hypertension, renal disorders, liver disorders, and lung diseases. The history should pay specific attention to complaints of bone pain, constitutional symptoms, neurological symptoms, and previous infections. A detailed neurologic exam should be included in the physical examination. The tests listed in Table 1.1 should be performed [23]. A complete blood count with a differential should be ordered and a peripheral blood smear should be evaluated for rouleaux formation and circulating plasma cells. The biochemistry screen should include calcium, albumin, creatinine, lactate dehydrogenase, beta-2 microglobulin, and C-reactive protein. In addition, liver function tests, electrolytes, and renal function tests may be required.

Table 1.1 Laboratory tests for multiple myeloma

History and physical examination
Complete blood count and differential; peripheral blood smear
Chemistry screen, including calcium and creatinine
Serum protein electrophoresis, immunofixation
Nephelometric quantification of serum immunoglobulins
Routine urinalysis, 24-h urine collection for electrophoresis and immunofixation
Bone marrow aspirate and/or biopsy
Cytogenetics (metaphase karyotype and FISH)
Radiologic skeletal bone survey, including spine, pelvis, skull, humeri, and femurs;
Magnetic resonance imaging in certain circumstances
Serum β_2-microglobulin and lactate dehydrogenase
Measurement of serum-free light chains

This research was originally published in *Blood*. Dimopoulos M, Kyle RA, Fermand J-P, et al. Consensus recommendations for standard investigative workup: report of the International Myeloma Workshop Consensus Panel 3 *Blood*. 2011;117:4701–4705. © the American Society of Hematology

Both serum and urine must be studied for the presence of a monoclonal protein. Agarose gel electrophoresis or capillary zone electrophoresis of serum and urine is preferred to screen for the presence of a monoclonal protein. Quantitation of serum immunoglobulins by nephelometry should also be done. Thus, results by both the densitometer tracing and nephelometry are recommended for measurement of the monoclonal protein. These two tests are complimentary, but nephelometric quantitation may be particularly useful for low levels of uninvolved immunoglobulins [24]. It should be pointed out that nephelometric quantitation oftentimes overestimates the monoclonal protein concentration when its value is elevated. The presence of a monoclonal protein must be confirmed by immunofixation to determine its heavy and light chain type. Immunofixation of the serum should also be performed in the presence of hypogammaglobulinemia or when the serum electrophoretic pattern appears normal if there is a suspicion of MM or a related disorder. Frequently light chain myeloma is associated with hypogammaglobulinemia or a normal-appearing electrophoretic pattern. If only a monoclonal light chain is detected and immunofixation is negative for IgG, IgA, or IgM, the possibility of IgD or IgE monoclonal immunoglobulin must be excluded. Thus, if only a monoclonal light chain is found, immunofixation for IgD and IgE is required and, if positive, quantitation of IgD or IgE must be done. Immunosubtraction has been performed instead of immunofixation electrophoresis, but it is less sensitive and is not recommended at present.

Measurement of serum albumin is essential because albumin is a major component of the International Staging System for multiple myeloma [25]. The most accurate method of measuring serum albumin is by nephelometry, but this approach is not commonly used. Serum albumin can be measured by densitometry from the electrophoretic strip, but its value can be affected by the size of the monoclonal protein. High concentrations of M-protein tend to overestimate the level of serum albumin [26]. Serum albumin can also be measured with bromcresol. This method provides good correlation with the "gold standard" nephelometric quantitation and is independent of the monoclonal protein level. It has been reported that all albumin methods perform similarly in predicting survival and therefore may be used in prognostication by the International Staging System [26].

The serum FLC assay is recommended in all newly diagnosed patients with plasma cell dyscrasias [27, 28]. Measurement of the FLC is very useful for patients with multiple myeloma with negative serum and urine with immunofixation (nonsecretory) and in those who secrete small, nonmeasurable amounts of M-protein (oligosecretory) in the serum or urine. The FLC assay is useful in patients with MGUS, smoldering multiple myeloma (SMM), and solitary plasmacytoma of bone because an abnormal value is associated with a higher risk of progression to symptomatic myeloma [29–31]. The serum FLC measurement is not a substitute for a 24-h urine evaluation for proteins. In addition, urine FLC assays should not be performed. The serum FLC analysis may be used in place of a 24-h urine collection in conjunction with serum protein electrophoresis and immunofixation for screening purposes only [28]. However, if a plasma cell proliferative disorder is identified, electrophoresis of an aliquot from a 24-h urine specimen and immunofixation are required.

The serum viscosity should be measured if the M-protein concentration is greater than 4 g/dL or there are symptoms suggestive of hyperviscosity. A unilateral bone marrow aspirate and biopsy should be performed when multiple myeloma or a related disorder is suspected. If possible, a CD138 stain should be used to determine the percentage of plasma cells in the bone marrow biopsy. Clonality of plasma cells is established by identification of a monoclonal immunoglobulin in the cytoplasm of plasma cells by immunoperoxidase staining or by immunofluorescence [32]. Immunophenotyping by flow cytometry is another option, but the technique may not be readily available and standardized for general use. In addition, the plasma cell percentage cannot be determined by flow cytometry of the bone marrow aspirate. A bone marrow aspirate alone may be sufficient for diagnosis, but a trephine biopsy is useful because it may provide a more reliable assessment of plasma cell infiltration and a repeat procedure is not necessary if the initial bone marrow aspirate is inadequate. If both procedures are used, the higher number of plasma cells obtained by either procedure is used for diagnosis [33].

All patients should have FISH, preferably after sorting the plasma cells, with probes that include chromosome 17p 13, t(4;14), and t(14;16) [34]. If possible, standard metaphase cytogenetics should also be done; however, only 20–25 % provide useful information.

Serum beta-2 microglobulin reflects tumor burden and is a critical test for the International Staging System. Serum lactate dehydrogenase should also be done because it is an independent prognostic factor [25, 35]. A metastatic bone survey with plain radiographs including the humeri and femurs should be performed in all patients. They should include a posteroanterior view of the chest, anteroposterior and lateral views of the cervical, thoracic and lumbar spine, humeri, and femora, anteroposterior and lateral views of the skull, and anteroposterior view of the pelvis. If patients have a normal bone survey but have bone pain or a neurologic deficit due to possible spinal cord compression, they require additional imaging studies.

MRI is a noninvasive technique that gives information about bone marrow involvement by myeloma cells [36]. An MRI of the spine and pelvis is indicated in all patients with a presumed solitary plasmacytoma of bone [37]. An MRI should also be considered in patients with SMM because it can detect occult lesions and predict for more rapid progression to symptomatic myeloma [38, 39]. An MRI is most useful in symptomatic patients who have a painful area of the skeleton or for evaluation of cord compression. It is helpful in determining whether a new collapsed vertebral body is due to osteoporosis or myelomatous involvement. If a focal lesion of myeloma is found in the vertebral body, the patient has symptomatic myeloma and requires systemic therapy.

The role of PET CT is not clearly defined in multiple myeloma. It is useful for detection of extraosseous soft tissue masses as well as evaluation of rib and appendicular bone lesions. It is also useful in patients suspected to have extramedullary plasmacytoma.

Diagnostic Criteria

The International Myeloma Working Group (IMWG) Criteria for the diagnosis of symptomatic MM emphasizes the importance of end-organ damage in making the diagnosis of symptomatic multiple myeloma [40, 41].

The presence of organ damage includes the serum calcium level, renal insufficiency, anemia, and lytic bone lesions (CRAB). These abnormalities must be related to the underlying plasma cell proliferative disorder. The presence of an M-protein in the serum and/or urine is critical. No specific level of M-protein is used as a cutoff. Nonsecretory myeloma as determined by immunofixation constitutes about 3 %, but the serum FLC ratio is abnormal in approximately two-thirds of these patients. The presence of 10 % or more clonal bone marrow plasma cells is considered diagnostic, but one must realize that 4 or 5 % of patients with symptomatic MM may have fewer than 10 % bone marrow plasma cells. Histopathologic confirmation of a soft tissue or skeletal plasmacytoma may also allow the diagnosis. Metastatic carcinoma, connective tissue disorders, lymphoma, and leukemia must be excluded in the differential diagnosis.

The presence of end-organ damage may depend upon the clinician's judgment concerning the presence of end-organ damage. There is no provision for the diagnosis of myeloma before the development of end-organ damage. Patients without end-organ damage but who will progress to symptomatic disease in a short period of time must be identified. For example, patients without end-organ damage, but who have 60 % or more clonal bone marrow plasma cells almost always progress to symptomatic MM within 2 years [42]. Therefore, most agree that these patients should be treated even before end-organ damage occurs.

Other markers that predict a high likelihood of progression are a FLC ratio ≥100, high levels of circulating plasma cells, fewer than 5 % normal plasma cells by immunophenotyping, high plasma cell proliferative rate by S phase on flow cytometry, ≥3 focal lesions on MRI, deletion of 17p on cytogenetic studies, significant increases in M-protein or light chain levels and an unexplained decrease in creatinine clearance by ≥25 %, and a rise in serum FLC levels or urinary M-protein.

Differential Diagnosis

It is essential that the physician distinguishes MM from asymptomatic plasma cell disorders such as MGUS or SMM that do not require therapy. [43–46] The diagnostic criteria for MM and the related plasma cell disorders that it must be differentiated from are given on Table 1.2.

Monoclonal Gammopathy of Undetermined Significance (MGUS)

The diagnostic criteria are (1) the presence of a serum M-protein <3 g/dL, (2) clonal bone marrow plasma cells <10 %, and (3) the absence of end-organ damage such as hypercalcemia, renal insufficiency, anemia, and bone lesions (CRAB) that can be attributed to the plasma cell proliferative disorder.

Table 1.2 Diagnostic criteria for multiple myeloma and related plasma cell disorders

Disorder	Disease definition
Monoclonal gammopathy of undetermined significance (MGUS)	All 3 criteria must be met • Serum monoclonal protein <3 g/dL • Clonal bone marrow plasma cells <10 % • Absence of end-organ damage such as hypercalcemia, renal insufficiency, anemia, and bone lesions (CRAB) that can be attributed to the plasma cell proliferative disorder; or in the case of IgM MGUS no evidence of anemia, constitutional symptoms, hyperviscosity, lymphadenopathy, or hepatosplenomegaly that can be attributed to the underlying lymphoproliferative disorder
Smoldering multiple myeloma (also referred to as asymptomatic multiple myeloma)	Both criteria must be met • Serum monoclonal protein (IgG or IgA) ≥3 g/dL and/or clonal bone marrow plasma cells 10–60 % • Absence of end-organ damage such as lytic bone lesions, anemia, hypercalcemia, or renal failure that can be attributed to a plasma cell proliferative disorder
Multiple myeloma	All criteria must be met except as noted • Clonal bone marrow plasma cells ≥10 % or biopsy-proven plasmacytoma • Evidence of end-organ damage that can be attributed to the underlying plasma cell proliferative disorder, specifically – Hypercalcemia: serum calcium ≥11.5 mg/dL – Renal insufficiency: serum creatinine >1.73 mmol/L (or >2 mg/dL) or estimated creatinine clearance less than 40 mL/min – Anemia: normochromic, normocytic with a hemoglobin value of >2 g/dL below the lower limit of normal or a hemoglobin value <10 g/dL – Bone lesions: lytic lesions, severe osteopenia, or pathologic fractures • In the absence of end-organ damage: clonal bone marrow plasma cells ≥60 %
IgM monoclonal gammopathy of undetermined significance (IgM MGUS)	All 3 criteria must be met • Serum IgM monoclonal protein <3 g/dL • Bone marrow lymphoplasmacytic infiltration <10 % • No evidence of anemia, constitutional symptoms, hyperviscosity, lymphadenopathy, or hepatosplenomegaly that can be attributed to the underlying lymphoproliferative disorder
Smoldering Waldenström's macroglobulinemia (also referred to as indolent or asymptomatic Waldenström's macroglobulinemia)	Both criteria must be met • Serum IgM monoclonal protein ≥3 g/dL and/or bone marrow lymphoplasmacytic infiltration ≥10 % • No evidence of anemia, constitutional symptoms, hyperviscosity, lymphadenopathy, or hepatosplenomegaly that can be attributed to the underlying lymphoproliferative disorder
Waldenström's macroglobulinemia	All criteria must be met • IgM monoclonal gammopathy (regardless of the size of the M-protein) • ≥10 % bone marrow lymphoplasmacytic infiltration (usually intertrabecular) by small lymphocytes that exhibit plasmacytoid or plasma cell differentiation and a typical immunophenotype (e.g., surface IgM^+, $CD5^{+/-}$, $CD10^-$, $CD19^+$, $CD20^+$, $CD23^-$) that satisfactorily excludes other lymphoproliferative disorders including chronic lymphocytic leukemia and mantle cell lymphoma • Evidence of anemia, constitutional symptoms, hyperviscosity, lymphadenopathy, or hepatosplenomegaly that can be attributed to the underlying lymphoproliferative disorder
Light chain MGUS	All criteria must be met • Abnormal FLC ratio (<0.26 or >1.65) • Increased level of the appropriate involved light chain (increased kappa FLC in patients with ratio >1.65 and increased lambda FLC in patients with ratio <0.26) • No immunoglobulin heavy chain expression on immunofixation • Absence of end-organ damage such as lytic bone lesions, anemia, hypercalcemia, or renal failure that can be attributed to a plasma cell proliferative disorder

(continued)

Table 1.2 (continued)

Disorder	Disease definition
Solitary plasmacytoma	All 4 criteria must be met • Biopsy-proven solitary lesion of bone or soft tissue with evidence of clonal plasma cells • Normal bone marrow with no evidence of clonal plasma cells • Normal skeletal survey and MRI of spine and pelvis (except for the primary solitary lesion) • Absence of end-organ damage such as hypercalcemia, renal insufficiency, anemia, or bone lesions (CRAB) that can be attributed to a lympho-plasma cell proliferative disorder
Systemic AL amyloidosis	All 4 criteria must be met • Presence of an amyloid-related systemic syndrome (such as renal, liver, heart, gastrointestinal tract, or peripheral nerve involvement) • Positive amyloid staining by Congo red in any tissue (e.g., fat aspirate, bone marrow, or organ biopsy) • Evidence that amyloid is light chain-related established by direct examination of the amyloid using mass spectrometry (MS)-based proteomic analysis, or immuno-electronmicroscopy • Evidence of a monoclonal plasma cell proliferative disorder (serum or urine M-protein, abnormal free light chain ratio, or clonal plasma cells in the bone marrow) *Note*: Approximately 2–3 % of patients with AL amyloidosis will not meet the requirement for evidence of a monoclonal plasma cell disorder listed above; the diagnosis of AL amyloidosis must be made with caution in these patients
POEMS syndrome	All 4 criteria must be met • Polyneuropathy • Monoclonal plasma cell proliferative disorder (almost always *lambda*) • Any one of the following 3 other *Major* criteria: 1. Sclerotic bone lesions 2. Castleman's disease 3. Elevated levels of vascular endothelial growth factor (VEGF)* • Any one of the following 6 minor criteria 1. Organomegaly (splenomegaly, hepatomegaly, or lymphadenopathy) 2. Extravascular volume overload (edema, pleural effusion, or ascites) 3. Endocrinopathy (adrenal, thyroid, pituitary, gonadal, parathyroid, pancreatic)** 4. Skin changes (hyperpigmentation, hypertrichosis, glomeruloid hemangiomata, plethora, acrocyanosis, flushing, white nails) 5. Papilledema 6. Thrombocytosis/polycythemia *Note*: Not every patient meeting the above criteria will have POEMS syndrome; the features should have a temporal relationship to each other and no other attributable cause. Anemia and/or thrombocytopenia are distinctively unusual in this syndrome unless Castleman disease is present *The source data do not define an optimal cutoff value for considering elevated VEGF level as a major criterion. We suggest that VEGF measured in the serum or plasma should be at least three to fourfold higher than the normal reference range for the laboratory that is doing the testing to be considered a major criteria ** In order to consider endocrinopathy as a minor criterion, an endocrine disorder other than diabetes or hypothyroidism is required since these two disorders are common in the general population

Modified from Kyle RA, Rajkumar SV. Leukemia 2009;23:3–9.

Patients with MGUS have a risk of progression to symptomatic multiple myeloma, AL amyloidosis, Waldenstrom's Macroglobulinemia, or related disorder [43, 44]. The major difference between MGUS and MM is the presence of end-organ damage in the latter.

Smoldering Multiple Myeloma (SMM)

SMM is characterized by serum monoclonal protein ≥3 g/dL and/or ≥10 % but <60 % clonal plasma cells in the bone marrow [42]. There is no hypercalcemia, renal insufficiency, anemia, or lytic bone lesions (end-organ damage). The risk of progression of SMM to symptomatic MM or AL amyloidosis is approximately 10 % per year during the first 5 years, 3 % per year in the next 5 years, and then 1–2 % per year thereafter resulting in a cumulative probability of progression of 73 % at 15 years [46]. The major risk factors for progression are the presence of a serum M-protein >3 g/dL, bone marrow plasma cells more than 10 %, and an abnormal FLC ratio <0.125 or more than 8 [30]. The probability of progression at 5 years was 25 % with one risk factor, 51 % with two risk factors and 76 % with three risk factors at the time of diagnosis. It has been reported that the presence of more than one focal lesion or diffuse marrow involvement on MRI are significantly associated with an increased risk of progression to symptomatic multiple myeloma [21]. If one is uncertain about the differentiation of MGUS or SMM from multiple myeloma and whether to begin chemotherapy immediately, it is better to wait and reevaluate the patient in 2 or 3 months. It is important to realize that patients with SMM may remain stable for years.

Solitary Plasmacytoma

The plasma cells of a plasmacytoma are identical to those of multiple myeloma and if they occur only in bone, they are called solitary plasmacytoma of bone and if they develop in soft tissues, they are called solitary extramedullary plasmacytomas. The diagnosis of solitary plasmacytomas are (1) Biopsy-proven plasmacytoma of bone or soft tissue consisting of clonal plasma cells, (2) No evidence of clonal plasma cells in the bone marrow aspirate or biopsy, (3) No lesions except for the initial solitary plasmacytoma on a complete skeletal survey and MRI of the spine and pelvis, (4) Absence of hypercalcemia, renal insufficiency, anemia, and lytic bone lesions as a result of the plasma cell disorder.

Waldenstrom's Macroglobulinemia

Waldenstrom's Macroglobulinemia (WM) is characterized by the presence of an IgM monoclonal protein of any size and a lymphoplasmacytic lymphoma involving the bone marrow. Usually it is easy to distinguish between WM and MM because of the clinical features and the presence of an IgM monoclonal protein in WM. However, some patients with MM and t(11;14) may have a lymphoplasmacytic proliferative process that resembles WM [47]. It should be emphasized that the t(11;14) translocation is not seen in WM.

AL Amyloidosis

AL Amyloidosis is characterized by a monoclonal plasma cell proliferative disorder producing light chains which deposit as amyloid in various organs resulting in the nephrotic syndrome, congestive heart failure, hepatomegaly, sensorimotor neuropathy, and renal insufficiency. AL amyloidosis is closely related to multiple myeloma. In one early report of 81 cases of AL, multiple myeloma was present in more than one-fourth of patients and abnormal plasma cells were found in all who had a bone marrow examination [48]. However, most patients with AL amyloidosis have fewer than 20 % plasma cells in the bone marrow, absence of lytic bone lesions, and modest amounts of Bence Jones proteinuria. Most importantly, a nephrotic syndrome is found in nearly one-third of patients with AL. In addition, cardiac involvement with infiltration of the myocardium and congestive heart failure are important features of AL. Multiple myeloma rarely develops in patients who initially have a diagnosis of AL amyloidosis. The presence of amyloid of the light chain type on biopsy solidifies the diagnosis of AL.

POEMS Syndrome

POEMS syndrome (osteosclerotic myeloma) is characterized by the presence of Polyneuropathy, Organomegaly, Endocrinopathy, Monoclonal protein, and Skin changes. This monoclonal plasma cell proliferative disorder has osteosclerotic lesions in virtually all cases. Castleman's disease is found in approximately 15 % of patients. Papilledema is common. Elevation of the serum VEGF (vascular endothelial growth factor) is found. The absence of anemia, hypercalcemia, pathologic fractures, and a high percentage of bone marrow plasma cells aid in the differentiation from MM.

Metastatic Carcinoma

The presence of lytic lesions in a patient with a monoclonal protein suggests multiple myeloma. One must remember that metastatic carcinoma from the kidney, breast, or lung can produce lytic lesions. Since malignancies occur in older patients it is not uncommon to have an unrelated MGUS. Patients with metastatic carcinoma oftentimes have constitutional symptoms and a modest-sized M-component and fewer than 10 % clonal plasma cells in the bone marrow. The diagnosis is made by demonstration of a metastatic carcinoma in biopsy.

Criteria for Response Assessment

The development of response criteria is essential for management of multiple myeloma. Response criteria have been developed by the Chronic Leukemia-Myeloma Task Force, Southwest Oncology Group (SWOG), and the Eastern Cooperative Oncology Group (ECOG), but they have been largely abandoned.

The European Group for Blood & Bone Marrow Transplant/International Bone Marrow Transplant Registry/American Bone Marrow Transplant Registry (EBMT/IBMTR/ABMTR) published criteria for the response and progression of MM treated by stem cell transplantation. These have been commonly referred to as the Blade Criteria or the EBMT criteria [49]. In 2006, the IMWG published uniform response criteria recommended for future clinical trials [50]. The IMWG uniform response criteria differed from the EBMT criteria because of the addition of FLC response, progression criteria for patients without measurable disease, modification of the definition for disease progression for patients in complete response (CR), the addition of very good partial response (VGPR), and stringent complete response (sCR) categories. They eliminated the mandatory 6-week wait time to confirm response and removed the minor response category. Additional clarifications and correction of errors were also made [50]. The IMWG response criteria supplement and clarify a number of the problems with the EBMT criteria and are now the standard that should be used in future clinical trials. It has also defined the criteria of progressive disease in patients achieving CR. Criteria for diagnosis, staging, risk stratification, and response assessment in multiple myeloma have been published (Table 1.3) [41].

We believe that patients with relapsed, refractory MM should retain the minor response category which consists of ≥25 % but <49 % reduction of serum M-protein and reduction of 24-h urine M-protein by 50–89 % which must exceed 200 mg/24 h. If extramedullary plasmacytomas are present at baseline there must be a 25–49 % reduction in the size of the soft tissue plasmacytomas. In addition, there must be no increase in size or number of lytic bone lesions. The development of compression fracture does not exclude response.

The VGPR category is a useful measure of depth of response. It distinguishes patients who have had a disappearance of their M-spike on electrophoresis but are still immunofixation positive from those patients who have had only a 50 % reduction in their serum M-spike. The VGPR category should be reported in clinical studies in order to compare different regimens more accurately.

The serum FLC assay is useful in patients who do not have measurable disease defined as a serum M-protein ≥1 g/100 mL or urine M-protein ≥200 mg/24 h. The baseline level of the involved FLC should be at least ≥100 mg/L and the FLC assay must have an abnormal ratio to indicate clonality. This assay consists of two separate determinations. One detects free kappa (normal

Table 1.3 International myeloma working group uniform response criteria for multiple myeloma

Response subcategory	Response criteria
Complete response (CR)[a]	• Negative immunofixation of serum and urine, and • Disappearance of any soft tissue plasmacytomas, and • <5 % plasma cells in bone marrow
Stringent complete response (sCR)[b]	CR as defined above plus • Normal FLC ratio, and • Absence of clonal PC by immunohistochemistry or 2–4 color flow cytometry
Very good partial response (VGPR)[a]	• Serum and urine M-component detectable by immunofixation but not on electrophoresis, or • ≥90 % or greater reduction in serum M-component plus urine M-component <100 mg per 24 h
Partial response (PR)	• ≥50 % reduction of serum M-protein and reduction in 24-h urinary M-protein by ≥90 % or to <200 mg per 24 h • If the serum and urine M-protein are unmeasurable a ≥50 % decrease in the difference between involved and uninvolved FLC levels is required in place of the M-protein criteria • If serum and urine M-protein are unmeasurable, and serum-free light assay is also unmeasurable, ≥50 % reduction in bone marrow plasma cells is required in place of M-protein, provided baseline percentage was ≥30 % • In addition to the above criteria, if present at baseline, ≥50 % reduction in the size of soft tissue plasmacytomas is also required
Stable disease (SD)	• Not meeting criteria for CR, VGPR, PR, or progressive disease
Progressive disease (PD)[b]	• Increase of 25 % from lowest response value in any one or more of the following – Serum M-component (absolute increase must be ≥0.5 g/dL)[c] and/or – Urine M-component (absolute increase must be ≥200 mg/24 h) and/or – Only in patients without measurable serum and urine M-protein levels: the difference between involved and uninvolved FLC levels (absolute increase must be >10 mg/L) – Only in patients without measurable serum and urine M-protein levels and without measurable disease by FLC levels, bone marrow plasma cell percentage (absolute % must be ≥10 %) • Definite development of new bone lesions or soft tissue plasmacytomas or definite increase in the size of existing bone lesions or soft tissue plasmacytomas • Development of hypercalcemia (corrected serum calcium >11.5 mg/dL) that can be attributed solely to the plasma cell proliferative disorder

Adapted with permission from Durie et al. International uniform response criteria for multiple myeloma. Leukemia 2006;20:1467–73; and Kyle RA, Rajkumar SV. Criteria for diagnosis, staging, risk stratification, and response assessment of multiple myeloma. Leukemia 2009;23:3–9

All response categories (CR, sCR, VGPR, PR, and PD) require two consecutive assessments made at anytime before the institution of any new therapy; complete response and PR and SD categories also require no known evidence of progressive or new bone lesions if radiographic studies were performed. VGPR and CR categories require serum and urine studies regardless of whether disease at baseline was measurable on serum, urine, both, or neither. Radiographic studies are not required to satisfy these response requirements. Bone marrow assessments need not be confirmed

[a]*Note clarifications to IMWG criteria for coding CR and VGPR in patients in whom the only measurable disease is by serum FLC levels*: CR in such patients a normal FLC ratio of 0.26–1.65 in addition to CR criteria listed above. VGPR in such patients requires in addition a >90 % decrease in the difference between involved and uninvolved free light chain FLC levels

[b]*Note clarifications to IMWG criteria for coding PD*: clarified than bone marrow criteria for progressive disease are to be used only in patients without measurable disease by M-protein and by FLC levels. Clarified that "25 % increase" refers to M-protein, FLC, and bone marrow results, and does not refer to bone lesions, soft tissue plasmacytomas, or hypercalcemia. Note that the "lowest response value" does not need to be a confirmed value

range 3.3–19.4 mg/L) and the other detects free lambda (normal 5.7–26.3 mg/L). The normal ratio of kappa/lambda light chain levels is 0.26–1.65. Those with a ratio <0.26 are defined as having a monoclonal lambda FLC and those with a ratio >1.65 are designated as having a monoclonal kappa FLC. The "involved" FLC isotype is the monoclonal light chain isotype while the opposite light chain type is the "uninvolved" FLC. The FLC levels increase with reduced renal function and thus do not represent monoclonal elevations. However, the difference in the level of the kappa and lambda (involved and uninvolved FLC) difference is useful in assessing response.

Acknowledgements This work was supported by National Cancer Institute grants CA168762, CA 107476, CA 100707, CA90297052, and CA 83724. Also supported in part by ECOG CA 21115T, the Jabbs Foundation (Birmingham, United Kingdom), and the Henry J. Predolin Foundation, USA.

References

1. Rajkumar SV, Gertz MA, Kyle RA, Greipp PR; Mayo Clinic Myeloma, Amyloid; Dysproteinemia Group. Current therapy for multiple myeloma.[see comment]. [Review] [89 refs]. Mayo Clin Proc. 2002; 77(8):813–22.
2. Kyle RA, Therneau TM, Rajkumar SV, Larson DR, Plevak MF, Melton LJ. Incidence of multiple myeloma in Olmsted County, Minnesota—trend over 6 decades. Cancer. 2004;101(11):2667–74.
3. Kyle RA, Gertz MA, Witzig TE, et al. Review of 1027 patients with newly diagnosed multiple myeloma. [see comment]. Mayo Clin Proc. 2003; 78(1):21–33.
4. Blade J, Kyle RA. Multiple myeloma in young patients: clinical presentation and treatment approach. [Review] [70 refs]. Leuk Lymphoma. 1998;30(5–6): 493–501.
5. Heilman RL, Velosa JA, Holley KE, Offord KP, Kyle RA. Long-term follow-up and response to chemotherapy in patients with light-chain deposition disease. Am J Kidney Dis. 1992;20(1):34–41.
6. Annesley TM, Burritt MF, Kyle RA. Artifactual hypercalcemia in multiple myeloma. Mayo Clin Proc. 1982;57(9):572–5.
7. Dispenzieri A, Kyle RA, Lacy MQ, et al. POEMS syndrome: definitions and long-term outcome. Blood. 2003;101(7):2496–506.
8. Fassas AB, Muwalla F, Berryman T, et al. Myeloma of the central nervous system: association with high-risk chromosomal abnormalities, plasmablastic morphology and extramedullary manifestations. Br J Haematol. 2002;117(1):103–8.
9. Chang H, Sloan S, Li D, Keith Stewart A. Multiple myeloma involving central nervous system: high frequency of chromosome 17p13.1 (p53) deletions. Br J Haematol. 2004;127(3):280–4. Prepublished on 2004/10/20 as doi:10.1111/j.1365-2141.2004.05199.x.
10. Gozzetti A, Cerase A, Lotti F, et al. Extramedullary intracranial localization of multiple myeloma and treatment with novel agents: a retrospective survey of 50 patients. Cancer. 2012;118(6):1574–84. Prepublished on 2011/09/21 as doi:10.1002/cncr.26447.
11. Talamo G, Cavallo F, Zangari M, et al. Hyperammonemia and encephalopathy in patients with multiple myeloma. Am J Hematol. 2007;82(5): 414–5. Prepublished on 2006/11/30 as doi:10.1002/ajh.20808.
12. Kyle RA, Maldonado JE, Bayrd ED. Plasma cell leukemia. Report on 17 cases. Arch Intern Med. 1974; 133(5):813–8.
13. Tiedemann RE, Gonzalez-Paz N, Kyle RA, et al. Genetic aberrations and survival in plasma cell leukemia. Leukemia. 2008;22(5):1044–52.
14. Drayson M, Tang LX, Drew R, Mead GP, Carr-Smith H, Bradwell AR. Serum free light-chain measurements for identifying and monitoring patients with nonsecretory multiple myeloma. Blood. 2001;97(9):2900–2. Prepublished on 2001/04/21.
15. Singhal S, Vickrey E, Krishnamurthy J, Singh V, Allen S, Mehta J. The relationship between the serum free light chain assay and serum immunofixation electrophoresis, and the definition of concordant and discordant free light chain ratios. Blood. 2009;114(1): 38–9. Prepublished on 2009/05/05 as doi:10.1182/blood-2009-02-205807.
16. Katzmann JA, Abraham RS, Dispenzieri A, Lust JA, Kyle RA. Diagnostic performance of quantitative kappa and lambda free light chain assays in clinical practice. Clin Chem. 2005;51(5):878–81.
17. Larson D, Kyle RA, Rajkumar SV. Prevalence and monitoring of oligosecretory myeloma. N Engl J Med. 2012;367(6):580–1. Prepublished on 2012/08/10 as doi:10.1056/NEJMc1206740.
18. Greipp PR, Leong T, Bennett JM, et al. Plasmablastic morphology—an independent prognostic factor with clinical and laboratory correlates: Eastern Cooperative Oncology Group (ECOG) myeloma trial E9486 report by the ECOG Myeloma Laboratory Group. Blood. 1998;91(7):2501–7.
19. Fonseca R, Bergsagel PL, Drach J, et al. International Myeloma Working Group molecular classification of multiple myeloma: spotlight review. Leukemia. 2009;23(12):2210–21. Prepublished on 2009/10/03 as doi:10.1038/leu.2009.174.
20. Lacy MQ, Gertz MA, Hanson CA, Inwards DJ, Kyle RA. Multiple myeloma associated with diffuse osteosclerotic bone lesions: a clinical entity distinct from osteosclerotic myeloma (POEMS syndrome). Am J Hematol. 1997;56(4):288–93.
21. Walker R, Barlogie B, Haessler J, et al. Magnetic resonance imaging in multiple myeloma: diagnostic and clinical implications. J Clin Oncol. 2007;25(9): 1121–8.
22. Bredella MA, Steinbach L, Caputo G, Segall G, Hawkins R. Value of FDG PET in the assessment of patients with multiple myeloma. AJR Am J Roentgenol. 2005;184(4):1199–204. Prepublished on 2005/03/25.

23. Dimopoulos M, Kyle R, Fermand JP, et al. Consensus recommendations for standard investigative workup: report of the International Myeloma Workshop Consensus Panel 3. Blood. 2011;117(18): 4701–5. Prepublished on 2011/02/05 as doi:10.1182/blood-2010-10-299529.
24. Kyle RA. Sequence of testing for monoclonal gammopathies. Arch Pathol Lab Med. 1999;123(2): 114–8.
25. Greipp PR, San Miguel J, Durie BGM, et al. International staging system for multiple myeloma. J Clin Oncol. 2005;23(15):3412–20.
26. Snozek CL, Saenger AK, Greipp PR, et al. Comparison of bromcresol green and agarose protein electrophoresis for quantitation of serum albumin in multiple myeloma. Clin Chem. 2007;53(6):1099–103.
27. Katzmann JA, Clark RJ, Abraham RS, et al. Serum reference intervals and diagnostic ranges for free kappa and free lambda immunoglobulin light chains: relative sensitivity for detection of monoclonal light chains. Clin Chem. 2002;48(9):1437–44.
28. Dispenzieri A, Kyle R, Merlini G, et al. International Myeloma Working Group guidelines for serum-free light chain analysis in multiple myeloma and related disorders. Leukemia. 2009;23(2):215–24.
29. Dingli D, Kyle RA, Rajkumar SV, et al. Immunoglobulin free light chains and solitary plasmacytoma of bone. Blood. 2006;108(6):1979–83.
30. Dispenzieri A, Kyle RA, Katzmann JA, et al. Immunoglobulin free light chain ratio is an independent risk factor for progression of smoldering (asymptomatic) multiple myeloma. Blood. 2008; 111(2):785–9.
31. Rajkumar SV, Kyle RA, Therneau TM, et al. Serum free light chain ratio is an independent risk factor for progression in monoclonal gammopathy of undetermined significance. Blood. 2005;106(3):812–7.
32. Kyle RA, Rajkumar SV. Multiple myeloma. N Engl J Med. 2004;351(18):1860–73.
33. Rajkumar SV, Fonseca R, Dispenzieri A, et al. Methods for estimation of bone marrow plasma cell involvement in myeloma: predictive value for response and survival in patients undergoing autologous stem cell transplantation. Am J Hematol. 2001;68(4):269–75.
34. Avet-Loiseau H. Role of genetics in prognostication in myeloma. Best Pract Res Clin Haematol. 2007;20(4):625–35. Prepublished on 2007/12/12 as doi:10.1016/j.beha.2007.08.005.
35. Dimopoulos MA, Barlogie B, Smith TL, Alexanian R. High serum lactate dehydrogenase level as a marker for drug resistance and short survival in multiple myeloma. Ann Intern Med. 1991;115(12):931–5. Prepublished on 1991/12/15.
36. Moulopoulos LA, Dimopoulos MA, Alexanian R, Leeds NE, Libshitz HI. Multiple myeloma: MR patterns of response to treatment. Radiology. 1994;193(2):441–6. Prepublished on 1994/11/01.
37. Moulopoulos LA, Dimopoulos MA, Weber D, Fuller L, Libshitz HI, Alexanian R. Magnetic resonance imaging in the staging of solitary plasmacytoma of bone. J Clin Oncol. 1993;11(7):1311–5. Prepublished on 1993/07/01.
38. Moulopoulos LA, Dimopoulos MA, Smith TL, et al. Prognostic significance of magnetic resonance imaging in patients with asymptomatic multiple myeloma. J Clin Oncol. 1995;13(1):251–6.
39. Mariette X, Zagdanski AM, Guermazi A, et al. Prognostic value of vertebral lesions detected by magnetic resonance imaging in patients with stage I multiple myeloma. Br J Haematol. 1999;104(4): 723–9.
40. International Myeloma Working Group. Criteria for the classification of monoclonal gammopathies, multiple myeloma and related disorders: a report of the International Myeloma Working Group. Br J Haematol. 2003;121(5):749–57.
41. Kyle RA, Rajkumar SV. Criteria for diagnosis, staging, risk stratification and response assessment of multiple myeloma. Leukemia. 2009;23(1):3–9.
42. Rajkumar SV, Larson D, Kyle RA. Diagnosis of smoldering multiple myeloma. N Engl J Med. 2011;365(5):474–5. Prepublished on 2011/08/05 as doi:10.1056/NEJMc1106428.
43. Kyle RA, Therneau TM, Rajkumar SV, Larson DR, Plevak MF, Melton III LJ. Long-term follow-up of 241 patients with monoclonal gammopathy of undetermined significance: the original Mayo Clinic series 25 years later. [see comment]. Mayo Clin Proc. 2004;79(7):859–66.
44. Kyle RA, Therneau TM, Rajkumar SV, et al. A long-term study of prognosis in monoclonal gammopathy of undetermined significance. [see comment]. N Engl J Med. 2002;346(8):564–9.
45. Kyle RA, Greipp PR. Smoldering multiple myeloma. N Engl J Med. 1980;302(24):1347–9.
46. Kyle RA, Remstein ED, Therneau TM, et al. Clinical course and prognosis of smoldering (asymptomatic) multiple myeloma. N Engl J Med. 2007;356(25): 2582–90.
47. Maldonado JE, Kyle RA, Brown Jr AL, Bayrd ED. "Intermediate" cell types and mixed cell proliferation in multiple myeloma: electron microscopic observations. Blood. 1966;27(2):212–26.
48. Kyle RA, Bayrd ED. "Primary" systemic amyloidosis and myeloma. Discussion of relationship and review of 81 cases. Arch Intern Med. 1961;107:344–53. Prepublished on 1961/03/01.
49. Blade J, Samson D, Reece D, et al. Criteria for evaluating disease response and progression in patients with multiple myeloma treated by high-dose therapy and haemopoietic stem cell transplantation. Myeloma Subcommittee of the EBMT. European Group for Blood and Marrow Transplant. Br J Haematol. 1998;102(5):1115–23.
50. Durie BG, Harousseau JL, Miguel JS, et al. International uniform response criteria for multiple myeloma. Leukemia. 2006;20(9):1467–73.

Detection of M Proteins

2

Jerry A. Katzmann

Introduction

Monoclonal plasma cell proliferative diseases such as multiple myeloma are characterized by the proliferation of a single clone of plasma cells which may produce and secrete a homogeneous monoclonal immunoglobulin. The monoclonal immunoglobulin is commonly referred to as an M protein. The M protein acts as a serological "tumor" marker that is useful for diagnosis and disease monitoring. The identification and quantitation of M proteins relies predominantly on the ability to differentiate between monoclonal and polyclonal immunoglobulins. This has traditionally been done with electrophoretic assays [1–3]. High-resolution agarose gel protein electrophoresis (PEL) and capillary zone electrophoresis (CZE) are relatively simple procedures that are used to detect and quantitate monoclonal proteins [4–6]. Immunofixation electrophoresis (IFE) in agarose and immuno-subtraction electrophoresis (ISE) in CZE are used to identify and characterize the immunoglobulin heavy and/or light chains. In the last few years additional methods have been developed that complement the electrophoretic assays [7, 8]. Quantitation of serum free light chains (FLC) by nephelometric immunoassays support some of the weaknesses of PEL and IFE, and international guidelines now include all three serum assays [9].

J.A. Katzmann, Ph.D. (✉)
Division of Clinical Biochemistry & Immunology, Department of Laboratory Medicine & Pathology, Mayo Clinic, 200 First Street, SW, Rochester, MN 55905, USA
e-mail: katzmann@mayo.edu

Assays for M Protein Detection

PEL separates proteins based on charge and size. Once the serum proteins have been separated by electrophoresis, the gel is stained for proteins and the distribution of the protein stain is captured by scanning the gel and obtaining an electropherogram (Fig. 2.1). Five serum fractions have traditionally been identified by PEL: albumin, alpha 1, alpha 2, beta, and gamma. The fractional areas in each part of the electropherogram can then be converted to serum concentrations by combining these results with the serum total protein (Table 2.1). In a normal serum the gamma fraction will have a broad, Gaussian distribution. The distribution of immunoglobulins through the gamma fraction is predominantly due to charge differences on the polyclonal immunoglobulins. In the IFE results illustrated in Fig. 2.1, the distribution seen in the IgG pattern corresponds to the PEL gamma fraction pattern. The quantitation of the gamma fraction provides information about hypogammaglobulinemia or hypergammaglobulinemia and the gamma fraction result should be similar to IgG quantitation by nephelometric assays. In a polyclonal hypergammaglobulinemic serum the gamma fraction would look similar but would have a larger fractional area. In the serum of a

M.A. Gertz and S.V. Rajkumar (eds.), *Multiple Myeloma: Diagnosis and Treatment*,
DOI 10.1007/978-1-4614-8520-9_2, © Mayo Foundation for Medical Education and Research 2014

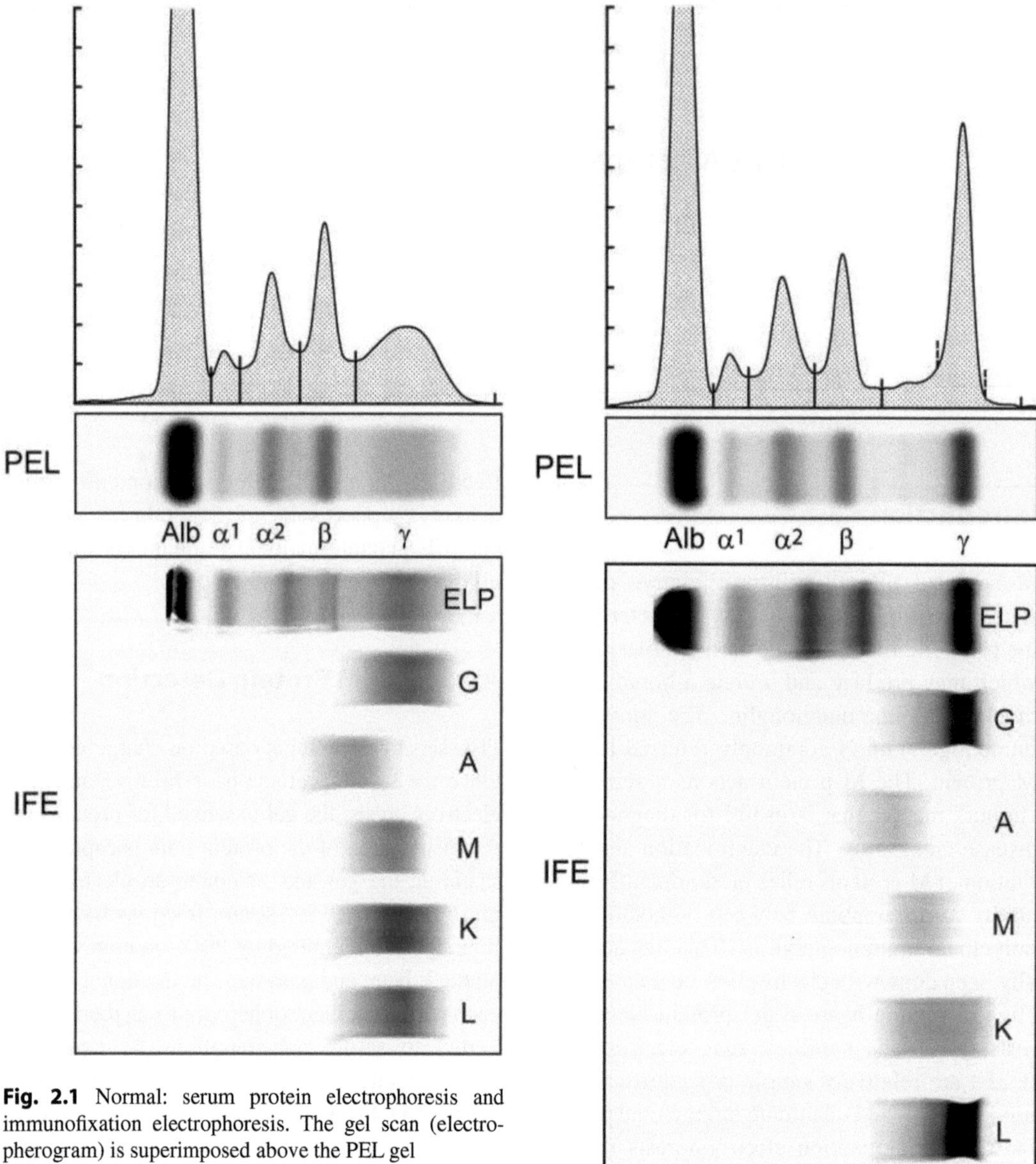

Fig. 2.1 Normal: serum protein electrophoresis and immunofixation electrophoresis. The gel scan (electropherogram) is superimposed above the PEL gel

Fig. 2.2 Monoclonal gammopathy: serum protein electrophoresis and immunofixation electrophoresis. The gel scan (electropherogram) is superimposed above the PEL gel. The *dashed lines* on both sides of the M protein indicate the M-spike fraction

Table 2.1 Quantitation of protein electrophoresis electropherogram fractions

	Area under the curve (%)	Fraction concentration (g/dL)	Reference values (g/dL)
Serum total protein		7.6	6.3–7.9
Albumin	56	4.2	3.4–4.7
Alpha 1	3	0.2	0.1–0.3
Alpha 2	9	0.8	0.6–1.0
Beta	12	0.9	0.7–1.2
Gamma	20	1.5	0.6–1.6

patient with a monoclonal gammopathy, the monoclonal immunoglobulin migrates in a restricted area of migration in the electrophoresis pattern (Fig. 2.2). All patients with a localized band on PEL require IFE or ISE to confirm the monoclonal protein and to determine the

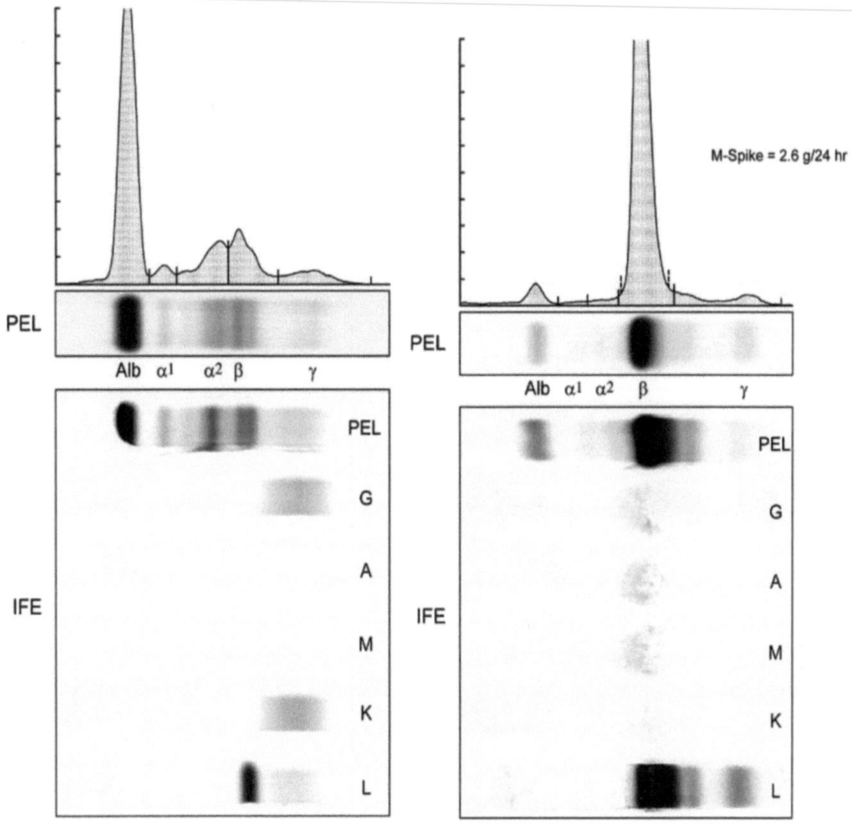

Fig. 2.3 Light chain multiple myeloma: serum (*left*) and urine (*right*) PEL and IFE

heavy chain class and/or light chain type. The IFE reactivity in Fig. 2.2 indicates that the restricted electrophoretic migration is a monoclonal immunoglobulin with a gamma heavy chain and an associated lambda light chain (IgG lambda). It is this restricted heavy chain migration on the gel and the associated migration of only one light chain type that identifies and characterizes the monoclonal immunoglobulin heavy and light chain type. The concentration of the monoclonal fraction (e.g., M-spike) from the serum PEL quantitates the amount of the monoclonal protein.

In many patients, the use of serum PEL and IFE for detection and quantitation of monoclonal proteins is very straightforward [10]. There are, however, some types of monoclonal proteins that are more of a challenge. Patients with light chain multiple myeloma (LCMM), for example, have lots of clonal plasma cells secreting monoclonal light chain, but the serum concentration may be low. The FLC has a low molecular weight and is quickly cleared into the urine. The PEL and IFE of serum and urine from a patient with LCMM is shown in Fig. 2.3. The serum IFE clearly shows a discrete lambda band with no corresponding gamma, alpha, or mu heavy chain. (A second IFE also showed no reactivity with delta or epsilon heavy chain.) Although the monoclonal lambda protein is detected in the serum, quantitation is not possible by the serum PEL. The 24 h urine PEL, however, shows a large lambda M-spike that is easily detected and quantitated. When we envision serum from a patient with MM, we picture large M spikes of intact immunoglobulin M protein: LCMM, however, represents 18–20 % of patients with MM, and because of the rapid clearance of monoclonal FLC from serum, it has been recommended to assay both serum and urine.

Patients with nonmalignant light chain diseases such as amyloid (AL) have serum and urine

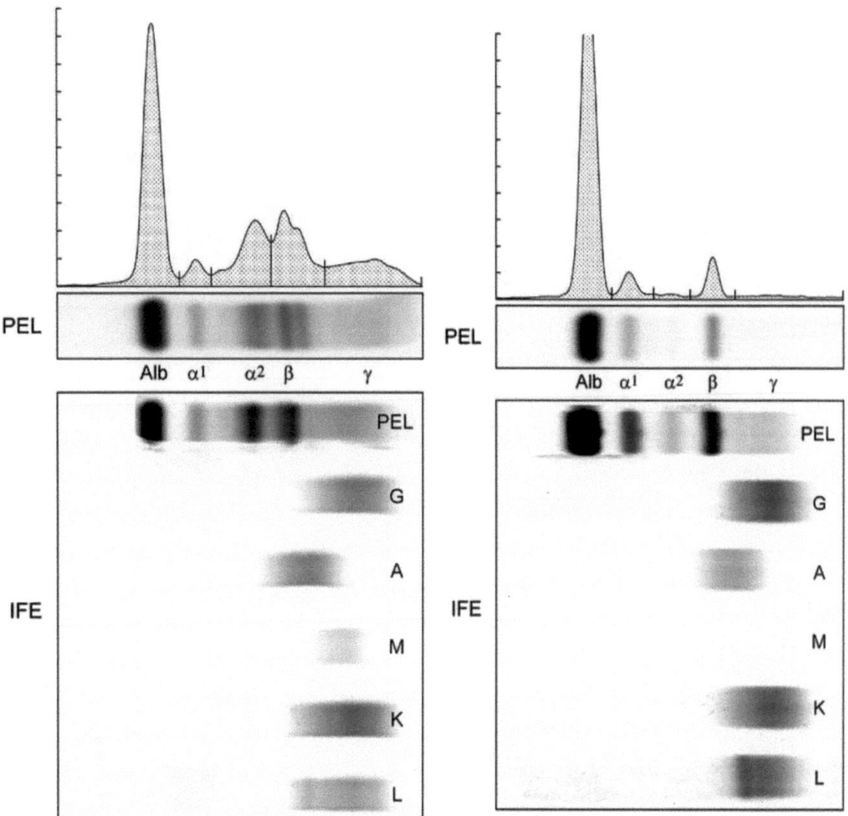

Fig. 2.4 Primary amyloid: serum (*left*) and urine (*right*) PEL and IFE

abnormalities that may be even more difficult for the laboratory to detect and quantitate. AL patients may have small numbers of bone marrow plasma cells and therefore also have small amounts of secreted monoclonal light chain. Examples of PEL and IFE of both serum and urine from an AL patient are illustrated in Fig. 2.4. Close examination reveals a faint monoclonal lambda band in the serum and urine. It is clear that if the concentration of the monoclonal lambda protein was lower, we would not be able to see the abnormality. In addition, there is no way to quantitate and therefore monitor the abnormality. The introduction of quantitative serum FLC immunoassays has helped identify these monoclonal FLC and has provided a quantitative measure to monitor the plasma cell disease.

The quantitative FLC assays use antisera directed against epitopes that are exposed only when the light chains are free (unbound to heavy chain) in solution [7]. These cryptic sites are involved in the very tight non-covalent binding of light chains to heavy chains. The antisera have a 10,000-fold preference for FLC compared to light chains contained within intact immunoglobulin molecules. That means that FLC immunoassays can be used to specifically quantitate FLC even in the presence of large concentrations of polyclonal immunoglobulins (e.g., in serum). The diagnostic approach is to measure the kappa FLC and the lambda FLC concentrations and use the ratio of kappa to lambda FLC to detect unbalanced light chain synthesis. This approach has proven surprisingly sensitive for detecting clonal FLC diseases. Abnormal serum FLC ratios have been detected in 100 % of patients with LCMM [11, 12], 90–95 % of AL patients [13–15], and 60–70 % of patients with nonsecretory multiple myeloma [12, 16]. Abnormal serum FLC ratios have also been detected in 90–95 % of patients with intact immunoglobulin MM [12, 17] and 40 % of monoclonal gammopathy of undetermined significance (MGUS) [18]. Since these two patient groups usually have easily detected M proteins by PEL and IFE, it is clear that not all monoclonal gammopathies secrete excess FLC and that a combination of tests is be needed for good diagnostic sensitivity.

Screening Panels for M Protein Detection

To identify the best approach for detection of monoclonal proteins, we performed a large study in which we identified Mayo patients with an assortment of plasma cell proliferative diseases who also had serum PEL, IFE, and FLC as well as urine PEL and IFE performed at the time of diagnosis [19]. This cohort consisted of 1,851 patients with various monoclonal gammopathies [MM, Waldenström's macroglobulinemia, smoldering multiple myeloma (SMM), MGUS, plasmacytoma, POEMS syndrome, primary amyloid (AL), and light chain deposition disease]. The data illustrated in Table 2.2 allows us to retrospectively determine which patients would have had M proteins detected by the various tests singly or in combination. In the three right-hand columns you can see that no single serum test is sensitive as a stand-alone assay. In the left-hand column you can see that using all five assays identifies almost all the patients but still misses 1.4 % of the cases. If urine assays are removed from the diagnostic panel, an additional 1.2 % of the cases are missed: 3 % of MGUS patients ($n=15$), 1 % of AL ($n=6$), 6 % of LCDD ($n=1$), and 10 % of extramedullary plasmacytoma ($n=1$). The elimination of urine from the diagnostic panel resulted in no decrease in sensitivity for patients with MM, macroglobulinemia, plasmacytoma, POEMS, or SMM. These and other studies [15, 20–23] have led the International Myeloma Working Group to recommend a screening panel of serum PEL, IFE, and FLC, and panels that include urine are only recommended if AL is suspected [9]. [Once an M protein has been detected, analysis of urine may be required as part of the diagnostic assessment.] Table 2.3 is a simplified illustration of this data. A diagnostic panel with no requirement for submission of a urine sample simplifies things for the patient and also reduces costs for the laboratory since there is a single sample to accession and no pre-analytic handling like centrifugation and concentration. Interestingly, removing serum IFE and using only serum PEL and FLC does not reduce sensitivity for detection of M protein in

Table 2.2 Diagnostic sensitivity of monoclonal gammopathy screening panels

	No. of samples	All serum and urine tests	Serum PEL+IFE+FLC (no urine)	Serum PEL+FLC+	Serum IFE	Serum PEL	Serum FLC
Diagnosis	No.	%	%	%	%	%	%
All	1,877	98.6	97.4	94.3	87.0	79.0	74.3
MM	467	100	100	100	94.4	87.6	98.6
WM	26	100	100	100	100	100	73.1
SMM	191	100	100	99.5	98.4	94.2	81.2
MGUS	524	100	97.1	88.7	92.8	81.9	42.4
Plasmacytoma	29	89.7	89.7	86.2	72.4	72.4	55.2
POEMS	31	96.8	96.8	74.2	96.8	74.2	9.7
Extramedullary MM	10	20.0	10.0	10.0	10.0	10.0	10.0
AL	581	98.1	97.1	96.2	73.8	65.9	88.3
LCDD	18	83.3	77.8	77.8	55.6	55.6	77.8

MM multiple myeloma, *WM* Waldenstrom macroglobulinemia, *SMM* smoldering multiple myeloma, *MGUS* monoclonal gammopathy of undetermined significance, *POEMS* POEMS syndrome, *AL* light chain amyloidosis, *LCDD* light chain deposition disease, *PEL* protein electrophoresis, *IFE* immunofixation, *FLC* free light chain

Table 2.3 Simplified summary of diagnostic sensitivity of monoclonal gammopathy screening panels

Diagnosis (*n*)	All serum and urine assays (%)	Serum PEL+IFE+FLC (3 serum assays) (%)	Serum PEL+FLC (2 serum assays) (%)
MM (*n*=467)	100	100	100
WM (*n*=26)	100	100	100
AL (*n*=581)	98.1	97.1	96.2

MM multiple myeloma, *WM* Waldenstrom macroglobulinemia, *AL* light chain amyloidosis, *PEL* protein electrophoresis, *IFE* immunofixation, *FLC* free light chain

MM and macroglobulinemia and results in only an additional 1 % decrease of sensitivity in AL. A diagnostic panel of serum PEL and FLC is probably the bare minimum screening panel that should be considered.

Monitoring M Proteins

Once an M protein has been detected and a specific diagnosis has been determined, the quantitation of the M protein can be used as a marker of the plasma cell clone's response to therapy or progression. A serum M-spike (Fig. 2.2) and/or urine M-spike (Fig. 2.3) may be present and easily quantitated. In addition, there are disease presentations in which there is significant suppression of polyclonal immunoglobulin synthesis (Fig. 2.5). In these cases the quantitation of immunoglobulin (IgG, IgA, or IgM) can also be used to monitor hematologic disease. Serum M-spike and immunoglobulin quantitation are not, however, always equivalent [24]. In general IgA monoclonal proteins give the same results with both methods. Monoclonal IgM protein concentrations are almost always higher by immuno-nephelometric quantitation then by PEL M-spike. It is therefore important to use the same method over time. Large IgG M-spikes are usually smaller than IgG quantitation, and this is likely due to saturation of stain on PEL. When monoclonal IgG m-spikes are greater than 3 g/dL, it is therefore important to also obtain IgG quantitation by immuno-nephelometry.

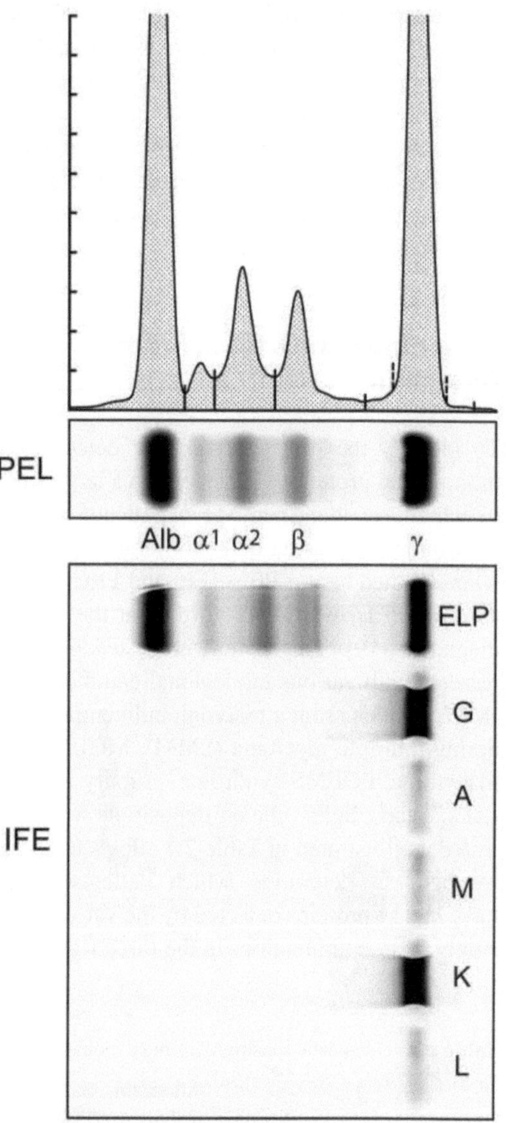

Fig. 2.5 Large M protein with suppressed polyclonal immunoglobulins

Not all patients can be monitored by PEL M-spikes or quantitative immunoglobulins. Some patients have small concentrations of M protein (Fig. 2.6). In these cases any attempt to quantitate the M protein will include substantial polyclonal immunoglobulins [25]. The M-spike will be more specific than quantitative IgG, but the M protein will still be a minority of the M-spike. As this M-spike gets smaller in response to therapy the

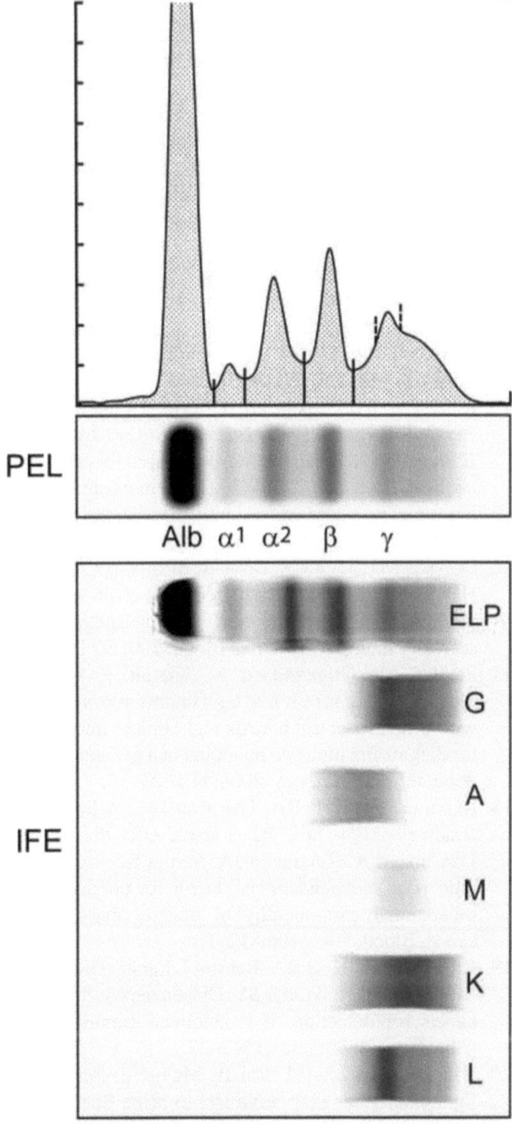

Fig. 2.6 Small M protein

laboratory has to make a judgment when to stop fractionating the M-spike. At that point we report the presence of a small monoclonal protein that we are unable to quantitate. New heavy-light chain reagents that can separately quantitate IgG kappa and IgG lambda, IgA kappa and IgA lambda, and IgM kappa and IgM lambda may be useful for these patients [26]. This heavy-light isotype-specific kappa to lambda ratio has been proposed as a potential monitoring method [27]. The use of the heavy-light chain ratio, however, has not yet been validated for patients with small M proteins.

The AL patient illustrated in Fig. 2.4 is an example of a case in which we were never able to quantitate the lambda M protein by using an M-spike and instead used quantitative FLC. The lambda FLC concentration was used to monitor this patient. The international guidelines for monitoring monoclonal gammopathies have usually suggested that the serum M-spike should be greater than 1 g/dL for accurate monitoring and that a 50 % decrease is a partial response [9]. The guidelines for urine M-spikes suggest they should be greater than 200 mg/24 h and that a 90 % decrease is a partial response. The guidelines for FLC quantitation suggest that the FLC ratio should be abnormal, the concentration of the monoclonal FLC should be greater than 10 mg/dL, and that a 50 % decrease in M protein concentration is a partial response. In order to test these guidelines we have studied long-term, sequential serum and urine samples in MM patients who have reached stable, partial remissions [28]. The analysis indicated that the biologic and disease-related variation in these stable patients was 8 % for serum M-spikes, 12 % for immunoglobulin quantitation, 28 % for serum monoclonal FLC concentrations, and 36 % for urine M-spikes. This variability data indicates that in order to have 95 % confidence in a decrease in M proteins, a serum M-spike should decrease by 28 %, FLC by 55 %, and urine M-spike by 63 %. The suggested criteria for partial response therefore make sense for serum M-spike (50 %) and urine M-spike (90 %). FLC quantitation, however, has variability that is similar to urine M-spike measurements and the urine criteria should probably be used for serum FLC.

Summary

Depending on the particular monoclonal protein the detection of M proteins may require serum PEL and IFE, urine PEL and IFE, and serum FLC quantitation. A diagnostic screening panel of serum PEL, IFE, and FLC has been recommended: if AL is suspected, urine PEL and IFE should be included as well. The use of this diagnostic panel also guides the clinician to the best approach to monitor disease.

References

1. Keren DF, Alexanian R, Goeken JA, Gorevic PD, Kyle RA, Tomar RH. Guidelines for clinical and laboratory evaluation of patients with monoclonal gammopathies. Arch Pathol Lab Med. 1999;123:106–7.
2. Keren D. Protein electrophoresis in clinical diagnosis. Chicago: ASCP Press; 2012.
3. Kyle RA. Sequence of testing for monoclonal gammopathies. Arch Pathol Lab Med. 1999;123:114–8.
4. Bienvenu J, Graziani MS, Arpin F, Bernon Blessum HC, Marchetti C, Righetti G, Somenzini M, Verga G, Aguzzi F. Multicenter evaluation of the Paragon CZE 2000 capillary zone electrophoresis system for serum protein electrophoresis and monoclonal protein typing. Clin Chem. 1998;44:599–605.
5. Katzmann JA, Clark R, Sanders E, Landers JP, Kyle RA. Prospective study of serum protein capillary zone electrophoresis and immunotyping of monoclonal proteins by immunosubtraction. Am J Clin Pathol. 1998;110:503–9.
6. Katzmann JA, Clark R, Wiegert E, Sanders E, Oda RP, Kyle RA, Namyst-Goldberg C, Landers JP. Identification of monoclonal proteins in serum: a quantitative comparison of acetate, agarose gel, and capillary electrophoresis. Electrophoresis. 1997;18(10):1775–80.
7. Bradwell AR, Carr-Smith HD, Mead GP, Tang LX, Showell PJ, Drayson MT, Drew R. Highly sensitive automated immunoassay for immunoglobulin free light chains in serum and urine. Clin Chem. 2001;47:637–80.
8. Katzmann JA, Clark RJ, Abraham RS, Bryant S, Lymp JF, Bradwell AR, Kyle RA. Serum reference intervals and diagnostic ranges for free κ and free λ immunoglobulin light chains: relative sensitivity for detection of monoclonal light chains. Clin Chem. 2002;48:1437–44.
9. Dispenzieri A, Kyle R, Merlini G, Miguel JS, Ludwig H, Hajek R, Palumbo A, et al. International Myeloma Working Group guidelines for serum-free light chain analysis in multiple myeloma and related disorders. Leukemia. 2009;23:215–24.
10. Kyle RA, Gertz MA, Witzig TE, Lust JA, Lacy MQ, Dispenzieri A, Fonseca R, Rajkumar SV, Offord JR, Larson DR, Plevak ME, Therneau TM, Greipp PR. Review of 1027 patients with newly diagnosed multiple myeloma. Mayo Clin Proc. 2003;78(1):21–33.
11. Bradwell AR, Mead GP, Carr-Smith HD, Drayson MT. Serum test for assessment of patients with Bence Jones myeloma. Lancet. 2003;361:489–91.
12. Katzmann JA, Abraham RS, Dispenzieri A, Lust JA, Kyle RA. Diagnostic performance of quantitative serum free light chain assays in clinical practice. Clin Chem. 2005;51:878–81.
13. Lachmann HJ, Gallimore R, Gillmore JD, Carr-Smith HD, Bradwell AR, Pepys MB, Hawkins PM. Outcome in systemic AL amyloidosis in relation to changes in concentration of circulating free immunoglobulin light chains following chemotherapy. Br J Haematol. 2003;122:78–84.
14. Bochtler T, Hegenbart U, Heiss C, Benner A, Cremer F, Volkmann M, Ludwig J, Perz JB, HO AD, Goldschmidt H, Schonland SO. Evaluation of the serum-free light chain test in untreated patients with AL amyloidosis. Haematologica. 2008;93(3):459–62.
15. Katzmann JA, Dispenzieri A, Kyle RA, Snyder MR, Plevak MF, Larson DR, Abraham RS, Lust JA, Melton JL, Rajkumar SV. Elimination of the need for urine studies in the screening algorithms for monoclonal gammopathies by using serum immunofixation and free light chain assays. Mayo Clin Proc. 2006;81(12):1575–8.
16. Drayson MT, Tang LX, Drew R, Mead GP, Carr-Smith HD, Bradwell AR. Serum free light-chain measurements for identifying and monitoring patients with nonsecretory multiple myeloma. Blood. 2001;97:2900–2.
17. Piehler AP, Gulbrandsen N, Kierulf P, Urdal P. Quantitation of serum free light chains in combination with protein electrophoresis and clinical information for diagnosing multiple myeloma in a general hospital population. Clin Chem. 2008;54:1823–30.
18. Rajkumar SV, Kyle RA, Therneau TM, Melton III LJ, Bradwell AR, Clark RJ, Larson DR, Plevak MF, Dispenzieri A, Katzmann JA. Serum free light chain ratio is an independent risk factor for progression in monoclonal gammopathy of undetermined significance. Blood. 2005;106:812–7.
19. Katzmann JA, Kyle RA, Benson J, Larson DR, Snyder MR, Lust JA, Rajkumar SV, Dispenzieri A. Screening panels for detection of monoclonal gammopathies. Clin Chem. 2009;55(8):1517–22.
20. Hill PG, Forsyth JM, Rai B, Mayne S. Serum free light chains: an alternative test to urine Bence Jones proteins when screening for monoclonal gammopathies. Clin Chem. 2006;52:1743–8.
21. Bakshi NA, Gulbranson R, Garstka D, Bradwell AR, Keren DF. Serum free light chain (FLC) measurement can aid capillary zone electrophoresis in detecting subtle FLC-producing M-proteins. Am J Clin Pathol. 2005;124:214–8.
22. Abadie JM, Bankson DD. Assessment of serum free light chain assays for plasma cell disorder screening in a veterans affairs population. Ann Clin Lab Sci. 2006;36:157–62.
23. Nowrousian MR, Brandhorst D, Sammet C, Kellert M, Daniels R, Schiett P, Poser M, Mueller S, Ebeling P, Welt A, Bradwell AR, Buttkereit U, Opalka B, Flasshove M, Moritz T, Seeber S. Serum free light chain analysis and urine immunofixation electrophoresis in patients with multiple myeloma. Clin Cancer Res. 2005;11(24):8706–14.

24. Murray DL, Ryu E, Snyder MR, Katzmann JA. Quantitation of serum monoclonal proteins: relationship between agarose gel electrophoresis and immunonephelometry. Clin Chem. 2009;55(8): 1523–9.
25. Murray DL, Seningen JL, Dispenzieri A, Snyder MR, Kyle RA, Rajkumar SV, Katzmann JA. Laboratory persistence and clinical progression of small monoclonal abnormalities. Am J Clin Pathol. 2012;138(4): 609–13.
26. Bradwell AR, Harding SJ, Fourrier NJ, Wallis GLF, Drayson MT, Carr-Smith HD, et al. Assessment of monoclonal gammopathies by nephelometric measurement of individual immunoglobulin kappa/lambda ratios. Clin Chem. 2009;55(9):1646–55.
27. Donato LJ, Zeldenrust SR, Murray DL, Katzmann JA. A 71-year-old woman with multiple myeloma status after stem cell transplantation. Clin Chem. 2011;57(12):1645–8.
28. Katzmann JA, Snyder MR, Rajkumar SV, Kyle RA, Therneau TM, Benson JT, Dispenzieri A. Long-term biological variation of serum protein electrophoresis M-spike, urine M-spike, and monoclonal serum free light chain quantification: implications for monitoring monoclonal gammopathies. Clin Chem. 2011;57(12): 1687–92.

Pathology of Multiple Myeloma

3

Dragan Jevremovic and William Morice

Introduction

Multiple myeloma (MM) and other plasma cell proliferative disorders (PCPD) are a group of systemic diseases which share as a unifying feature the presence of clonal plasma cells. As described in previous chapters, bone marrow is the most common tissue involved, but the neoplastic plasma cells may be found in virtually any tissue/organ.

While serum protein electrophoresis and free light chain analysis are essential in early detection and follow-up, the pathologic diagnosis of MM and other PCPD is made on the bone marrow aspirate and biopsy specimen [1]. The goal of the pathologic examination of the bone marrow is to: (a) quantify bone marrow plasma cells (necessary WHO criteria for the diagnosis of MM); (b) establish PC clonality; (c) distinguish MM from lymphoplasmacytic lymphoma (LPL) and other B-cell lymphomas with plasmacytic differentiation; (d) analyze prognostic factors; (e) detect amyloid deposits; and (f) detect other potential pathologic processes, in lymphoid and myeloid compartments.

D. Jevremovic, M.D., Ph.D. (✉) • W. Morice, M.D., Ph.D.
Division of Hematology, Mayo Clinic, 200 First Street, SW, Rochester, MN 55905, USA
e-mail: jevremovic.dragan@mayo.edu; morice.william@mayo.edu

Quantification of Bone Marrow Plasma Cells

The standard of care for PC quantification is still morphologic assessment of the bone marrow aspirate and biopsy (Fig. 3.1). Flow cytometry immunophenotyping (FCIP) is not a reliable method for PC quantification as studies have shown that the FCIP tends to underestimate the percentage of PCs. This is due to a number of factors such as exclusion of lipid phase-associated disease component and ex vivo loss of antigens used for PC identification [2, 3]. In addition, the Ficoll separation process used in some laboratories for mononuclear cell enrichment makes FCIP quantification of plasma cells even more problematic. Although FCIP does not supplant morphologic marrow assessment, multiparametric PC analysis by this method is an important part of the diagnostic evaluation, enabling separation of neoplastic (monoclonal) from background (polyclonal) PC population, which is not possible by morphologic assessment [4]. This feature is utilized in characterization of plasma cells for clonality, calculation of proliferation fraction, and minimal residual disease (MRD) analysis (see below). In addition to Wright-Giemsa stain of the bone marrow aspirate, evaluation of the bone marrow core biopsy by morphology (Hematoxylin-Eosin stain) or by immunohistochemistry (IHC: CD138, MUM-1/IRF-4, immunoglobulin light chains) is necessary to exclude sampling error; it is not uncom-

M.A. Gertz and S.V. Rajkumar (eds.), *Multiple Myeloma: Diagnosis and Treatment*,
DOI 10.1007/978-1-4614-8520-9_3, © Mayo Foundation for Medical Education and Research 2014

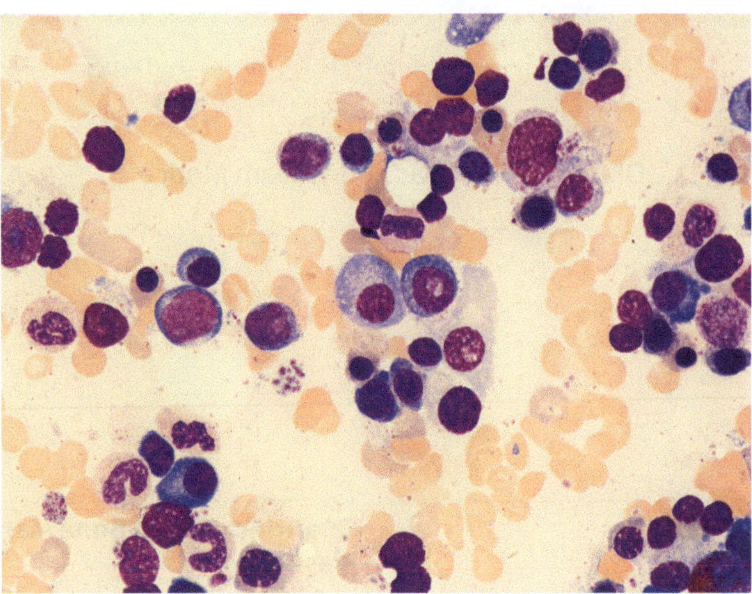

Fig. 3.1 Wright-Giemsa stain of the bone marrow aspirate (×600). Plasma cells are large with abundant blue cytoplasm, perinuclear hof, and round nuclei with checkered chromatin. Atypical plasma cell in the center right shows intranuclear Dutcher body (cytoplasmic invagination)

mon to observe aspirates with very few plasma cells and encounter sheets of PCs associated with fibrosis in the biopsy specimen. Normal bone marrow aspirate contains approximately 1–2 % PCs, and the defined threshold for the diagnosis of myeloma is 10 %, as defined by WHO guidelines [1]. Reactive marrow PCs may be increased above this threshold in a number of conditions, however, therefore establishing PC clonality is essential.

Establishment of Plasma Cell Clonality

Clonality of PCs is inferred by showing of monotypic immunoglobulin light chain expression (kappa or lambda) and/or abnormal patterns of antigen expression. Rarely, the clonal PCs lack detectable immunoglobulin expression (Ig-negative). FCIP, IHC, and in situ hybridization (ISH) are commonly used methods for establishing PC clonality. FCIP has an advantage of multiparametric analysis of plasma cells, up to 8 or 10 antigens in clinical laboratories, enabling a more precise separation of neoplastic PCs (CD19 and CD45-negative, CD56-positive) from normal PCs (CD19 and CD45-positive, CD56-negative) (Fig. 3.2). FCIP collection of large number of events (500,000 per specimen) enables a high sensitivity evaluation (0.01 %) for the presence of clonal PCs in the bone marrow aspirate. This is especially important for the detection of MRD after treatment. If aspirate is of poor quality due to technical difficulties or marrow fibrosis, IHC or ISH can be performed on the bone marrow biopsy specimen. These methodologies may also be helpful in older specimens, as PCs become more difficult to detect by FCIP in BM aspirates after 72 h.

Differential Diagnosis

A number of B-cell neoplasms may exhibit plasmacytic differentiation, the quintessential entity being LPL. In LPL the neoplastic cells exhibit a cytologic spectrum of small lymphocytes, plasmacytoid lymphocytes, and plasma cells. LPL commonly involves bone marrow or lymph nodes, and sometimes spleen and other tissues. It is usually associated with secretion of IgM class of immunoglobulin in the blood. Due to high molecular weight of IgM pentamer molecule, blood viscosity can be increased, leading to syndrome of

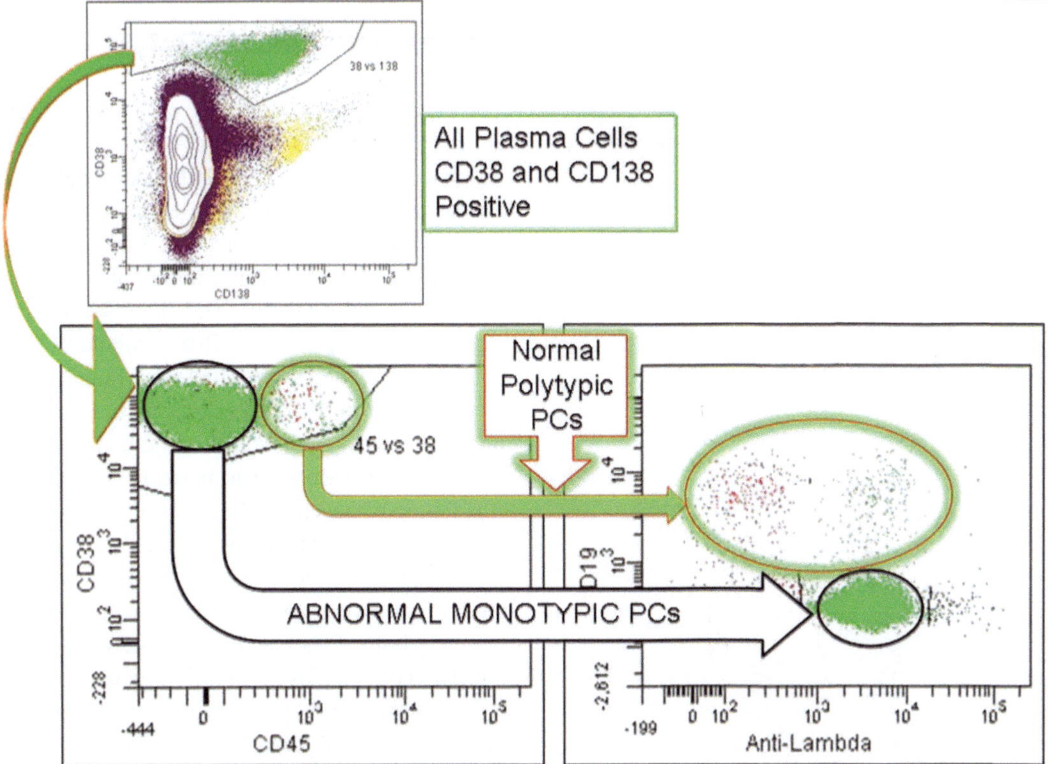

Fig. 3.2 Flow cytometry immunophenotyping of plasma cells. Plasma cells are identified by bright expression of CD38 and CD138. Normal plasma cells are positive for CD19 and CD45 and show polytypic immunoglobulin light chain expression (*green/red circle*). Myeloma PCs are negative for CD19 and CD45 and show lambda light chain restriction (*black circle*)

Waldenström macroglobulinemia (WM). Bone marrow examination helps differentiating LPL from MM, which is important for both therapeutic and prognostic purposes. In MM, a monomorphic plasma cell population is usually pure without associated lymphoid component, whereas in LPL typically small lymphocytes and plasmacytoid lymphocytes predominate. LPL may infiltrate the marrow in a nodular or interstitial pattern and the plasma cells and lymphocytes may be intimately admixed, such as with lymphoid nodules rimmed by plasma cells, or physically separate (Fig. 3.3). FCIP in LPL typically reveals monotypic B-cells, which may be CD5 positive. The plasma cells in LPL are variably well detected by FCIP, express the same light chain as the B-cell component, and typically retain expression of CD19 and CD45 (unlike in MM); they are never positive for CD56 and cyclin D1 [5, 6]. Clinical features are also helpful, including the presence of lymphadenopathy, the absence of bone lytic lesions, and the presence of IgM paraprotein. It is important to emphasize that IgM paraprotein can be associated with other B-cell neoplasms, including marginal zone lymphoma (MZL) and chronic lymphocytic leukemia (CLL). MZL can be particularly difficult to distinguish from LPL on bone marrow biopsy, as both entities can have plasmacytic differentiation. Very rarely, MM can also secrete IgM; IgM myeloma may have lymphoplasmacytoid cytology and be CD19 positive; in such cases detection of cyclin D1 overexpression in IgM myeloma and the presence of bony disease is critical in distinguishing it from LPL [7].

In addition to distinguishing MM from LPL or other lymphomas, bone marrow biopsy can help in the diagnosis of POEMS (polyneuropathy, organomegaly, endocrinopathy, M-protein, skin changes) syndrome. POEMS syndrome is usually represented in the bone marrow by a relatively small proportion of monoclonal lambda plasma

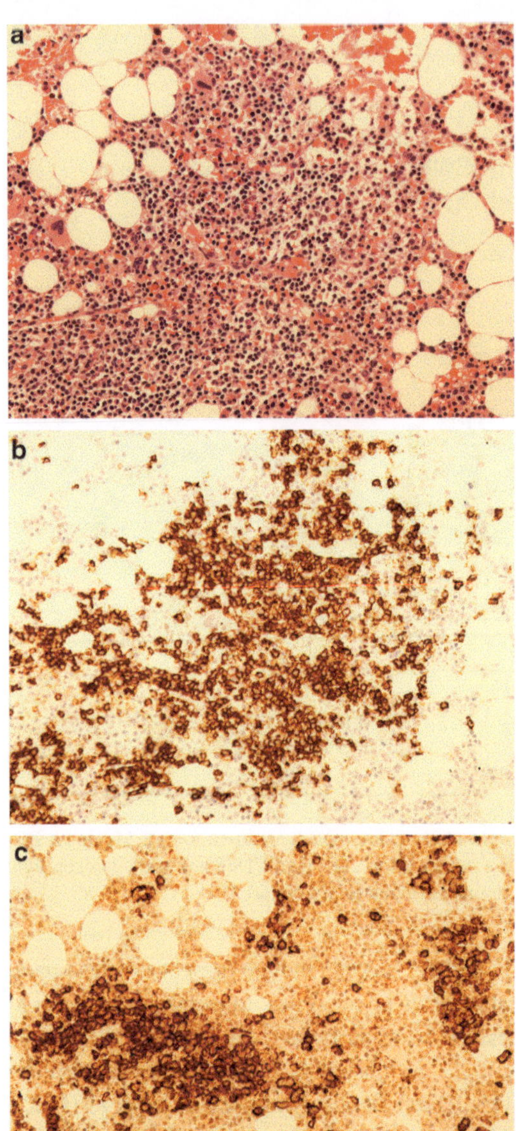

Fig. 3.3 Lymphoplasmacytic lymphoma involving the bone marrow (×200). (**a**) H&E stain shows nodular infiltrate of a mixture of small lymphocytes, plasmacytoid lymphocytes and plasma cells. (**b**) CD20 stain shows that small lymphocytes and plasmacytoid lymphocytes are of B-cell lineage. (**c**) CD138 stain shows associated plasma cells

cells (associated with increased polyclonal plasma cells), reactive lymphoid aggregates surrounded by plasma cells, megakaryocytic hyperplasia, and varying levels of bone sclerosis [8].

Analysis of Prognostic Factors

The most important laboratory prognostic factors are proliferation rate of neoplastic plasma cells and cytogenetic findings [9, 10]. Additional prognostic factors, including gene expression profiling, have also been described [11]. Older methods for determining PC proliferation rate included BrdU DNA pulse labeling and fluorescent staining of the aspirate with anti-BrdU antibodies [12]. Clinical correlation studies have shown that BrdU incorporation in >3 % of cells is associated with poor prognosis. However, this method is labor-intensive and is difficult to perform. It has been supplanted by recently developed FCIP methods for measuring S-phase of neoplastic PCs by detection of DAPI nuclear staining (Fig. 3.4). This method has several advantages: (1) neoplastic and non-neoplastic PCs can be accurately discriminated and their relative proportions calculated; (2) it enables measuring proliferation rate of neoplastic PCs only (separate from polytypic background); (3) it is highly sensitive and shows great precision in calculating S-phase of PCs; (4) it can detect aneuploid and polyploid populations adding to prognostic factors; and (5) it enables detection of small clones based on their DNA content. Clinical studies validating the S-phase cut-off value for this method are still in progress, but are likely to be between 1.5 and 3 %.

As mentioned in earlier chapters, several cytogenetic findings have been shown to be associated with poor prognosis, including t(4:14), t(14;16), del(13), and del(17p) by fluorescence in situ hybridization (FISH) and hypodiploidy by karyotype analysis [9, 10].

Amyloid Deposition

Amyloid is insoluble and enzyme-resistant form of a misfolded protein. Its accumulation in extracellular space leads to multiple organ dysfunction, including heart, peripheral nerves, esophagus, spleen, and kidney. Many proteins can form amyloid, but the most common one is immunoglobulin light chain (primary or AL

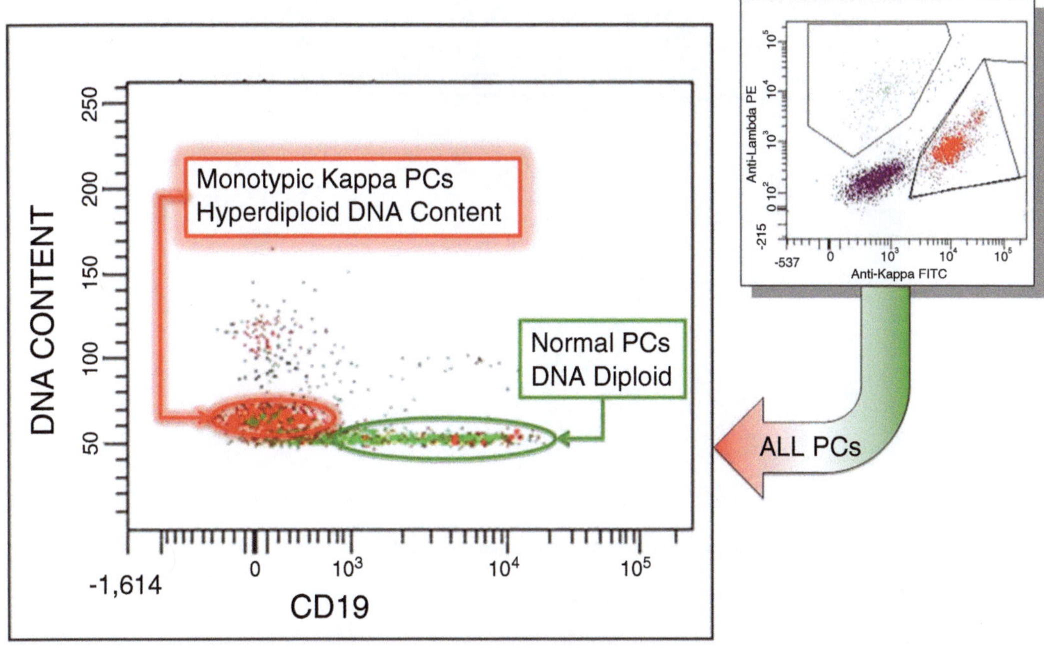

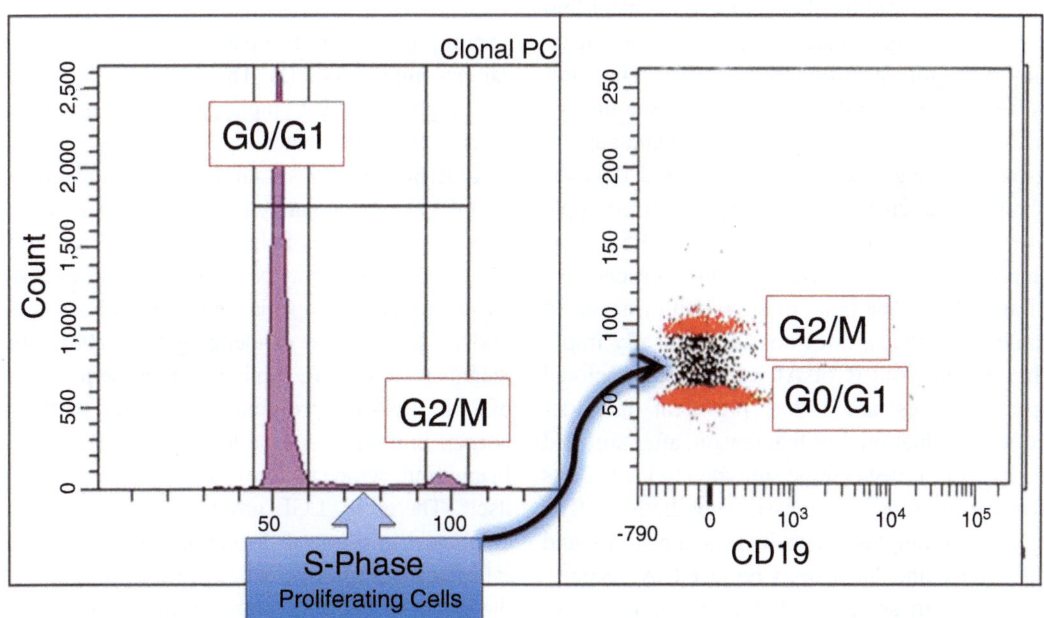

Fig. 3.4 Plasma cell proliferation assay by FCIP. (**a**) Monotypic kappa, CD19-negative plasma cells (*red circle*) are compared to polytypic (normal) CD19-positive plasma cells (*green circle*) for DNA content based on DAPI nuclear staining. In this example, monotypic kappa plasma cells show hyperdiploid DNA content. (**b**) Determining the proliferative fraction of plasma cells (S-phase of the cell cycle) based on DAPI staining

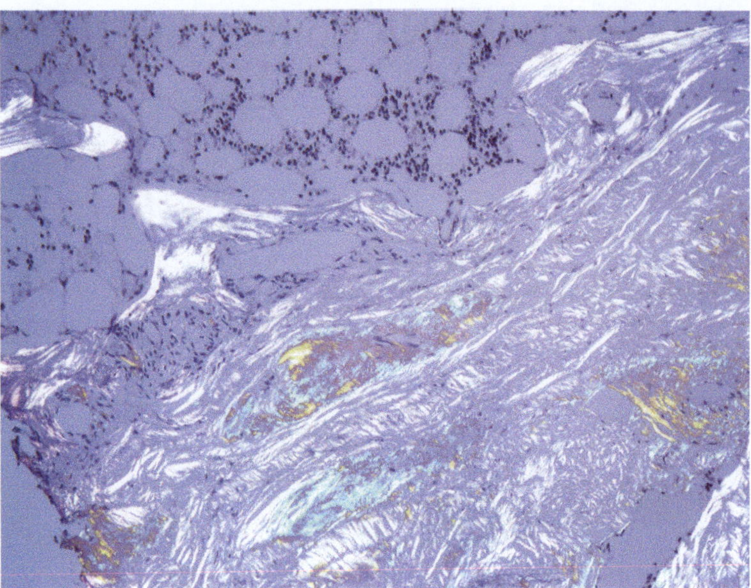

Fig. 3.5 Amyloid deposition in periosteal blood vessels (Congo red, ×100)

amyloid). The misfolding of amyloidogenic protein results in antiparallel beta pleated-sheets that give amyloid its chemical and physical features, including resistance to enzymatic digestion and light transmission properties. The latter is used in amyloid detection in the tissue biopsy, including bone marrow and subcutaneous fat aspirate: Congo Red stain of amyloid deposits shows characteristic birefringence (red-apple green) under polarized light (Fig. 3.5). It is important to emphasize that the presence of clonal PCs in the bone marrow, with associated amyloid deposits, does not automatically imply that the amyloid is of AL type, as monoclonal gammopathies are rather prevalent in older patient population. For that reason, after amyloid is detected, it needs to be subtyped to identify its forming protein. The classical methods of IHC staining of amyloid deposits lack sensitivity and specificity and have been replaced by recently developed mass spectrometry proteomic methods [13]. This method shows a remarkable ability to precisely identify protein forming amyloid; more than a hundred different amyloidogenic proteins have been identified so far using proteomic tools.

Other Pathologic Processes

There is a wide range of pathologic processes that can accompany PCPDs. The most common ones are Large Granular Lymphocyte (LGL) proliferations and therapy-related myeloid neoplasms.

LGL proliferations (LGL leukemias) are monoclonal or oligoclonal lymphoproliferative disorders of cytotoxic lymphocytes (T or NK-cells). These expansions may be associated with cytopenias (anemia, neutropenia, and/or thrombocytopenia) [14]. It can be challenging to establish the diagnosis of an LGL proliferation in the presence of PCPD, as LGL proliferations can be a part of a normal immune response to emerging PC clone. In addition, cytopenias are often a feature of PCPD itself. Therefore, LGL proliferations are usually diagnosed in cases of disproportionate lymphoid infiltrates and cytopenias that are not explained by the extent of PC involvement of the bone marrow or M-protein concentration. However, criteria for establishing the diagnosis of LGL proliferation in the presence of PCPD are not well-defined.

Therapy for MM includes cytotoxic drugs such as melphalan. The well-known side effect of these

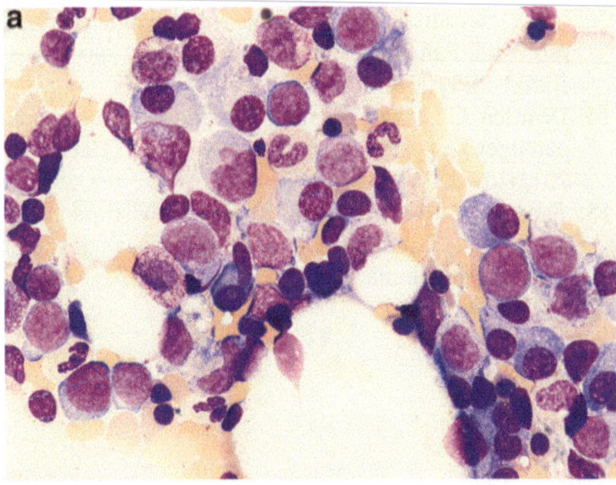

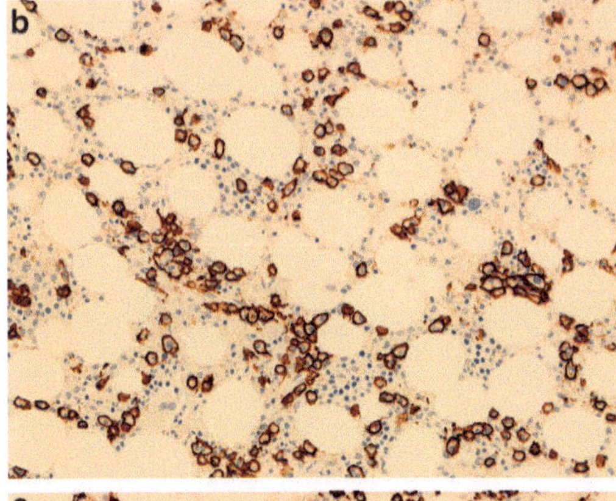

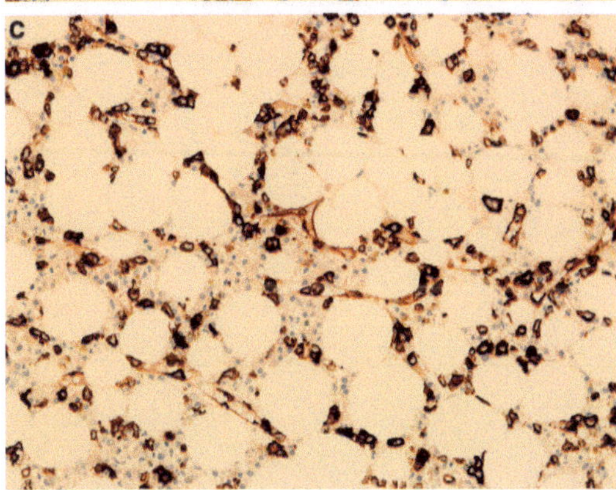

Fig. 3.6 Secondary acute myeloid leukemia developing in a patient with treated MM. (**a**) Wright-Giemsa stain of the bone marrow aspirate shows increased plasma cells and blasts (×600). (**b**) CD138 stain on the biopsy specimen shows increased plasma cells. (**c**) CD34 stain shows increased myeloid blasts

drugs is DNA damage in normal hematopoietic cells. The accumulation of DNA damage can lead to secondary, therapy-related, myeloid neoplasms such as myelodysplastic syndrome (MDS) and acute myeloid leukemia (AML) [15] (Fig. 3.6). Careful examination of bone marrow specimen for early signs of therapy-related changes is necessary in any MM patient on therapy.

References

1. McKenna RW, Kyle RA, Kuehl WM, Grogan TM, Harris NL, Coupland RW. Plasma cell neoplasms. In: Swerdlow SH, Campo E, Harris NL, Jaffe ES, Pileri SA, Stain H, Thiele J, Vardiman JW, editors. WHO classification of tumours of haematopoietic and lymphoid tissue. Lyon: IARC; 2008. p. 200–13.
2. Morice WG, Hanson CA, Kumar S, Frederick LA, Lesnick CE, Greipp PR. Novel multi-parameter flow cytometry sensitively detects phenotypically distinct plasma cell subsets in plasma cell proliferative disorders. Leukemia. 2007;21:2043–6.
3. Nadav L, Katz BZ, Baron S, et al. Diverse niches within multiple myeloma bone marrow aspirates affect plasma cell enumeration. Br J Haematol. 2006;133:530–2.
4. Kumar S, Kimlinger T, Morice W. Immunophenotyping in multiple myeloma and related plasma cell disorders. Best Pract Res Clin Haematol. 2010;23:433–51.
5. Morice WG, Chen D, Kurtin PJ, Hanson CA, McPhail ED. Novel immunophenotypic features of marrow lymphoplasmacytic lymphoma and correlation with Waldenstrom's macroglobulinemia. Mod Pathol. 2009;22:807–16.
6. Swerdlow SH, Berger F, Pileri SA, Harris NL, Jaffe ES, Stain H. Lymphoplasmacytic lymphoma. In: Swerdlow SH, Campo E, Harris NL, Jaffe ES, Pileri SA, Stain H, Thiele J, Vardiman JW, editors. WHO classification of tumours of haematopoietic and lymphoid tissues. Lyon: IARC; 2008. p. 194–5.
7. Schuster SR, Rajkumar SV, Dispenzieri A, et al. IgM multiple myeloma: disease definition, prognosis, and differentiation from Waldenstrom's macroglobulinemia. Am J Hematol. 2010;85:853–5.
8. Dao LN, Hanson CA, Dispenzieri A, Morice WG, Kurtin PJ, Hoyer JD. Bone marrow histopathology in POEMS syndrome: a distinctive combination of plasma cell, lymphoid, and myeloid findings in 87 patients. Blood. 2011;117:6438–44.
9. Fonseca R, Bergsagel PL, Drach J, et al. International Myeloma Working Group molecular classification of multiple myeloma: spotlight review. Leukemia. 2009;23: 2210–21.
10. Munshi NC, Anderson KC, Bergsagel PL, et al. Consensus recommendations for risk stratification in multiple myeloma: report of the International Myeloma Workshop Consensus Panel 2. Blood. 2011; 117:4696–700.
11. Kumar SK, Uno H, Jacobus SJ, et al. Impact of gene expression profiling-based risk stratification in

patients with myeloma receiving initial therapy with lenalidomide and dexamethasone. Blood. 2011;118: 4359–62.

12. Greipp PR, Lust JA, O'Fallon WM, Katzmann JA, Witzig TE, Kyle RA. Plasma cell labeling index and beta 2-microglobulin predict survival independent of thymidine kinase and C-reactive protein in multiple myeloma. Blood. 1993;81:3382–7.
13. Vrana JA, Gamez JD, Madden BJ, Theis JD, Bergen III HR, Dogan A. Classification of amyloidosis by laser microdissection and mass spectrometry-based proteomic analysis in clinical biopsy specimens. Blood. 2009;114:4957–9.
14. Dearden C. Large granular lymphocytic leukaemia pathogenesis and management. Br J Haematol. 2011;152:273–83.
15. Thomas A, Mailankody S, Korde N, Kristinsson SY, Turesson I, Landgren O. Second malignancies after multiple myeloma: from 1960s to 2010s. Blood. 2012;119:2731–7.

4 Pathogenesis of Multiple Myeloma

Marta Chesi and P. Leif Bergsagel

Introduction

Multiple myeloma (MM) is monoclonal tumor of antibody secreting plasma cells (PC) in the bone marrow (BM), that is often diagnosed by the presence of a typical M-spike by serum protein electrophoresis (SPEP), or by free light chains in the urine. Its symptomatic phase is associated with significant end organ damage including lytic bone lesions, anemia, loss of kidney function, immunodeficiency, and amyloid deposits in various tissues [1]. MM incidence is higher in blacks than whites, and in men than women [2], for a total estimate of 21,700 cases and 10,710 deaths in the United States in 2012 [3]. Although MM continues to be considered an incurable disease, thanks to the recent therapeutic advances, the 5-year survival rate reported in the SEER database has increased from 28 % (1987–1989) to 43 % (2002–2008) [2]. Notably, a subset of patients with cytogenetically defined low-risk MM, initially treated in 1999 were reported having a 10-year survival rate of 75 % [4], with presumably even better results possible for patients starting treatment today. MM cells are the malignant counterpart of post-germinal center (GC) long-lived PCs, characterized by strong BM dependence, somatic hypermutation (SHM) of immunoglobulin (Ig) genes, and isotype class switch resulting in the absence of IgM expression in all but 1 % of tumors [5]. However, MM cells differ from healthy PCs because they retain the potential for a low rate of proliferation (1–3 % of cycling cells).

Multi-step Clinical Course of Multiple Myeloma

Virtually every case of MM is preceded by a premalignant PC tumor called monoclonal gammopathy of undetermined significance (MGUS) [6, 7] that, like MM, produces a typical M-spike (almost always non-IgM) by SPEP or free light chain in the urine. It has to be distinguished from an IgM-secreting lymphoid MGUS, a precursor phase of chronic lymphocytic leukemia, lymphoplasmacytoma, and Waldenstrom's macroglobulinemia. PC MGUS is age-dependent, is present in about 4 % of individuals over the age of 50 [8, 9], and can progress to MM at average rates of 1 % per year to and MM. MGUS is distinguished from MM by having an M-spike of <30 g/L, with no more than 10 % of BM mononuclear cells being tumor cells, and no end organ damage or other symptoms. Progression of MGUS to smoldering MM and symptomatic MM is associ-

M. Chesi, Ph.D.
Division of Biochemistry and Molecular Biology, Mayo Clinic Arizona, 13400 E Shea Blvd, Scottsdale, AZ 85259, USA
e-mail: Chesi.Marta@mayo.edu

P.L. Bergsagel, M.D. (✉)
Division of Hematology Research and Division of Hematology/Oncology, Mayo Clinic Arizona, 13400 E Shea Blvd, Scottsdale, AZ 85259, USA
e-mail: Bergsagel.Leif@mayo.edu

M.A. Gertz and S.V. Rajkumar (eds.), *Multiple Myeloma: Diagnosis and Treatment*,
DOI 10.1007/978-1-4614-8520-9_4, © Mayo Foundation for Medical Education and Research 2014

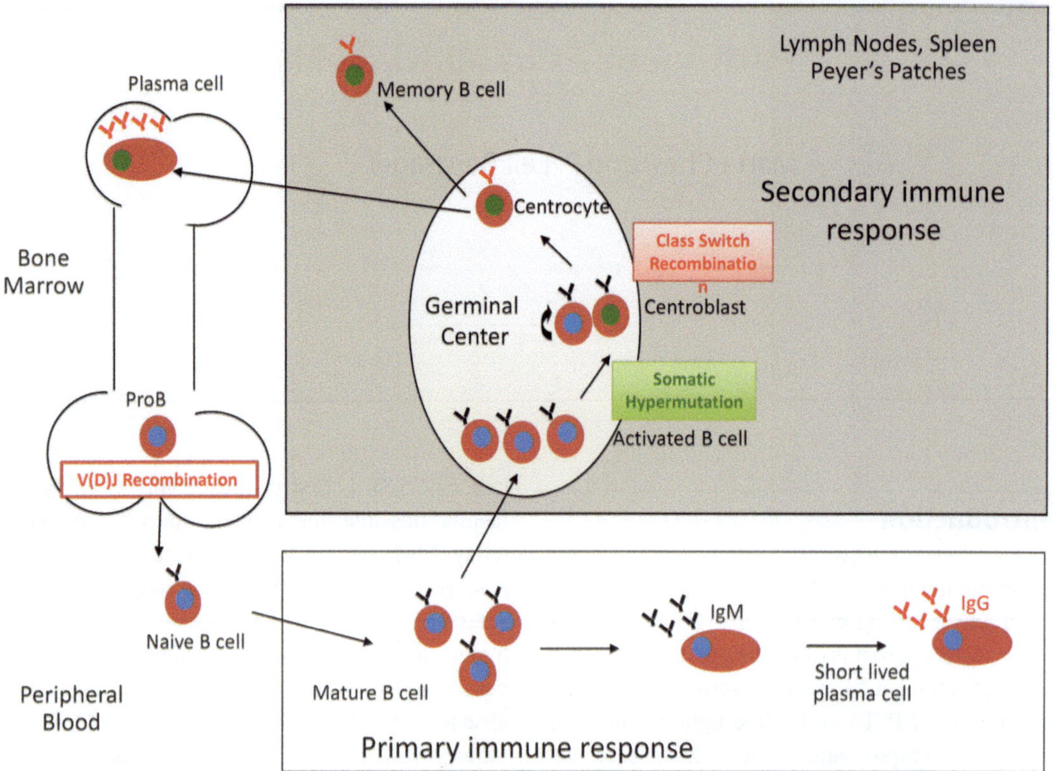

Fig. 4.1 Normal plasma cell development. Pre-germinal center B cells expressing surface immunoglobulin can enter germinal centers where the immunoglobulin genes undergo repeated rounds of somatic hypermutation followed by IgH isotype switch recombination. In MM, IgH translocations occur as a result of errors in these two physiologic DNA modification processes (10 % and 90 %, respectively). Post-GC B cells can generate plasmablast that home to the bone marrow where stromal cells facilitate differentiation into long-lived PC. Normal PC express surface CD138, CD19, and CD45, whereas MM cells express CD138, only 10 % express CD19, 99 % are CD45- or dim, and 70 % express CD56

ated with an expanding BM tumor mass and increasingly severe organ impairment or symptoms [1]. Despite the recent advances in the understanding of the MM pathogenesis, it is still largely impossible to predict which MGUS patient will and which one will never progress to MM. Although MM cells are characterized by a strong dependence on the BM tumor microenvironment, at late stages of the disease the more aggressive tumor may sometimes extends to extramedullary locations, such as spleen, liver, and extracellular spaces. *Extramedullary* MM (EMM) can also present with a leukemic phase, that is classified as secondary or primary *plasma cell leukemia* (PCL), depending on whether or not a preceding intramedullary MM was recognized. Most of the available human MM cell lines (HMCLs) have been generated from EMM or PCL tumors [10, 11] and represent a renewable repository of the oncogenic events involved in initiation and progression of the most aggressive end-stage MM tumors.

Origins of MM

During a secondary immune response, activated lymphocytes migrate into GCs were they undergo antigen selection by multiple rounds of SHM and IgH class switch recombination (CSR). Cells whose B cell receptor loses affinity for the antigen are counterselected and undergo apoptosis, while positively selected cells are rescued from apoptosis by expression of BCL2 and differentiate into either memory cells or plasma blasts (PB) before homing to the BM as long-lived PC (Fig. 4.1).

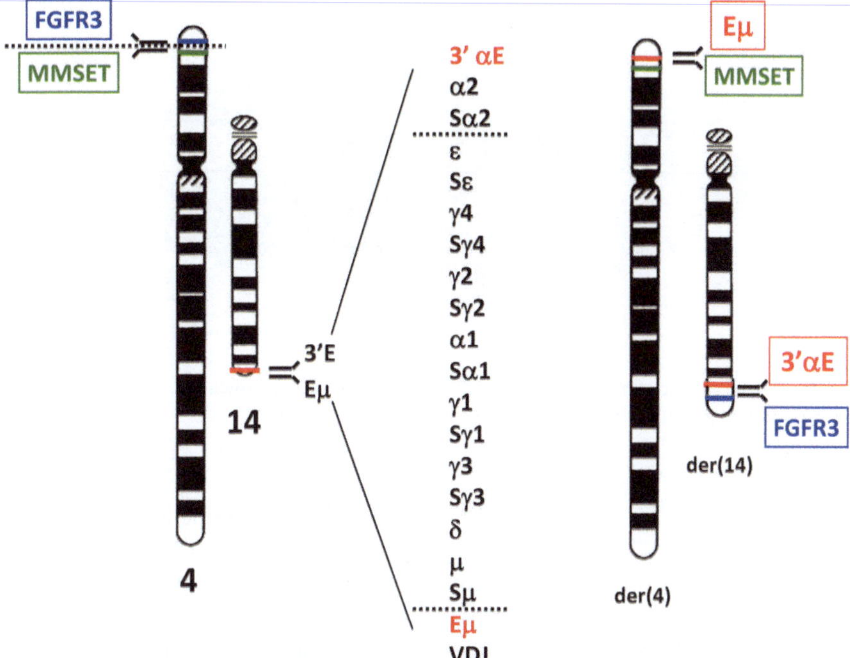

Fig. 4.2 Anatomy of t(4;14)(p16.3; q32) chromosome translocation. An IgH locus that has completed VDJ recombination can undergo productive switch recombination (S) as a result of targeted double-strand breaks (DSB) in switch regions that are upstream of constant regions; sequences between the two switch regions are lost. Rarely, a t(4;14) translocation occurs when DSB occur in switch regions and in the 5′ end of the MMSET gene, and there is heterologous joining of the DSB to form two derivative chromosomes, der(14) and der(4) that contain the respective centromeres. The FGFR3 oncogene is dysregulated on der(14) by the 3′Eα enhancer, and der(4) produces a hybrid Ig-MMSET transcript, which contains only MMSET codons, and is dysregulated by the Eμ enhancer

Although pre-GC short-lived PCs can also be generated during primary immune response, the presence of somatic mutations in the immunoglobulin genes without further remodeling clearly indicates a post-GC origin for MM.

Primary IgH Translocations

Translocations involving the IgH locus (14q32) or one of the IgL loci (κ, 2p12 or λ, 22q11) are present in at least half of MM cases and are thought to result from errors during the physiological process of CSR or SHM since the breakpoints are usually located near or within IgH switch regions, but sometimes near VDJ sequences [12]. It is presumed that these translocations represent primary—perhaps initiating—oncogenic events as normal B cells pass through GCs. In fact, although clonal heterogeneity has been identified in MM as in many other cancers, the primary chromosome translocations continue to mark the tumor clone throughout disease progression. As in other B cell tumors, these translocations result in dysregulated expression of an oncogene that is juxtaposed to the strong Ig enhancers. However, translocations involving an IgH switch region uniquely dissociate the intronic (Emu) from one or both 3′ IgH enhancers (3′E), so that two putative oncogenes can become dysregulated on the two derivative chromosomes. This is exemplified by the t(4;14) translocation that simultaneously dysregulate FGFR3 on der(14) and MMSET on der(4) in MM (Fig. 4.2).

These IgH translocations are efficiently detected by fluorescent in situ hybridization (FISH) analyses. Large studies from several groups show that the prevalence of IgH translocations increase with disease stage: about 50 % in MGUS or SMM, 55–70 % for intramedullary MM, 85 % in PCL, and >90 % in HMCL [13, 14]. Limited studies indicate that IgL translocations

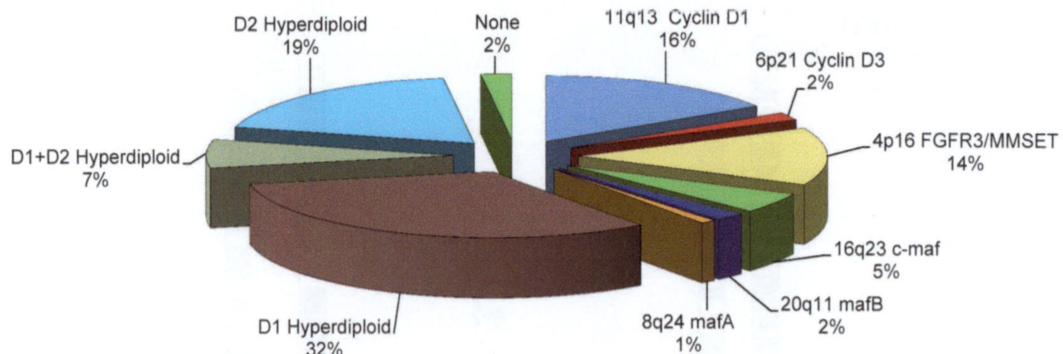

Fig. 4.3 Distribution of genetic subtypes of untreated MM using the TC classification. A pie chart shows the relative frequency of the different genetic subgroups of MM using the TC classification

are present in about 10 % of MGUS/SMM tumors, and about 15–20 % of intramedullary MM tumors and HMCL [11]. Translocations involving an IgK locus are rare, occurring in only 1–2 % of MM tumors and HMCL [11].

There are three recurrent primary IgH translocation groups, with the chromosomal sites, target oncogenes, and approximate prevalence in MM (~40 % prevalence for all three groups) as follows: CYCLIN D (11q13-*CYCLIN D1*-15 %; 12p13-*CYCLIN D2*- <1 %; 6p25-*CYCLIN D3*-2 %); MAF (16q23-*MAF*-5 %; 20q12-MAFB-2 %; 8q24.3-*MAFA*-<1 %); MMSET/(FGFR3)-4p16-(*MMSET* in all but also *FGFR3* in 80 % of these tumors)-15 % (Fig. 4.3). With the exception perhaps of FGFR3, it is interesting to note that none of the primary translocations causes dysregulation of strong oncogenes, suggesting that perhaps this would be incompatible with terminal differentiation of PCs and their homing to the BM. Also IgH translocation groups are mutually exclusive, although double translocations have been reported in HMCLs (e.g., KMS11 carries both an MAF and FGFR3 translocation on the two IgH alleles).

It is thought that CYCLIN D translocations only dysregulate expression of a CYCLIN D gene. By contrast MAF translocations, dysregulate expression of an MAF transcription factor that causes increased expression of many genes, including CYCLIN D2 and adhesion molecules that are thought to enhance the ability of the tumor cell to interact with the BM microenvironment [15, 16]. The contributions of the two genes dysregulated by t(4;14) remain controversial. MMSET is a chromatin-remodeling factor that is over-expressed in all tumors with a t(4;14), whereas about 20 % of tumors lack der(14) and FGFR3 expression. The rare acquisition of FGFR3 activating mutations during progression confirms a role for FGFR3 in MM pathogenesis. Although an activated mutant FGFR3 can be oncogenic, it recently was shown that wild-type FGFR3 (as is found in most t[4;14]) can contribute to B cell oncogenesis [17]. It remains to be determined if FGFR3 is critical early in pathogenesis but becomes dispensable during progression of t(4;14) MM, especially in the presence of RAS-BRAF activating mutations that, like mutated FGFR3, also lead to constitutive phosphorylation of ERK1-2. Preclinical studies suggest that tyrosine kinase inhibitors are active only against t(4;14) HMCL with activating mutations of FGFR3, whereas anti-FGFR3 monoclonal antibodies that inhibit FGFR3 signaling but also elicit antibody-dependent cell-mediated cyotoxicity are active against HMCLs expressing wild type FGFR3 [18, 19]. Definitive results about the clinical activity of FGFR3-targeted therapy have not been reported yet. Despite an apparently indispensable role in t(4;14) MM, it remains to be determined how MMSET contributes to MM pathogenesis. There are some clues. It is a histone methyltransferase for H3K36me2, and when over-expressed results in a global increase in H3K36 methylation, and a decrease in H3K27 methylation, which most likely is the cause of the many changes in gene expression observed in t(4;14) tumors [15, 20–22]. In addition, it recently has been determined that MMSET has a role in DNA repair. Following DNA damage MMSET is phosphorylated on Ser102 by ATM and is recruited to sites of double-strand breaks (DSB) where it results in methylation of H4K20 that is required for recruitment of p53 binding protein (53BP1). 53BP1 is required for p53 accumulation, G2/M checkpoint arrest, and the intra-S-phase checkpoint in response to ionizing radiation. Approximately half of the translocation breakpoints in t(4;14) MM result in a truncated MMSET that lacks Ser102 and cannot be recruited to DSBs, resulting in a failure to recruit 53BP1 and a loss of the normal DNA damage response pathway. It is not known whether this biologic difference results in a different clinical outcome for t(4;14) MM patients with a truncated versus full-length MMSET [23]. Importantly, loss of MMSET expression alters adhesion, suppresses growth, and results in apoptosis of HMCLs, suggesting that it is an attractive therapeutic target [21].

Hyperdiploidy

There is a consensus that chromosome content reflects at least two pathways of pathogenesis. Nearly half of MGUS and MM tumors are hyperdiploid (HRD), with 48–75 (mostly 49–56) chromosomes, usually with extra copies of three or more specific chromosomes (3,5,7,9,11,15,19, 21). Non-hyperdiploid (NHRD) tumors have <48 and/or >75 chromosomes. Strikingly, HRD tumors rarely (~10 %) have a primary IgH translocation, whereas NHRD tumors usually (~70 %) have an IgH translocation [24] (Fig. 4.4). Although it has been proposed that NHRD and HRD tumors represent different pathways of pathogenesis, the timing, mechanism, and molecular consequences of hyperdiploidy is unknown. In any case, HRD patients seem to have a better prognosis than NHRD patients. Curiously, EMM tumors and HMCLs nearly always have an NHRD genotype, suggesting that HRD tumors are more stromal cell-dependent than NHRD tumors. Alternatively it is possible that HRD is selected against in proliferating cells. In fact, a few cell lines derived from HRD patients have lost the extra chromosomes (unpublished observation). Interestingly, in patients with t(4;14), t(14;16), t(14;20), or del17p the presence of one or more trisomies are associated with a substantially better prognosis than the absence of trisomies. This suggests that the phenotype associated with trisomies may be dominant [25].

Cyclin Ds and MM Progression

Almost all cases of plasma cell neoplasm starting from the MGUS stage and independently on the chromosome content aberrantly express one or more of the CYCLIN D genes and it has been proposed that dysregulation of a CYCLIN D gene provides a unifying, early oncogenic event in MGUS and MM (Fig. 4.4). Remarkably though this is not associated with increased proliferation, as the PC labeling index in MGUS, like in normal PCs, remain virtually =0. Yet the expression level of cyclin D1, cyclin D2, or cyclin D3 mRNA in MM and MGUS is distinctly higher than in normal PCs. This results from several mechanisms including a direct *cis*-dysregulation in MM tumors with a CYCLIN D gene translocation [i.e., t(11;14), t(6;14), or t(12;14)] or a *trans-dysregulation* in tumors with a translocation of MAF [t(14;16)], encoding a transcription factor that directly bind to the CYCLIN D2 promoter. Although MMSET/FGFR3 tumors express moderately high levels of CYCLIN D2, the cause of increased CYCLIN D2 expression remains unknown. The majority of HRD tumors express CYCLIN D1 bi-allelically, perhaps because they contain a trisomic chromosome 11, whereas most other tumors express increased levels of CYCLIN D2 by unknown mechanism. Only a few percent of MM tumors do not express any CYCLIN D gene, but have been shown to contain a high level of contamination with normal cells. Another fraction of cyclin D negative samples show bi-allelic deletion of RB1, the cell cycle inhibitor directly targeted by CYCLIN D, therefore bypassing the need for CYCLIN D gene.

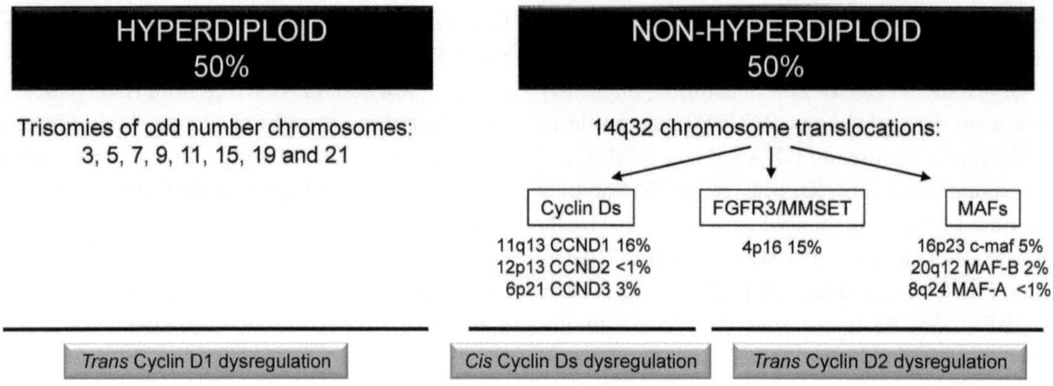

HYPERDIPLOID
50%

Trisomies of odd number chromosomes:
3, 5, 7, 9, 11, 15, 19 and 21

NON-HYPERDIPLOID
50%

14q32 chromosome translocations:

Cyclin Ds
11q13 CCND1 16%
12p13 CCND2 <1%
6p21 CCND3 3%

FGFR3/MMSET
4p16 15%

MAFs
16p23 c-maf 5%
20q12 MAF-B 2%
8q24 MAF-A <1%

Trans Cyclin D1 dysregulation

Cis Cyclin Ds dysregulation

Trans Cyclin D2 dysregulation

Fig. 4.4 Cyclin Ds dysregulation in MM. MGUS and MM karyotypes can be divided into hyperdiploid and non-hyperdiploid based on chromosomal content. Almost all hyperdiploid tumors have bi-allelic cyclin D1 trans-dysregulation. Non-hyperdiploid tumors often have t(14q32) translocations affecting the indicated loci (frequency is shown). In about 25 % of them, one of the D type cyclins is cis-dysregulated by a 14q32 translocation, in the other non-hyperdiploid tumors cyclin D2 expression is trans-dysregulated

Molecular Classification of MM

The patterns of spiked expression of genes deregulated by primary IgH translocations and the universal over-expression of *CCNDs* genes led to the Translocations and Cyclin D (TC) classification that includes eight groups: those with primary translocations (designated 4p16, 11q13, 6p21, MAF), those that over-expressed *CCND1* and *CCND2* either alone or in combination (D1, D1&D2, D2), and the rare cases that do not over-express any CCND genes ("none") (Table 4.1) [15]. Greater than 95 % of tumors in the D1 group are HRD. In addition, most of the patients with HRD MM and trisomy 11 fall within the D1 and D1&D2 groups, while those without trisomy 11 fall within the D2 group, although a majority of the D2 group are NHRD. This classification system is derived from a supervised analysis of gene expression data based on the different mechanisms that dysregulate a *CCND* gene as an early and unifying event in pathogenesis.

An MM classification based on an unsupervised analysis of microarray gene expression profiling from the UAMS identified seven tumor groups characterized by the co-expression of unique gene clusters [26]. This classification was partially replicated in an independent unsupervised analysis of a combined HOVON-GMMG dataset that identified ten tumor groups with considerable overlap with the UAMS groups [27]. Interestingly, these clusters partially overlap with the subgroups of the TC classification corresponding to the different primary translocations and HRD. Importantly, however, they also highlight other secondary events that become dominant during MM progression that can occur independently in each subtype of MM: proliferation (PR), expression of NFkB target genes (NFkB), cancer-testis antigens (CTA), and the phosphatase *PTP4A3/PRL3* (PRL3). In addition to insights into the molecular biology of the disease, these classifications are prognostically relevant because, together with other cytogenetic markers (i.e., 17p deletion) they help stratifying patients into high and low risk. The CD-1 and CD-2 groups represent subgroups of patients with t(11;14) and t(6;14), with the former characterized by argino-succinate synthetase 1 expression, and the later by expression of B cell antigens (*CD20*, *VPREB*, *CD79A*). Interestingly they identify patients with markedly different clinical outcomes. Of all the molecular subgroups, CD-1 has the quickest onset and highest frequency of CR (90 %), whereas CD-2 has the slowest onset, and lowest frequency of CR (45 %), when treated with Total Therapy 3. However, after the MF, the CD-1 have the shortest CR duration (77 % at 2 years), whereas the CD-2 have the longest (100 % at 2 years) [28].

Table 4.1 Comparison of different molecular classifications in multiple myeloma

Group	TC	Gene	%	CYCLIN D	UAMS	HOVON-GMMG
Cyclin D translocation	11q13	CCND1	15	CYCLIN D1	CD-1	CD-1 CD-2
	12p13	CCND2	<1	CYCLIN D2	CD-2	
	6p25	CCND3	2	CYCLIN D3		
MAF translocation	16q23	MAF	5	CYCLIN D2	MF	MF
	20q12	MAFB	2	CYCLIN D2		
	8q24	MAFA	<1	CYCLIN D2		
MMSET translocation	4p16	MMSET/FGFR3	15	CYCLIN D2	MS	MS
Hyperdiploid with trisomy 11	D1		33	CYCLIN D1	HY	HY CD-1 NFkB CTA PRL3
	D1+D2		7	CYCLIN D1 and D2	PR	PR CTA
Hyperdiploid without trisomy 11 and others	D2		18	CYCLIN D2	LB	LB CTA PRL3
Other	None	RB1 bi-allelic deletion	2	No CYCLIN D	PR	PR CTA

MGUS to MM Progression

A plethora of mutations have been identified in MM patients, which can occur at different frequency independently in the different disease groups and are thought to promote disease progression.

MYC Dysregulation

There is increased expression of c-*MYC* in most newly diagnosed MM tumors compared to MGUS tumors [29]. Recently, it was shown that sporadic activation of an *MYC* transgene in GC B cells in an MGUS prone mouse strain led to the universal development of MM tumors [30, 31]. Hence, increased *MYC* expression seems to be responsible for progression from MGUS to MM. Complex translocations involving *MYC* (c-*MYC*≫N-*MYC*>L-*MYC*) appear to be secondary progression events that often do not involve Ig loci [32]. They are rare or absent in MGUS, but occur in 15 % of newly diagnosed tumors, 50 % of advanced tumors, and 90 % of HMCLs [11, 33]. A recent report suggests that a small molecule inhibitor of BRD4 can inhibit *MYC* RNA expression in MM, with therapeutic effect [34].

Chromosome 13 Deletion

A recent study concludes that chromosome 13 deletion can be an early event in MGUS (e.g., in *MAF*, *MMSET* tumors) or a progression event (e.g., in t(11;14) tumors) [35]. The pathogenic effect of this chromosome deletion is unknown, though it is possible that haploinsufficiency of *RB1* promotes tumorigenesis [13]. A recent genome-wide sequencing study identified mutations of DIS3, a gene of unknown function on 13q, in about 10 % of MM. Although only very few mutations have been reported to date, it has been suggested that DIS3 mutation occur in parallel with deletions of RB1 [36], suggesting a possible dependence between these two events. Although del13 was initially reported to be an independent prognostic factor, it is now accepted only when detected by conventional cytogenetic in the more proliferative cells.

Activating Mutations of *RAS* and *BRAF*

The prevalence of activating *NRAS* or *KRAS* mutations is about 15–18 % each in newly diagnosed and relapsed MM tumors [13, 37], but substantially higher in tumors that express *CCND1* compared to tumors that express *CCND2*. For MGUS tumors, the prevalence of *NRAS* mutations is 7 %, but *KRAS* mutations have not been described [38]. This is consistent with increasing evidence that *NRAS* and *KRAS* mutations have overlapping but nonidentical effects [39] and also the hypothesis that *KRAS* mutations provide a molecular mark of the transition of MGUS to MM [40, 41]. MM tumors depend on the continued expression of activated but not wild type *RAS* [42]. Recently, *BRAF* mutations were described in 4 % of MM tumors, suggesting a possible role for BRAF inhibitors in these cases [43].

Activating Mutations of NFkappaB Pathway

Extrinsic ligands (APRIL and BAFF) produced by BM stromal cells provide critical survival signals to long-lived PCs by stimulating TACI, BCMA, and BAFF receptors to activate the NFKB pathways [44]. Most MGUS and MM tumors highly express NFKB target genes, suggesting a continued role of extrinsic signaling in PC tumors [45, 46] and at least in part explaining the constant dependency of MM cells on the BM microenvironment. Activating mutations in positive regulators and inactivating mutations in negative regulators of the NFKB pathway have been identified in at least 20 % of untreated MM tumors and ~50 % of HMCLs, rendering the cells less dependent on ligand-mediated NFKB activation (Fig. 4.5) [43] and most likely contributing to extramedullary spread of the disease. Interestingly, the NFKB negative regulator TRAF3 located on 14q32 is inactivated in >10 % MM tumors, suggesting that at least in the presence of RAS/BRAF compensating mutation there may be an advantage for t(4;14) MM to lose the der(14) containing FGFR3 in favor of activating the NFKB pathway. Small molecules that inhibit extrinsic signaling (including TACI.Fc, IKKβ, and NIK (MAP3K14)) are being developed as potential therapeutic agents [47, 48]. There is also some evidence suggesting that cells addicted to constitutive NFKB activation may be particularly sensitive to proteasome inhibition [46].

Chromosome 17p Loss and Abnormalities of *TP53*

Deletions that include the *TP53* locus occur in ~10 % of untreated MM tumors, and the prevalence increases with disease stage [13, 49]. *TP53* mutations were present in 37 % of untreated MM tumors with del17p, but not in patients without del17p [50]. Even in the absence of TP53 mutations, del17p remains a strong independent negative predictor for survival of MM patients, although it remains to be determined if the poor prognosis is due to haploinsufficiency or to predisposition to complete inactivation of TP53 eventually occurring with tumor progression. Recently, decreased expression of microRNAs miR-199, -192, and -215 in MM was reported to increase MDM2, an inhibitor of *TP53* [51], contributing to loss of p53 activity.

Gain of Chromosome 1q and Loss of Chromosome 1p

These genomic events frequently occur together in MM, and each of them is associated with a poor prognosis [13, 52]. The relevant genes on 1q are unclear at this time although the anti-apoptotic gene MCL1 has been suggested as a potential driver of the adverse survival. By contrast, there are potential targets on two regions of 1p that are associated with a poor prognosis: *CDKN2C* (p18INK4c) at 1p32.3 and *FAM46C* at 1p12 [53, 54]. Homozygous deletion of the cell cycle regulator *CDKN2C*, which is present in about 30 % of HMCL and about 5 % of untreated MM tumors, is associated with increased proliferation and a poor prognosis, whereas monoallelic deletion is not. Mutations of *FAM46C*—often with hemizygous deletion—were identified in 3.4 and 13 % of MM tumors in two studies, and in 25 % of 16 HMCL, although the function of this gene is still unknown [43, 53].

Other Pathogenic Events

Secondary Ig translocations, including most IgK and IgL translocations and IgH translocations not

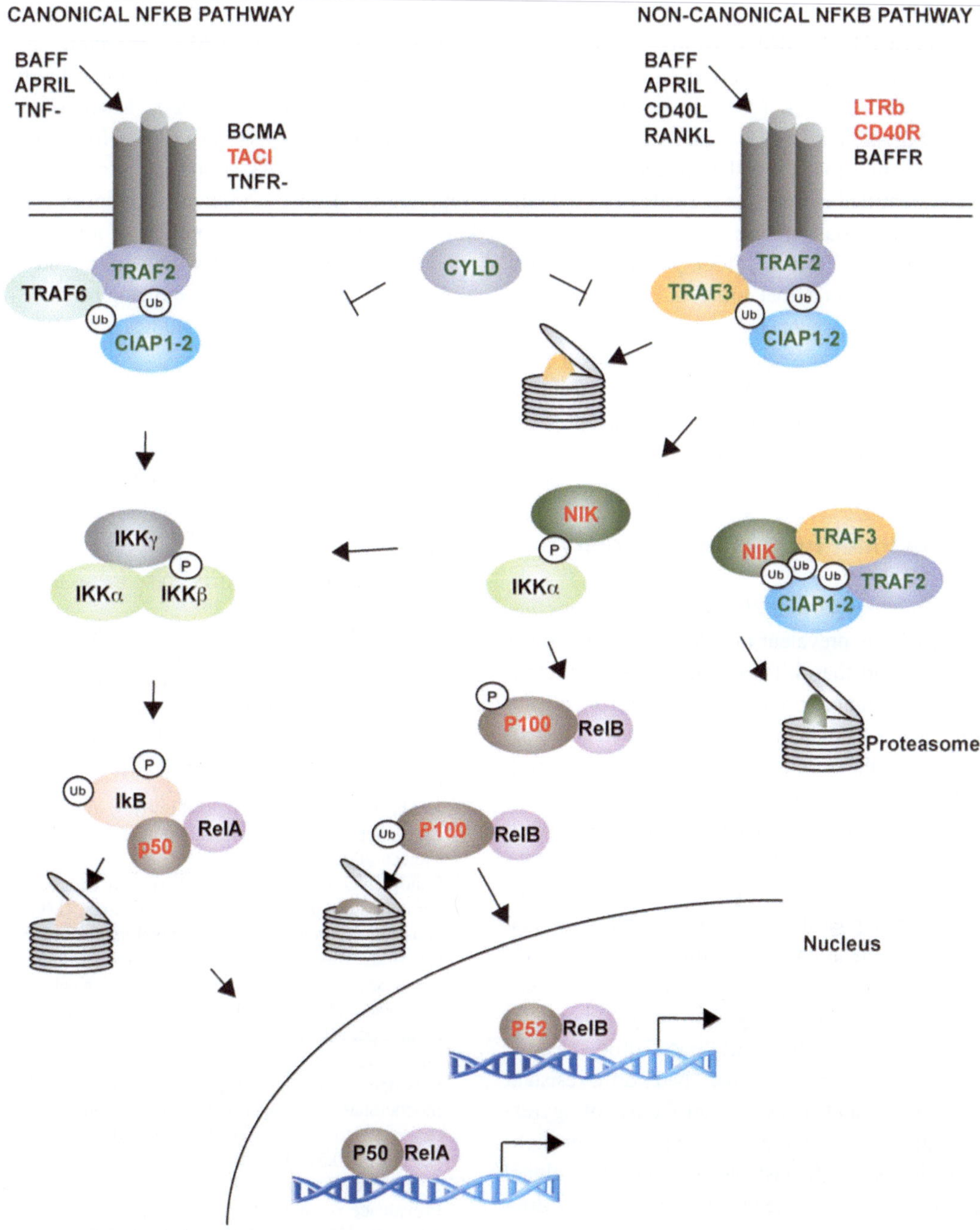

Fig. 4.5 Mutations of the NF κB pathway in MM. Molecular components and processing events for the classical and alternative NFkB pathways are depicted, both of which result in the translocation of an active NFkB transcription factor into the nucleus. Both pathways can be activated by a variety of stimuli, including the interaction of external factors with PC receptors. Positive regulatory proteins (*red*) and negative regulatory proteins (*green*) are targets for mutations that constitutively activate NFkB during the progression of some MM tumors

involving one of the seven primary partners, can occur at all stages of disease, and with a similar frequency in HRD and NHRD tumors, but apart from MYC, few partner loci have been identified [11]. Other genomic rearrangements are frequent, but only a few specific target genes have been identified [52, 55, 56]. Changes in DNA methylation are frequent, with one study suggesting that a marked increase in hypomethylation is associated with the MGUS to MM transition [57], whereas a second study suggests only a small increase in hypomethylation for MM compared to MGUS [58]. Mutations in seven genes regulating RNA metabolism, protein translation, and homeostasis were identified in 16 of 38 patients [43]. In addition to previous studies implicating roles for *MMSET* and *KDM6A* (UTX), genomic sequencing studies found that other histone modifying enzymes are frequent targets of mutation, although the epigenetic consequences are unknown [43]. Similarly, changes in microRNA expression at different stages have been identified, but more extensive studies are needed [51, 59].

Intra-Clonal Tumor Heterogeneity

Recent evidences indicate suggest that tumor heterogeneity is prevalent in MM, as in many other cancers, and that different subclones are present within the tumor population, characterized by distinct genetic mutations that contributed independently to the tumor progression [36, 56, 60]. Recently a high level of intra-clonal tumor heterogeneity has been described in some patients with high-risk MM [36, 56, 60] associated in one case with alternating clonal dominance under therapeutic selective pressure, observations with important clinical implications. The findings suggest a competition between subclones for limited resources and raise the possibility that early, suboptimal treatment may eradicate the "good" drug-sensitive clone, making room for the "bad" drug-resistant clone to expand. They support the use of aggressive multidrug combination approaches for high-risk disease with unstable genomes and clonal heterogeneity, and sequential one or two drug approaches for low-risk disease with stable genomes and lacking clonal heterogeneity.

Summary

Significant progress has been made is understanding the molecular pathogenesis and biology of MM. Oncogenic pathways can be activated through cell intrinsic or extrinsic mechanisms. Similar to other cancers, MM is characterized by multistage accumulation of genetic abnormalities deregulating different pathways. Much of this knowledge is already being utilized for diagnosis, prognosis, and risk-stratification of patients. Importantly, from a clinical standpoint, this knowledge has led to development of novel therapeutic strategies, some of which are already in clinical use, and many others showing promise in preclinical and early clinical studies.

References

1. Malpas JS, Bergsagel DE, Kyle R, Anderson K. Multiple myeloma: biology and management. Oxford: Oxford University Press; 2004.
2. Howlader N, Noone AM, Krapcho M, et al. SEER cancer statistics review 1975–2009. Bethesda, MD: National Cancer Institute; 2012.
3. Siegel R, Naishadham D, Jemal A. Cancer statistics, 2012. CA Cancer J Clin. 2012;62(1):10–29.
4. Avet-Loiseau H, Attal M, Campion L, et al. Long-term analysis of the IFM 99 trials for myeloma: cytogenetic abnormalities [t(4;14), del(17p), 1q gains] play a major role in defining long-term survival. J Clin Oncol. 2012;30(16):1949–52.
5. Kuehl WM, Bergsagel PL. Multiple myeloma: evolving genetic events and host interactions. Nat Rev Cancer. 2002;2(3):175–87.
6. Landgren O, Kyle RA, Pfeiffer RM, et al. Monoclonal gammopathy of undetermined significance (MGUS) consistently precedes multiple myeloma: a prospective study. Blood. 2009;113(22):5412–7.
7. Weiss BM, Abadie J, Verma P, Howard RS, Kuehl WM. A monoclonal gammopathy precedes multiple myeloma in most patients. Blood. 2009;113(22):5418–22.
8. Dispenzieri A, Katzmann JA, Kyle RA, et al. Prevalence and risk of progression of light-chain monoclonal gammopathy of undetermined significance: a retrospective population-based cohort study. Lancet. 2010;375(9727):1721–8.
9. Kyle RA, Therneau TM, Rajkumar SV, et al. Prevalence of monoclonal gammopathy of undetermined significance. N Engl J Med. 2006;354(13):1362–9.
10. Drexler HG, Matsuo Y. Malignant hematopoietic cell lines: in vitro models for the study of multiple myeloma and plasma cell leukemia. Leuk Res. 2000;24(8):681–703.
11. Gabrea A, Martelli ML, Qi Y, et al. Secondary genomic rearrangements involving immunoglobulin or MYC loci show similar prevalences in hyperdiploid and nonhyperdiploid myeloma tumors. Genes Chromosomes Cancer. 2008;47(7):573–90.

12. Bergsagel PL, Kuehl WM. Chromosome translocations in multiple myeloma. Oncogene. 2001;20(40):5611–22.
13. Fonseca R, Bergsagel PL, Drach J, et al. International Myeloma Working Group molecular classification of multiple myeloma: spotlight review. Leukemia. 2009;23(12):2210–21.
14. Avet-Loiseau H, Facon T, Daviet A, et al. 14q32 translocations and monosomy 13 observed in monoclonal gammopathy of undetermined significance delineate a multistep process for the oncogenesis of multiple myeloma. Intergroupe Francophone du Myelome. Cancer Res. 1999;59(18):4546–50.
15. Bergsagel PL, Kuehl WM, Zhan F, Sawyer J, Barlogie B, Shaughnessy Jr J. Cyclin D dysregulation: an early and unifying pathogenic event in multiple myeloma. Blood. 2005;106(1):296–303.
16. Hurt EM, Wiestner A, Rosenwald A, et al. Overexpression of c-maf is a frequent oncogenic event in multiple myeloma that promotes proliferation and pathological interactions with bone marrow stroma. Cancer Cell. 2004;5(2):191–9.
17. Zingone A, Cultraro CM, Shin D-M, et al. Ectopic expression of wild-type FGFR3 cooperates with MYC to accelerate development of B-cell lineage neoplasms. Leukemia. 2010;24(6):1171–8.
18. Qing J, Du X, Chen Y, et al. Antibody-based targeting of FGFR3 in bladder carcinoma and t(4;14)-positive multiple myeloma in mice. J Clin Invest. 2009;119(5):1216–29.
19. Trudel S, Li ZH, Wei E, et al. CHIR-258, a novel, multitargeted tyrosine kinase inhibitor for the potential treatment of t(4;14) multiple myeloma. Blood. 2005;105(7):2941–8.
20. Marango J, Shimoyama M, Nishio H, et al. The MMSET protein is a histone methyltransferase with characteristics of a transcriptional corepressor. Blood. 2008;111(6):3145–54.
21. Martinez-Garcia E, Popovic R, Min D-J, et al. The MMSET histone methyl transferase switches global histone methylation and alters gene expression in t(4;14) multiple myeloma cells. Blood. 2011;117(1):211–20.
22. Kuo AJ, Cheung P, Chen K, et al. NSD2 links dimethylation of histone H3 at lysine 36 to oncogenic programming. Mol Cell. 2011;44(4):609–20.
23. Pei H, Zhang L, Luo K, et al. MMSET regulates histone H4K20 methylation and 53BP1 accumulation at DNA damage sites. Nature. 2011;470(7332):124–8.
24. Fonseca R, Debes-Marun CS, Picken EB, et al. The recurrent IgH translocations are highly associated with nonhyperdiploid variant multiple myeloma. Blood. 2003;102(7):2562–7.
25. Kumar S, Fonseca R, Ketterling RP, et al. Trisomies in multiple myeloma: impact on survival in patients with high-risk cytogenetics. Blood. 2012;119(9):2100–5.
26. Zhan F, Huang Y, Colla S, et al. The molecular classification of multiple myeloma. Blood. 2006;108(6):2020–8.
27. Broyl A, Hose D, Lokhorst H, et al. Gene expression profiling for molecular classification of multiple myeloma in newly diagnosed patients. Blood. 2010;116(14):2543–53.
28. Nair B, van Rhee F, Shaughnessy JD, et al. Superior results of Total Therapy 3 (2003–33) in gene expression profiling-defined low-risk multiple myeloma confirmed in subsequent trial 2006–66 with VRD maintenance. Blood. 2010;115(21):4168–73.
29. Chng WJ, Huang GF, Chung T-H, et al. Clinical and biological implications of MYC activation: a common difference between MGUS and newly diagnosed multiple myeloma. Leukemia. 2011;25(6):1026–35.
30. Chesi M, Robbiani DF, Sebag M, et al. AID-dependent activation of a MYC transgene induces multiple myeloma in a conditional mouse model of post-germinal center malignancies. Cancer Cell. 2008;13(2):167–80.
31. Chesi M, Matthews GM, Garbitt VM, et al. Drug response in a genetically engineered mouse model of multiple myeloma is predictive of clinical efficacy. Blood. 2012;120(2):376–85.
32. Dib A, Gabrea A, Glebov OK, Bergsagel PL, Kuehl WM. Characterization of MYC translocations in multiple myeloma cell lines. J Natl Cancer Inst. 2008;39:25–31.
33. Avet-Loiseau H, Gerson F, Magrangeas F, Minvielle S, Harousseau JL, Bataille R. Rearrangements of the c-myc oncogene are present in 15% of primary human multiple myeloma tumors. Blood. 2001;98(10):3082–6.
34. Delmore JE, Issa GC, Lemieux ME, et al. BET bromodomain inhibition as a therapeutic strategy to target c-Myc. Cell. 2011;146(6):904–17.
35. Chiecchio L, Dagrada GP, Ibrahim AH, et al. Timing of acquisition of deletion 13 in plasma cell dyscrasias is dependent on genetic context. Haematologica. 2009;94(12):1708–13.
36. Walker BA, Wardell CP, Melchor L, et al. Intraclonal heterogeneity and distinct molecular mechanisms characterize the development of t(4;14) and t(11;14) myeloma. Blood. 2012;120(5):1077–86.
37. Chng WJ, Gonzalez-Paz N, Price-Troska T, et al. Clinical and biological significance of RAS mutations in multiple myeloma. Leukemia. 2008;22(12):2280–4.
38. Zingone A, Kuehl WM. Pathogenesis of monoclonal gammopathy of undetermined significance and progression to multiple myeloma. Semin Hematol. 2011;48(1):4–12.
39. Haigis KM, Kendall KR, Wang Y, et al. Differential effects of oncogenic K-Ras and N-Ras on proliferation, differentiation and tumor progression in the colon. Nat Genet. 2008;40(5):600–8.
40. Rasmussen T, Haaber J, Dahl IM, et al. Identification of translocation products but not K-RAS mutations in memory B cells from patients with multiple myeloma. Haematologica. 2010;95(10):1730–7.
41. Rasmussen T, Kuehl M, Lodahl M, Johnsen HE, Dahl IMS. Possible roles for activating RAS mutations in the MGUS to MM transition and in the intramedullary to extramedullary transition in some plasma cell tumors. Blood. 2005;105(1):317–23.

42. Steinbrunn T, Stuhmer T, Gattenlöhner S, et al. Mutated RAS and constitutively activated Akt delineate distinct oncogenic pathways, which independently contribute to multiple myeloma cell survival. Blood. 2011;117(6):1998–2004.
43. Chapman MA, Lawrence MS, Keats JJ, et al. Initial genome sequencing and analysis of multiple myeloma. Nature. 2011;471(7339):467–72.
44. Elgueta R, de Vries VC, Noelle RJ. The immortality of humoral immunity. Immunol Rev. 2011;236:139–50.
45. Annunziata CM, Davis RE, Demchenko Y, et al. Frequent engagement of the classical and alternative NF-kappaB pathways by diverse genetic abnormalities in multiple myeloma. Cancer Cell. 2007;12(2):115–30.
46. Keats JJ, Fonseca R, Chesi M, et al. Promiscuous mutations activate the noncanonical NF-kappaB pathway in multiple myeloma. Cancer Cell. 2007;12(2):131–44.
47. Demchenko YN, Glebov OK, Zingone A, Keats JJ, Bergsagel PL, Kuehl WM. Classical and/or alternative NF-kappaB pathway activation in multiple myeloma. Blood. 2010;115(17):3541–52.
48. Rossi JF, Moreaux J, Hose D, et al. Atacicept in relapsed/refractory multiple myeloma or active Waldenström's macroglobulinemia: a phase I study. Br J Cancer. 2009;101(7):1051–8.
49. Tiedemann RE, Gonzalez-Paz N, Kyle RA, et al. Genetic aberrations and survival in plasma cell leukemia. Leukemia. 2008;22(5):1044–52.
50. Lode L, Eveillard M, Trichet V, et al. Mutations in TP53 are exclusively associated with del(17p) in multiple myeloma. Haematologica. 2010;95(11):1973–6.
51. Pichiorri F, Suh S-S, Rocci A, et al. Downregulation of p53-inducible microRNAs 192, 194, and 215 impairs the p53/MDM2 autoregulatory loop in multiple myeloma development. Cancer Cell. 2010;18(4):367–81.
52. Walker BA, Leone PE, Chiecchio L, et al. A compendium of myeloma-associated chromosomal copy number abnormalities and their prognostic value. Blood. 2010;116(15):e56–65.
53. Boyd KD, Ross FM, Walker BA, et al. Mapping of chromosome 1p deletions in myeloma identifies FAM46C at 1p12 and CDKN2C at 1p32.3 as being genes in regions associated with adverse survival. Clin Cancer Res. 2011;17(24):7776–84.
54. Dib A, Peterson TR, Raducha-Grace L, et al. Paradoxical expression of INK4c in proliferative multiple myeloma tumors: bi-allelic deletion vs increased expression. Cell Div. 2006;1:23.
55. Avet-Loiseau H, Li C, Magrangeas F, et al. Prognostic significance of copy-number alterations in multiple myeloma. J Clin Oncol. 2009;27(27):4585–90.
56. Keats JJ, Chesi M, Egan JB, et al. Clonal competition with alternating dominance in multiple myeloma. Blood. 2012;120(5):1067–76.
57. Walker BA, Wardell CP, Chiecchio L, et al. Aberrant global methylation patterns affect the molecular pathogenesis and prognosis of multiple myeloma. Blood. 2011;117(2):553–62.
58. Salhia B, Baker A, Ahmann G, Auclair D, Fonseca R, Carpten J. DNA methylation analysis determines the high frequency of genic hypomethylation and low frequency of hypermethylation events in plasma cell tumors. Cancer Res. 2010;70(17):6934–44.
59. Pichiorri F, Suh SS, Ladetto M, et al. MicroRNAs regulate critical genes associated with multiple myeloma pathogenesis. Proc Natl Acad Sci U S A. 2008;105(35):12885–90.
60. Magrangeas F, Avet-Loiseau H, Gouraud W, et al. Minor clone provides a reservoir for relapse in multiple myeloma. Leukemia. 2013;27:473–81.

Staging of Multiple Myeloma

5

Vivek Roy and Philip R. Greipp

Introduction

Multiple myeloma is a heterogeneous disease characterized by proliferation of neoplastic clonal plasma cells and a range of clinical manifestations including skeletal destruction, hypercalcemia, anemia, renal failure, immune suppression, and hyperviscosity syndrome [1]. Outcome of patients with myeloma is very variable with survival ranging from a few months to several years depending on the biology of the disease as well as the health status of the patient, which in turn may be largely affected by disease burden.

The heterogeneity of the disease presents a challenge for the patient, clinician as well as the research community. Accurate prediction of the clinical course is important in treatment planning. Many treatment options that have different likelihood of response and carry different levels of risk of toxicity may be available for a given patient. Having a reliable prediction of disease prognosis allows both the patient and physician to choose therapy commensurate with the predicted natural history of the disease. Patients with disease that is expected to have a more aggressive course may be offered, and they may be willing to accept, therapy that offers higher probability of response even if it carries more risks of side effects whereas patients predicted to have slowly progressive disease may be candidates for less aggressive therapy. Availability of a standardized prediction system also allows for comparisons across different clinical trials by providing a means to ensure equivalent patient populations in the trials. Similarly, efficacy of different therapies developed over time can be better compared. An ideal staging system would utilize objective and reproducible factors that are easily obtainable and commonly used in clinical practice. The staging system should be applicable across the spectrum of the disease and segregate patients into roughly equal groups (Table 5.1).

Over the years, various clinical and laboratory factors have been shown to correlate with disease outcome (Table 5.2). These factors reflect the pathophysiology of the disease, extent of disease, end organ damage, health status of the patient, or a combination of these factors. As the underlying biology of the disease has been better understood, there has been greater appreciation of the critical role of cytogenetic and molecular alterations causing dysregulation of intracellular pathways in determining the clinical course and prognosis of myeloma. The cytogenetics and molecular risk stratification of myeloma will be discussed in detail elsewhere in the book and will not be further addressed here.

Early studies in 1960s and 1970s identified a number of clinical and laboratory parameters

V. Roy, M.D. (✉)
Division of Hematology and Oncology, Mayo Clinic, Jacksonville, FL, USA
e-mail: roy.vivek@mayo.edu

P.R. Greipp, M.D.
Division of Hematology, Mayo Clinic, 200 First Street, SW, Rochester, MN 55905, USA

M.A. Gertz and S.V. Rajkumar (eds.), *Multiple Myeloma: Diagnosis and Treatment*,
DOI 10.1007/978-1-4614-8520-9_5, © Mayo Foundation for Medical Education and Research 2014

Table 5.1 Desirable characteristics of a staging system

- Based on widely and easily obtainable parameters
- Parameters are objective and reproducible
- Parameters relatively specific and unique to the disease
- Segregates patients into roughly equal groups
- Applicable across the spectrum of disease and treatment

Table 5.2 Prognostic factors and myeloma

Factors associated with prognosis in multiple myeloma
Patient-related
Age
Gender
Performance status
Laboratory parameters
Hemoglobin
Platelet count
Albumin
Calcium
BUN/creatinine
Beta2 microglobulin
C-reactive protein
LDH
Disease-specific
Type of paraprotein
Light chain myeloma
Abnormal free light chain ratio
Plasmablastic morphology
PCLI
Rapid response
Primary resistance to therapy
Cytogenetic features
Hypodiploidy
del 13 (by cytogenetics)
t(14;16), t (14;20)
del 17p

associated with survival in multiple myeloma including performance status, hemoglobin level, serum calcium, renal function, albumin, type of myeloma protein, bone lesions, and percent of plasma cells in the marrow [2–7]. In a cooperative group study by Acute Leukemia Group B (ALGB) and Eastern Cooperative Oncology Group (ECOG) a combination of four clinical and laboratory factors were used to categorize patients into "good risk" (BUN less than 30, calcium ≤ 12, absence of significant infection, WBC$\geq$4,000/mm^3, and estimated survival >2 months) and "poor risk" groups (not meeting the above mentioned good risk criteria). Patients in the good risk group had more than twice the response rate and longer survival [2].

Durie–Salmon Staging System

More elaborate predictive models were developed in the 1970s and 1980s and validated in clinical trials. Salmon et al. showed in 1970 that immunoglobulin synthesis and total tumor cell number could be correlated with clinically observable parameters in IgG multiple myeloma [8]. They proposed a staging system, Durie and Salmon staging (DSS) based on clinical and laboratory features including hemoglobin level, extent of bone lesions, serum calcium, and monoclonal protein levels in the serum and urine. These features were used to predict myeloma cell mass (multiple myeloma cells $\times 10^{12}$/m^2 body surface area) and correlated with response to chemotherapy and survival [7]. Patients were categorized as stage I, II, or III depending on predicted low, intermediate, or high plasma cell burden. Each stage was further subdivided into A or B depending on the serum creatinine level <2 or $\geq$2 mg/dL. The median duration of survival for IA patients was approximately 5 years whereas that of stage III B patients was 14.7 months. The system permitted relatively easy categorization of multiple myeloma patient and led to better interpretation of therapeutic trials because patient populations in clinical trials could be compared. However, it had significant shortcomings particularly in evaluating and scoring bone lesions and it did not take into account more important biological features such as a proliferative rate of multiple myeloma cells. Nonetheless, the system was validated in subsequent studies by other investigators and shown to predict median survival in large cohorts of patients [5, 9–12]. It was widely adopted and remained in common use for over 30 years.

Modifications to Durie Salmon Staging

Over time there have been attempts to improve Durie–Salmon staging systems by adding additional stratifying variables. Cavo et al. showed in a study of 163 patient's that addition of platelet count improved the discriminating power of Durie–Salmon staging system and segregated high risk (stage II and III) groups into smaller subgroups of patients with platelet count less than 150,000/cmm who had median survival of 9 months whereas patients with stage II and III disease and platelet count ≥150,000/cmm had median survival of 48 months [13]. One of the shortcomings of Durie–Salmon staging system is that the classification is based on the number and extent of bone lesions found on plain X-rays and observer-dependent parameter. With the availability of more sensitive bone imaging techniques, MRI and PET scans, a modified staging system Durie-Salmon Plus has been proposed. This system integrated MRI and whole-body FDG PET scan into the DSS system and was shown to further discriminate early stage disease patients as well as identify higher risk subgroups of patients with stage II and III disease [14]. This modified system however has not gained broad acceptability.

The Medical Research Council (MRC) of the UK analyzed determinants of prognosis in a large cohort of 485 patients entered in the MRC's third therapeutic trial. This study confirmed many previously identified prognostic factors including better outcome in females. They proposed blood urea, hemoglobin, and clinical performance status as the three major determinants of prognosis. Based on these factors patients could be grouped into three risk categories. Good risk group had blood urea ≤8 mmol, hemoglobin ≥100 g/L, and no or minimal symptoms. This group comprised 22 % of patients in the trial and had survival probability of 76 % after median follow-up of 36 months. The poor prognosis group defined by blood urea >10 mmol, hemoglobin ≤75 g/L and restricted clinical activity comprised 22 % of patients and had survival probability of only 9 %. The rest of the patients (56 %) who did not meet the poor or good prognosis criteria were placed in the intermediate prognosis group and had survival probability of 50 % after median follow-up of 36 months [15].

Merlini, Waldenstrom, and Jayakar evaluated eight common multiple myeloma-related clinical and laboratory parameters to identify factors most significantly associated with survival in a cohort of 173 patients. Multiple regression analysis showed that survival of IgG and Bence Jones myeloma patients could be best predicted by combination of serum creatinine, serum calcium, and bone marrow plasma cell percentage (MWJ system). Survival predictions for individual patients could be made by inserting individual patient's parameters into survival graphs and multiple regression equations [10]. Patients were segregated into roughly equal groups; 50 patients in stage III, 30 in stage II and 43 in stage I. The relative death rates approximately doubled between the stages with median survival of 12, 41, and 76 months in stage III, II, and I, respectively.

These three staging systems, DSS, MRC, and MWJ, prevalent in the 1970s and 1980s were evaluated by other investigators. Bataille et al. correlated the presenting features of 147 newly diagnosed multiple myeloma patients with survival duration using multiple regression analysis [16]. In addition to the variables utilized by the three staging systems, the study also evaluated two new variables: Serum beta2 microglobulin (B2m) and instantaneous rate of bone resorption using a calcitonin-induced hypocalcemia that had been shown to be a marker of myeloma activity and previous studies [17]. The study found that all three systems gave significant discrimination of high risk patients from others although each system gave different distribution of patients. The Durie–Salmon system was found to be the most valuable for stratification of patients and added significantly to the survival predictions provided by either MRC or MWJ. A similar study evaluated the prognostic significance of different presenting parameters in 180 patients with multiple myeloma. Eight predictive variables were isolated in univariate analysis but only blood urea and serum albumin were found to have significance and in multivariate model and could successfully segregate patients into high risk and low risk groups [18]. The authors also compared the three major myeloma staging systems (DSS, MRC, and MWJ) in this cohort of patients and found that only the MRC system showed prognostic validity [18]. Another study that compared staging systems in use in the 1970s and 1980s found significant differences in the predicted ability of the systems. It was noted that none of the systems were clearly superior to single risk factors, especially creatinine and hemoglobin [19].

Prognostic Factors Relevant to Staging

In the 1980s and 1990s, other prognostic factors were identified including serum albumin, beta2 microglobulin, C-reactive protein, and proliferative activity of bone marrow plasma cells.

Beta2 microglobulin, a low molecular weight protein, is the light chain component of the HLA class I antigen complex and synthesized by all nucleated cells. It is normally excreted in the urine and blood levels of beta2 microglobulin increase with impairment of renal function. It was recognized as an important independent prognostic factor in multiple myeloma in 1980s [20–22]. Serum levels of beta2 microglobulin correlate strongly with tumor burden and also reflect renal impairment which itself is an adverse prognostic marker in myeloma. Moreover, the fact that serum beta2 microglobulin level predicts survival regardless of DS stage suggests that it reflects more than just tumor burden and renal function but possibly also other biological properties such as proliferation rate. Beta2 microglobulin alone had a strong predictive value surpassing that of MRC or MWJ or their combination. The addition of beta2 microglobulin to Durie–Salmon further enhanced its discriminative value. Combination of beta2 microglobulin and albumin, parameters that were not part of DSS, MRC or MWJ staging systems, was more predictive than any of the staging systems and was the best model to predict survival in the study by Bataille et al. [16].

Interleukin-6 (IL-6) is potent growth and survival factor for multiple myeloma cells [23, 24]. C-reactive protein concentration reflects IL-6 activity. There is a close correlation between their serum concentrations and their predictive value for multiple myeloma prognosis largely overlap [25]. Because of the ease of measurement CRP has been commonly used as a surrogate marker for IL-6 in clinical use. The predictive value of CRP is independent of beta2 microglobulin and their combination was shown to be able to stratify multiple myeloma patients into low, intermediate, and high risk groups with median survival of 54, 27, and 6 months, respectively [26]. It is important to remember that CRP is an acute phase reactant and the prognostic utility of elevated CRP level is probably only applicable in the absence of other causes of CRP elevation such as infection or inflammation.

Proliferative characteristics of plasma cells in multiple myeloma correlate with clinical outcomes [27, 28]. Plasma cell labeling index (PCLI) test identifies the proportion of clonal plasma cells in S phase in a rapid and reproducible manner [29]. Bone marrow cells are incubated with 5-bromo-2-deoxyuridine. Clonal plasma cells are identified by reactivity to kappa or lambda light chain reagent. Cells in S phase in the clonal population are detected using BU-1 antibody. Most of the factors used in myeloma staging systems reflect the effect of disease on the patient. In contrast, PCLI is a direct measure of the tumor proliferation. It was shown to be a powerful independent predictor of survival in a study that evaluated a number of prognostic factors in 107 patients with newly diagnosed multiple myeloma. Univariate analysis showed prognostic significance for thymidine kinase level, C-reactive protein, beta2 microglobulin, albumin, age, and PCLI. However, only beta2 microglobulin and PCLI retained independent prognostic significance in multivariate analysis [30]. Low levels of these factors predicted for excellent outcome with 8 of 9 patients aged less than 65 (who otherwise had stage distribution similar to other patients in the cohort) with low PCLI and B2m survived more than 6 years.

International Staging System

These studies established beta2 microglobulin, either by itself or in combination with another parameter, as a strong predictive marker of survival duration in multiple myeloma. However, there was no consensus as to the optimal use of any one or combination of factors or about the cut off levels. An international effort was launched to develop a consensus staging system that would be based on widely available objective parameters used around the world. A panel of international experts gathered data on 10,750 patients from 15 Asian, European, and North American institutions and groups between 1981 through

Table 5.3 International staging system for myeloma

Stage	Criteria	Median survival (months)
I	Serum β2-microglobulin <3.5 mg/dL Serum albumin ≥3.5 g/dL	62
II	Not stage I or II	44
III	Serum β2-microglobulin ≥5.5 mg/dL	29

There are two categories of stage II: serum β2-microglobulin <3.5 mg/dL but serum albumin <3.5 g/dL; or serum β2-microglobulin 3.5 to <5.5 mg/dL irrespective of the serum albumin level

2002. Of these patients, 7,430 (69 %) came from clinical trial data. Extensive demographic, patient and myeloma-related laboratory data including standard cytogenetics, FISH, and proliferative activity of plasma cells was collected. Univariate and multivariate survival analyses were performed. Prognostic factors identified in prior studies including low platelet count, age more than 65 years, serum creatinine ≥2 mg/dL, LDH, hemoglobin less than 10, poor performance status, bone marrow plasma cell percent ≥33 %, light chain myeloma, and non-IgA isotype were confirmed. Beta2 microglobulin and albumin emerged as the most consistent, broadly applicable prognostic factors correlated with survival duration. Based on these two factors a three stage system, International Staging System (ISS) [31], was developed that provided highly statistically significant stratification (Table 5.3).

There were roughly a third of patients in each of the three stages and median survival was 62, 44, and 29 months in stages I, II, and III, respectively. The ISS was shown to have comparable discriminatory efficacy in patients from different geographical regions of the world, patients from individual institutions or cooperative groups, and both younger (<65 years) or older patients. The staging system discriminated similarly for patients treated with standard dose therapy or high-dose therapy with autologous hematopoietic cell transplant.

The authors also compared ISS with DS system and found that the ISS provided more uniform distribution of patients across the three stages. The survival of ISS stage I corresponded exactly to DS stage IA with median survival of 62 months. Survival of DS stage IIA patients (58 m) was also similar to ISS stage I while survival of ISS stage II patients was similar to DS stage III A patients (45 months). Notably, the poor risk group (substage B) off all the DS stages could be grouped together in ISS stage III. ISS has been rapidly and widely adopted because it is easy to compute, has objective parameters that eliminate inter-observer variability, and provides for more uniform distribution of patients across the three stages. It has subsequently been validated in other independent studies [32].

ISS was compared to other staging system for its ability to predict the outcomes of recipients of autologous stem cell transplant. A Korean study evaluated whether staging at the time of diagnosis could influence survival of multiple myeloma patients undergoing stem cell transplant as first-line therapy. Patients (N= 152) were followed for a median of 22.6 months after transplant. Progression-free and overall survival could be predicted by ISS but not by DS system. Staging at the time of diagnosis was a better predictor of survival than staging at the time of transplant [33].

ISS and DSS were also compared for their ability to predict outcomes of autologous transplant recipients in a retrospective study by Center for International Blood and Marrow Transplant Research (CIBMTR) [34]. Patients (N=729) who underwent transplant within 12 months of diagnosis were staged by both the systems at diagnosis and at transplant. Median follow was 56 months. There was only 36 % concordance between the two staging systems. Relative risks of PFS and OS were significantly different for stage I versus II and stage II versus III for DSS but only for stage II versus III for ISS. It is not clear whether the ability to undergo transplant or the transplant itself overrode the differences in ISS early stage patients.

Summary

Multiple myeloma is a heterogeneous disease with very variable outcomes depending on the disease as well as patient characteristics. There is a need to develop predictive staging systems to facilitate clinical care of patient as well as help with developing and interpreting clinical trials. Many staging systems have been developed over time and ISS is currently the most commonly used because of its simplicity and efficacy. However, none of the systems fully account for the variability of outcome. There remains a need for further refinement, a goal likely to be achieved by incorporating other more sensitive and biologically relevant markers such as MRI, PET, cytogenetic information, and gene expression profiling. The challenge is to devise staging system that is highly predictive and yet simple and based on easily available clinical parameters.

References

1. Kyle RA, Rajkumar SV. Multiple myeloma. N Engl J Med. 2004;351:1860–73.
2. Costa G, Engle RL, Schilling A, et al. Melphalan and prednisone: an effective combination ofor the treatment of multiple myeloma. Am J Med. 1973;54:589–99.
3. Peto R. Urea, albumin, and response rates. Br Med J. 1971;2:324.
4. Dawson AA, Ogston D. Factors influencing the prognosis in myelomatosis. Postgrad Med J. 1971;47:635–8.
5. Alexanian R, Balcerzak S, Bonnet JD, et al. Prognostic factors in multiple myeloma. Cancer. 1975;36: 1192–201.
6. Carbone PP, Kellerhouse LE, Gehan EA. Plasmacytic myeloma. A study of the relationship of survival to various clinical manifestations and anomalous protein type in 112 patients. Am J Med. 1967;42:937–48.
7. Durie BG, Salmon SE. A clinical staging system for multiple myeloma. Correlation of measured myeloma cell mass with presenting clinical features, response to treatment, and survival. Cancer. 1975;36:842–54.
8. Salmon SE, Smith BA. Immunoglobulin synthesis and total body tumor cell number in IgG multiple myeloma. J Clin Invest. 1970;49:1114–21.
9. Woodruff RK, Wadsworth J, Malpas JS, Tobias JS. Clinical staging in multiple myeloma. Br J Haematol. 1979;42:199–205.
10. Merlini G, Waldenstrom JG, Jayakar SD. A new improved clinical staging system for multiple myeloma based on analysis of 123 treated patients. Blood. 1980;55:1011–9.
11. Bergsagel DE, Bailey AJ, Langley GR, MacDonald RN, White DF, Miller AB. The chemotherapy on plasma-cell myeloma and the incidence of acute leukemia. N Engl J Med. 1979;301:743–8.
12. Belpomme D, Simon F, Pouillart P, et al. Prognostic factors and treatment of multiple myeloma: interest of a cyclic sequential chemohormonotherapy combining cyclophosphamide, melphalan, and prednisone. Recent Results Cancer Res. 1978;65:28–40.
13. Cavo M, Galieni P, Grimaldi M, et al. Improvement of Durie & Salmon staging for multiple myeloma by adding platelet count as a stratifying variable: a multivariate regression analysis of 163 untreated patients. Eur J Haematol Suppl. 1989;51:99–104.
14. Durie BG. The role of anatomic and functional staging in myeloma: description of Durie/Salmon plus staging system. Eur J Cancer. 2006;42:1539–43.
15. Medical Research Council's Working Party on Leukemia in Adults. Prognostic features in the third MRC myelomatosis trial. Medical Research Council's Working Party on Leukaemia in Adults. Br J Cancer. 1980;42:831–40.
16. Bataille R, Durie BG, Grenier J, Sany J. Prognostic factors and staging in multiple myeloma: a reappraisal. J Clin Oncol. 1986;4:80–7.
17. Bataille R, Legendre C, Sany J. Acute effects of salmon calcitonin in multiple myeloma: a valuable method for serial evaluation of osteoclastic lesions and disease activity—a prospective study of 125 patients. J Clin Oncol. 1985;3:229–36.
18. Blade J, Rozman C, Cervantes F, Reverter JC, Montserrat E. A new prognostic system for multiple myeloma based on easily available parameters. Br J Haematol. 1989;72:507–11.
19. Gassmann W, Pralle H, Haferlach T, et al. Staging systems for multiple myeloma: a comparison. Br J Haematol. 1985;59:703–11.
20. Durie BG, Stock-Novack D, Salmon SE, et al. Prognostic value of pretreatment serum beta 2 microglobulin in myeloma: a Southwest Oncology Group Study. Blood. 1990;75:823–30.
21. Bataille R, Vincent C, Revillard JP, Sany J. Serum beta-2-microglobulin binding activity in monoclonal gammopathy: correlative study and clinical significance. Eur J Cancer Clin Oncol. 1983;19:1075–80.
22. Child JA, Crawford SM, Norfolk DR, O'Quigley J, Scarffe JH, Struthers LP. Evaluation of serum beta 2-microglobulin as a prognostic indicator in myelomatosis. Br J Cancer. 1983;47:111–4.
23. Kawano M, Hirano T, Matsuda T, et al. Autocrine generation and requirement of BSF-2/IL-6 for human multiple myelomas. Nature. 1988;332:83–5.
24. Klein B, Zhang XG, Jourdan M, et al. Paracrine rather than autocrine regulation of myeloma-cell growth and differentiation by interleukin-6. Blood. 1989;73: 517–26.
25. Tienhaara A, Pulkki K, Mattila K, Irjala K, Pelliniemi TT. Serum immunoreactive interleukin-6 and C-reactive protein levels in patients with multiple myeloma at diagnosis. Br J Haematol. 1994;86: 391–3.
26. Bataille R, Boccadoro M, Klein B, Durie B, Pileri A. C-reactive protein and beta-2 microglobulin produce a simple and powerful myeloma staging system. Blood. 1992;80:733–7.
27. San Miguel JF, Garcia-Sanz R, Gonzalez M, et al. A new staging system for multiple myeloma based on the number of S-phase plasma cells. Blood. 1995;85: 448–55.

28. Latreille J, Barlogie B, Johnston D, Drewinko B, Alexanian R. Ploidy and proliferative characteristics in monoclonal gammopathies. Blood. 1982;59:43–51.
29. Greipp PR, Katzmann JA, O'Fallon WM, Kyle RA. Value of beta 2-microglobulin level and plasma cell labeling indices as prognostic factors in patients with newly diagnosed myeloma. Blood. 1988;72:219–23.
30. Greipp PR, Lust JA, O'Fallon WM, Katzmann JA, Witzig TE, Kyle RA. Plasma cell labeling index and beta 2-microglobulin predict survival independent of thymidine kinase and C-reactive protein in multiple myeloma. Blood. 1993;81:3382–7.
31. Greipp PR, San Miguel J, Durie BG, et al. International staging system for multiple myeloma. J Clin Oncol. 2005;23:3412–20.
32. Hungria VT, Maiolino A, Martinez G, et al. Confirmation of the utility of the International Staging System and identification of a unique pattern of disease in Brazilian patients with multiple myeloma. Haematologica. 2008;93:791–2.
33. Kim H, Sohn HJ, Kim S, et al. New staging systems can predict prognosis of multiple myeloma patients undergoing autologous peripheral blood stem cell transplantation as first-line therapy. Biol Blood Marrow Transplant. 2006;12:837–44.
34. Hari PN, Zhang MJ, Roy V, et al. Is the International Staging System superior to the Durie-Salmon staging system? A comparison in multiple myeloma patients undergoing autologous transplant. Leukemia. 2009; 23:1528–34.

Molecular Classification and Risk Stratification

6

Shaji Kumar, Rafael Fonseca, and Keith Stewart

Introduction

Studies over the past decade have greatly improved our understanding of the molecular basis of multiple myeloma and mechanisms of disease progression. Initial studies in myeloma, as with other hematological malignancies, depended solely on metaphase cytogenetics [1–5]. While this methodology was critical in the early studies of the disease, less than a third of the patients had bone marrow cytogenetic studies that were informative, primarily a reflection of the low proliferative state of the malignant plasma cells [6–8]. This was followed by the development of interphase FISH (fluorescent in situ hybridization), which did not depend on dividing cells for detection of abnormalities [9, 10]. With universal adoption of FISH studies, it became clear that nearly all patients with myeloma had genetic abnormalities that could be detected using FISH [11, 12]. Further refinement of the FISH techniques allowed simultaneous detection of the plasma cells, either by using markers for plasma cells or by performing FISH testing on sorted plasma cells, thus ensuring that the abnormality detected was unique to the plasma cells. Development of high-density oligonucleotide arrays allowed assessment of gene expression in tumor cells, and development of this technology provided an unprecedented look into the plasma cell biology, and better appreciation of the genetic heterogeneity that is the hallmark of this disease [13–18]. More recently, cutting edge genomic techniques including RNA sequencing, array CGH, SNP arrays, and whole genome sequencing have all been applied to myeloma allowing us to dissect the molecular complexity of this disease. A better appreciation of the heterogeneity uncovered by these assays have in turn led to several attempts at classifying the disease into groups that have implications on the disease outcome as well as best decisions regarding the best treatment approaches [19].

S. Kumar, M.D. (✉)
Division of Hematology, Mayo Clinic,
200 First Street, SW, Rochester, MN 55905, USA
e-mail: kumar.shaji@mayo.edu

R. Fonseca, M.D.
Center for Individualized Medicine,
Mayo Clinic Cancer Center, 13400 East Shea Boulevard, Collaborative Research Building, 1-105,
Scottsdale, AZ 85259-5494, USA

Division of Hematology, Mayo Clinic,
200 First Street, SW, Rochester, MN 55905, USA
e-mail: fonseca.rafael@mayo.edu

K. Stewart, M.B. Ch.B.
Division of Hematology, Mayo Clinic,
200 First Street, SW, Rochester, MN 55905, USA

Mayo Clinic in Arizona, 13400 East Shea Boulevard,
Scottsdale, AZ 85259, USA
e-mail: stewart.keith@mayo.edu

M.A. Gertz and S.V. Rajkumar (eds.), *Multiple Myeloma: Diagnosis and Treatment*,
DOI 10.1007/978-1-4614-8520-9_6, © Mayo Foundation for Medical Education and Research 2014

Molecular Classification

FISH-Based Classification

Nearly all patients with myeloma have genetic abnormalities detected by FISH and can be broadly classified into numeric abnormalities (mostly trisomies and monosomies) and structural abnormalities (translocations and deletions) (Fig. 6.1) [11, 12]. Patients can carry more than one class of abnormalities with significant overlap in terms of the abnormalities seen [9, 10, 20]. Trisomies are typically seen in the odd-numbered chromosomes, most commonly trisomies of 3, 5, 7, 9, 11, 15, 19, and 21. The most common monosomy seen in myeloma is monosomy 13; with the others including monosomy 14 and monosomy 17 (Table 6.1). The trisomies of odd-numbered chromosomes results in a hyperdiploid clone and can be observed in 40–50 % of the patients. Translocations typically involve the immunoglobulin heavy chain region on chromosome and one of a set of recurrent partner chromosomes. There are five recurrent chromosomal partners (oncogenes) that are involved in IgH translocations in MGUS and MM: 4p16 (MMSET and usually FGFR3), 6p21 (CCN D3), 11q13 (CCN D1), 16q23 (c-MAF), and 20q11 (MAFB). In a proportion of patients with translocations involving the IgH locus on chromosome 14, the partner chromosome cannot be identified. Finally, deletions of the long or short arms may involve several chromosomes with the most commonly observed ones being chromosomes 1, 13, and 17.

It is thought that the trisomies and translocations represent primary abnormalities seen in the plasma cell clone [20–22]. When observed on FISH studies, it is believed that all the plasma cells in the clone carry these primary genetic abnormalities. In contrast, structural abnormalities such as amplification/duplication of chromosome 1q and deletions of 1p and 17p may not be seen at the time of diagnosis and can be acquired during the course of the disease [23–30]. In contrast to the primary abnormalities, abnormalities such as del17p may be seen only in a proportion of the myeloma cells, a finding that may influence the prognostic value of this abnormality.

TC Classification

While the majority of the myeloma cells are not actively dividing at any given time, the level of cyclin D1, cyclin D2, or cyclin D3 mRNA in virtually all myeloma cells is relatively high compared with healthy BM PCs. Various mechanisms

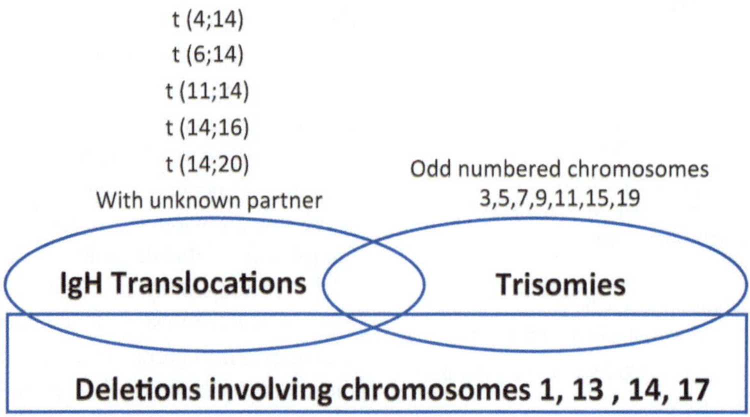

Fig. 6.1 Fish abnormalities in myeloma

Table 6.1 Distribution of FISH abnormalities in patients with multiple myeloma [11]

FISH abnormality	Frequency (%)
Trisomy(ies) without IgH abnormality	201 (42 %)
IgH abnormality without trisomy(ies)	146 (30 %)
t(11;14)	74 (18)
t(4;14)	28 (10)
t(14;16)	19 (5)
t(14;20)	1 (<1)
Unknown partner/deletion of IgH region	24 (5)
IgH abnormality with trisomy(ies)	74 (15 %)
t(11;14)	12 (18)
t(4;14)	19 (10)
t(14;16)	5 (5)
t(6;14)	3 (<1)
Unknown partner/deletion of IgH region	35
Monosomy 14 in absence of IgH translocations or trisomy(ies)	22 (4.5 %)
Other cytogenetic abnormalities in absence of IgH translocations or trisomy(ies) or monosomy 14 (primarily monosomy 13 and p53 abnormalities)	26 (5.5 %)
Normal	15 (3 %)

have been proposed for the elevated cyclin [21, 22] expression in the myeloma cells in different contexts, but appear to be a common phenomenon in the myeloma patients. In approximately 25 % of MM an IgH translocation directly dysregulates CCND1 (11q13), CCND3 (6p21), or a MAF gene (cMAF, 16q23 or MAFB, 20q11) encoding a transcription factor that targets cyclin D2. Similar degree of elevated cyclin D expression can also be observed in the other translocations (4;14) as well as in hyperdiploid tumors; but the mechanism of increased expression is clearly different. Irrespective of the associated primary abnormality and the exact mechanism involved, cyclin overexpression appears to be a unifying and early event. It has been hypothesized that the dysregulation of a cyclin D gene may render the cells more susceptible to proliferative stimuli, resulting in selective expansion as a result of interaction with the BM microenvironment including the stromal and/or endothelial cells as well as the plethora of growth promoting cytokines such as interleukin-6.

Based on these early studies, Bergsagel and Keuhl proposed a TC (Translocation and Cyclin D) classification [21]. This classification utilizes gene expression profiling to provide information regarding overexpression of the different cyclins. The specific translocations present may be identified by using FISH or by overexpression of the oncogenes dysregulated by the five recurrent IgH translocations: 11q13 (CCN D1); 6p21 (CCN D3); 4p16 (MMSET and usually FGFR3); 16q23 (maf); and 20q11 (mafB). These groups (Table 6.2) can be distinguished on the basis of the IgH translocation and the level and type of cyclin D expression: 11q13 (16 %) and 6p21 tumors (3 %) express high levels of either cyclin D1 or cyclin D3; D1 tumors (34 %) ectopically express low to moderate levels of cyclin D1 despite the absence of a t(11;14) translocation. The D1 + D2 group (6 %) expresses cyclin D2 in addition to D1; D2 tumors (17 %) do not fall into one of the other groups, and express cyclin D2; None (1 %) expresses no D-type cyclins. 4p16 group (15 %) expresses high levels of cyclin D2 as a result of the t(4;14) translocation; maf group (7 %) expresses the highest levels of cyclin D2, potentially regulated by high levels of either c-maf or mafB. Supervised hierarchical cluster analysis of gene expression profiles demonstrates that this classification identifies homogeneous groups of tumors with distinctive patterns of gene expression that correlates with specific clinical phenotypes.

GEP-Based Classification

Zhan et al. proposed a gene expression-based classification, based on unsupervised hierarchical clustering of mRNA expression profiles of CD138-enriched plasma cells from 414 newly diagnosed patients receiving high-dose therapy and tandem stem cell transplants in the total therapy protocols (Table 6.3) [31]. The training set consisted of 256 cases enrolled on total therapy 2 (TT2). The test set comprised 158 patients enrolled in total therapy 3 (TT3) and served to validate the gene expression model generated based on the TT2 patients. The unsupervised analysis resulted in arrangement of the samples into seven distinct groups. *Group 1* was characterized by the overexpression of numerous cell

Table 6.2 TC classification [21]

Group	Primary translocation	Gene at breakpoint	D-cyclin	Ploidy	Proliferation index	Frequency (%)
6p21	*6p21*	*CCND3*	D3	NH	Average	3
11q13	*11q13*	*CCND1*	D1	D, NH	Average	16
D1	None	None	D1	H	Low	34
D1+D2	None	None	D1 and D2	H	High	6
D2	None	None	D2	H, NH	Average	17
None	None	None	None	NH	Average	2
4p16	*4p16*	*FGFR3/MMSET*	D2	NH>H	Average	15
maf	*16q23* *20q11*	*c-maf* *mafB*	D2	NH	High	5

Table 6.3 GEP-based classification of Zhan et al.

	Group 1 (PR Group)	Group 2 (LB Group)	Group 3 (MS Group)	Group 4 (HY Group)	Group 5 (CD1 Group)	Group 6 (CD2 Group)	Group 7 (MF Group)
B2M≥339 nM	64	37	30	30	35	42	49
LDH≥190 U/L	51	26	31	23	29	36	42
Albumin≤35 g/L	49	34	60	40	26	32	27
Cytogenetic abnormalities	74	29	49	42	34	12	38
MRI focal lesions≥3	78	27	55	59	69	60	42

cycle- and proliferation-related genes, was associated with a higher gene expression-defined proliferation index (PI), and hence was designated as proliferation (PR) subgroup. The PR group had a PI similar to that of human MM cell lines and as expected had a higher proportion of metaphase cytogenetic abnormalities compared with other groups. Both hyperdiploid and non-hyperdiploid cases were equally common in the PR group. *Group 2* was characterized by the elevated expression of endothelin 1(EDN1), a negative regulator of DKK1 expression. Group 2 expressed relatively high levels of the IL6LR and low levels of the WNT signaling antagonists FRZB and DKK1 relative to the other groups. Clinically, group 2 had a significantly lower number of magnetic resonance imaging (MRI)—defined focal lesions than seen in the other groups and was termed as low bone disease (LB) group. *Group 3* consisted primarily of patients with increased MMSET expression, driven by the reciprocal t(4;14)(p16;q32) translocation typically resulting in the hyperactivation of both the FGFR3 and MMSET genes. Since the MMSET spike was the dominant feature of group 3, this group was designated as the MS (MMSET) group. *Group 4* (HY group) was characterized by the presence of a hyperdiploid signature, being associated with hyperdiploid karyotypes in more than 90 % of the cases. Two of the common translocations seen in myeloma lead to increased expression of cyclin D family members: cyclin D1 by the t(11;14)(q13;q32) in 17 % and CCND3 by t(6;14)(p21;q32) in 2 %. In the hierarchical analysis, samples with CCND1 and CCND3 spikes clustered together pointing towards dysregulation of common downstream transcriptional programs. These samples with increased expression of CCND1 and CCND3 each were contained in two distinct groups and were termed CD-1 (*group 5*) and CD-2 (*group 6*). Finally, *group 7* consisted of patients with the t(14;16)(q32;q23) and t(14;20)(q32;q11) translocations, which result in activation of c-MAF and MAFB proto-oncogenes, respectively. MAF and MAFB spikes clustered together, again pointing towards dysregulation of common downstream targets, and was designated as the MF group (MAF/MAFB).

A similar approach was undertaken by the HOVON group, who examined gene expression profiles of purified CD138+ plasma cells from 320 newly diagnosed myeloma patients included in the Dutch-Belgian/German HOVON-65/ GMMG-HD4 trial [32]. In this study hierarchical clustering identified ten subgroups; six corresponded to clusters described in the previously described classification by Zhan et al., PR (4.7 %), MS (1.3 %), HY (24.1 %), CD-1 (4.1 %), CD-2 (1.6 %), and MF (1.0 %). The LB group, however, was identified as a subcluster of the MF group (4.7 %). One subgroup (12.2 %) showed a myeloid signature. Three novel subgroups were defined: one characterized by high expression of genes involved in the NF-kB pathway (11.6 %), second group characterized by overexpression of cancer testis antigens without overexpression of proliferation genes (6.9 %), and a third group with up-regulation of protein tyrosine phosphatases PRL-3 and PTPRZ1 as well as SOCS3 (2.8 %).

Future Directions

Evaluation of the myeloma cell with the modern genomic tools has unveiled alterations in nearly every known aspect of the genetic make up of the cell. Whole genome sequencing approaches have provided clear evidence of the genetic chaos seen in the myeloma cells. Serial studies using sequencing approaches have provided unequivocal proof of the genetic evolution associated with disease progression, with clonal evolution marked by genomic instability leading to acquisition of new abnormalities, waxing and waning of different tumor clones under therapeutic pressure, and emergence of multidrug-resistant clones present in the beginning, but at very low numbers. While these changes are likely similar to that happening in all tumors, it also highlights the complexity of developing classification and risk stratification systems based on changes at genomic level. While these studies will continue to unravel the genetic alterations at various levels, the approach to classification should continue to balance practicality with complexity and comprehensiveness and should continue to be based on clinical utility, particularly the selection of therapy approaches.

Risk Stratification

Improved understanding of the genetic underpinnings of the disease not only serves to classify them in terms of their biology and clinical manifestations, but also to predict outcomes. The molecular approaches to classification of myeloma have also resulted in several risk stratification systems.

Cytogenetic Risk Stratification

From a clinical standpoint FISH-based risk stratification systems remain the best validated and most easily available for clinical practice [4, 11, 12, 19, 33–36]. Among the primary abnormalities previously described, a hyperdiploid karyotype characterized by trisomies is associated with the best outcome among patients with multiple myeloma. Among the various translocations, those with a t(11;14) appear to have similar outcomes as those with the trisomies. In contrast, the t(4;14), t(14; 16), and t(14;20) have been associated with shorter time to progression after different available therapies and also a poor overall survival from diagnosis. However, in patients with overlapping abnormalities, the presence of trisomies has been shown to negate the poor risk associated with these translocation, at least in a patient population predominantly treated with IMiD-based regimens [11]. Among the numeric abnormalities, monosomy 13 is seen in nearly 50 % of the patients and was initially considered a high-risk marker [37]. However, it soon became clear that the deleterious effect of monosomy 13 was related to an enrichment of other high-risk marker in this group and not an independent effect. Finally, among the remaining commonly seen abnormalities, deletion 17p and abnormalities of chromosome 1 (del1p or amplification of 1q) have been associated with poor outcome when detected at the time of diagnosis or acquired the disease course. Deletion 17p, or less commonly

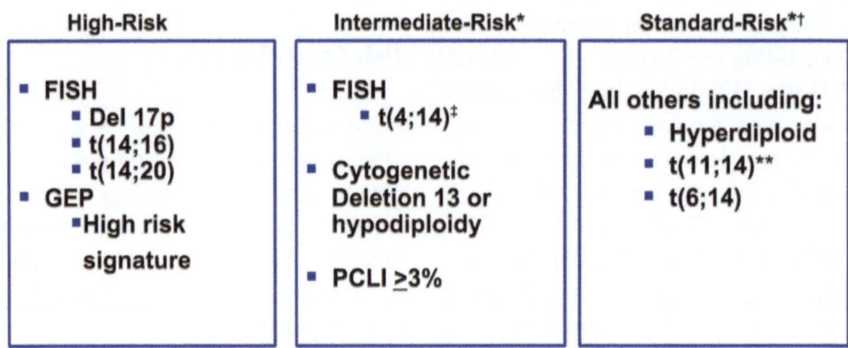

Fig. 6.2 mSMART 2.0: classification of active MM

monosomy 17, leads to loss of the *TP53* gene, commonly referred to as guardian of the genome. While mutations of the *TP53* gene is associated with drug resistance and poor outcome in various tumors, it is not clear if the mechanisms underlying the poor prognosis associated with this lesion are similar in myeloma. Mutations of the *TP53* gene are relatively uncommon except in the very late stages, thus leaving an intact *TP53* locus in the majority of patients with this abnormality. Similarly, the mechanisms underlying the poor prognosis associated with chromosome 1 abnormalities remain to be defined. While detection of metaphase abnormalities is possible in less than a third of the patients with myeloma given the low proliferative nature of the plasma cells, when plasma cell-specific abnormalities are detected they are associated with a poor outcome irrespective of the nature of the specific abnormalities. Thus, the presence of any cytogenetic abnormality on metaphase cytogenetics is typically associated with a poor outcome in patients with myeloma, and as expected there is a significant overlap between the high-risk abnormalities seen by FISH as described above and the presence of abnormalities on metaphase cytogenetics [3, 38, 39].

However, risk stratification systems are dynamic in nature in face of changing therapeutic landscapes. This is particularly evident in myeloma, where availability of new drugs during the past decade has led to a paradigm shift in the treatment approaches to the disease and resulting in considerably improved survival [40]. The FISH and cytogenetics-based risk stratification proposed by the Mayo group; the mSMART approach represents such a dynamic prognostic model (Fig. 6.2) [19]. Patients with trisomies (hyperdiploid myeloma) and t(11;14) have the best survival outcomes with current treatment approach and are considered standard risk. Patients with del17p, t(14;16), and t (14;20), who have the poorest survival with the best available therapies, are considered as having high-risk myeloma. Features that have historically been associated with a poor outcome, but has shown significant improvement in the recent years with the novel therapies have been grouped together as intermediate risk (t(4;14), and those with high proliferation rates). Clearly, heterogeneity exists within these groups as highlighted by several studies. Patients with the high-risk markers who also had trisomies had a better outcome than one would otherwise anticipate. Patients with t(4;14) have been shown to have different outcomes based on B2M levels and the degree of anemia [41]. Thus, it is clear that the FISH-based risk

Table 6.4 Combinations of ISS- and FISH-based risk stratification systems

	IMWG				*MRC IX*			
	%	ISS stage	FISH abnormalities (t(4;14) OR del17p)	4-year OS (%)	%	ISS stage	FISH abnormalities (t(4;14), t(14;16), t(14,20), +1q21, and del(17p13))	Median OS (months)
Low risk	51	I	None	71	38	I	≤1 Abnormality	67.8
		II	None			II	None	
Intermediate risk	29	I	Present	45	48	I	≥2 Abnormality	41.3
		III	None			II	≥1 Abnormality	
						III	≤1 Abnormality	
High risk	20	II	Present	33	14	II	≥2 Abnormality	19.4
		III	Present			III	≥2 Abnormality	

stratification clearly has disadvantages in terms of heterogeneity, but remains the most accessible in routine clinical practice, has the advantage of the ease of interpretation, allows clear delineation into nonoverlapping groups, and can help dictate therapy.

International Staging System

The International Staging System (ISS) was developed nearly a decade ago, based on two simple and easily available measurements, serum beta2 microglobulin (B2M) and serum albumin [42]. Classifying patients based on these two parameters allowed development of three distinct stages with very different outcomes. Patients with a serum albumin ≥3.5 g/dL and a B2M<3.5 mg/L were classified as ISS stage 1, those with B2M>5.5 mg/L as stage 3, and the remaining patients were classified as stage 2. Recent studies in contemporary cohorts have confirmed that this classification system has stood the test of time. More recently, the International Myeloma Working Group has attempted to merge the FISH-based risk stratifications system with ISS in order to develop a more comprehensive risk stratification system (Table 6.4) [35]. This study included 2,642 patients with multiple myeloma analyzed at diagnosis for β2-microglobulin and albumin and had FISH data available. The derived model included presence of t(4;14) and del17p as poor risk FIH markers. The ISS-iFISH group I was defined by patients with ISS stage I or II with neither t(4;14) nor del(17p); group II was defined as either ISS stage III, with neither t(4;14) nor del(17p), or ISS stage I, with either t(4;14) or del(17p). Finally, group III was defined as ISS stage II or III with either t(4;14) or del(17p). The patient distribution was 51 % in group I, 29 % in group II, and 20 % were in group III. The 4-year OS estimates were 71, 45, and 33 % for ISS-FISH groups I, II, and III, respectively.

Others have also combined the ISS staging system with FISH results to develop risk stratification models. In an analysis of over 1,000 patients enrolled in the MRC IX clinical trial, the ISS stage was significantly associated with survival, with a median OS that was not reached for ISS I, 47.7 months for ISS II, and 35.7 months for ISS III [43]. Both the high-risk FISH markers (t(4;14), t(14;16), t(14,20), +1q21, and del(17p13)) and ISS were independently associated with PFS and OS. When the two systems were combined, three distinct risk groups were identified. Patients with ISS I or II and no adverse FISH abnormality, or ISS I and one adverse abnormality, had excellent outcomes with median OS of 67.8 months. In contrast, patients with ISS II or III in the presence of >1 adverse lesion (13.8 %) had a median OS of only 19.4 months. The remaining patients were placed into an intermediate risk group consisting of patients with ISS I and >1 adverse lesion, ISS II and one adverse lesion and ISS III with 0–1 adverse lesions, and was associated with a median OS of 41.3 months.

Gene Expression Profiling

The extensive use of gene expression profiling studies in myeloma has in turn resulted in development of several GEP-based risk stratification system. The GEP70 signature developed by the Arkansas group represents the first of these attempts [14]. The investigators at Arkansas performed microarray analysis on tumor cells from 532 newly diagnosed patients treated on two separate total therapy protocols. They identified 70 genes that were linked to early disease-related death. Thirty percent of the genes were on chromosome 1 with most up-regulated genes mapping to chromosome 1q and down-regulated genes mapping to chromosome 1p. They developed a score based on the ratio of mean expression levels of up-regulated to down-regulated genes, and using a cutoff defined 13 % of patients as having high-risk MM. These patients had shorter durations of complete remission, event-free survival, and overall survival. In addition, they also identified a shorter list of 17 genes that predicted outcome almost as well as the 70-gene model. This risk model has since been validated in a large number of datasets including patients treated with IMiD-based regimens or bortezomib-based regimens, with or without high-dose therapy.

The French IFM group as well as the HOVON groups using patient samples from different clinical trials has carried out similar studies. In the French study, gene expression profiles were generated for 250 newly diagnosed patients enrolled in the IFM 99 trials [16]. This study developed a 15-gene signature that identified patients at the highest risk of early death following diagnosis of multiple myeloma. As expected, the high-risk group (15-gene model quartile 4) was significantly associated with deletion of 13q, deletion of 17p, gain of 1q, and translocation t(4;14). In contrast, the very low-risk group (15-gene model quartiles 1 and 2) was enriched in hyperdiploid MM patients. Majority of the genes in this signature were those involved in cell cycle regulation. More recently, the Dutch group developed another signature for identification of high-risk patients [15]. GEPs obtained from newly diagnosed patients enrolled in the HOVON65/GMMG-HD4 trial ($n=290$) were used to develop a prognostic signature of 92 genes (EMC-92-gene signature). To define a high-risk population, the cutoff threshold of the GEP score was decided based on the proportion of patients with less than a 2-year survival. This signature was then validated in several different datasets. As expected, poor prognostic genetic markers such as 1q gain, del(17p), t(4;14), t(14;16), t(14;20), and del(13q) were enriched in the high-risk populations.

While the GEP-based risk stratification systems may provide more discriminatory ability to identify the real poor actors, there are several hurdles to its universal application. From a biological standpoint, there are considerable differences between the signatures in terms of the actual genes included. Most of these studies have been done in the setting of clinical trial and feasibility and logistics of performing these tests in routine clinical practice remain unclear. As technology evolves, it is likely that gene expression-based approaches to risk stratification will become more commonplace and will determine therapy.

Conclusion

It is clear that multiple myeloma is characterized by significant heterogeneity in terms of outcome. It is clearly important to be able to identify these patients ahead of time not only to provide better estimates of outcome, but more importantly to direct therapy in a fashion that would alter the outcomes favorable. Currently FISH-based systems and ISS remain the most practical approaches in routine clinical practice. Ongoing studies should explore better tools to identify patients more precisely in terms of their outcomes as well as unique responsiveness to specific therapies.

References

1. Drach J, Angerler J, Schuster J, et al. Interphase fluorescence in situ hybridization identifies chromosomal abnormalities in plasma cells from patients with monoclonal gammopathy of undetermined significance. Blood. 1995;86(10):3915–21.

2. Tricot G, Sawyer JR, Jagannath S, et al. Unique role of cytogenetics in the prognosis of patients with myeloma receiving high-dose therapy and autotransplants. J Clin Oncol. 1997;15(7):2659–66.
3. Rajkumar S, Fonseca R, Lacy M, et al. Abnormal cytogenetics predict poor survival after high-dose therapy and autologous blood cell transplantation in multiple myeloma. Bone Marrow Transplant. 1999; 24(5):497–503.
4. Avet-Loiseau H. Role of genetics in prognostication in myeloma. Best Pract Res Clin Haematol. 2007;20(4):625–35.
5. Fonseca R, Ahmann GJ, Juneau AL, et al. Cytogenetic abnormalities in multiple myeloma and related plasma cell disorders: a comparison of conventional cytogenetics to fluorescent in situ hybridization with simultaneous cytoplasmic immunoglobulin staining. Blood. 1997;90 Suppl 1:349a.
6. Seong C, Delasalle K, Hayes K, et al. Prognostic value of cytogenetics in multiple myeloma. Br J Haematol. 1998;101(1):189–94.
7. Smadja NV, Fruchart C, Isnard F, et al. Chromosomal analysis in multiple myeloma: cytogenetic evidence of two different diseases. Leukemia. 1998;12(6): 960–9.
8. Fonseca R, Coignet LJ, Dewald GW. Cytogenetic abnormalities in multiple myeloma. Hematol Oncol Clin North Am. 1999;13(6):1169–80, viii.
9. Fonseca R, Barlogie B, Bataille R, et al. Genetics and cytogenetics of multiple myeloma: a workshop report. Cancer Res. 2004;64(4):1546–58.
10. Fonseca R, Bergsagel PL, Drach J, et al. International Myeloma Working Group molecular classification of multiple myeloma: spotlight review. Leukemia. 2009;23(12):2210–21.
11. Kumar S, Fonseca R, Ketterling RP, et al. Trisomies in multiple myeloma: impact on survival in patients with high-risk cytogenetics. Blood. 2012;119(9):2100–5.
12. Avet-Loiseau H, Attal M, Moreau P, et al. Genetic abnormalities and survival in multiple myeloma: the experience of the Intergroupe Francophone du Myelome. Blood. 2007;109(8):3489–95.
13. Shaughnessy Jr J, Zhan F, Barlogie B, Stewart AK. Gene expression profiling and multiple myeloma. Best Pract Res Clin Haematol. 2005;18(4):537–52.
14. Shaughnessy Jr JD, Zhan F, Burington BE, et al. A validated gene expression model of high-risk multiple myeloma is defined by deregulated expression of genes mapping to chromosome 1. Blood. 2007;109(6): 2276–84.
15. Kuiper R, Broyl A, de Knegt Y, et al. A gene expression signature for high-risk multiple myeloma. Leukemia. 2012;26(11):2406–13.
16. Decaux O, Lode L, Magrangeas F, et al. Prediction of survival in multiple myeloma based on gene expression profiles reveals cell cycle and chromosomal instability signatures in high-risk patients and hyperdiploid signatures in low-risk patients: a study of the Intergroupe Francophone du Myelome. J Clin Oncol. 2008;26(29):4798–805.
17. Zhan F, Barlogie B, Mulligan G, Shaughnessy Jr JD, Bryant B. High-risk myeloma: a gene expression based risk-stratification model for newly diagnosed multiple myeloma treated with high-dose therapy is predictive of outcome in relapsed disease treated with single-agent bortezomib or high-dose dexamethasone. Blood. 2008;111(2):968–9.
18. Kumar SK, Uno H, Jacobus SJ, et al. Impact of gene expression profiling-based risk stratification in patients with myeloma receiving initial therapy with lenalidomide and dexamethasone. Blood. 2011; 118(16):4359–62.
19. Kumar SK, Mikhael JR, Buadi FK, et al. Management of newly diagnosed symptomatic multiple myeloma: updated Mayo Stratification of Myeloma and Risk-Adapted Therapy (mSMART) Consensus Guidelines. Mayo Clin Proc. 2009;84(12):1095–110.
20. Bergsagel PL, Kuehl WM. Chromosome translocations in multiple myeloma. Oncogene. 2001;20(40): 5611–22.
21. Bergsagel PL, Kuehl WM. Molecular pathogenesis and a consequent classification of multiple myeloma. J Clin Oncol. 2005;23(26):6333–8.
22. Bergsagel PL, Kuehl WM, Zhan F, Sawyer J, Barlogie B, Shaughnessy Jr J. Cyclin D dysregulation: an early and unifying pathogenic event in multiple myeloma. Blood. 2005;106(1):296–303.
23. Avet-Loiseau H, Li JY, Godon C, et al. P53 deletion is not a frequent event in multiple myeloma. Br J Haematol. 1999;106(3):717–9.
24. Elnenaei MO, Gruszka-Westwood AM, A'Hernt R, et al. Gene abnormalities in multiple myeloma; the relevance of TP53, MDM2, and CDKN2A. Haematologica. 2003;88(5):529–37.
25. Chang H, Qi C, Yi QL, Reece D, Stewart AK. p53 gene deletion detected by fluorescence in situ hybridization is an adverse prognostic factor for patients with multiple myeloma following autologous stem cell transplantation. Blood. 2005;105(1):358–60.
26. Gertz MA, Lacy MQ, Dispenzieri A, et al. Clinical implications of t(11;14)(q13;q32), t(4;14)(p16.3;q32), and -17p13 in myeloma patients treated with high-dose therapy. Blood. 2005;106(8):2837–40.
27. Gonzalez-Paz N, Chng WJ, McClure RF, et al. Tumor suppressor p16 methylation in multiple myeloma: biological and clinical implications. Blood. 2007;109(3):1228–32. doi:10.1182/blood-2006-05-024661.
28. Nemec P, Zemanova Z, Greslikova H, et al. Gain of 1q21 is an unfavorable genetic prognostic factor for multiple myeloma patients treated with high-dose chemotherapy. Biol Blood Marrow Transplant. 2010; 16(4):548–54.
29. Balcarkova J, Urbankova H, Scudla V, et al. Gain of chromosome arm 1q in patients in relapse and progression of multiple myeloma. Cancer Genet Cytogenet. 2009;192(2):68–72.
30. Qazilbash MH, Saliba RM, Ahmed B, et al. Deletion of the short arm of chromosome 1 (del 1p) is a strong predictor of poor outcome in myeloma patients

undergoing an autotransplant. Biol Blood Marrow Transplant. 2007;13(9):1066–72.
31. Zhan F, Huang Y, Colla S, et al. The molecular classification of multiple myeloma. Blood. 2006;108(6): 2020–8.
32. Broyl A, Hose D, Lokhorst H, et al. Gene expression profiling for molecular classification of multiple myeloma in newly diagnosed patients. Blood. 2010; 116(14):2543–53.
33. Fonseca R, Blood E, Rue M, et al. Clinical and biologic implications of recurrent genomic aberrations in myeloma. Blood. 2003;101(11):4569–75.
34. Fonseca R, Stewart AK. Targeted therapeutics for multiple myeloma: the arrival of a risk-stratified approach. Mol Cancer Ther. 2007;6(3):802–10.
35. Avet-Loiseau H, Durie BG, Cavo M, et al. Combining fluorescent in situ hybridization data with ISS staging improves risk assessment in myeloma: an International Myeloma Working Group collaborative project. Leukemia. 2013;27(3):711–7.
36. Avet-Loiseau H, Soulier J, Fermand JP, et al. Impact of high-risk cytogenetics and prior therapy on outcomes in patients with advanced relapsed or refractory multiple myeloma treated with lenalidomide plus dexamethasone. Leukemia. 2010;24(3):623–8.
37. Avet-Louseau H, Daviet A, Sauner S, Bataille R, Intergroupe Francophone du Myélome. Chromosome 13 abnormalities in multiple myeloma are mostly monosomy 13. Br J Haematol. 2000;111(4):1116–7.
38. Chiecchio L, Protheroe RK, Ibrahim AH, et al. Deletion of chromosome 13 detected by conventional cytogenetics is a critical prognostic factor in myeloma. Leukemia. 2006;20(9):1610–7.
39. Zhou Y, Nair B, Shaughnessy Jr JD, et al. Cytogenetic abnormalities in multiple myeloma: poor prognosis linked to concomitant detection in random and focal lesion bone marrow samples and associated with high-risk gene expression profile. Br J Haematol. 2009;145(5):637–41.
40. Kumar SK, Rajkumar SV, Dispenzieri A, et al. Improved survival in multiple myeloma and the impact of novel therapies. Blood. 2008;111(5):2516–20.
41. Moreau P, Attal M, Garban F, et al. Heterogeneity of t(4;14) in multiple myeloma. Long-term follow-up of 100 cases treated with tandem transplantation in IFM99 trials. Leukemia. 2007;21(9):2020–4.
42. Greipp PR, San Miguel J, Durie BG, et al. International staging system for multiple myeloma. J Clin Oncol. 2005;23(15):3412–20.
43. Boyd KD, Ross FM, Chiecchio L, et al. A novel prognostic model in myeloma based on co-segregating adverse FISH lesions and the ISS: analysis of patients treated in the MRC Myeloma IX trial. Leukemia. 2012;26(2):349–55.

Monoclonal Gammopathies of Undetermined Significance and Smoldering Multiple Myeloma

7

John A. Lust, Diane F. Jelinek, and Kathleen A. Donovan

Introduction

Monoclonal gammopathy of undetermined significance (MGUS) is an asymptomatic, premalignant clonal plasma cell proliferative disorder [1–4]. It was initially referred to as *essential hyperglobulinemia* by Jan Waldenström, as well as several other terms such as benign, idiopathic, asymptomatic, nonmyelomatous, discrete, cryptogenic, and rudimentary monoclonal gammopathy; dysimmunoglobulinemia; lanthanic monoclonal gammopathy; idiopathic paraproteinemia; and asymptomatic paraimmunoglobulinemia [5, 6]. However, since there is an indefinite risk of progression to multiple myeloma (MM) or related disorder such as macroglobulinemia (WM) or amyloidosis (AL), the term MGUS is now the accepted nomenclature [1, 2, 7, 8]. Smoldering multiple myeloma (SMM) is a clinically defined premalignant stage between MGUS and MM [9, 10]. MGUS and SMM must be differentiated from MM, and from a number of related plasma cell disorders using the criteria listed in see Table 1.2 in Chap. 1 [8, 11].

J.A. Lust, M.D., Ph.D. (✉) • K.A. Donovan, Ph.D.
Division of Hematology, Mayo Clinic, 200 First Street, SW, Rochester, MN 55905, USA
e-mail: lust.john@mayo.edu; donovan.kathleen2@mayo.edu

D.F. Jelinek, Ph.D.
Division of Hematology, Department of Immunology, Mayo Clinic, 200 First Street SW, Rochester, MN 55905, USA
e-mail: jelinek.diane@mayo.edu

Monoclonal Gammopathy of Undetermined Significance Definition

MGUS is defined by the presence of a serum M-protein <3 g/dL, bone marrow plasma cells <10 %, and the absence of anemia, hypercalcemia, lytic bone lesions, or renal failure that can be attributed to the plasma cell proliferative disorder (see Table 1.2 in Chap. 1: Criteria for Diagnosis and Response) [12, 13]. In the case of IgM MGUS, there should be no evidence of lymphadenopathy or organomegaly attributable to the clonal lymphoid/plasma cell proliferative disorder. A new subtype of MGUS termed light chain MGUS is defined by the presence of an abnormal FLC ratio (<0.26 or >1.65), elevated level of involved FLC, no immunoglobulin heavy chain expression on immunofixation, bone marrow plasma cells <10 %, and absence of anemia, hypercalcemia, lytic bone lesions, or renal failure that can be attributed to the plasma cell proliferative disorder [4].

Pathophysiology

MM is almost always preceded by the asymptomatic premalignant MGUS stage [14, 15]. The screening arm of the nationwide population-based prospective prostate, lung, colon, ovarian (PLCO) cancer screening trial allowed for collection of annual blood samples from 77,469

M.A. Gertz and S.V. Rajkumar (eds.), *Multiple Myeloma: Diagnosis and Treatment*,

DOI 10.1007/978-1-4614-8520-9_7,

healthy adults. From this cohort, a joint study by the National Cancer Institute and the Mayo Clinic identified 71 individuals who developed MM during the course of the study. Serial serum samples from these patients (up to 6) obtained 2.0–9.8 years prior to MM diagnosis were then analyzed. The study found that an asymptomatic MGUS phase always preceded MM and was found in 100 % of cases 6 years prior to MM [14].

The events responsible for malignant transformation of MGUS to MM or a related plasma cell proliferative disorder are unknown. Genetic changes, bone marrow angiogenesis, modulation of cytokine cascades inducing clonal proliferation, and infectious agents may play a role in the progression of MGUS to MM or a related disorder [16, 17]. However, the specific role of these alterations is not well understood.

Clonal origin: The precise sequence of events that leads to the initiation of the MGUS clone is not known. However antigenic stimulation and/or immunosuppression are thought to be predisposing factors. Toll-like receptors (TLRs) are normally expressed by B lymphocytes and are essential for these cells to recognize infectious agents and pathogen-associated molecular patterns (PAMP) which then initiates the host-defense response [18–20]. The aberrant expression of TLRs by plasma cells may be an initiating event that causes these cells to respond abnormally to TLR-specific ligands resulting in increased MM cell proliferation, survival, and resistance to apoptosis, mediated in part by autocrine interleukin-6 production [18, 19].

Immunosuppression may also contribute to the initiation of monoclonal gammopathies inhibiting tumor surveillance. Monoclonal proteins are known to arise in the context of immunosuppressive states such as bone marrow or stem cell transplantation (SCT), organ transplantation, and human immunodeficiency virus (HIV) infection [21–25]. Moreover, patients undergoing renal transplantation develop monoclonal proteins dependent on the level of immunosuppression that they are subjected to post-transplant [24].

Cytogenetic abnormalities: Cytogenetic changes are common in MM and in MGUS. On the basis of fluorescence in situ hybridization studies, almost all patients with MM have either immunoglobulin heavy chain (IgH) translocations involving chromosome 14q32 or trisomies. These cytogenetic changes referred to as "primary cytogenetic abnormalities" are also present in MGUS [26]. Thus, approximately 50 % of patients with MGUS have primary translocations on chromosome 14q32 (IgH translocated MGUS/SMM) [26, 27]. The most common partner chromosome loci are: 11q13, 4p16.3, 6p21, 16q23, and 20q11 [28–30]. These translocations lead to the dysregulation of oncogenes such as cyclin D1 (11q13), *FGFR3*/MMSET (fibroblastic growth factor receptor 3/MM SET domain) (4p16.3), cyclin D3 (6p21), *C-MAF* (16q23), and MAF-B (20q11). The dysregulation of these oncogenes is thought to be critical for the initiation of the MGUS clone rather than progression of MGUS to MM. Approximately 40 % of patients (40 %) with MGUS have trisomies of odd-numbered chromosomes leading to hyperdiploidy (IgH non-translocated MGUS). In a small subset, there is likely both IgH translocations and trisomies, and in some neither abnormality can be detected.

Deletions of chromosome 13 have been found to have an adverse prognostic value in MM. However, this cytogenetic abnormality occurs early in the disease pathogenesis and is also present in the MGUS stage [31, 32]. Although deletions of chromosome 13 confer an adverse effect on MM, there are no data that the rate of progression from MGUS to MM is accelerated because of this abnormality. In contrast, whereas K- and N-*ras* mutations and deletion of 17p are common in MM, these abnormalities are typically absent in MGUS [33].

Angiogenesis: Bone marrow angiogenesis is increased in MM and has prognostic value [34]. In a study of 400 patients with a spectrum of plasma cell disorders, the median microvessel density (in vessels per high-power field) was 1.3 in the 42 normal controls, 1.7 in AL, 3 in MGUS, 4 in SMM, 11 in MM, and 20 in relapsed MM [35]. Thus bone marrow angiogenesis increases progressively from the premalignant MGUS stage to advanced MM. Using a chick embryo chorioallantoic membrane angiogenesis assay, Vacca et al. reported that 76 % of MM bone marrow samples had increased angiogenic potential compared with 20 % of MGUS samples [36]. Their findings suggest that increased angiogenesis may play a role in progression of MGUS to MM.

Cytokines: Interleukin-6 has been shown to be an autocrine growth factor for human myeloma cells [37]. Myeloma cells freshly isolated from patients produce IL-6 and express its receptor. Exogenous IL-6 augments the in vitro growth of myeloma cells and anti-IL-6 antibody inhibits their growth [37]. Animal studies utilizing IL-6 knockout mice have shown that IL-6 is an essential requirement for the development of B lineage neoplasms [38]. A myeloma cell line U266 expresses mRNA for both IL-6 and IL-6R. The proliferation of this cell line can be inhibited using anti-IL-6 antibody or anti-sense IL-6 oligonucleotides further supporting the critical role of IL-6 in the growth of these cells [39]. Significantly elevated serum IL-6 levels have been detected in 3 % of MGUS/SMM patients, 35 % of overt myeloma patients, and in 100 % of a plasma cell leukemia group [40]. RT-PCR studies on CD38+ sorted MM plasma cells confirmed the production of IL-6 in plasma cells from MM patients [41]. Using an anti-bromodeoxyuridine monoclonal antibody to specifically count myeloma cells in S-phase (i.e., the labeling index), the IL-6 responsiveness of myeloma cells in vitro correlates with their labeling index in vivo, and hence to the severity of the disease emphasizing the importance of IL-6 in driving the proliferating MM plasma cell [42]. An antibody to IL-6 administered in vivo has been shown to dramatically decrease the labeling index of the tumor cells in patients with aggressive multiple myeloma [43]. Alterations in IL-6R alpha chain (CD126) expression demonstrated in MGUS stage plasma cells appears to be one of the first steps in this IL-6 driven proliferative pathway in MM [44].

The source of the IL-6 in this disease is both autocrine (especially in advanced stage MM) and paracrine in nature. The paracrine IL-6 has been demonstrated to be induced by aberrant IL-1 production driving stromal cell secretion of large amounts of IL-6 [45, 46] as well as by other IL-1-induced cytokines such as TNF-α and MIP-1α [47]. Studies on normal bone marrow cells underscore the importance of IL-6 as a key growth factor for plasmablasts. Anti-IL-6 antibodies prevented Ig secretion and cell differentiation of normal plasmablasts obtained from patients with reactive plasmacytoses by inducing apoptosis of the plasmablasts [48].

The IL-6 receptor consists of an 80-kD IL-6 binding molecule (gp80) and a 130-kD signal-transducing chain (gp130) [49]. Gp130 also serves as the signal-transducing chain for leukemia inhibitory factor (LIF), oncostatin M (OSM), ciliary neurotophic factor (CNTF), and IL-11 [50]. Therefore, all of these factors have been shown to stimulate myeloma cell growth [51, 52]. However, the observed responsiveness of most myeloma cells to these growth factors is variable when compared to IL-6 because the ligand-binding receptors for these cytokines are not as consistently expressed on myeloma cells as the IL-6 binding gp80 receptor.

Other cytokines such as insulin-like growth factor I, IL-10, and hepatocyte growth factor have also been shown to stimulate myeloma cell line growth [53–55]. Myeloma cells produce vascular endothelial growth factor (VEGF) that can stimulate IL-6 in a paracrine fashion leading to myeloma cell growth [56]. Another study showed that proliferation of purified myeloma cells from patients was induced by interleukin-6 in six of ten patients but not to GM-CSF, G-CSF, M-CSF, interleukin-1α, interleukin-1β, interleukin-2, or interleukin-4 [57].

Studies on the IL-1/IL-6 axis in the pathogenesis of myeloma: IL-6 has clearly been shown to be one of the central growth factors driving myeloma cell proliferation whose levels and activity can be monitored through the high-sensitivity CRP assay and the plasma cell labeling index (PCLI). We have investigated the differences in IL-6 and IL-1β expression in monoclonal plasma cells from patients with MGUS or MM and concluded that aberrant IL-1 expression appeared to distinguish

MGUS from MM better than IL-6 expression [41, 58]. We developed a functional assay that measures the IL-1-induced IL-6 production by bone marrow stromal cells that serves as a highly sensitive surrogate marker for IL-1β functional activity in BM samples from patients with monoclonal plasma proliferative disorders. We hypothesized that patients with MM or SMM at risk for progression to active MM may have higher IL-1β bioactivity than patients with stable SMM or MGUS. IL-1β bioactivity was determined by quantitating IL-1β specific IL-6 production by cultured bone marrow stromal cells, in the presence or absence of an IL-1 inhibitor, using an IL-6 ELISA [46]. Using this IL-1β bioassay, myeloma patient bone marrow cells stimulated a higher level of IL-6 when compared with normal or MGUS patients. The degree of IL-1 specificity for each patient was determined by inhibiting the IL-6 production with IL-1 inhibitors such as IL-1 receptor antagonist (IL-1Ra). The results demonstrated that the in vitro stromal cell IL-6 production induced by bone marrow cells from patients with active disease was IL-1-mediated. Most importantly, the SMM/IMM patients that eventually progressed to active disease induced a higher level of IL-6 compared with the SMM/IMM patients with stable disease [46]. This study divided SMM patients into two groups based on paracrine IL-6 production and emphasized the importance of inhibiting the proliferating myeloma cells at this stage of disease [46].

Correlation IL-1β production and the clinical features of MM: The biologic effects of IL-1β closely parallel several of the clinical features of human myeloma. IL-1β has potent osteoclast activating factor activity, can increase the expression of adhesion molecules, and can induce paracrine IL-6 production [46, 58, 59]. The increased production of adhesion molecules could explain why myeloma cells are found predominantly in the bone marrow. Subsequently, these "fixed" monoclonal plasma cells could now stimulate osteoclasts through the production of IL-1β and paracrine generation of IL-6 resulting in osteolytic disease. The paracrine generation of IL-6 by marrow stromal cells may further support the growth and survival of the myeloma cells. The importance of IL-1β in myeloma pathogenesis is a result of its ability to induce IL-6. Because femtogram amounts of IL-1β can stimulate IL-6 production [46], IL-1β may act as a "trigger" to induce IL-6 and other cytokine cascades, resulting in progression to active myeloma. This paracrine model of IL-6 production also suggests a rational therapeutic approach for myeloma prevention, i.e., inhibit the IL-1β-induced IL-6 production with a potent IL-1β inhibitor.

Epidemiology

Prevalence: The prevalence of MGUS has been estimated in a large population-based study that included 21,463 of the 28,038 enumerated residents (77 %) of Olmsted County, Minnesota, who were 50 years or older [3]. MGUS was identified in 694 (3.2 %) of these subjects. Age-adjusted rates were greater in men than in women, 4.0 % vs. 2.7 % ($P<0.001$). The prevalence of MGUS was 5.3 % among persons 70 years or older and 7.5 % among those 85 years or older. Several other studies have reported similar prevalence estimates [60]. In addition, approximately 1 % of the general population over the age of 50 has light chain MGUS [4].

The incidence of M-proteins is higher in blacks than in whites. In the study by Cohen et al., the prevalence of an M-protein was 8.4 % in 916 blacks and 3.6 % in whites [61]. Landgren et al., in a study of four million African American and white males admitted to Veterans Affairs Hospitals, found that the prevalence of MGUS was 0.98 % in African Americans and 0.4 % in whites [62]. The age-adjusted prevalence ratio of MGUS in African Americans compared with was 3.0 (95 % confidence interval, 2.7–3.3). The increase of MGUS in blacks may be related to genetic or environmental factors. A population-based study found that the increased risk of MGUS seen in African Americans was also seen in blacks in Ghana, suggesting that the racial disparity may be due more to genetic factors [63]. Further, a study of women in the southern part of the United States found that the racial disparity between blacks and whites persisted even after adjusting for socioeconomic status, again suggesting that the differences were more likely genetic rather than environmental [64].

One study found that only 2.7 % of elderly Japanese patients had a monoclonal gammopathy [65]. A subsequent population-based study in Japan found that the risk of MGUS was lower compared with the white population of Olmsted County [66].

Incidence: The annual incidence of MGUS in males is estimated to be 120/100,000 at age 50, and rises to 530/100,000 at age 90 years [67]. The rates for women are 60/100,000 at age 50, and 370/100,000 at age 90. The fact that the increased prevalence of MGUS with rising age is not just related to accumulation of new cases but due to an actual increase in incidence suggests that an age-related cumulative damage model is at play in the pathogenesis of MGUS.

Risk factors: The incidence and prevalence of MGUS rises with age [3, 67]. MGUS is also more common in males. Blacks have a higher risk of MGUS than whites as discussed above [61–64, 68]. Besides age, race, and gender, there are other risk factors that have been identified, both genetic and environmental. First-degree relatives of patients with MGUS and MM have a two- to threefold higher risk of MGUS compared to those with no known affected relatives [69–71]. Obesity and immunosuppression are also known risk factors for MGUS [24, 25, 64].

Clinical Features

MGUS is an asymptomatic condition. It is typically detected as an incidental finding when electrophoresis and immunofixation of the serum and/or urine or the serum FLC assay are performed during the work-up of suspected MM or WM. Thus, MGUS is usually detected during the work-up of unexplained weakness or fatigue, increased erythrocyte sedimentation rate, anemia, unexplained back pain, osteoporosis, osteolytic lesions or fractures, hypercalcemia, proteinuria, renal insufficiency, or recurrent infections. MGUS is also detected during work-up of patients with symptoms suggestive of AL amyloidosis such as unexplained sensorimotor peripheral neuropathy, carpal tunnel syndrome, refractory congestive heart failure, nephrotic syndrome, orthostatic hypotension, malabsorption, weight loss, change in the tongue or voice, paresthesias, numbness, increased bruising, bleeding, and steatorrhea.

Most cases of MGUS remain undiagnosed due to the asymptomatic nature of the condition. At age 60, the proportion of prevalent cases that are clinically recognized is only 13 % [67]. This rate rises to 33 % at age 80. When MGUS is first diagnosed, it is estimated that the condition has already been present in an undiagnosed form for a median duration of over10 years [67]. For example, it is estimated that 56 % of women age 70 diagnosed with MGUS have had the condition for over 10 years, including 28 % for over 20 years. Corresponding values for men are 55 % and 31 %, respectively.

Prognosis

Mayo Clinic referral population: The prognosis of MGUS was first established in a study of 241 patients seen at the Mayo Clinic from 1956 through 1970 [1]. The actuarial rate of progression to MM or related disorder at 10 years was 17 %; at 20 years, 34 %; and at 25 years, 39 % [72]. Of the 64 patients with progression, 44 (69 %) had MM.

Southeastern Minnesota Study: The risk of progression has also been estimated in a larger population-based study of 1,384 persons with MGUS who resided in the 11 counties of southeastern Minnesota; the risk of progression of MGUS to MM or related disorder was found to be 1 % per year [2]. The median age at diagnosis of MGUS was 72 years. The M-protein level at diagnosis ranged from unmeasurable to 3.0 g/dL. On the basis of the heavy-chain type of immunoglobulins, 70 % of the M-proteins were IgG, 12 % IgA, and 15 % IgM. A biclonal gammopathy was found in 45 patients (3 %). The light chain type was κ in 61 % and λ in 39 %. A reduction of uninvolved (normal or background) immunoglobulins was found in 38 % of 840 patients in whom quantitation of immunoglobulins was determined. The 1,384 patients in this study were followed up for a total of 11,009 person-years (median, 15.4 years; range, 0–35 years). During follow-up, MM, primary AL, lymphoma with an IgM serum M-protein, WM, plasmacytoma, or chronic lymphocytic leukemia developed in 115 patients (8 %). The cumulative probability of progression to one of these disorders was 10 % at 10 years, 21 % at 20 years, and 26 % at 25 years. Patients were at risk for progression even after 25 years or more of stable MGUS. Although the risk of progression is 1 % per year, it must be emphasized that this does not take into account other competing causes of death in elderly patients. After adjusting for competing causes of death, the true lifetime probability of progression of MGUS for the average patient is only approximately 10 %.

Prognostic Factors

No findings at diagnosis of MGUS can reliably distinguish patients whose condition will remain stable indefinitely from those in whom MM or related malignancy develops. However, there are several known prognostic factors that assist in estimation of the risk of progression for appropriate counseling and management.

Size of M-protein: The size of the M-protein at recognition of MGUS is one of the most important predictors for the risk of progression. In the study of 1,384 patients from Southeastern Minnesota, the risk of progression to MM or a related disorder 10 years after diagnosis of MGUS was 6 % for patients with an initial M-protein level of 0.5 g/dL or less, 7 % for 1 g/dL, 11 % for 1.5 g/dL, 20 % for 2 g/dL, 24 % for 2.5 g/dL, and 34 % for 3.0 g/dL [2]. Corresponding rates for progression at 20 years were 14 %, 16 %, 25 %, 41 %, 49 %, and 64 %, respectively. The risk of progression in a patient with an M-protein level of 1.5 g/dL was almost twofold greater than that in a patient with an M-protein level of 0.5 g/dL, and the risk of progression in a patient with an M-protein level of 2.5 g/dL was 4.6 times that of a patient with a 0.5-g/dL spike.

Type of M-protein: Patients with an IgM or IgA M-protein have a higher risk of progression compared with those with an IgG M-protein [2]. IgM MGUS is a unique subtype of MGUS in which patients are at risk of progression to Waldenström macroglobulinemia rather than MM [73]. Due to confusion in terminology, some patients with Waldenström macroglobulinemia are referred to as having non-Hodgkin lymphoma or lymphoplasmacytic lymphoma (a term commonly used by pathologists to describe the bone marrow findings of patients with Waldenström macroglobulinemia). Rarely patients with IgM MGUS evolve into IgM MM [74]. Among 213 patients in the southeastern Minnesota MGUS study, 23 developed "non-Hodgkin's lymphoma" or Waldenström macroglobulinemia, three developed chronic lymphocytic leukemia, and three developed AL amyloidosis [73]. The risk of progression was 1.5 % per year. The risk of progression of light chain MGUS relative to IgA, IgG, or IgM MGUS is not known.

Bone marrow plasma cells: MGUS patients who have 5–9 % bone marrow plasma cells have a higher risk of progression compared with those with <5 % bone marrow plasma cells [75]. Of 1,104 patients with MGUS in this study, at a median follow-up of 65 months, 64 MGUS cases (5.8 %) evolved to MM or related plasma cell disorder. Patients with greater than 5 % marrow plasmacytosis had a significantly higher risk of progression compared to those with 5 % or fewer plasma cells, 1.35 vs. 0.64 per 100 person-years, respectively, $P=0.004$.

Abnormal serum FLC ratio: An abnormal FLC ratio is an independent risk factor for progression of MGUS. In a study of 1,148 patients with MGUS, 379 (33 %) had an abnormal FLC ratio [76]. The risk of progression in patients with an abnormal FLC ratio was significantly higher than that in patients with a normal ratio (hazard ratio 3.5; $P<0.001$) and was independent of the size and type of serum M-protein.

Table 7.1 Risk-stratification model to predict progression of monoclonal gammopathy of undetermined significance to myeloma or related disorders

Risk group	No. of patients	Relative risk	Absolute risk of progression at 20 years (%)	Absolute risk of progression at 20 years accounting for death as a competing risk (%)
Low-risk (serum M-protein <1.5 g/dL, IgG subtype, normal FLC ratio (0.26–1.65))	449	1	5	2
Low-intermediate-risk (any one factor abnormal)	420	5.4	21	10
High-intermediate-risk (any two factors abnormal)	226	10.1	37	18
High-risk (all three factors abnormal)	53	20.8	58	27

From Rajkumar SV et al., Serum-free light chain ratio is an independent risk factor for progression in monoclonal gammopathy of undetermined significance (MGUS) Blood. 2005; 106;812–817. © The American Society of Hematology

Risk-Stratification

A risk-stratification model can be used to predict risk of progression in MGUS and is useful for management [76]. The model is based on the size and type of the M-protein and the FLC ratio (Table 7.1). Patients with all three risk factors consisting of an abnormal serum FLC ratio, IgA or IgM MGUS, and an increased serum M-protein value (≥1.5 g/dL) have a risk of progression at 20 years of 58 %, whereas the risk is 37 % with any two risk factors present, 21 % with one risk factor present, and 5 % when none of the risk factors are present. When competing causes of death were taken into account, the risk of progression in the low-risk group is only 2 % at 20 years.

Life Expectancy and Cause of Death

In the Mayo Clinic study of 241 patients with MGUS, survival was shorter compared with an age- and sex-adjusted 1980 US population (13.7 vs. 15.7 years) [77]. Similarly, in the population-based study of 1,384 patients with MGUS in Southeastern Minnesota, median survival was 8.1 years compared with the expected median of 11.8 years for Minnesota residents of matched age and sex ($P<0.001$) [2]. In the study by van de Poel et al. [78], the long-term survival of 334 patients with MGUS was slightly shorter than the expected survival of an age- and sex-adjusted population. However, it is not clear from these studies if there is an excess risk of death from MGUS once the deaths due to malignant progression are accounted for.

Management

The differentiation between MGUS and MM and other related disorders is based on the strict criteria (see Table 1.2 in Chap. 1: Criteria for Diagnosis and Response) [8]. At the time of initial diagnosis all patients need a complete blood count (CBC), serum calcium, and serum creatinine, and a radiographic survey of the skeleton. A bone marrow aspiration and biopsy is also recommended for most patients, and cytogenetic studies should be done at baseline on the bone marrow sample. Although a bone marrow biopsy is required for the definition of MGUS, not all patients need to have such an examination if the clinical picture is otherwise consistent with MGUS, and the patient is at low risk by the risk-stratification model shown in Table 7.1 [76]. If available, peripheral blood flow cytometry for circulating plasma cells should be done.

Once the diagnosis is made, the CBC, serum calcium, creatinine, and serum protein electrophoresis (and serum FLC if light chain MGUS) must be repeated in 6 months [79]. If stable, then in patients with low-risk MGUS, an assessment of the M-protein level is needed only if symptoms worrisome for progression develop. This recommendation is based on the fact that the progression risk is very low in these patients, and that there are no data that monitoring can prevent complications in a timely manner [80]. In all other patients with MGUS, a lifelong annual follow-up of the M-protein is recommended.

No single factor can differentiate a patient with a benign monoclonal gammopathy from one in whom a malignant plasma cell disorder develops subsequently. However, the presence of a high plasma cell proliferative rate, circulating plasma cells, or other concerning clinical or laboratory features in a patient with MGUS needs to be followed up frequently for other evidence of progression.

Smoldering Multiple Myeloma

Definition

SMM is defined by the presence of a serum M-protein ≥3 g/dL and/or bone marrow plasma cells 10–60 %, and absence of anemia, hypercalcemia, lytic bone lesions, or renal failure that can be attributed to the plasma cell proliferative disorder (see Table 1.2 in Chap. 1: Criteria for diagnosis and response) [12, 13].

Epidemiology

SMM accounts for approximately 15 % of all cases of newly diagnosed MM [81]. In a study conducted at the M.D. Anderson Cancer Center, 95 (15 %) of 638 patients with MM were considered to have asymptomatic MM [82]. Other investigators have found a higher proportion of patients with SMM, but the sample size in these studies is small [83, 84]. The prevalence estimates for SMM are distorted because many reports include asymptomatic patients with lytic bone lesions on skeletal survey. Some exclude patients with bone lesions on skeletal survey but include patients who have lytic lesions on magnetic resonance imaging. Calculation of the true prevalence of SMM on the basis of strict criteria is not available.

Pathophysiology

SMM is not a unique biologic entity [16, 17, 85]. It is heterogeneous entity created primarily for clinical purposes to identify a group of patients with asymptomatic plasma cell dyscrasia that have a much higher risk of progression than MGUS (10 % per year) so that these patients can be monitored more closely [10, 16, 86]. From a biologic standpoint, SMM includes patients with premalignancy (biological MGUS) and patients with early asymptomatic malignancy (MM) [17, 87]. Unfortunately, at present, histopathologic and other laboratory methods cannot distinguish SMM patients with premalignant MGUS from those who have early MM since there is no clear marker of malignancy that can distinguish a clonal premalignant plasma cell from a clonal malignant MM cell.

Clinical Features

As with MGUS, SMM is asymptomatic and is diagnosed during the routine work-up for a variety of symptoms and signs [79, 86]. SMM should be differentiated from related plasma cell disorders using strict criteria (see Table 1.2 in Chap. 1; Criteria for Diagnosis and Response) [8].

Prognosis

The risk of progression of SMM is much higher compared with MGUS, 10 % per year compared with 1 % per year. In a study of 276 patients with SMM, the risk of progression was 10 % per year for the first 5 years, 5 % per year for the next 3 years, and then 1–2 % per year thereafter [10]. This pattern of progression in which there is a plateau after 10 years is consistent with the heterogeneous nature of SMM; in the first 10 years, the subset of patients with early MM declare themselves with symptomatic disease, while after 10 years, the remaining cohort of patients is identical to MGUS in biology and clinical behavior. A subset of patients can remain free of progression for several years [9]. Another study has reported a lower rate of progression of only 20 % at 6 years [75]. However, the definition of SMM used in this study was different; it considered patients to have SMM only if they had no disease progression after 1 year of follow-up.

Prognostic Factors

The assessment of prognostic factors for SMM is hampered by varying diagnostic criteria used to define the cohort. Several studies also include patients with lytic lesions. Future studies of SMM need to use more uniformly accepted criteria so that results can be compared.

Extent of bone marrow involvement: The natural history of SMM in the literature is based almost exclusively on data from patients with bone marrow plasma cells of less than 60 %. In studies describing the diagnosis, natural history, and progression of SMM, no upper limit of bone marrow involvement was defined [10]. In a study of 276 patients with SMM only 6 of 276 patients (2 %) had a bone marrow plasma cell percentage of ≥60 % [88]. Four of these six patients progressed to symptomatic MM between 3 and 9 months following diagnosis of SMM. The median progression-free survival was 7.7 months. In a separate cohort of 655 patients with SMM seen from1996 to 2010 at the Mayo Clinic, only 21 patients (3.2 %) had a bone marrow plasma cell percentage of ≥60 %. Ninety-five percent of patients with ≥60 % bone marrow plasma cells progressed to MM within 2 years of diagnosis, with a median time to progression (TTP) of 7 months. Patients with SMM who have bone marrow involvement of 60 % or greater almost invariably progress to MM within 2 years, and we now recommend that such patients be considered as MM regardless of the presence or absence of end-organ damage and be initiated on therapy [87, 88]. The prognostic value of levels of bone marrow involvement from 10 to 60 % needs further study.

Circulating plasma cells: The ability of plasma cells to escape from the bone marrow microenvironment and circulate in the peripheral blood ("marrow emancipation") is a likely hallmark of aggressive disease as well as malignant transformation. Except for the small subset of solitary plasmacytoma, most MM patients present with lytic bone lesions in multiple bones, suggesting hematogenous dissemination once a malignant transformation has occurred. Patients with abnormal peripheral blood monoclonal plasma cell studies, defined as an increase in the number or proliferative rate of circulating plasma cells by immunofluorescent assays, are at higher risk for earlier progression to MM. In a study of 57 patients, it was found that the median TTP was 9 months for those with abnormal circulating plasma cell values on a slide-based immunofluorescent assay vs. 30 months for those with normal results ($P<0.01$) [89]. In a more recent study of 91 patients diagnosed with SMM at the Mayo Clinic, Bianchi et al. found that the level of circulating plasma cells could be used to identify patients with a high risk of progression to MM within the first 2 years [90]. Patients with a high level of circulating plasma cells on an immunofluorescent assay (absolute peripheral blood plasma cells $>5{,}000\times10^6$/L and/or >5 % cytoplasmic immunoglobulin positive plasma cells per 100 peripheral blood mononuclear cells) were significantly more likely to progress to active disease within 2 years compared with patients without high circulating plasma cells, 71 % vs. 25 %, respectively, $P=0.001$. Corresponding rates for progression within 3 years were 86 % vs. 35 %, respectively, $P<0.001$. The slide-based immunofluorescent method is not widely available, and these results can be more practically applied by detecting and quantifying circulating plasma cells using a six-color flow cytometric assay. In the flow assay, circulating plasma cells can be detected with high sensitivity by counting 150,000 mononuclear cell events and can be used to calculate the absolute number of blood plasma cells per microliter in SMM patients.

Magnetic resonance imaging: Patients who undergo magnetic resonance imaging often have abnormalities detected even when the skeletal survey shows no lytic lesions [81, 91]. Abnormal focal lesions on magnetic resonance imaging are associated with a shortened TTP in SMM [92, 93].

Serum-free light chain assay: The serum FLC ratio can predict risk of progression in MGUS [76]. Similarly, among 116 patients with solitary plasmacytoma, an abnormal FLC ratio was associated with higher risk of progression to MM ($P=0.039$) [94]. In a study of 273 patients with SMM, an FLC ratio of ≤0.125 or ≥8 was an independent risk factor for progression (HR, 2.3; 95 % CI: 1.6–3.2). Patients identified as high risk based on this assay had a 25 % per year risk of progression in the first 2 years [95].

Absence of normal plasma cells on multiparametric flow cytometry: Certain immunophenotypic markers distinguish MM cells from normal PCs with a high degree of accuracy [96]. A Spanish study defines abnormal (MM-type) plasma cell immunophenotype as lack of expression of CD19 and/or CD45, expression of CD56, or weak expression of CD38. In SMM, if >95 % plasma cells in the bone marrow have an abnormal immunophenotype, there is a 17-fold increased risk of progression [97]. In other words, the presence of <5 % normal bone marrow plasma cells in a patient with SMM is associated with a significantly higher risk of progression.

Cytogenetic abnormalities: The prognostic value of cytogenetic abnormalities in SMM has not been fully evaluated. In general, the presence of MYC abnormalities, 17p deletion, and *RAS* mutations, particularly *K-RAS*, are markers of malignant transformation and are likely associated with higher risk of progression in SMM [33].

Plasma cell proliferative rate: A cardinal feature distinguishing MGUS from MM is the proliferative rate of the clonal plasma cell population. Indeed, using a slide-based immunofluorescent assay, there are preliminary data that high PCLI values (≥1) identify patients with SMM who progress within 2 years with high specificity [98]. A six-color flow cytometric assay, currently in clinical practice, offers greater sensitivity and reproducibility. Further studies are needed to investigate the flow cytometry-based proliferative rate as a biomarker that can distinguish SMM patients with malignant transformation from those who have MGUS.

Interleukin-1 levels: Using the IL-1β bioassay described above, patients with active myeloma induced quantitative higher levels of IL-1β-induced IL-6 production when compared with MGUS patients. The bioassay distinguished two groups of SMM patients, those who were high producers, similar to patients with active MM, and those who were low producers, comparable to MGUS patients. The SMM patients that eventually progressed to active disease induced a higher level of IL-6 compared with the SMM patients with stable disease. IL-1 antagonists in vitro inhibited the paracrine IL-6 production by >90 % in the majority of patients with elevated levels [46].

Management

The current standard of care in SMM is close follow-up once every 3–6 months without chemotherapy [79, 86]. Two trials done prior to the arrival of thalidomide, lenalidomide, and bortezomib found no significant improvement in OS in patients who received immediate treatment with melphalan plus prednisone compared with those who received treatment at progression for stage I or asymptomatic MM. Hjorth et al. randomly assigned 50 patients with asymptomatic stage I MM to observation vs. chemotherapy with melphalan and prednisone [99]. No differences were observed in OS between the two groups. Grignani et al. reported similar survival time with immediate or deferred therapy in a series of 44 patients with asymptomatic MM [100]. However, these trials were underpowered, and more data are needed [87]. The recommendation to observe closely without treatment until progression is also based on the possible short-term and long-term side effects of therapy, and the fact that in some patients SMM may not progress for months to years.

More recently, clinical trials have found that thalidomide may delay TTP, but there are long-term side effects associated with this treatment that may make it unsuitable for intervention in an asymptomatic population [101, 102]. In a randomized trial, Witzig et al. compared thalidomide plus zoledronic acid vs. zoledronic acid alone in patients with SMM [103]. The TTP was superior for patients treated with thalidomide plus zoledronic acid ($n=35$) compared with zoledronic acid alone ($n=33$); median TTP 2.4 years (95 % CI: 1.4–3.6) vs. 1.2 years (95 % CI: 0.7–2.5), respectively, $P = 0.02$. Lenalidomide plus dexamethasone has also shown promising activity in high-risk SMM. A recent randomized trial of lenalidomide plus dexamethasone in high-risk SMM is an excellent example of this strategy, in which the investigators demonstrated a significant prolongation of TTP, and preliminary evidence of a survival benefit [104]. An ECOG trial is comparing lenalidomide vs. observation in this patient population.

In a Phase II trial using Interleukin-1 receptor antagonist (IL-1Ra) and low-dose dexamethasone, the median PFS for the 47 SMM/IMM patients treated in the trial was 3.1 years [105]. IL-1Ra led to a decrease in both the high-sensitivity C reactive protein (hs-CRP), a surrogate marker for plasma cell IL-6 levels, and correspondingly, the PCLI, a measure of the myeloma cell proliferative rate in responsive patients [105]. Statistical analysis using a partitioning algorithm showed that the median PFS for patients without ($n = 12$) and with ($n = 35$) $a \geq 15$ % decrease in the baseline hs-CRP (comparing baseline and 6 month values) was 6 months and >3 years, respectively ($P = 0.002$). Patients with IMM were more likely to progress. Twenty percent of the 35 patients with a hs-CRP decrease presented with IMM whereas 50 % of the 12 patients without a hs-CRP decrease had IMM. Stability of the M-protein also separated the two groups. The median PFS for patients with ($n = 19$) and without ($n = 28$) $a \geq 5$ % increase in the M-protein from baseline (comparing baseline and 6 month values) was 6 months and >3 years, respectively ($P < 0.0001$) [105].

Myeloma cell resistance to dexamethasone-induced apoptosis is a well-recognized in vitro and in vivo phenomenon. It occurs because of increased production of IL-6 in the myeloma microenvironment [106–108]. The combination of IL-1Ra and dexamethasone minimized this problem because IL-1Ra was highly effective at inhibiting IL-6 production (Fig. 7.1) and retained an apoptosis-susceptible tumor cell clone. The clinical trial results paralleled in vitro findings in that there was little effect of the IL-1Ra alone on the M-protein because IL-1Ra does not induce myeloma cell apoptosis [105]. The addition of dexamethasone synergized with the IL-1Ra by inducing myeloma cell apoptosis (Fig. 7.1). Dexamethasone targeted the non-proliferating myeloma compartment that appeared to be producing the IL-1 in addition to the secreted M-protein, while IL-1Ra reduced the elevated IL-6 levels in the microenvironment and inhibited the IL-6 responsive proliferating myeloma cell subset (Fig. 7.1).

The IL-1Ra and dexamethasone induce a chronic disease state in responsive patients with SMM/IMM at high risk for progression. In responding patients, the PCLI and CRP have remained low, along with a stable M-protein. The goal of this study was to delay or prevent the development of active myeloma and therefore minor responses or the induction of stable disease are important in this disease group. Patients with low numbers of plasma cells may be controlled with IL-1Ra alone whereas patients with ≥20 % plasma cells typically require the addition of dexamethasone. Targeting the myeloma proliferative component with IL-1Ra leads to a reduced growth rate of the proliferating plasma cells and potentially slows the acquisition of harmful genetic changes.

The in vitro biologic studies and the in vivo clinical trial results demonstrate that it may be possible to delay/prevent progression to active myeloma in responsive patients by targeting the IL-1β-induced IL-6 production that stimulates the myeloma proliferative component. The importance of the PCLI as a prognostic factor has been reported in several myeloma studies where patients with a high labeling index have a shortened overall survival [109–113]. The results from this trial may suggest that, in addition to the M-protein, it will be essential to monitor the proliferative myeloma population and utilize the hs-CRP to aid as predictors of progression. Currently, the M-protein is the major clinical parameter utilized as the measure of response for clinical trials and also for the selection of new therapeutic agents. Current therapies are highly effective at targeting the monoclonal antibody producing non-proliferative myeloma cell. However, their effect on the proliferative myeloma subset is less clear. It has been suggested that myeloma remains

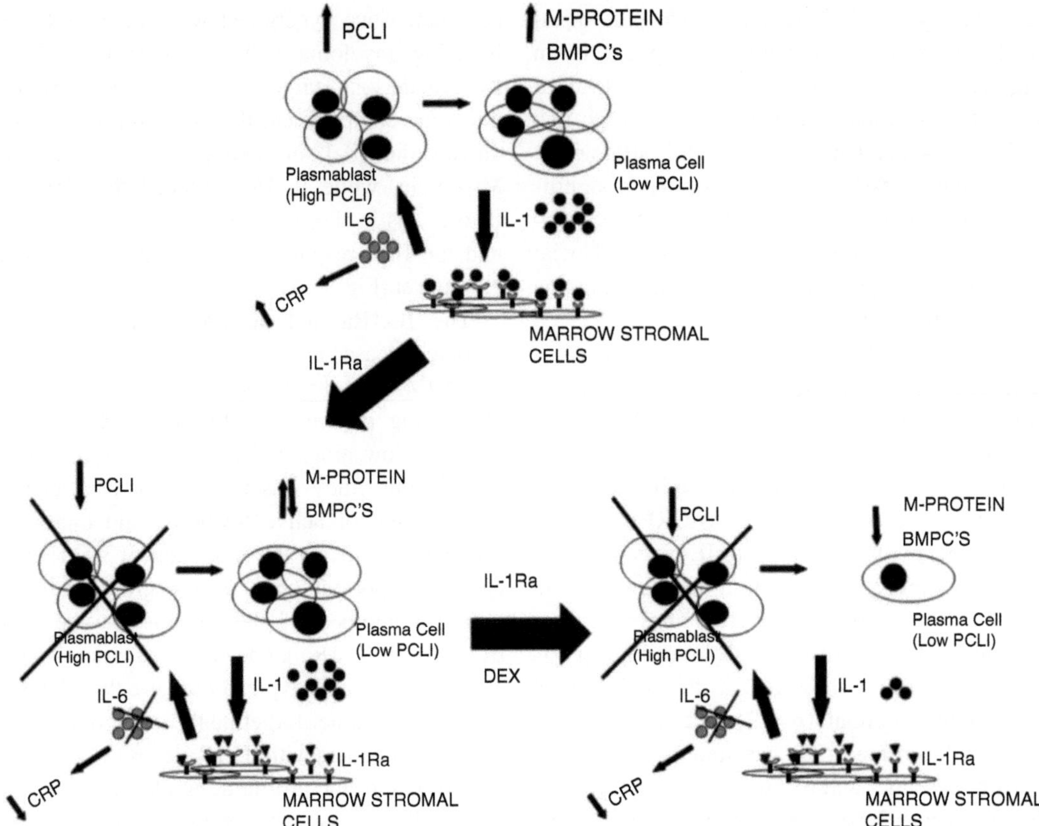

Fig. 7.1 Schematic of the role of IL-1Ra and dexamethasone in the myeloma microenvironment. Bone marrow cells from patients with progressive SMM/IMM produce IL-1**β** that stimulates stromal cells to make IL-6 which can be monitored by the hs-CRP (*upper panel*). The IL-6 can then stimulate the growth of the proliferative myeloma component resulting in an elevated plasma cell labeling index. IL-1Ra selectively targets the proliferative myeloma component resulting in a decrease in the hs-CRP and the PCLI. The proliferative component is crossed out (*lower left*) because it is unknown whether these cells are induced into a non-proliferative state or eliminated. Dexamethasone complements IL-1Ra biologic activity by inducing myeloma cell apoptosis and decreasing the percent bone marrow plasma cells, M-protein, and myeloma cell-produced IL-1 levels (*lower right*). Taken from Lust et al. [105]

incurable because the stem cell/proliferative component is not adequately targeted by current therapies [114]. The IL-1Ra treatment study clearly separates the responsiveness of the proliferative vs. the nonproliferative components of this disease. It is also important to note that there is evidence to suggest that some of the newer therapies may be worsening the proliferative subset resulting in terminal disease with a high growth rate [115]. Future myeloma therapies may need to employ agents that target both the IL-1β-driven IL-6 responsive myeloma proliferative population as well as the IL-1β producing non-proliferative components. Targeting the proliferative myeloma component is likely to result in improved overall survival not only in patients with high-risk SMM/IMM but also in patients with active disease. Of interest, the importance of the IL-1 model has been confirmed using a mathematical analysis between normal and malignant cells [116]. Carefully weighing the results of predictive biomarkers for progression to active myeloma and the risk vs. benefits of any given treatment still needs to be evaluated within the SMM patient population given the wide range of progression observed within this group.

References

1. Kyle RA. Monoclonal gammopathy of undetermined significance. Natural history in 241 cases. Am J Med. 1978;64:814–26.
2. Kyle RA, Therneau TM, Rajkumar SV, et al. A long-term study of prognosis of monoclonal gammopathy of undetermined significance. N Engl J Med. 2002;346:564–9.
3. Kyle RA, Therneau TM, Rajkumar SV, et al. Prevalence of monoclonal gammopathy of undetermined significance. N Engl J Med. 2006;354:1362–9.
4. Dispenzieri A, Katzmann JA, Kyle RA, et al. Prevalence and risk of progression of light-chain monoclonal gammopathy of undetermined significance: a retrospective population-based cohort study. Lancet. 2010;375:1721–8.
5. Waldenstrom J. Studies on conditions associated with disturbed gamma globulin formation (gammopathies). Harvey Lect. 1961;56:211–31.
6. Axelsson U, Bachmann R, Hallen J. Frequency of pathological proteins (M-components) om 6,995 sera from an adult population. Acta Med Scand. 1966;179:235–47.
7. Rajkumar SV, Kyle RA, Buadi FK. Advances in the diagnosis, classification, risk stratification, and management of monoclonal gammopathy of undetermined significance: implications for recategorizing disease entities in the presence of evolving scientific evidence. Mayo Clin Proc. 2010;85:945–8.
8. Kyle RA, Rajkumar SV. Criteria for diagnosis, staging, risk stratification and response assessment of multiple myeloma. Leukemia. 2009;23:3–9.
9. Kyle RA, Greipp PR. Smoldering multiple myeloma. N Engl J Med. 1980;302:1347–9.
10. Kyle RA, Remstein ED, Therneau TM, et al. Clinical course and prognosis of smoldering (asymptomatic) multiple myeloma. N Engl J Med. 2007;356:2582–90.
11. Rajkumar SV. Plasma cell disorders. In: Goldman L, Schafer AI, editors. Cecil textbook of medicine. 24th ed. Philadelphia: Elsevier; 2012. p. 1233–43.
12. Kyle RA, Rajkumar SV. Plasma cell disorders. In: Goldman L, Ausiello D, editors. Cecil textbook of medicine. 22nd ed. Philadelphia: W. B. Saunders; 2004. p. 1184–95.
13. Rajkumar SV. MGUS and smoldering multiple myeloma: update on pathogenesis, natural history, and management. Hematology Am Soc Hematol Educ Program. 2005;2005:340–5.
14. Landgren O, Kyle RA, Pfeiffer RM, et al. Monoclonal gammopathy of undetermined significance (MGUS) consistently precedes multiple myeloma: a prospective study. Blood. 2009;113:5412–7.
15. Weiss BM, Abadie J, Verma P, Howard RS, Kuehl WM. A monoclonal gammopathy precedes multiple myeloma in most patients. Blood. 2009;113:5418–22.
16. Rajkumar SV. Prevention of progression in monoclonal gammopathy of undetermined significance. Clin Cancer Res. 2009;15:5606–8.
17. Rajkumar SV. Preventive strategies in monoclonal gammopathy of undetermined significance and smoldering multiple myeloma. Am J Hematol. 2012;87:453–4.
18. Jego G, Bataille R, Geffroy-Luseau A, Descamps G, Pellat-Deceunynck C. Pathogen-associated molecular patterns are growth and survival factors for human myeloma cells through Toll-like receptors. Leukemia. 2006;20:1130–7.
19. Bohnhorst J, Rasmussen T, Moen SH, et al. Toll-like receptors mediate proliferation and survival of multiple myeloma cells. Leukemia. 2006;20:1138–44.
20. Mantovani A, Garlanda C. Inflammation and multiple myeloma: the Toll connection. Leukemia. 2006;20:937–8.
21. Zent CS, Wilson CS, Tricot G, et al. Oligoclonal protein bands and Ig isotype switching in multiple myeloma treated with high-dose therapy and hematopoietic cell transplantation. Blood. 1998;91:3518–23.
22. Amara S, Dezube BJ, Cooley TP, Pantanowitz L, Aboulafia DM. HIV-associated monoclonal gammopathy: a retrospective analysis of 25 patients [see comment]. Clin Infect Dis. 2006;43:1198–205.
23. Dezube BJ, Aboulafia DM, Pantanowitz L. Plasma cell disorders in HIV-infected patients: from benign gammopathy to multiple myeloma. AIDS Read. 2004;14:372–4.
24. Passweg J, Thiel G, Bock HA. Monoclonal gammopathy after intense induction immunosuppression in renal transplant patients. Nephrol Dial Transplant. 1996;11:2461–5.
25. Zemble RM, Takach PA, Levinson AI. The relationship between hypogammaglobulinemia, monoclonal gammopathy of undetermined significance and humoral immunodeficiency: a case series. J Clin Immunol. 2011;31:737–43.
26. Fonseca R, Barlogie B, Bataille R, et al. Genetics and cytogenetics of multiple myeloma: a workshop report. Cancer Res. 2004;64:1546–58.
27. Kyle RA, Rajkumar SV. Multiple myeloma. N Engl J Med. 2004;351:1860–73.
28. Kuehl WM, Bergsagel PL. Multiple myeloma: evolving genetic events and host interactions. Nat Rev Cancer. 2002;2:175–87.
29. Bergsagel PL, Kuehl WM. Chromosome translocations in multiple myeloma. Oncogene. 2001;20: 5611–22.
30. Fonseca R, Bailey RJ, Ahmann GJ, et al. Genomic abnormalities in monoclonal gammopathy of undetermined significance. Blood. 2002;100:1417–24.
31. Kaufmann H, Ackermann J, Baldia C, et al. Both IGH translocations and chromosome 13q deletions are early events in monoclonal gammopathy of undetermined significance and do not evolve during transition to multiple myeloma. Leukemia. 2004;18: 1879–82.
32. Konigsberg R, Ackermann J, Kaufmann H, et al. Deletions of chromosome 13q in monoclonal gammopathy of undetermined significance. Leukemia. 2000;14:1975–9.

33. Chng WJ, Gonzalez-Paz N, Price-Troska T, et al. Clinical and biological significance of RAS mutations in multiple myeloma. Leukemia. 2008;22: 2280–4.
34. Rajkumar SV, Leong T, Roche PC, et al. Prognostic value of bone marrow angiogenesis in multiple myeloma. Clin Cancer Res. 2000;6:3111–6.
35. Rajkumar SV, Mesa RA, Fonseca R, et al. Bone marrow angiogenesis in 400 patients with monoclonal gammopathy of undetermined significance, multiple myeloma, and primary amyloidosis. Clin Cancer Res. 2002;8:2210–6.
36. Vacca A, Ribatti D, Presta M, et al. Bone marrow neovascularization, plasma cell angiogenic potential, and matrix metalloproteinase-2 secretion parallel progression of human multiple myeloma. Blood. 1999;93:3064–73.
37. Kawano M, Hirano T, Matsuda T, et al. Autocrine generation and requirement of BSF-2/IL-6 for human multiple myelomas. Nature. 1988;332:83–5.
38. Hilbert DM, Kopf M, Mock BA, Kohler G, Rudikoff S. Interleukin 6 is essential for in vivo development of B lineage neoplasms. J Exp Med. 1995;182: 243–8.
39. Schwab G, Siegall CB, Aarden LA, Neckers LM, Nordan RP. Characterization of an interleukin-6-mediated autocrine growth loop in the human multiple myeloma cell line, U266. Blood. 1991;77: 587–93.
40. Bataille R, Jourdan M, Zhang XG, Klein B. Serum levels of interleukin 6, a potent myeloma cell growth factor, as a reflect of disease severity in plasma cell dyscrasias. J Clin Invest. 1989;84:2008–11.
41. Donovan KA, Lacy MQ, Kline MP, et al. Contrast in cytokine expression between patients with monoclonal gammopathy of undetermined significance or multiple myeloma. Leukemia. 1998;12:593–600.
42. Zhang XG, Klein B, Bataille R. Interleukin-6 is a potent myeloma-cell growth factor in patients with aggressive multiple myeloma. Blood. 1989;74: 11–3.
43. Bataille R, Barlogie B, Lu ZY, et al. Biologic effects of anti-interleukin-6 murine monoclonal antibody in advanced multiple myeloma. Blood. 1995;86: 685–91.
44. Rawstron AC, Fenton JA, Ashcroft J, et al. The interleukin-6 receptor alpha-chain (CD126) is expressed by neoplastic but not normal plasma cells. Blood. 2000;96:3880–6.
45. Carter A, Merchav S, Silvian-Draxler I, Tatarsky I. The role of interleukin-1 and tumour necrosis factor-alpha in human multiple myeloma. Br J Haematol. 1990;74:424–31.
46. Xiong Y, Donovan KA, Kline MP, et al. Identification of two groups of smoldering multiple myeloma patients who are either high or low producers of interleukin-1. J Interferon Cytokine Res. 2006;26: 83–95.
47. Dinarello CA. Biologic basis for interleukin-1 in disease. Blood. 1996;87:2095–147.
48. Jego G, Bataille R, Pellat-Deceunynck C. Interleukin-6 is a growth factor for nonmalignant human plasmablasts. Blood. 2001;97:1817–22.
49. Kishimoto T, Akira S, Taga T. Interleukin-6 and its receptor: a paradigm for cytokines. Science. 1992; 258:593–7.
50. Hirano T, Matsuda T, Nakajima K. Signal transduction through gp130 that is shared among the receptors for the interleukin 6 related cytokine subfamily. Stem Cells. 1994;12:262–77.
51. Westendorf JJ, Jelinek DF. Growth regulatory pathways in myeloma. Evidence for autocrine oncostatin M expression. J Immunol. 1996;157:3081–8.
52. Zhang XG, Gu JJ, Lu ZY, et al. Ciliary neurotropic factor, interleukin 11, leukemia inhibitory factor, and oncostatin M are growth factors for human myeloma cell lines using the interleukin 6 signal transducer gp130. J Exp Med. 1994;179:1337–42.
53. Lu ZY, Zhang XG, Rodriguez C, et al. Interleukin-10 is a proliferation factor but not a differentiation factor for human myeloma cells. Blood. 1995;85: 2521–7.
54. Borset M, Hjorth-Hansen H, Seidel C, Sundan A, Waage A. Hepatocyte growth factor and its receptor c-met in multiple myeloma. Blood. 1996;88: 3998–4004.
55. Freund GG, Kulas DT, Mooney RA. Insulin and IGF-1 increase mitogenesis and glucose metabolism in the multiple myeloma cell line, RPMI 8226. J Immunol. 1993;151:1811–20.
56. Dankbar B, Padro T, Leo R, et al. Vascular endothelial growth factor and interleukin-6 in paracrine tumor-stromal cell interactions in multiple myeloma. Blood. 2000;95:2630–6.
57. Anderson KC, Jones RM, Morimoto C, Leavitt P, Barut BA. Response patterns of purified myeloma cells to hematopoietic growth factors. Blood. 1989;73:1915–24.
58. Lacy MQ, Donovan KA, Heimbach JK, Ahmann GJ, Lust JA. Comparison of interleukin-1 beta expression by in situ hybridization in monoclonal gammopathy of undetermined significance and multiple myeloma. Blood. 1999;93:300–5.
59. Lust JA, Donovan KA. The role of interleukin-1 beta in the pathogenesis of multiple myeloma. Hematol Oncol Clin North Am. 1999;13:1117–25.
60. Wadhera RK, Rajkumar SV. Prevalence of monoclonal gammopathy of undetermined significance: a systematic review. Mayo Clin Proc. 2010;85: 933–42.
61. Cohen HJ, Crawford J, Rao MK, Pieper CF, Currie MS. Racial differences in the prevalence of monoclonal gammopathy in a community-based sample of the elderly. [Erratum appears in Am J Med 1998 Oct;105(4):362]. Am J Med. 1998;104:439–44.
62. Landgren O, Gridley G, Turesson I, et al. Risk of monoclonal gammopathy of undetermined significance (MGUS) and subsequent multiple myeloma among African American and white veterans in the United States. Blood. 2006;107:904–6.

63. Landgren O, Katzmann JA, Hsing AW, et al. Prevalence of monoclonal gammopathy of undetermined significance among men in Ghana. Mayo Clin Proc. 2007;82:1468–73.
64. Landgren O, Rajkumar SV, Pfeiffer RM, et al. Obesity is associated with an increased risk of monoclonal gammopathy of undetermined significance (MGUS) among African-American and Caucasian women. Blood. 2010;116:1056–9.
65. Bowden M, Crawford J, Cohen HJ, Noyama O. A comparative study of monoclonal gammopathies and immunoglobulin levels in Japanese and United States elderly. J Am Geriatr Soc. 1993;41:11–4.
66. Iwanaga M, Tagawa M, Tsukasaki K, Kamihira S, Tomonaga M. Prevalence of monoclonal gammopathy of undetermined significance: study of 52,802 persons in Nagasaki City, Japan. Mayo Clin Proc. 2007;82:1474–9.
67. Therneau TM, Kyle RA, Melton III LJ, et al. Incidence of monoclonal gammopathy of undetermined significance and estimation of duration before first clinical recognition. Mayo Clin Proc. 2012; 87(11):1071–9.
68. Greenberg AJ, Vachon CM, Rajkumar SV. Disparities in the prevalence, pathogenesis and progression of monoclonal gammopathy of undetermined significance and multiple myeloma between blacks and whites. Leukemia. 2012;26(4):609–14.
69. Greenberg AJ, Rajkumar SV, Vachon CM. Familial monoclonal gammopathy of undetermined significance and multiple myeloma: epidemiology, risk factors, and biological characteristics. Blood. 2012;119:4771–9.
70. Vachon CM, Kyle RA, Therneau TM, et al. Increased risk of monoclonal gammopathy in first-degree relatives of patients with multiple myeloma or monoclonal gammopathy of undetermined significance. Blood. 2009;114:785–90.
71. Greenberg AJ, Rajkumar SV, Larson DR, et al. Increased prevalence of light chain monoclonal gammopathy of undetermined significance (LC-MGUS) in first-degree relatives of individuals with multiple myeloma. Br J Haematol. 2012;157:472–5.
72. Kyle RA, Therneau TM, Rajkumar SV, Larson DR, Plevak MF, Melton III LJ. Long-term follow-up of 241 patients with monoclonal gammopathy of undetermined significance: the original Mayo Clinic series 25 years later [see comment]. Mayo Clin Proc. 2004;79:859–66.
73. Kyle RA, Therneau TM, Rajkumar SV, et al. Long-term follow-up of IgM monoclonal gammopathy of undetermined significance. Blood. 2003;102:3759–64.
74. Schuster S, Rajkumar SV, Dispenzieri A, et al. IgM multiple myeloma: disease definition, prognosis, and differentiation from Waldenstrom's macroglobulinemia. Am J Hematol. 2010;85:853–5.
75. Cesana C, Klersy C, Barbarano L, et al. Prognostic factors for malignant transformation in monoclonal gammopathy of undetermined significance and smoldering multiple myeloma. J Clin Oncol. 2002;20:1625–34.
76. Rajkumar SV, Kyle RA, Therneau TM, et al. Serum free light chain ratio is an independent risk factor for progression in monoclonal gammopathy of undetermined significance (MGUS). Blood. 2005;106: 812–7.
77. Kyle RA. "Benign" monoclonal gammopathy—after 20 to 35 years of follow-up. Mayo Clin Proc. 1993;68:26–36.
78. van de Poel MH, Coebergh JW, Hillen HF. Malignant transformation of monoclonal gammopathy of undetermined significance among out-patients of a community hospital in southeastern Netherlands. Br J Haematol. 1995;91:121–5.
79. Kyle RA, Durie BGM, Rajkumar SV, et al. Monoclonal gammopathy of undetermined significance (MGUS) and smoldering (asymptomatic) multiple myeloma: IMWG consensus perspectives risk factors for progression and guidelines for monitoring and management. Leukemia. 2010;24: 1121–7.
80. Bianchi G, Kyle RA, Colby CL, et al. Impact of optimal follow-up of monoclonal gammopathy of undetermined significance (MGUS) on early diagnosis and prevention of myeloma-related complications. Blood. 2010;116:2019–25.
81. Dimopoulos MA, Moulopoulos LA, Maniatis A, Alexanian R. Solitary plasmacytoma of bone and asymptomatic multiple myeloma. Blood. 2000;96: 2037–44.
82. Dimopoulos MA, Moulopoulos A, Smith T, Delasalle KB, Alexanian R. Risk of disease progression in asymptomatic multiple myeloma. Am J Med. 1993;94:57–61.
83. Riccardi A, Gobbi PG, Ucci G, et al. Changing clinical presentation of multiple myeloma. Eur J Cancer. 1991;27:1401–5.
84. Wisloff F, Andersen P, Andersson TR, et al. Incidence and follow-up of asymptomatic multiple myeloma. The myeloma project of health region I in Norway. II. Eur J Haematol. 1991;47:338–41.
85. Lust JA, Donovan KA. Smoldering multiple myeloma. Emerg Cancer Ther. 2010;1:261–82.
86. Blade J, Dimopoulos M, Rosinol L, Rajkumar SV, Kyle RA. Smoldering (asymptomatic) multiple myeloma: current diagnostic criteria, new predictors of outcome, and follow-up recommendations. J Clin Oncol. 2010;28:690–7.
87. Rajkumar SV, Merlini G, San Miguel JF. Redefining myeloma. Nat Rev Clin Oncol. 2012;9:494–6.
88. Rajkumar SV, Larson D, Kyle RA. Diagnosis of smoldering multiple myeloma. N Engl J Med. 2011;365:474–5.
89. Witzig TE, Kyle RA, O'Fallon WM, Greipp PR. Detection of peripheral blood plasma cells as a predictor of disease course in patients with smoldering multiple myeloma. Br J Haematol. 1994;87:266–72.
90. Bianchi G, Kyle RA, Larson DR, et al. High levels of peripheral blood circulating plasma cells as a specific risk factor for progression of smoldering multiple myeloma. Leukemia. 2013;27(3):680–5.

91. Moulopoulos LA, Dimopoulos MA, Smith TL, et al. Prognostic significance of magnetic resonance imaging in patients with asymptomatic multiple myeloma. J Clin Oncol. 1995;13:251–6.
92. Weber DM, Dimopoulos MA, Moulopoulos LA, Delasalle KB, Smith T, Alexanian R. Prognostic features of asymptomatic multiple myeloma. Br J Haematol. 1997;97:810–4.
93. Mariette X, Zagdanski AM, Guermazi A, et al. Prognostic value of vertebral lesions detected by magnetic resonance imaging in patients with stage I multiple myeloma. Br J Haematol. 1999;104:723–9.
94. Dingli D, Kyle RA, Rajkumar SV, et al. Immunoglobulin free light chains and solitary plasmacytoma of bone. Blood. 2006;108:1979–83.
95. Dispenzieri A, Kyle RA, Katzmann JA, et al. Immunoglobulin free light chain ratio is an independent risk factor for progression of smoldering (asymptomatic) multiple myeloma. Blood. 2008; 111:785–9.
96. Rawstron AC, Orfao A, Beksac M, et al. Report of the European Myeloma Network on multiparametric flow cytometry in multiple myeloma and related disorders. Haematologica. 2008;93:431–8.
97. Pérez-Persona E, Mateo G, García-Sanz R, et al. Risk of progression in smouldering myeloma and monoclonal gammopathies of unknown significance: comparative analysis of the evolution of monoclonal component and multiparameter flow cytometry of bone marrow plasma cells. Br J Haematol. 2009;148:110–4.
98. Madan S, Kyle RA, Greipp PR. Plasma cell labeling index in the evaluation of smoldering (asymptomatic) multiple myeloma. Mayo Clin Proc. 2010;85:300.
99. Hjorth M, Hellquist L, Holmberg E, Magnusson B, Rodjer S, Westin J. Initial versus deferred melphalan-prednisone therapy for asymptomatic multiple myeloma stage I—a randomized study. Myeloma Group of Western Sweden. Eur J Haematol. 1993;50:95–102.
100. Grignani G, Gobbi PG, Formisano R, et al. A prognostic index for multiple myeloma. Br J Cancer. 1996;73:1101–7.
101. Rajkumar SV, Gertz MA, Lacy MQ, et al. Thalidomide as initial therapy for early-stage myeloma. Leukemia. 2003;17:775–9.
102. Weber D, Rankin K, Gavino M, Delasalle K, Alexanian R. Thalidomide alone or with dexamethasone for previously untreated multiple myeloma. J Clin Oncol. 2003;21:16–9.
103. Witzig TE, Laumann KM, Lacy MQ, et al. A phase III randomized trial of thalidomide plus zoledronic acid versus zoledronic acid alone in patients with asymptomatic multiple myeloma. Leukemia. 2013; 27(1):220–5.
104. Mateos M-V, Lopez-Corral L, Hernandez M, et al. Smoldering multiple myeloma (SMM) at high-risk of progression to symptomatic disease: a phase III, randomized, multicenter trial based on lenalidomide-dexamethasone (Len-Dex) as induction therapy followed by maintenance therapy with len alone vs no treatment. In: ASH Annual Meeting Abstracts 2011;118:991.
105. Lust JA, Lacy MQ, Zeldenrust SR, et al. Induction of a chronic disease state in patients with smoldering or indolent multiple myeloma by targeting interleukin 1β-induced interleukin 6 production and the myeloma proliferative component. Mayo Clin Proc. 2009;84:114–22.
106. Grigorieva I, Thomas X, Epstein J. The bone marrow stromal environment is a major factor in myeloma cell resistance to dexamethasone. Exp Hematol. 1998;26:597–603.
107. Hardin J, MacLeod S, Grigorieva I, et al. Interleukin-6 prevents dexamethasone-induced myeloma cell death. Blood. 1994;84:3063–70.
108. Rowley M, Liu P, Van Ness B. Heterogeneity in therapeutic response of genetically altered myeloma cell lines to interleukin 6, dexamethasone, doxorubicin, and melphalan. Blood. 2000;96:3175–80.
109. Greipp PR, Witzig TE, Gonchoroff NJ, et al. Immunofluorescence labeling indices in myeloma and related monoclonal gammopathies. Mayo Clin Proc. 1987;62:969–77.
110. Greipp PR, Katzmann JA, O'Fallon WM, Kyle RA. Value of beta 2-microglobulin level and plasma cell labeling indices as prognostic factors in patients with newly diagnosed myeloma. Blood. 1988;72: 219–23.
111. Greipp PR, Kyle RA. Clinical, morphological, and cell kinetic differences among multiple myeloma, monoclonal gammopathy of undetermined significance, and smoldering multiple myeloma. Blood. 1983;62:166–71.
112. Greipp PR, Lust JA, O'Fallon WM, Katzmann JA, Witzig TE, Kyle RA. Plasma cell labeling index and beta 2-microglobulin predict survival independent of thymidine kinase and C-reactive protein in multiple myeloma [see comment]. Blood. 1993;81:3382–7.
113. Greipp PR, Lust JA. Pathogenetic relation between monoclonal gammopathies of undetermined significance and multiple myeloma. Stem Cells. 1995;2:10–21.
114. Huff CA, Matsui W, Smith BD, Jones RJ. The paradox of response and survival in cancer therapeutics. Blood. 2006;107:431–4.
115. Balleari E, Ghio R, Falcone A, Musto P. Possible multiple myeloma dedifferentiation following thalidomide therapy: a report of four cases. Leuk Lymphoma. 2004;45:735–8.
116. Dingli D, Chalub FACC, Santos FC, Van Segbroeck S, Pacheco JM. Cancer phenotype as the outcome of an evolutionary game between normal and malignant cells. Br J Cancer. 2009;101:1130–6.

Treatment of Newly Diagnosed Multiple Myeloma

8

Shaji Kumar and Steven J. Russell

Introduction

The past decade has witnessed a revolution in the treatment of multiple myeloma as a result of introduction of several new effective drugs, which in conjunction with increased use of autologous stem cell transplantation and improved supportive care strategies have resulted in significantly improved survival outcomes for these patients. The survival of patients with myeloma has more than doubled in the past decade, a success story unparalleled by any other cancer. In addition to the improved armamentarium of therapeutic options, there has been a better understanding of the basic disease biology as well as the heterogeneity seen in the disease, in particular the genetic heterogeneity. This has led to development of risk stratifications systems that is increasingly allowing us to individualize the therapy of patients with multiple myeloma. The general approach to treatment of patients with myeloma can be grouped into seven discrete steps as shown in Table 8.1. A systematic approach to the treatment allows us to judiciously use the available therapeutic options allowing the best possible outcomes for these patients.

S. Kumar, M.D. (✉)
Division of Hematology, Mayo Clinic,
200 First Street, SW, Rochester, MN 55905, USA
e-mail: kumar.shaji@mayo.edu

S.J. Russell, M.D., Ph.D.
Division of Hematology and Department of Molecular Medicine, Mayo Clinic,
Rochester, MN, USA

Diagnosis

The diagnosis of multiple myeloma is essentially a two-step process, the first to establish the presence of a monoclonal plasma cell process and the second to make the determination that it represents active disease requiring therapy. While the first step is more objective based on clear results from a set of laboratory tests, the latter can be more subjective and sometimes challenging.

The diagnosis of a plasma cell proliferative disorder rests on the ability to demonstrate one or more of the following, namely, a monoclonal protein in the serum or urine, and/or the presence of monoclonal plasma cells in the bone marrow, peripheral blood, or discrete soft tissue masses. The demonstration of the monoclonal protein may require one or more of protein electrophoresis performed on serum or urine, immunofixation of serum or urine, and serum free light chain assay. The protein electrophoresis involves charge-based separation of the serum or urine proteins on a gel, which allows detection of the presence of a monoclonal protein. The monoclonal immunoglobulin protein typically migrates to the gamma region, but IgA monoclonal protein and light chains can migrate to the beta region, causing confusion. This test lacks sensitivity and can miss small monoclonal proteins and presence of monoclonal light chain. The next step in the process of monoclonal protein assessment is an immunofixation study, performed on the serum or urine, involving staining with antibodies

M.A. Gertz and S.V. Rajkumar (eds.), *Multiple Myeloma: Diagnosis and Treatment*,
DOI 10.1007/978-1-4614-8520-9_8, © Mayo Foundation for Medical Education and Research 2014

Table 8.1 Steps to treatment of multiple myeloma

1. Diagnosis and determination of need for therapy (distinguishing from MGUS and smoldering myeloma)
2. Staging and risk stratification
3. Induction therapy
4. Consolidation therapy
5. Maintenance therapy
6. Monitoring, identification, and treatment of disease relapse
7. Supportive care

directed against each of the heavy chains and the kappa and lambda light chains. This allows identification of the type of monoclonal protein in terms of their heavy chains and light chain isotype, as well as detection of small amounts of monoclonal protein otherwise not detected on protein electrophoresis. However, unlike the SPEP or UPEP, IFE is not quantitative. In 0–15 % of patients, both these tests can be negative, a condition previously referred to as nonsecretory myeloma. However, the introduction of the serum free light chain assay allows us to quantitate monoclonal free light chain, kappa or lambda light chain that circulates unbound to the heavy chain, by virtue of its reactivity against epitopes normally hidden when they are bound to the heavy chain. The FLC assay signals the presence of a clonal process when the ratio between the kappa and the lambda FLC is skewed, and more importantly allows quantitation of the clonal chain allowing serial disease monitoring. Between the three tests, over 98 % of patients can be demonstrated to have a monoclonal protein leaving behind a very small minority, who are truly nonsecretory in that they do not secrete any monoclonal protein.

The other component of the diagnosis is demonstration of monoclonal plasma cells, the hallmark of the disease. The plasma cells normally reside in the bone marrow, which is where the clonal plasma cells are typically detected, through a bone marrow aspirate of trephine biopsy. The bone marrow examination gives an estimate of the tumor cell burden in the average patients and can vary anywhere from a normal looking marrow to a marrow almost completely replaced by clonal plasma cells. Unfortunately the marrow involvement in myeloma can be patchy resulting in sampling variations. However, varying numbers of plasma cells can also be detected in circulation in the vast majority of myeloma patients, especially with the use of multiparameter flow cytometry (MFC). Finally, a small proportion of patients will present with soft tissue masses, in association with an area of bone destruction or otherwise, which on biopsy typically shows sheets of monoclonal plasma cells. The demonstration of clonality in the plasma cells depends on their exclusive expression of the kappa or lambda light chain detected by immunohistochemistry, immunofluorescence, or in situ hybridization.

Demonstration of the presence of a monoclonal process is clearly the first step, but even more important is the determination of the need for therapy. MM is but a part of the spectrum of monoclonal disorders that includes MGUS, smoldering multiple myeloma, and symptomatic myeloma. Determination of where it lies in that spectrum determines the course of action, whether to observe or to institute therapy. The entities of MGUS and smoldering myeloma have been described in previous chapters and will not be discussed further. The diagnosis of symptomatic myeloma requiring therapy hinges on the demonstration of end-organ damage from myeloma, which typically includes presence of hyper*C*alcemia, *R*enal insufficiency, *A*nemia, and/or *B*one lesions, referred to by the acronym CRAB.

Risk Stratification

Once it has been determined that a patient has myeloma that requires therapy, the next step is to assess the risk status. Risk stratification has become an integral part of the myeloma evaluation as with other cancers and in playing an increasingly important role in the treatment decisions. Various prognostic factors and the different approaches to risk stratification have already been detailed in the previous chapters. From a therapy standpoint, three risk factors play an important role in the selection of treatment; namely the age/performance status, renal function, and the presence or absence of high-risk genetic abnormalities.

Initial Therapy (Induction Therapy)

The initial approach to myeloma has seen the most change in the past decade with the advent of the new drugs. While the tools employed have undergone a radical transformation, the basic underlying principles remain same. The goals of the initial therapy are to control the disease process as rapidly as possible and reversing the complications of the disease, while minimizing the toxicity and allowing collection of stem cells for autologous stem cell transplantation when considered appropriate. The early and rapid control of disease without significant toxicity plays an important role in reducing the early mortality that used to be seen previously. Despite the uniform goals, substantial differences exist in terms of the approaches to initial therapy of myeloma, and unfortunately limited data is available from randomized trials to provide firm guidance. We have over the years developed a consensus approach to initial management of myeloma based on a combination of best available data and expert opinion where data is lacking. These guidelines have been published and are freely available on the web at www.msmart.org and are revised several times a year when new and relevant data becomes available (Fig. 8.1).

Traditionally, the initial therapy of myeloma has been based on whether patients would be considered eligible for autologous stem cell transplantation. This approach was taken to reduce the likelihood of compromised stem cell collection as a result of the use of drugs such as melphalan. However, the determination of transplant eligibility varies significantly across different centers and groups. While the randomized trials have typically included only patients under 65 years of age, there is a wealth of data highlighting the safety and efficacy of SCT in older patients. Over the past decade, the newer drugs have been systematically incorporated into the traditional regimens used in both transplant-eligible and transplant-ineligible patients. In fact, many of the currently used regimens do not significantly impact the ability to collect stem cells and as a result the need to classify patients based on the transplant eligibility has diminished over time. The commonly used regimens along with the response rates and survival outcomes with these regimens are as shown in Table 8.2; the most relevant ones are discussed in more detail below. Results of major randomized trials in transplant-eligible and transplant-ineligible patients are shown in Tables 8.3 and 8.4, respectively.

Lenalidomide/Dexamethasone (Rd)

In previously untreated patients with active MM, initial therapy with Rd results in overall response rates of 91–95 %, with very good partial response (VGPR) or better in 32–38 % [1, 2]. Rajkumar et al. [1] treated 34 patients with lenalidomide 25 mg orally days 1–21 and dexamethasone 40 mg days 1–4, 9–12, and 17–20, both repeated every 28 days. The overall response rate was 91 %, with 6 % achieving complete response and 32 % VGPR. The most common toxicity was neutropenia and fatigue. The 2-year progression-free survival rates for patients proceeding to SCT and patients remaining on Rev-Dex were 83 % and 59 %, respectively; the OS rates were 92 % and 90 % at 2 years and 92 % and 85 % at 3 years, respectively [3]. This was followed by a randomized controlled trial comparing lenalidomide with standard dexamethasone (RD; days 1–4, 9–12, and 17–20 of a 28 day schedule) with lenalidomide with reduced intensity dexamethasone (Rd; weekly dexamethasone) [4]. After 4 months of therapy, 79 % of the RD patients and 68 % of the Rd patients had achieved a partial response or better; however, at 1 year, OS was superior in the Rd arm as compared to the RD arm (92 % versus 87 %, $P=0.0002$). The trial was stopped early due to this finding concern, and patients on RD were crossed over to lower dose dexamethasone regimen (Rd). Grade 3–4 AEs and early deaths were higher in the RD group with the most common serious toxicities being DVT, infections, and fatigue.

Based on these trials, Rd has been adopted by as an effective first-line therapy for treatment of newly diagnosed disease. Long-term studies of Rd combination suggest excellent outcomes, with good tolerability and ability to continue on therapy for long periods. The OS of a cohort of 286 patients receiving first-line Rd therapy was

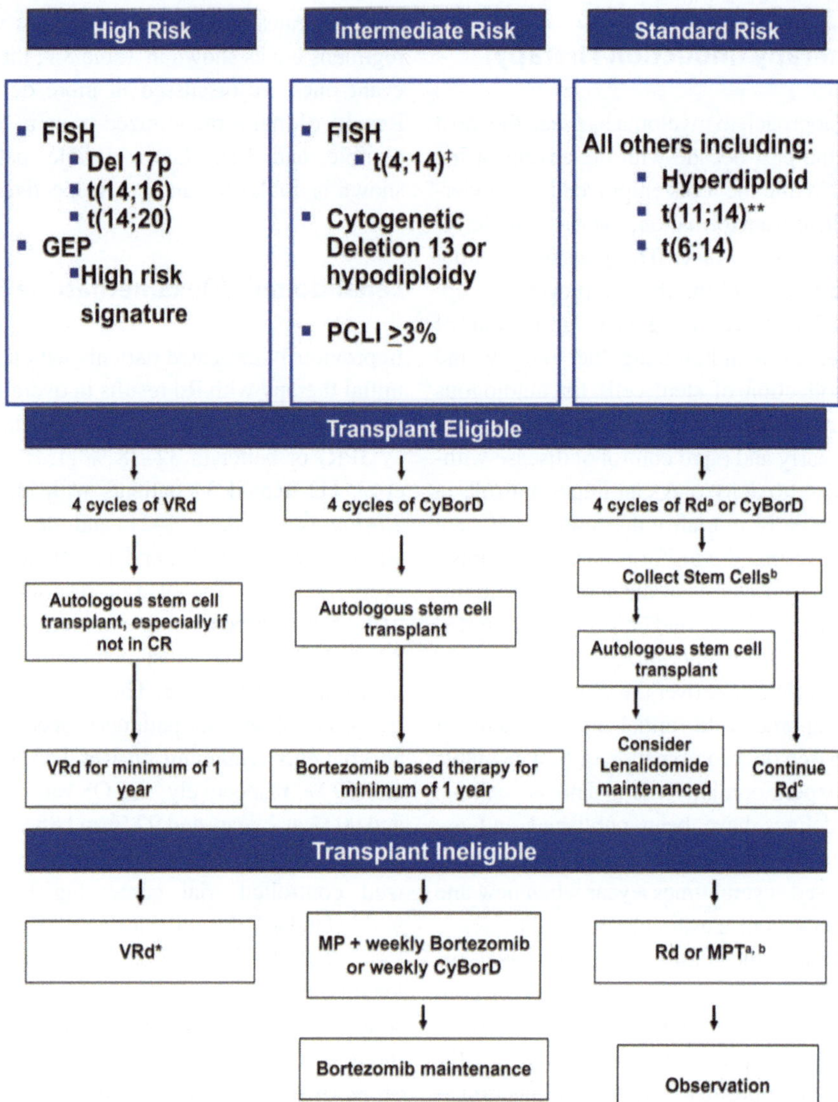

Fig. 8.1 Risk stratification-based approach to management of myeloma. *Note that a subset of patients with these factors will be classified as high-risk by GEP. †LDH > ULN and beta-2M > 5.5 may indicate worse prognosis. ‡Prognosis is worse when associated with high beta-2M and anemia. **t(11;14) may be associated with plasma cell leukemia. [a]Bortezomib containing regimens preferred in renal failure or if rapid response needed. [b]If age >65 or >4 cycles of Rd, consider G-CSF plus cytoxan or plerixafor. [c]Continuing Rd is optional for patients responding to Rd and with low toxicities; Dex is usually discontinued after first year. [d]Consider risks and benefits; If used, consider limited duration 12–24 months

nearly 80 % at 5 years. The outcomes among the transplant-eligible patients have been comparable whether or not they proceeded to an early autologous stem cell transplant or chose to have an SCT at the time of their relapse. Moreover, in the non-transplant-eligible patients, the outcomes with Rd as primary therapy have been excellent compared to the historical results.

Bortezomib and Dexamethasone (VD)

Bortezomib was studied as a single agent in the a small phase 2 study by Jagannath et al., with dexamethasone added for lack of adequate response [5]. While Bortezomib as a single agent achieved a 40 % response rate (>PR), the RR

Table 8.2 Phase 2 induction regimens

References	Regimen	CR (%)	VGPR (%)	PR (%)	OR (%)	PFS	OS
Offidani et al. [38]	ThaDD	34	24	30	88	3-yr 57 %	3-yr 74 %
Rajkumar [1]	RD	6	32	53	91	NA	NA
Niesvizky et al. [2]	BiRD	25	18	53	95	2-yr 75 %	NA
Kumar et al. [31]	CRD	13	34	38	85	28 mo	2-yr OS 87
Jagannath et al. [5, 23]	Bortez	3	9	28	40	21 mo	4-yr 67 %
Richardson et al. [24]	Bortez	3	8	23	41	17 mo	1-yr 92 %
Dispenzieri et al. [25]	Bortez	0	10	38	48	8 mo	2-yr 76 %
Harousseau et al. [26]	Bortez-Dex	20	0	47	67	NA	NA
Reeder [7]	CyBorD	39	22	17	88	NA	NA
Reeder et al. [28]	mCyBorD	43	17	33	93	NA	NA
Kumar et al. [10]	VCD	22	19	34	75	1-yr 93 %	1-yr 100 %
Kumar et al. [10]	mVCD	47	6	47	100	1-yr 100 %	1-yr 100 %
Oakavee et al. [33, 34]	PAD	24	0	71	95	29 mo	2-yr 95 %
Popat et al. [34, 35]	LD-PAD	11	28	50	89	24 mo	2-yr 73 %
Berenson et al. [36]	VDD	20	9	43	72	NA	NA
Ghosh et al. [27]	VT	10	20	43	73	17 mo	3-yr 74 %
Hussein et al. [37]	DVd-T	36	13	34	83	28 mo	NA
Zervas et al. [39]	T-DVD	10	0	64	74	1-yr 70 %	1-yr 80 %
Wang et al. [30]	VTD	19	0	73	92		
Richardson et al. [9]	VRD	29	40	33	66	1-yr 75 %	1.5-yr 97 %
Kumar et al. [10]	VRD	24	27	34	85	1-yr 83 %	1-yr 100 %
Jakubowiak et al. [40]	RVDD	44	23	29	96	2-yr 70 %	2-yr 75 %
Kumar et al. [10]	VDRC	25	33	30	88	1-yr 86 %	1-yr 92 %
Jakubowiak et al. [32]	CarRd	42	39	17	98	1-yr 97 %	NA

BiRD biaxin, lenalidomide, and dexamethasone; *bortez* bortezomib; *CarRd* carfilzomib, lenalidomide, and dexamethasone; *CRD* cyclophosphamide, lenalidomide, and dexamethasone; *CR* complete response; *CyBorD* cyclophosphamide, bortezomib, and dexamethasone; *dex* dexamethasone; *EFS* event-free survival; *LD-PAD* low-dose PAD: N, number of patients; *NA* not available; *OR* overall response rate; *OS* overall survival; *PFS* progression-free survival; *PR* partial response; *ThaDD* thalidomide, pegylated doxorubicin, and dexamethasone; *mo* months; *thal* thalidomide; *mCyBorD* modified CyBoD; *MDT* MD and thalidomide; *MPR* melphalan, prednisone and lenalidomide; *mVCD* modified VCD; *PAD* bortezomib, doxorubicin, and dexamethasone; *RVDD* lenalidomide, bortezomib, doxorubicin, and dexathasone; *ThaDD* thalidomide, pegylated doxorubicin, and dexamethasone; *T-DVd* thalidomide, pegylated doxorubicin, vincristine, and dexamethasone; *ThaDD* thalidomide, doxorubicin, and dexamethasone; *VCD* bortezomib, cyclophosphamide, and dexamethasone; *VDD* bortezomib, doxorubicin, and dexamethasone; *VDRC* bortezomib, dexamethasone, lenalidomide, and cyclophosphamide; *VDT* bortezomib, pegylated liposomal doxorubicin, and thalidomide; *VGPR* very good partial response; *VMP* MP and bortezomib; *yr* year; *VRD* bortezomib, lenalidomide, and dexamethasone; *VT* bortezomib and thalidomide

further increased to 88 % in combination with dexamethasone. The combination was also compared to VAD as induction therapy prior to SCT in a phase 3 trial, resulting in deeper responses and reduced need for tandem ASCT as well as improved PFS post SCT [6]. In the current era, bortezomib tend to be used more in combination with cyclophosphamide or lenalidomide as described below.

Cyclophosphamide, Bortezomib, and Dexamethasone (CyBorD or VCD)

The new drugs have been combined with alkylators, both cyclophosphamide and melphalan, with excellent results [7, 10, 28, 29]. Reeder et al. treated 33 patients with newly diagnosed MM with four 28 day cycles of bortezomib 1.3 mg/m^2 intravenously on days 1, 4, 8, and 11, cyclophosphamide

Table 8.3 Phase 3 randomized controlled trials

		Post-induction response (%)		Post-ASCT(s)/ maintenance response (%)			
References	Regimen[a]	Overall	≥VGPR (CR)	Overall	≥VGPR (CR)	Median PFS/EFS	Median OS
Barlogie et al. [41]	TT2 no thal	40	(10)	78	(43)[c]	44 % 5-year[c]	63 % 5-year
	TT2+thal	60	(19)	86	(62)[c]	56 % 5-year [c]	64 % 5-year
MAG/macro [42]	VAD	NA	7 (NA)	NA	42 (NA)	NA	NA
	Thal-dex	NA	25 (NA)	NA	44 (NA)	NA	NA
IFM 2005-1 [43]	VAD+DCEP	63[c]	15 (6)[c]	79	37 (18)[c]	30 months	77 % 3-year
	BD+DCEP	79[c]	38 (15)[c]	84	54 (35)[c]	36 months	81 % 3 year
GIMEMA [44]	VTD+VTD/D	93[c]	62 (19)[c]	96	89 (58)[c]	68 % 3-year[c]	86 % 3-year
	TD+TD/D	79[c]	28 (5)[c]	89	74 (4)[c]	56 % 3-year[c]	84 % 3-year
HOVON50 [45]	VAD+IFN	57[c]	18 (2) [c]	79[c]	54 (23)[c]	25[c]	60
	TAD+Thal	71[c]	37 (3)[c]	88[c]	66 (31)[c]	34[c]	73
MRC IX [46]	CVAD+Thal or P	71	27 (8)	90	62 (37)	25 months	57 % 4-year
	CTD+Thal or P	82	43 (13)	92	74 (50)	27 months	62 % 4-year
HOVON-65/	VAD+IFN	54[c]	14 (2)[c]	83[c]	56 (24)[c]	28 months	55 % 5 year[c]
GMMG-HD4 [47]	PAD+Velcade	78[c]	42 (7)[c]	90[c]	76 (36)[c]	35 months	61 % 5-year[c]
PETHEMA/	VTD	85	60 (35)[c]	NA	NA (46)[c]	56 months[c]	74 % 4-year
GEM05MEN0S65 [48]	TD	62	29 (14)[c]	NA	NA (24)[c]	28 months[c]	65 % 4-year
	VBMCP/BVAD/B	75	36 (21)[c]	NA	NA (38)[c]	35 months[c]	70 % 4-year
IFM 2007–02 [49]	VD	81	36 (12) [c]	86	58 (31)[c]	30 months	No difference
	vtD	88	49 (13)[c]	89	74 (29)[c]	26 months	
E1A00 [50]	TD	63[c]	NA (4)	NA	NA	NA	1-year 82
	D	41[c]	NA (0)	NA	NA	NA	1-year 82
E4A03 [4]	Rd	70[c]	26 (4)[c]	NA	NA	25 months[c]	2-year 87 %
	RD	81[c]	33 (5)[c]	NA	NA	19 months[c]	2-year 75 %
S0232 [51]	RD	78[c]	63 (26)[c]	NA	NA	3-year 52 %[c]	3-year 79 %
	D	48[c]	16 (4)[c]	NA	NA	3-year 32 %[c]	3-year 73 %

[a]Regimens listed as "induction" + "consolidation/maintenance"
[b]ASCT was not a predetermined part of these trials, so data includes both patients who did and did not undergo ASCT
[c]Statistically significant difference between arms

300 mg/m^2 orally on days 1, 8, 15, and 22 and dexamethasone 40 mg orally on days 1–4, 9–12, and 17–20 on a 28-day cycle for four cycles [7]. Responses were rapid with an overall response rate of 88%, and 39 % achieving complete/near complete response. Peripheral neuropathy rate was high at 66 %, with 7 % grade 3. A modified dose schedule of the trial used weekly bortezomib at 1.5 mg/m^2 IV on days 1, 8, 15, and 22 and dexamethasone modified to 40 mg once weekly after cycle 2 [28]. Response rates were comparable but with significantly less neuropathy. In another study Kropff et al. treated 30 patients with three 21-day cycles of bortezomib 1.3 mg/m^2 on days 1, 4, 8, 11 plus dexamethasone 40 mg on the day of bortezomib injection and the day after plus cyclophosphamide at 900, 1,200, or 1,500 mg/m^2 on day 1 [8]. The maximum tolerated dose of cyclophosphamide was defined as 900 mg/m^2. Overall response rate was 77 %, with a 10 % CR rate.

Bortezomib, Lenalidomide, and Dexamethasone (VRD)

Richardson studied 66 previously untreated patients in a phase 1/2 study using the combination of bortezomib, lenalidomide, and dexamethasone [9]. Patients received eight 3-week cycles and either proceeded to transplantation or maintenance with bortezomib given at a reduced frequency. All patients responded, with 67 % achieving a VGPR or better. With median follow-up of 21 months, the estimated 18-month PFS

Table 8.4 Randomized trials in non-transplant patients

Study	Regimen	CR (%)	P	≥PR (%)	P	Median PFS/EFS (months)	P	Overall survival (months)	P
Facon (IFM 95–01) [52]	Dex	1	NS	42	<0.001	12	With M versus no M, P<0.001	33	NS
	Dex-IFN	1		43		15		32	
	MP	1		41		21		34	
	MD	3		70		23		40	
Ludwig [53]	Thal-Dex	2	NS	68	0.002	17	NS	2-year 61 %	NS
	MP	2		52		21		2-year 70 %	
IFM99-06 [13] [a]	MPT	13	<0.001	76	<0.001	28	<0.001	52	0.0006
	MP	2		35		18		33	
IFM01-01 [14]	MPT	7	<0.001	62	<0.001	24	0.001	45	0.03
	MP	1		31		19		28	
GIMEMA [15, 16]	MPT	15	<0.001	60	NA	22	0.004	45	NS
	MP	2		45		14		48	
NMSG #12 [17]	MPT	13	<0.001	57	<0.001	15	NS	29	NS
	MP	4		40		14		32	
HOVON 49 [54]	MPT	23	<0.001	66	<0.001	13	<0.001	40	0.05
	MP	8		45		9		31	
TMSG [55]	MPT	9	NS	58	0.03	21	NS	26	NS
	MP	9		37		14		28	
MRC IX–non-intensive [56]	CTDa	13	NA	64	<0.001	13	0.01	33	NS
	MP	2		33		12		31	
MM-015 [18]	MPR-R	33	NA	77	0.002	31	<0.001	3-year 70 %	NS
	MPR	33		68		14		3-year 62 %	
	MP	12		50		13		3-year 66 %	
VISTA [19, 20]	VMP	30	<0.001	71	<0.001	24.0 m	<0.001	3-year 68 %	0.008
	MP	4		35		16.6 m		3-year 54 %	
PETHEMA/GEM [57]	VMP	20	NS	80	NS	34 m	NS	3-year 74 %	NS
	VTP	28		81		25 m		3-year 65 %	
VMPT+VT [58]	VMP	24	<0.001	81	NS	3-year 41 %	0.008	3-year 87 %	NS
	VMPT+VT	38		89		3-year 56 %		3-year 89 %	
E4A08≥70 [4, 59]	Rd	NA	NA	74	NS	22	0.1	2-year 90 %	0.03
	RD			75		16		2-year 69 %	
THAL-MM-003 [60]	TD	8	NS	63	<0.001	15	<0.001	2-year 69 %	NS
	D	3		46		6		2-year 63 %	

CR complete response; *MP* melphalan and prednisone; *MPT* melphalan, prednisone, thalidomide; *NA* not available; *OS* overall survival; *PFS/EFS* event-free survival or progression-free survival; *VMP* bortezomib, melphalan, and prednisone; *VMPT* bortezomib, melphalan, prednisone, and thalidomide

and OS for the entire cohort regardless of the use of transplant were 75 % and 97 %, respectively. Sensory neuropathy occurred in 80 % of patients and 32 % reported neuropathic pain.

Another phase 2 study (EVOLUTION) randomized patients to receive either bortezomib, dexamethasone, cyclophosphamide, and lenalidomide (VDCR), bortezomib, dexamethasone, and lenalidomide (VRD), or two different regimens of VCD in 140 previously untreated patients has been reported [10]. A maximum of eight 21-day cycles followed by maintenance bortezomib (1.3 mg/m^2 every other week for 24 weeks) was administered. The bortezomib was administered as 1.3 mg/m^2 days 1, 4, 8, and 11 and the dexamethasone was administered as 40 mg days 1, 8, and 15 for all patients. The VRD patients received lenalidomide 25 mg days 1–14, whereas the VDCR patients received lenalidomide 15 mg days 1–14 and cyclophosphamide 500 mg/m^2 days 1 and 8. The VCD patients received cyclophosphamide 500 mg/m^2 days 1 and 8, whereas the VCD-mod patients received cyclophosphamide 500 mg/m^2 days 1, 8, and 15. Nearly all patients responded and the VGPR or better (CR) rates were 58 % (25 %), 51 % (24 %), 41 % (22 %), and 53 % (47 %) for patients on VDCR, VDR, VCD, and VCD-mod, respectively. The corresponding 1-year progression-free survival was 86, 83, 93, and 100 %. However, the toxicity was significantly higher in the four-drug arm.

Unfortunately, the different studies have provided therapies for varying durations with or without use of stem cell transplantation making it difficult to compare the survival outcomes associated with specific regimens, and more importantly, the comparison between these regimens. The incorporation of the novel drugs such as IMiDs and the proteasome inhibitors have led to unprecedented response rates and response depth compared to older alkylator and steroid-based therapies. Moreover, combination regimens that include an IMiD and a proteasome inhibitor have led to very high response rates, but at the cost of higher toxicity rates compared to combinations with one or the other. So the debate as to whether to use a combination of both classes of drugs or one or the other, combination versus sequential therapy, continues in the absence of definitive data. One can argue that the endpoints used for assessing the induction therapy should include in addition to the response rates, the associated toxicities and most importantly the benefit in terms of early mortality. However, with the subsequent therapies (such as use of transplant) clouding the long-term outcomes such as overall survival and improvement in short-term outcomes such as avoidance of early death being maximized by any regimen containing at least one of the new drug, it has become difficult to derive conclusion from the available data. Hopefully, as the data matures from the current generation of randomized trials, we will have more definitive answers. In contrast to the question of combination versus sequential therapy, more clarity and consensus exists with respect to use of specific agents in the context of specific high-risk factors (Fig. 8.1). As was discussed in the risk stratification chapter, myeloma can be grouped onto a standard, intermediate, and high-risk categories based primarily on the genetic abnormalities. Our approach, as outlined in the mSMART strategy, is shown in Fig. 8.1.

Transplant-Ineligible Patients

The combination of melphalan and prednisone (MP) has been studied extensively in the non-transplant population and was the standard therapy until the advent of the new drugs [11, 12]. Response rates are from different studies varied from 40 to 60 % and median survival was around 3 years. With the introduction of the new drugs and initial studies showing excellent efficacy when combined with alkylating drugs, a series of phase 3 trials were undertaken examining the impact of adding thalidomide, lenalidomide, or bortezomib to melphalan and prednisone.

Melphalan, Prednisone, and Thalidomide (MPT)

Overall six randomized trials have been reported to date examining the value of adding thalidomide to MP. While all have shown improved response rates and four have shown improved PFS, only three have demonstrated an OS advantage. Meta-analysis of the different trials suggest a clear PFS and OS advantage to the combination; however, the benefit of the combination comes at the cost of considerable increased toxicity.

The initial IFM 99-06 study [13] randomized 447 patients to twelve 6-week cycles of either of MP (melphalan 0.25 mg/kg per day and prednisone 2 mg/kg/day days 1–4 every 6 weeks) or MPT (MP plus 200–400 mg of thalidomide daily) or to two sequential mini-autologous peripheral blood stem cell transplants (MEL100). The thalidomide was not continued past the 12th cycle of therapy. Higher response rates and longer PFS as well as OS were seen with the MPT as compared to either the MP or MEL100 groups. The IFM01-01 [14] in contrast studied patients over the age of 75, who were randomized to twelve 6-week cycles of either of MP (melphalan 0.2 mg/kg per day and prednisone 2 mg/kg/day days 1–4 every 6 weeks) or MPT (MP plus 50–100 mg of thalidomide daily). The combinations resulted in improved PFS and OS, but with increased rates of hematological toxicity as well as neuropathy. In the GIMEMA trial, patients were randomized to either standard dose oral MP for 6 months or to MP for 6 months with concurrent thalidomide, which was then continued indefinitely [15, 16]. Overall response rates were significantly higher with the MPT than the MP, which translated into improved PFS, but long-term results did not confirm the initially observed OS advantage. In the HOVON-49 trial, patients were randomized to either 8 cycles of MP (melphalan 0.25 mg/kg per day and prednisone 2 mg/kg/day days 1–5 every 4 weeks) or MPT (MP plus 200 mg/day thalidomide). The 2 year PFS was higher with MPT (33 % versus 21 %), and OS with MPT was also superior (40 versus 31 months, $P<0.05$). In the Nordic study [17], 357 patients were randomized to MP (4 days of melphalan 0.25 mg/kg per day and prednisone 100 mg/day every 6 weeks) or MPT (MP plus 200–400 mg/day thalidomide). Treatment was continued to plateau and the thalidomide was continued until relapse. Although there were superior CR and PR rates in the MPT arm, this did not result in any improvement in PFS or OS between the two groups.

Melphalan, Prednisone, and Lenalidomide (MPR)

MP has also been compared to the combination of melphalan, prednisone, and lenalidomide in a three-arm phase 3 trial [18]: MP versus MP with lenalidomide (MPR) versus MPR with lenalidomide maintenance (MPR-R). Four hundred and fifty-nine patients were randomized to MP (nine 4 week cycles of melphalan 0.18 mg/kg/day and prednisone 2 mg/kg/day days 1–4), MPR (nine 4 week cycles of MP plus lenalidomide 10 mg days 1–21), or nine cycles of MPR with indefinite lenalidomide maintenance (10 mg days 1–21 every 4 weeks). While addition of lenalidomide to MP led to higher response rates, and improved PFS when lenalidomide maintenance was used, there was no difference in the OS between the arms. Toxicity was substantially higher in the lenalidomide arms.

Melphalan, Prednisone, and Bortezomib (VMP)

The VISTA trial [19] compared MP to bortezomib and MP (VMP), with patients receiving nine 6-week cycles of either melphalan (at a dose of 9 mg/m^2) and prednisone (60 mg/m^2) on days 1–4, alone or in combination with bortezomib (1.3 mg/m^2) on days 1, 4, 8, 11, 22, 25, 29, and 32 during cycles 1–4 and on days 1, 8, 22, and 29 during cycles 5–9. Median PFS was 24 months with VMP as compared to 17 months with MP, and 3-year OS was higher for VMP at 68 % compared to 54 % [20]. Grade 3–4 adverse events, however, were more frequent in patients receiving VMP (46 % versus 36 %).

Subsequent trials have sought to build upon the VMP regimen by adding thalidomide to the combination (VMPT) with or without prolonged maintenance therapy. Palumbo and colleagues randomized patients to receive either nine 5-week cycles of VMP or nine 5-week cycles of VMPT, and continued maintenance thalidomide along with alternate week bortezomib. While response rates and PFS were higher in the four-drug combination with maintenance, the OS was not different. Toxicity was significantly higher using the four-drug regimen with more neutropenia, cardiac events, and thromboembolic events. During the course of the trial, the treatment schedule for bortezomib was changed from twice weekly to once weekly, allowing a comparison of the two approaches. It was found that the cumulative dose of bortezomib administered was similar with the two approaches, but with significant reduction in severe sensory peripheral neuropathy from 16 to 3 %. As a result of this study, bortezomib is increasingly being used once weekly as part of different drug combinations.

Consolidation and Maintenance

While the goals of the initial therapy were to rapidly control the disease, reverse the disease-related complications, and ready the patient for stem cell transplantation when indicated, consolidation approaches by definition aim to further build on the gains of the initial therapy. While the concept of consolidation therapy is not as clearly delineated in myeloma as it is with other hematological malignancies like acute leukemia, the broad goals remain the same. Various approaches have been employed as consolidation therapy in myeloma. Traditionally, transplant-eligible patients received 4–6 months of induction therapy with one of the commonly used induction regimens and then received autologous stem cell transplantation, while the transplant-ineligible patients continued on the initial therapy for 12–18 cycles.

For the transplant-eligible patients, SCT has been shown to improve overall survival in several studies when compared to no transplantation. Application of SCT following induction therapy significantly improved the depth of response following the initial therapy, leading to improved progression-free survival as well as overall survival. Based on the results from a series of phase 3 trials, SCT had been considered the standard of care for the younger transplant-eligible patients. Subsequent trials examined the concept of a tandem autologous stem cell transplant compared to a single transplant and showed benefit in a subgroup of patients, where the first transplant failed to achieve a VGPR or better. The results of the various studies and the current concepts regarding SCT in myeloma have been discussed in other chapters.

The distinction between these phases of treatment (induction, consolidation, and maintenance) has increasingly become blurred over the past decade with increasing efficacy of induction regimens with the incorporation of new drugs and more widespread use of maintenance therapy in the post-transplant setting. Prior to the advent of new drugs, the traditional induction regimens, primarily steroid-based, were associated with overall response rates of 40–60 % and complete response rates of less than 10 %, which improved to over 90 % and 30 %, respectively, for overall and complete response with the use of SCT. However, the newer regimens, especially those incorporating both IMiDs and proteasome inhibitors, have led to response rates hitherto only seen in the context on high-dose therapy. Given these results, SCT is increasingly being delayed and used a salvage therapy at the time of disease relapse following initial therapy with various combinations containing the new drugs. These patients, comprising an increasing proportion of patients with myeloma, continue on the initial therapy for prolonged periods reaching the same level of response as would have been seen with a transplant-based consolidation approach with or without maintenance. Based on the data available, this approach has not compromised the overall survival of patients with myeloma, thus shifting the role of SCT from a "consolidation therapy" for all eligible patients to another "treatment regimen" for nearly half of the patients with myeloma who elect to delay the SCT. Along with this, recent trails have shown survival benefit with the use of these new drugs as maintenance approaches following SCT further blurring the lines between these phases of therapy. The pros and cons of maintenance approaches used post SCT have been discussed in depth elsewhere. Finally, the use of prolonged "maintenance approaches both following SCT as well as following non-SCT-based new drug regimens in the transplant-eligible as well as non-transplant-eligible patients have led a remarkable convergence in the treatment approaches across the board for all patients with multiple myeloma in current era."

Supportive Care

The improvements in the supportive care for MM have significantly contributed towards the improved outcome in patients with myeloma. While this topic is covered more extensively in other sections, it is important to highlight certain aspects of the supportive care approach in myeloma. The most important has been the results of the randomized trials demonstrating a distinct advantage for the use of bisphosphonates in not only reducing the risk of skeletal events, but also improving the overall survival of patients with myeloma. It has become clear that patients with myeloma should be initiated on bisphosphonates at diagnosis irrespective of the presence of bone disease. Aggressive approaches to disease control have led to improvement in renal function early on after diagnosis and clearly contribute to better outcomes. Finally, while randomized trials have failed to demonstrate a benefit for prophylactic antibiotics, aggressive treatment of infections in the early stages after diagnosis is likely to have contributed to better outcomes.

Current Controversies and Critical Questions

One of the most controversial areas with respect to the goals of therapy in myeloma, especially in the context of initial treatment of myeloma, has been the duration of therapy and the depth of response that needs to be attained. While the overall goal is undoubtedly to maximize the survival of patients with myeloma, the optimal way to employ the available tools to reach this goal remains a point of considerable debate supported by limited randomized controlled data and shadowed by a variety of differing "expert" opinions.

The benefit of continued therapy (maintenance or prolonged initial therapy) seen in the recent trials has raised an important question regarding the optimal duration of therapy in patients receiving initial therapy for myeloma. The initial approach had been that a limited duration of therapy is appropriate for these patients, with new regimens as induction followed by transplant in the younger patients, and limited duration of melphalan-based regimen for the older patients. This approach had been primarily driven by the results seen with melphalan-based regimens, where long-term therapy has been associated with leukemogenesis and the potential effects of therapy-related side effects on quality of life has been of concern. With the newer therapies these concerns have been mitigated to a great extent and many of the recent trials have allowed patients to continue on initial therapy until disease progression. In the Mayo Clinic phase 2 trial of lenalidomide in newly diagnosed myeloma [3], long-term therapy with intent to SCT at relapse was associated with increasing depth of response up to 12–18 months ultimately reaching a VGPR rate of 67 %. Arguments in favor of continued therapy till progression is that any let up in therapy may lead to reemergence of disease which then may be more difficult to control, while continuous therapy raise concerns about long-term side effects of the new drugs that we might not be aware of, as well as the possibility of selecting drug-resistant tumor clones. Unfortunately, there is no evidence to support continuous therapy to progression versus repeated therapy based on disease activity.

Another bone of contention has been the goal of therapy with respect to the depth of response to be achieved. Clearly, the new multidrug combinations have contributed to unprecedented response depths as indicated by the high rates of VGPR and CRs seen in the more recent trials. The wealth of available data suggest improved outcomes associated with achievement of complete response, but this has to be viewed in the context of what CR really defines as well as the data linking CR achievement and long-term outcome. CR as defined currently represents only a modest reduction in the tumor burden as is clear from the studies' inferior outcomes with the presence of residual disease detected by OCR or flow cytometry-based methods. However, the available evidence does not allow us to discern whether the improvement in outcome is related more to the disease biology that allows a patient to get into a CR or whether the therapeutic approach that resulted in the CR is more important. Treatment approaches such as stem cell transplantation in the past have led to increased CR rates and improved survival, and among patients getting the same treatment CR has been associated with improved survival reflecting the impact of disease biology. Similarly in patients with preexisting MGUS and those with an MGUS-like gene expression signature appear to be less likely to obtain a CR with intensive approaches like total therapy [21, 22], with no adverse impact on their outcome. In contrast, the patients who appear to derive the maximum benefit of obtaining a CR with these therapies are those with high-risk disease by gene expression profile. It is likely that a significant proportion of patients with myeloma have a more "indolent" type of disease where achievement of a CR may be difficult with all the current therapies and persisting with this goal will result in unnecessary toxicity, while the patients with more aggressive disease require such a focused approach to maximize clonal eradication and prevention of early relapses and development of resistance.

References

1. Rajkumar SV, Hayman SR, Lacy MQ, et al. Combination therapy with lenalidomide plus dexamethasone (Rev/Dex) for newly diagnosed myeloma. Blood. 2005;106(13):4050–3.
2. Niesvizky R, Jayabalan DS, Christos PJ, et al. BiRD (Biaxin [clarithromycin]/Revlimid [lenalidomide]/dexamethasone) combination therapy results in high complete- and overall-response rates in treatment-naive symptomatic multiple myeloma. Blood. 2008;111(3):1101–9.
3. Lacy MQ, Gertz MA, Dispenzieri A, et al. Long-term results of response to therapy, time to progression, and survival with lenalidomide plus dexamethasone in newly diagnosed myeloma. Mayo Clin Proc. 2007;82(10):1179–84.
4. Rajkumar SV, Jacobus S, Callander NS, et al. Lenalidomide plus high-dose dexamethasone versus lenalidomide plus low-dose dexamethasone as initial therapy for newly diagnosed multiple myeloma: an open-label randomised controlled trial. Lancet Oncol. 2010;11(1):29–37.
5. Jagannath S, Durie BG, Wolf J, et al. Bortezomib therapy alone and in combination with dexamethasone for previously untreated symptomatic multiple myeloma. Br J Haematol. 2005;129(6):776–83.
6. Harousseau JL, Mathiot C, Attal M, et al. VELCADE/dexamethasone (Vel/D) versus VAD as induction treatment prior to autologous stem cell transplantion (ASCT) in newly diagnosed multiple myeloma (MM): updated results of the IFM 2005/01 trial. ASH Annual Meeting Abstracts. 2007;110(11):450.
7. Reeder CB, Reece DE, Kukreti V, et al. Cyclophosphamide, bortezomib and dexamethasone induction for newly diagnosed multiple myeloma: high response rates in a phase II clinical trial. Leukemia. 2009;23(7):1337–41.
8. Kropff M, Liebisch P, Knop S, et al. DSMM XI study: dose definition for intravenous cyclophosphamide in combination with bortezomib/dexamethasone for remission induction in patients with newly diagnosed myeloma. Ann Hematol. 2009;88(11):1125–30.
9. Richardson PG, Weller E, Lonial S, et al. Lenalidomide, bortezomib, and dexamethasone combination therapy in patients with newly diagnosed multiple myeloma. Blood. 2010;116(5):679–86.
10. Kumar S, Flinn I, Richardson PG, et al. Randomized, multicenter, phase 2 study (EVOLUTION) of combinations of bortezomib, dexamethasone, cyclophosphamide, and lenalidomide in previously untreated multiple myeloma. Blood. 2012;119(19):4375–82.
11. Alexanian R, Bonnet J, Gehan E, et al. Combination chemotherapy for multiple myeloma. Cancer. 1972;30(2):382–9.
12. Costa G, Engle RL, Schilling A, et al. Melphalan and prednisone: an effective combination for the treatment of multiple myeloma. Am J Med. 1973;54:589–99.
13. Facon T, Mary JY, Hulin C, et al. Melphalan and prednisone plus thalidomide versus melphalan and prednisone alone or reduced-intensity autologous stem cell transplantation in elderly patients with multiple myeloma (IFM 99–06): a randomised trial. Lancet. 2007;370(9594):1209–18.
14. Hulin C, Facon T, Rodon P, et al. Efficacy of melphalan and prednisone plus thalidomide in patients older than 75 years with newly diagnosed multiple myeloma: IFM 01/01 trial. J Clin Oncol. 2009;27(22):3664–70.
15. Palumbo A, Bringhen S, Caravita T, et al. Oral melphalan and prednisone chemotherapy plus thalidomide compared with melphalan and prednisone alone in elderly patients with multiple myeloma: randomised controlled trial. Lancet. 2006;367(9513):825–31.
16. Palumbo A, Bringhen S, Liberati AM, et al. Oral melphalan, prednisone, and thalidomide in elderly patients with multiple myeloma: updated results of a randomized, controlled trial. Blood. 2008;112(8):3107–14.
17. Waage A, Gimsing P, Fayers P, et al. Melphalan and prednisone plus thalidomide or placebo in elderly patients with multiple myeloma. Blood. 2010;116(9):1405–12.
18. Palumbo A, Hajek R, Delforge M, et al. Continuous lenalidomide treatment for newly diagnosed multiple myeloma. N Engl J Med. 2012;366(19):1759–69.
19. San Miguel JF, Schlag R, Khuageva NK, et al. Bortezomib plus melphalan and prednisone for initial treatment of multiple myeloma. N Engl J Med. 2008;359(9):906–17.
20. Mateos MV, Richardson PG, Schlag R, et al. Bortezomib plus melphalan and prednisone compared with melphalan and prednisone in previously untreated multiple myeloma: updated follow-up and impact of subsequent therapy in the phase III VISTA trial. J Clin Oncol. 2010;28(13):2259–66.
21. Zhan F, Barlogie B, Arzoumanian V, et al. Gene-expression signature of benign monoclonal gammopathy evident in multiple myeloma is linked to good prognosis. Blood. 2007;109(4):1692–700.
22. Kumar SK, Dingli D, Lacy MQ, et al. Outcome after autologous stem cell transplantation for multiple myeloma in patients with preceding plasma cell disorders. Br J Haematol. 2008;141(2):205–11.
23. Jagannath S, Durie BG, Wolf JL, et al. Extended follow-up of a phase 2 trial of bortezomib alone and in combination with dexamethasone for the frontline treatment of multiple myeloma. Br J Haematol. 2009;146(6):619–26.
24. Richardson PG, Xie W, Mitsiades C, et al. Single-agent bortezomib in previously untreated multiple myeloma: efficacy, characterization of peripheral

neuropathy, and molecular correlations with response and neuropathy. J Clin Oncol. 2009;27(21):3518–25.

25. Dispenzieri A, Jacobus S, Vesole DH, Callandar N, Fonseca R, Greipp PR. Primary therapy with single agent bortezomib as induction, maintenance and re-induction in patients with high-risk myeloma: results of the ECOG E2A02 trial. Leukemia. 2010;24(8):1406–11.
26. Harousseau JL, Attal M, Coiteux V, et al. Bortezomib (VELCADE®) plus dexamethasone as induction treatment prior to autologous stem cell transplantation in patients with newly diagnosed multiple myeloma: preliminary results of an IFM Phase II Study. *ASCO*. 2005:#6653.
27. Ghosh N, Ye X, Ferguson A, Huff CA, Borrello I. Bortezomib and thalidomide, a steroid free regimen in newly diagnosed patients with multiple myeloma. Br J Haematol. 2011;152(5):593–9.
28. Reeder CB, Reece DE, Kukreti V, et al. Once- versus twice-weekly bortezomib induction therapy with CyBorD in newly diagnosed multiple myeloma. Blood. 2010;115(16):3416–7.
29. Bensinger WI, Jagannath S, Vescio R, et al. Phase 2 study of two sequential three-drug combinations containing bortezomib, cyclophosphamide and dexamethasone, followed by bortezomib, thalidomide and dexamethasone as frontline therapy for multiple myeloma. Br J Haematol. 2010;148(4):562–8.
30. Wang M, Giralt S, Delasalle K, Handy B, Alexanian R. Bortezomib in combination with thalidomide-dexamethasone for previously untreated multiple myeloma. Hematology. 2007;12(3):235–239.
31. Kumar SK, Lacy MQ, Hayman SR, et al. Lenalidomide, cyclophosphamide and dexamethasone (CRd) for newly diagnosed multiple myeloma: results from a phase 2 trial. Am J Hematol. 2011;86(8):640–5.
32. Jakubowiak AJ, Dytfeld D, Griffith KA, et al. A phase 1/2 study of carfilzomib in combination with lenalidomide and low-dose dexamethasone as a frontline treatment for multiple myeloma. Blood. 2012;120(9): 1801–9.
33. Oakervee HE, Popat R, Curry N, et al. PAD combination therapy (PS-341/bortezomib, doxorubicin and dexamethasone) for previously untreated patients with multiple myeloma. Br J Haematol. 2005;129(6): 755–62.
34. Popat R, Oakervee HE, Hallam S, et al. Bortezomib, doxorubicin and dexamethasone (PAD) front-line treatment of multiple myeloma: updated results after long-term follow-up. Br J Haematol. 2008;141(4):512–6.
35. Popat R, Oakervee HE, Curry N, et al. Reduced dose PAD combination therapy (PS-341/bortezomib, adriamycin and dexamethasone) for previously untreated patients with multiple myeloma. ASH Annual Meeting Abstracts. 2005;106(11):2554.
36. Berenson JR, Yellin O, Chen CS, et al. A modified regimen of pegylated liposomal doxorubicin, bortezomib and dexamethasone (DVD) is effective and well tolerated for previously untreated multiple myeloma patients. Br J Haematol. 2011;155(5):580–7.
37. Hussein MA, Baz R, Srkalovic G, et al. Phase 2 study of pegylated liposomal doxorubicin, vincristine, decreased-frequency dexamethasone, and thalidomide in newly diagnosed and relapsed-refractory multiple myeloma. Mayo Clin Proc. 2006;81(7):889–95.
38. Offidani M, Corvatta L, Piersantelli MN, et al. Thalidomide, dexamethasone, and pegylated liposomal doxorubicin (ThaDD) for patients older than 65 years with newly diagnosed multiple myeloma. Blood. 2006;108(7):2159–2164.
39. Zervas K, Dimopoulos MA, Hatzicharissi E, et al. Primary treatment of multiple myeloma with thalidomide, vincristine, liposomal doxorubicin and dexamethasone (T-VAD doxil): a phase II multicenter study. Ann Oncol. 2004;15(1):134–8.
40. Jakubowiak AJ, Griffith KA, Reece DE, et al. Lenalidomide, bortezomib, pegylated liposomal doxorubicin, and dexamethasone in newly diagnosed multiple myeloma: a phase 1/2 Multiple Myeloma Research Consortium trial. Blood. 2011;118(3): 535–43.
41. Barlogie B, Tricot G, Anaissie E, et al. Thalidomide and hematopoietic-cell transplantation for multiple myeloma. N Engl J Med. 2006;354(10):1021–30.
42. Macro M, Divine M, Uzunhan Y, et al. Dexamethasone+thalidomide (Dex/Thal) compared to VAD as a pre-transplant treatment in newly diagnosed multiple myeloma (MM): a randomized trial. ASH Annual Meeting Abstracts. 2006;108(11):57.
43. Harousseau JL, Attal M, Avet-Loiseau H, et al. Bortezomib plus dexamethasone is superior to vincristine plus doxorubicin plus dexamethasone as induction treatment prior to autologous stem-cell transplantation in newly diagnosed multiple myeloma: results of the IFM 2005–01 phase III trial. J Clin Oncol. 2010;28(30):4621–9.
44. Cavo M, Tacchetti P, Patriarca F, et al. Bortezomib with thalidomide plus dexamethasone compared with thalidomide plus dexamethasone as induction therapy before, and consolidation therapy after, double autologous stem-cell transplantation in newly diagnosed multiple myeloma: a randomised phase 3 study. Lancet. 2010;376(9758):2075–85.
45. Lokhorst HM, van der Holt B, Zweegman S, et al. A randomized phase 3 study on the effect of thalidomide combined with adriamycin, dexamethasone, and high-dose melphalan, followed by thalidomide maintenance in patients with multiple myeloma. Blood. 2010;115(6):1113–20.
46. Morgan GJ, Davies FE, Gregory WM, et al. Cyclophosphamide, thalidomide, and dexamethasone as induction therapy for newly diagnosed multiple myeloma patients destined for autologous stem-cell transplantation: MRC Myeloma IX randomized trial results. Haematologica. 2012;97(3):442–50.
47. Sonneveld P, Schmidt-Wolf IG, van der Holt B, et al. Bortezomib induction and maintenance treatment in patients with newly diagnosed multiple myeloma: results of the randomized phase III HOVON-65/GMMG-HD4 trial. J Clin Oncol. 2012;30(24):2946–55.

48. Rosinol L, Oriol A, Teruel AI, et al. Superiority of bortezomib, thalidomide, and dexamethasone (VTD) as induction pretransplantation therapy in multiple myeloma: a randomized phase 3 PETHEMA/GEM study. Blood. 2012;120(8):1589–96.
49. Moreau P, Avet-Loiseau H, Facon T, et al. Bortezomib plus dexamethasone versus reduced-dose bortezomib, thalidomide plus dexamethasone as induction treatment before autologous stem cell transplantation in newly diagnosed multiple myeloma. Blood. 2011;118(22):5752–8; quiz 5982.
50. Rajkumar SV, Blood E, Vesole D, Fonseca R, Greipp PR. Phase III clinical trial of thalidomide plus dexamethasone compared with dexamethasone alone in newly diagnosed multiple myeloma: a clinical trial coordinated by the Eastern Cooperative Oncology Group. J Clin Oncol. 2006;24(3):431–6.
51. Zonder JA, Crowley J, Hussein MA, et al. Lenalidomide and high-dose dexamethasone compared with dexamethasone as initial therapy for multiple myeloma: a randomized Southwest Oncology Group trial (S0232). Blood. 2010;116(26):5838–41.
52. Facon T, Mary JY, Pegourie B, et al. Dexamethasone-based regimens versus melphalan-prednisone for elderly multiple myeloma patients ineligible for high-dose therapy. Blood. 2006;107(4):1292–8.
53. Ludwig H, Hajek R, Tothova E, et al. Thalidomide-dexamethasone compared to melphalan-prednisolone in elderly patients with multiple myeloma. Blood. 2009;113(15):3435–42.
54. Wijermans P, Schaafsma M, Termorshuizen F, et al. Phase III study of the value of thalidomide added to melphalan plus prednisone in elderly patients with newly diagnosed multiple myeloma: the HOVON 49 Study. J Clin Oncol. 2010;28(19):3160–6.
55. Beksac M, Haznedar R, Firatli-Tuglular T, et al. Addition of thalidomide to oral melphalan/prednisone in patients with multiple myeloma not eligible for transplantation: results of a randomized trial from the Turkish Myeloma Study Group. Eur J Haematol. 2011;86(1):16–22.
56. Morgan GJ, Davies FE, Gregory WM, et al. Cyclophosphamide, thalidomide, and dexamethasone (CTD) as initial therapy for patients with multiple myeloma unsuitable for autologous transplantation. Blood. 2011;118(5):1231–8.
57. Mateos MV, Oriol A, Martinez-Lopez J, et al. Bortezomib, melphalan, and prednisone versus bortezomib, thalidomide, and prednisone as induction therapy followed by maintenance treatment with bortezomib and thalidomide versus bortezomib and prednisone in elderly patients with untreated multiple myeloma: a randomised trial. Lancet Oncol. 2010; 11(10):934–41.
58. Palumbo A, Bringhen S, Rossi D, et al. Bortezomib-melphalan-prednisone-thalidomide followed by maintenance with bortezomib-thalidomide compared with bortezomib-melphalan-prednisone for initial treatment of multiple myeloma: a randomized controlled trial. J Clin Oncol. 2010;28(34):5101–9.
59. Vesole DH, Jacobus S, Rajkumar SV, et al. Lenalidomide plus low-dose dexamethasone (Ld): superior one and two year survival regardless of age compared to lenalidomide plus high-dose dexamethasone (LD). ASH Annual Meeting Abstracts. 2010; 116(21):308.
60. Rajkumar SV, Rosinol L, Hussein M, et al. Multicenter, randomized, double-blind, placebo-controlled study of thalidomide plus dexamethasone compared with dexamethasone as initial therapy for newly diagnosed multiple myeloma. J Clin Oncol. 2008;26(13):2171–7.

Approach to Relapsed Refractory Myeloma

9

Joseph Mikhael, Shaji Kumar, and S. Vincent Rajkumar

Introduction

Despite tremendous advances in the initial management of patients with myeloma, now translating to at least a doubling of median overall survival in the last decade, this disease remains incurable in nearly all patients [1]. Although time to first relapse has been extended with superior induction, consolidation, and maintenance strategies, relapse is inevitable. With the emergence of many novel agents in the relapsed setting, options for providers and patients have dramatically increased. The optimal sequencing, combination, and dosing of these agents have yet to be determined. Indeed, with so many therapeutic options available, the clinician must have a rational, risk stratified and feasible to approaching patients in relapse.

This chapter provides an approach to therapy for the myeloma patient with relapsed and/or refractory disease. The detailed discussion of the data for the various treatment options in relapsed disease, including Stem Cell Transplantation, New Agents, and Biologic Therapy, is covered in subsequent chapters (see Chaps. 10–13). The purpose of this chapter is to provide an overall strategy for the management of relapsed refractory disease and to help guide clinicians in selecting the most appropriate therapy for their patient. This approach emphasizes the heterogeneity of both the disease and the patient.

The biology of multiple myeloma is highly variable, with very indolent and aggressive forms [2]. Furthermore, with subsequent relapses and clonal selection, the disease may evolve significantly over time [3]. Patient variables such as age, renal status, preference, side effect profile, and comorbid disease must also be incorporated in the selection of relapsed therapy.

Definitions

Definitions used in relapsed myeloma have been established by the International Myeloma Workshop Consensus Panel [4]. Relapsed *and* refractory myeloma is defined as disease that is nonresponsive while *on* salvage therapy, or progresses within 60 days of stopping last therapy in patients who have achieved at least a minimal response (MR) or better at some point in the past. Primary refractory myeloma is defined as disease that is nonresponsive in patients who have never achieved MR or better with any therapy. It includes patients who never achieve MR or better

J. Mikhael, M.D. (✉)
Division of Hematology and Medical Oncology, Mayo Clinic Arizona, 13400 East Shea Boulevard, Scottsdale, AZ 85259-5494, USA
e-mail: mikhael.joseph@mayo.edu

S. Kumar, M.D.
Division of Hematology, Mayo Clinic, 200 First Street, SW, Rochester, MN 55905, USA

S.V. Rajkumar, M.D.
Myeloma Amyloidosis Dysproteinemia Group, Division of Hematology, Mayo Clinic, Rochester, MN, USA

M.A. Gertz and S.V. Rajkumar (eds.), *Multiple Myeloma: Diagnosis and Treatment*,
DOI 10.1007/978-1-4614-8520-9_9, © Mayo Foundation for Medical Education and Research 2014

in whom there is no significant change in M protein and no evidence of clinical progression (nonresponding–nonprogressive) as well as patients who meet criteria for progressive disease despite any therapy (progressive). The general term "relapsed myeloma" is defined as previously treated myeloma that progresses and requires the initiation of salvage therapy but does not meet criteria for either "primary refractory myeloma" or "relapsed-and-refractory myeloma" categories [4].

Indications for Therapy

A critical question that must be addressed is the need to treat patients immediately. With such a spectrum of disease from MGUS to smoldering myeloma to active myeloma, myeloma does not always need to be immediately treated. Once a patient has established myeloma the decision to retreat at time of relapse tends to be more liberal than in a patient who has never been treated—in initial therapy there is usually evidence of end organ damage in the form of CRAB (Calcium elevation, Renal insufficiency, Anemia or Bone disease), whereas in the context of retreatment one may not wait until there is concrete evidence of end organ damage. This is important clinically as the treated relapsed patient will likely be on therapy indefinitely, and before committing them to the risks of that therapy it should be clear that it is warranted. Many patients have a very "slow" biochemical relapse and may not need immediate treatment but close monitoring. By contrast, some patients may not meet formal criteria for relapse but are clearly requiring intervention.

To help guide the clinician, attempts have been made to standardize the definition for relapsed disease. In general, relapses can be classified as clinical or biochemical. Clinical relapse in myeloma is defined as worsening end organ damage such as new or expanding bone lesions, plasmacytomas, renal failure, anemia, or hypercalcemia using the definition of clinical relapse in the International Myeloma Working Group (IMWG) Criteria [5]. Patients with clinical relapse clearly need institution of therapy for relapsed disease. Biochemical relapses occur when there is an increase in the monoclonal protein component that meets the definitions of progression as per the IMWG Criteria, without any evidence of clinical relapse. Not all patients with biochemical relapse need therapy. In the setting of a pure biochemical relapse, the International Myeloma Workshop Consensus Panel recommends therapy at a minimum for all patients in whom there is a doubling of the M-component in two consecutive measurements separated by less than or equal to 2 months; or an increase in the absolute levels of serum M protein by more than or equal to 1 g/dL, or urine M protein by more than or equal to 500 mg/24 h, or involved FLC level by more than or equal to 20 mg/dL (plus an abnormal FLC ratio) in two consecutive measurements separated by less than or equal to 2 months [4]. In such patients, myeloma therapy should be restarted in clinical practice, even if signs and symptoms of new end organ damage are not yet apparent. Additionally, there may be patients with biochemical relapse who do not meet the minimal threshold set by the Consensus Panel, in whom the decision to initiate therapy needs to be individualized.

Choice of Therapy

Myeloma is characterized by multiple relapses and remissions. With each successive regimen, the depth and duration of response diminishes [6]. Patients who have an indolent relapse can be treated first with regimens such as lenalidomide plus dexamethasone (Rd) or bortezomib, cyclophosphamide, or dexamethasone (VCD). In contrast, patients with more aggressive relapse often require therapy with more aggressive combinations such as bortezomib, lenalidomide, dexamethasone (VRD) or bortezomib, liposomal doxorubicin, dexamethasone (VDD), or bendamustine [7]. Patients with multiple plasmacytomas or plasma cell leukemia at relapse may require therapy with a multidrug regimen such as bortezomib, dexamethasone, thalidomide, cisplatin, doxorubicin, cyclophosphamide, and etoposide (VDT-PACE) [8].

The depth and the duration of response to initial therapy play a critical role in deciding choice of therapy at relapse. Patients who achieve a very deep response, in particular with very good partial response (VGPR) or greater with a particular regimen in the past, will benefit from repeating the same therapy at relapse. Historically, 50–60 % of patients have responded to repeat treatment with the same regimen if relapse occurred after unmaintained remission [9]. Modern studies also confirm the efficacy of retreatment [10]. Among patients treated with immunomodulatory agents, of 113 evaluable patients, 50 (44 %) achieved at least a partial response with retreatment at time of relapse. In a chronic disease in which most patients will be sequentially treated with multiple regimens, being able to reemploy therapies provides for a longer term approach, especially with many patients now living longer than 10 years. In patients with standard-risk disease, even minor responses may of clinical benefit if they are prolonged, so re-treating in that context may also be of benefit.

The toxicity associated with prior treatments also influences the choice of therapy at the time of relapse. When limited options were available in myeloma, many adverse events secondary to drugs such as melphalan (cytopenias, infections), vincristine (neuropathy), thalidomide (neuropathy, constipation, thrombosis) simply had to be tolerated. However, with the emergence of many novel agents, the ability to limit those toxicities has been achieved. When selecting treatment at relapse, it is important to take into account residual toxicities from earlier therapies in order not to exacerbate previous or ongoing symptoms, especially when they may become permanent. Furthermore, care must be taken to not expose patients to cumulative toxicities (such as myelosuppression) that may further limit future therapeutic options later in the disease course.

The main areas of concern include neuropathy (sensory, motor, associations with pain), myelotoxicity, rash, fatigue, and others. Simple measures such as administering bortezomib once weekly via the subcutaneous route instead of twice weekly intravenously can greatly reduce the risk of severe neuropathy [11–13].

Standard Treatment Options

There are at least five commonly used drug-classes that are useful in the treatment of multiple myeloma: alkylating agents (melphalan, cyclophosphamide, bendamustine), corticosteroids (prednisone, dexamethasone, methylprednisolone), immunomodulatory agents (thalidomide, lenalidomide, and pomalidomide), proteasome inhibitors (bortezomib, carfilzomib,), and anthracyclines (doxorubicin and liposomal doxorubicin) [7]. Data with newer agents will be reviewed in a subsequent chapter (see Chap. 12). Data on thalidomide, bortezomib, and lenalidomide are reviewed below.

Thalidomide

Thalidomide has a response rate of 25 % in heavily pretreated patients with relapsed and refractory disease [14]. The median duration of response is approximately 1 year. Thalidomide can be given in combination with other drugs such as dexamethasone (TD) or cyclophosphamide plus dexamethasone (CTD). Response rates in relapsed disease are about 50 % with TD, and over 65 % with CTD [15–17]. The use of thalidomide in pregnancy is absolutely contraindicated and the System for Thalidomide Education and Prescribing Safety Program (STEPS) must be followed to prevent teratogenicity [18]. The incidence of deep vein thrombosis (DVT) is 1–3 % in patients receiving thalidomide alone, 10–15 % in patients receiving thalidomide in combination with dexamethasone, and 25 % in combination with other cytotoxic chemotherapeutic agents, particularly doxorubicin [19–23].

Bortezomib

Approximately one-third of patients with relapsed myeloma respond to bortezomib as a single agent, with an average response duration of 1 year [24, 25]. The dose used in initial trials was 1.3 mg/m^2 given twice weekly on days 1, 4,

8, and 11 every 21 days. However, bortezomib is now administered subcutaneously in a once-weekly schedule to minimize neurotoxicity. Several combinations such as bortezomib dexamethasone (VD), bortezomib, thalidomide, dexamethasone (VTD), VCD (also referred to as CyBorD), and VRD have been developed and are all active in patients with relapsed disease [26]. Patients who fail an alkylator-based combination such as VCD can respond to an immunomodulatory agent-based regimen such as VRD. VTD is particularly useful in renal failure.

Lenalidomide

As a single agent approximately 25 % of relapsed or refractory patients respond to lenalidomide. Two large phase III trials have compared lenalidomide plus dexamethasone (RD) compared to placebo plus dexamethasone in relapsed multiple myeloma [27, 28]. In these trials, RD was associated with improved survival. Typical dosing of lenalidomide for myeloma is 25–30 mg per day on days 1–21 of a 28 day cycle, with dose adjustments based on toxicity.

Liposomal Doxorubicin

In a phase trial, median time to progression was superior with bortezomib plus liposomal doxorubicin compared with bortezomib alone, 9.3 versus 6.5 months, respectively, $P<0.001$ [29]. OS at 15 months was also superior, 76 % compared with 65 %, respectively, $P=0.03$. Overall, liposomal doxorubicin has modest activity in relapsed myeloma.

Glucocorticoids and Alkylating Agents

Dexamethasone or intravenous methylprednisolone are active in relapsed myeloma, but are usually given in combination with other active agents [30, 31]. Intravenous melphalan at a dose of 25 mg/m^2 is another active regimen, but usually requires transfusion and growth factor support.

Stem Cell Transplantation

The use of autologous stem cell transplant as an option for the treatment of relapsed myeloma has been extensively investigated. Patients who have cryopreserved stem cells early in the disease course can derive significant benefit from ASCT as salvage therapy [32]. Similarly, eligible patients who have had a transplant with a response duration of more than 18–24 months can undergo the procedure again especially if additional stem cells have been cryopreserved.

Risk Stratification

Many of the prognostic factors that are relevant at the time of initial diagnosis continue to be important at the time of relapse. These include the International Staging System, the plasma cell proliferation rate, serum LDH, performance status, refractory status with respect to various drugs, and the presence of circulating cells or extramedullary disease [33]. In addition to these, perhaps the most important determinants of risk status are molecular cytogenetic findings [34]. Of particular importance may be the acquisition of new abnormalities, including the p53 deletion which portends a poor outcome. Knowing the patient's risk status may influence therapeutic choices. In general, high-risk patients will require more aggressive combinations for prolonged periods of time. Intermediate-risk patients will benefit from bortezomib-based approaches, while standard-risk patients will benefit from a more "sequential" approach to relapse.

Other Factors

There are no "standard" second-line, third-line, fourth-line, etc., approach in myeloma. The appropriate sequence of therapies, although unknown, is based on numerous disease (such as risk stratification) and patient factors. These patient factors must be well considered in evaluating the patient in relapse. Although it is impossible to list all of these factors, the following are of particular importance in myeloma:

- Age—dose reducing most agents is necessary.
- Renal insufficiency—preference given to thalidomide, bortezomib, carfilzomib, and possibly pomalidomide.
- Cost—although not usually the only factor, the direct to patient and system cost should be considered.
- Convenience—some patients may not be able to travel to obtain parenteral therapies and oral regimens may be preferred.

Clinical Trials

Until myeloma is a curable disease in all patients, clinical trials will play a critical role in the treatment of these patients. Clinicaltrials.gov reveals that there are usually over 150 active trials in multiple myeloma at any given time, the majority of which relate to relapsed disease. With many novel agents in development (see Chap. 12), there will surely be a pipeline of trials for many years to come. The most promising new drugs include elotuzumab, antibodies targeting CD38, cyclin D inhibitors, and ARRY-520. A clinical trial should always be considered when evaluating a patient with relapsed myeloma.

References

1. Rajkumar SV. Multiple myeloma: 2013 update on diagnosis, risk-stratification, and management. Am J Hematol. 2013;88:225–35.
2. Fonseca R, Bergsagel PL, Drach J, et al. International Myeloma Working Group molecular classification of multiple myeloma: spotlight review. Leukemia. 2009; 23:2210–21.
3. Keats JJ, Chesi M, Egan JB, et al. Clonal competition with alternating dominance in multiple myeloma. Blood. 2012;120:1067–76.
4. Rajkumar SV, Harousseau JL, Durie B, et al. Consensus recommendations for the uniform reporting of clinical trials: report of the International Myeloma Workshop Consensus Panel 1. Blood. 2011;117:4691–5.
5. Durie BGM, Harousseau J-L, Miguel JS, et al. International uniform response criteria for multiple myeloma. Leukemia. 2006;20:1467–73.
6. Kumar SK, Therneau TM, Gertz MA, et al. Clinical course of patients with relapsed multiple myeloma. Mayo Clin Proc. 2004;79:867–74.
7. Rajkumar SV. Treatment of multiple myeloma. Nat Rev Clin Oncol. 2011;8:479–91.
8. Tiedemann RE, Gonzalez-Paz N, Kyle RA, et al. Genetic aberrations and survival in plasma cell leukemia. Leukemia. 2008;22(5):1044–52.
9. Alexanian R, Gehan E, Haut A, Saiki J, Weick J. Unmaintained remissions in multiple myeloma. Blood. 1978;51:1005–11.
10. Madan S, Lacy MQ, Dispenzieri A, et al. Efficacy of retreatment with immunomodulatory drugs (IMiDs) in patients receiving IMiDs for initial therapy of newly diagnosed multiple myeloma. Blood. 2011; 118:1763–5.
11. Mateos MV, Oriol A, Martinez-Lopez J. Bortezomib/melphalan/prednisone (VMP) versus bortezomib/thalidomide/prednisone (VTP) as induction therapy followed by maintenance treatment with bortezomib/thalidomide (VT) versus bortezomib/prednisone (VP): a randomised trial in elderly untreated patients with multiple myeloma older than 65 years. Lancet Oncol. 2010;11:934–41.
12. Palumbo A, Bringhen S, Rossi D, et al. Bortezomib-melphalan-prednisone-thalidomide followed by maintenance with bortezomib-thalidomide compared with bortezomib-melphalan-prednisone for initial treatment of multiple myeloma: a randomized controlled trial. J Clin Oncol. 2010;28:5101–9.
13. Moreau P, Pylypenko H, Grosicki S, et al. Subcutaneous versus intravenous administration of bortezomib in patients with relapsed multiple myeloma: a randomised, phase 3, non-inferiority study. Lancet Oncol. 2011;12:431–40.
14. Singhal S, Mehta J, Desikan R, et al. Antitumor activity of thalidomide in refractory multiple myeloma [see comments]. N Engl J Med. 1999;341:1565–71.
15. Dimopoulos MA, Hamilos G, Zomas A, et al. Pulsed cyclophosphamide, thalidomide and dexamethasone: an oral regimen for previously treated patients with multiple myeloma. Hematol J. 2004;5:112–7.
16. Garcia-Sanz R, Gonzalez-Fraile MI, Sierra M, Lopez C, Gonzalez M, San Miguel JF. The combination of thalidomide, cyclophosphamide and dexamethasone (ThaCyDex) is feasible and can be an option for relapsed/refractory multiple myeloma. Hematol J. 2002;3:43–8.
17. Kropff MH, Lang N, Bisping G, et al. Hyperfractionated cyclophosphamide in combination with pulsed dexamethasone and thalidomide (HyperCDT) in primary refractory or relapsed multiple myeloma. Br J Haematol. 2003;122:607–16.
18. Zeldis JB, Williams BA, Thomas SD, Elsayed ME. S.T.E.P.S.: a comprehensive program for controlling and monitoring access to thalidomide. Clin Ther. 1999;21:319–30.

19. Barlogie B, Desikan R, Eddlemon P, et al. Extended survival in advanced and refractory multiple myeloma after single-agent thalidomide: identification of prognostic factors in a phase 2 study of 169 patients. Blood. 2001;98:492–4.
20. Osman K, Comenzo R, Rajkumar SV. Deep vein thrombosis and thalidomide therapy for multiple myeloma. N Engl J Med. 2001;344:1951–2.
21. Zangari M, Anaissie E, Barlogie B, et al. Increased risk of deep-vein thrombosis in patients with multiple myeloma receiving thalidomide and chemotherapy. Blood. 2001;98:1614–5.
22. Zangari M, Siegel E, Barlogie B, et al. Thrombogenic activity of doxorubicin in myeloma patients receiving thalidomide: implications for therapy. Blood. 2002;100:1168–71.
23. Dimopoulos MA, Anagnostopoulos A, Weber D. Treatment of plasma cell dyscrasias with thalidomide and its derivatives. J Clin Oncol. 2003;21: 4444–54.
24. Richardson PG, Barlogie B, Berenson J, et al. A phase 2 study of bortezomib in relapsed, refractory myeloma. N Engl J Med. 2003;348:2609–17.
25. Richardson PG, Sonneveld P, Schuster MW, et al. Bortezomib or high-dose dexamethasone for relapsed multiple myeloma [see comment]. N Engl J Med. 2005;352:2487–98.
26. Richardson PG, Laubach J, Mitsiades C, et al. Tailoring treatment for multiple myeloma patients with relapsed and refractory disease. Oncology. 2010;24:22–9.
27. Dimopoulos M, Spencer A, Attal M, et al. Lenalidomide plus dexamethasone for relapsed or refractory multiple myeloma. N Engl J Med. 2007;357:2123–32.
28. Weber DM, Chen C, Niesvizky R, et al. Lenalidomide plus dexamethasone for relapsed multiple myeloma in North America. N Engl J Med. 2007;357:2133–42.
29. Orlowski RZ, Nagler A, Sonneveld P, et al. Randomized phase III study of pegylated liposomal doxorubicin plus bortezomib compared with bortezomib alone in relapsed or refractory multiple myeloma: combination therapy improves time to progression. J Clin Oncol. 2007;25:3892–901.
30. Alexanian R, Barlogie B, Dixon D. High-dose glucocorticoid treatment of resistant myeloma. Ann Intern Med. 1986;105:8–11.
31. Gertz MA, Garton JP, Greipp PR, Witzig TE, Kyle RA. A phase II study of high-dose methylprednisolone in refractory or relapsed multiple myeloma. Leukemia. 1995;9:2115–8.
32. Gertz MA, Lacy MQ, Inwards DJ, et al. Early harvest and late transplantation as an effective therapeutic strategy in multiple myeloma. Bone Marrow Transplant. 1999;23:221–6.
33. Russell SJ, Rajkumar SV. Multiple myeloma and the road to personalised medicine. Lancet Oncol. 2011;12:617–9.
34. Mikhael JR, Dingli D, Roy V, et al. Management of newly diagnosed symptomatic multiple myeloma: updated Mayo Stratification of Myeloma and Risk-Adapted Therapy (mSMART) consensus guidelines 2013. Mayo Clin Proc. 2013;88:360–76.

Autologous Stem Cell Transplantation in the Management of Multiple Myeloma

10

Morie A. Gertz and Craig B. Reeder

Introduction

Autologous stem cell transplantation has been shown to improve the survival in patients with multiple myeloma. Seven randomized clinical trials have been reported demonstrating the superiority of stem cell transplantation in inducing disease responses, increasing complete remissions, and prolonging event-free survival (Table 10.1).

Three trials demonstrated significant prolongation of median survival in newly diagnosed patients [1]. The largest of these trials enrolled 401 patients and, compared with standard therapy, prolonged median survival by almost 1 year [2]. The available therapies in the era of these trials, however, did not include the novel agents, thalidomide, lenalidomide, and bortezomib, and some have questioned the rationale for stem cell transplantation with the advent of novel agents.

A meta-analysis on 575 patients randomly assigned to high-dose or conventional therapy with 104 months of median follow-up did not significantly prolong long-term survival. However, there was significant improvement in quality of life as measured by a mean gain of 14.5 months in TWIST (time without symptoms of disease or toxicity of treatment) [3]. With advances in supportive care, fluoroquinolone antibiotics, and enhanced techniques to improve CD34 cell yield, outpatient peripheral blood stem cell transplantation is now being done routinely. More than 60 % of patients are manageable as outpatients provided a caregiver is available [4]. At Mayo Clinic, the determinants of the likelihood of remaining an outpatient during stem cell transplantation are age (> or <65) and serum creatinine (> or <1.7 mg/dL). Overall, only 40 % of patients are hospitalized for a median of 7 days. Despite the ability to perform stem cell transplant as an outpatient, the procedure takes a toll. A quality of life study shows that symptom means are mild at baseline, intensify during conditioning, peak at leukocyte nadir, and decrease by day 30. Symptoms associated with stem cell transplantation include anorexia, fatigue, weakness, nausea, altered sleep habits, and diarrhea [5].

Patient Selection

Patients are considered eligible for stem cell transplantation based on performance status and organ function. In the United States, age alone is not a factor in deciding transplant eligibility, at least up to age 78. However, in many other countries patients over the age of 65 are not considered candidates for transplantation.

M.A. Gertz, M.D., M.A.C.P. (✉)
Division of Hematology, Mayo Clinic,
200 First Street, SW, Rochester, MN 55905, USA
e-mail: gertz.morie@mayo.edu

C.B. Reeder, M.D.
Division of Hematology and Oncology,
Mayo Clinic Arizona, 13400 East Shea Boulevard,
Scottsdale, AZ 85259, USA
e-mail: reeder.craig@mayo.edu

M.A. Gertz and S.V. Rajkumar (eds.), *Multiple Myeloma: Diagnosis and Treatment*,
DOI 10.1007/978-1-4614-8520-9_10, © Mayo Foundation for Medical Education and Research 2014

Table 10.1 Randomized studies comparing conventional chemotherapy vs. high-dose therapy [17]

Author	No. of patients	Age (y)	Median follow-up	CR rate (%) CC	CR rate (%) HDT	Median EFS (mo) CC	Median EFS (mo) HDT	Median OS (mo) CC	Median OS (mo) HDT
Attal et al.	200	<65	7 y	5[a]	22[a]	18[a]	28[a]	44[a]	57[a]
Fermand et al.	190	55–65	56 mo	5[a]	19[a]	19[a]	24[a]	50	55
Bladé et al.	164	<65	44 mo	11[a]	30[a]	33	42	66	61
Palumbo et al.	195	<70	39 mo	6[a]	25[a]	15.6[a]	28[a]	42[a]	58[a]
Child et al.	407	<65	42 mo	8[a]	44[a]	19[a]	31[a]	42[a]	54[a]
Fermand et al.	190	55–65	10 y	20 CR + VGPR[a]	48 CR + VGPR[a]	19[b]	25[b]	48	48
Barlogie et al.	516	≤70	76 mo	15	17	7 y 14 %	7 y 17 %	7 y 38 %	7 y 38 %

y indicates years, *CR* complete response, *EFS* event-free survival, *OS* overall survival, *CC* conventional chemotherapy, *HDT* high-dose therapy, *mo* months, *VGPR* very good partial response
[a]Significant
[b]Borderline significance

Renal Failure

Stem cell transplantation is feasible in myeloma patients with renal failure. Renal failure is seen in 22 % of myeloma patients at diagnosis. In one study, patients were divided into three groups: (1) those that had normal renal function at diagnosis and transplant, (2) those that had renal failure at diagnosis but had normalized at the completion of induction therapy, and (3) those that had persistent renal insufficiency following induction therapy. Among 20 patients with persistent renal insufficiency at the time of transplant, ten had normalized post-transplant. However, patients with renal failure had significantly longer hospitalization, increased use of blood products, and an increased number of infections. The reported transplant-related mortality was 17 % in this cohort. Eight patients were on dialysis during transplant, and four died within the first 100 days post-transplant. Patients in need of dialysis at time of transplant must be carefully evaluated before considering high-dose chemotherapy [6]. The outcome of high-dose chemotherapy was evaluated retrospectively in 27 patients with myeloma. Twenty-three patients were on dialysis at the time of transplant. Thirty-seven percent received Mel-200. The median conditioning dose was 140 mg/m^2. Five patients died of transplant-related toxicity before day 100. The response rate was 70 %. The median time to disease progression was 32 months. The median time to best response was 6.5 months. Twenty-four percent became dialysis-independent 5 months post stem cell transplantation. At a median follow-up of 70 months, 7 of 23 were alive and 3 of 7 had progressive disease. High-dose therapy is feasible with renal failure; 5-year survival is seen in approximately one-third [7]. When the dose of melphalan in patients with renal failure is reduced to 100 mg/m^2, the regimen was less toxic but was equally efficient and improved the prognosis in this group of patients with no difference in treatment-related mortality compared with counterparts with normal renal function. Stem cell transplantation with renal failure is feasible, but dose reduction of melphalan is strongly recommended [8]. Forty-six patients with myeloma and renal failure defined by a creatinine >2 mg/dL were reported. The complete and partial response rates were 75 %. The treatment-related mortality was 4 %. Significant improvement in renal function, a GFR (glomerular filtration rate) improvement of 25 %, was seen in 32 %. The 3-year progression-free and overall survival was 36 % and 64 %, respectively. Stem cell transplantation should be offered to patients with renal failure. Renal function will improve in one-third. The dose of melphalan can be reduced without compromising response [9].

Elderly Patients

Autologous stem cell transplantation is also safe and feasible in elderly patients with multiple myeloma. Twenty-six patients over the age of 70 received melphalan conditioning. Complete and partial responses were seen in 77 %, 19 % complete. The median progression-free survival was 24 months. Median overall survival was not reached. The day 100, all-cause mortality was zero. The 3-year progression-free and overall survival was 39 % and 65 %, respectively. Predictors of a shorter progression-free survival included a low serum albumin, relapsed disease at transplant, and over 12 months between diagnosis and transplant [10]. In an update of 84 patients over the age of 70, the day 100 non-relapse mortality was 3 %. The overall response rate at day 100 was 85 %, 18 % complete. The estimated progression-free and overall survival at 5 years was 27 % and 67 %, respectively. Age alone should not be an exclusion criterion for auto stem cell transplantation.

In an effort to determine whether high-dose therapy is beneficial to the elderly with the advent of novel drug combinations, a study compared outcomes of a regimen that included thalidomide, dexamethasone, and pegylated liposomal doxorubicin with maintenance therapy to a similar induction with stem cell transplantation. This was a non-randomized study where 62 patients ineligible for transplant received six induction courses followed by maintenance with thalidomide and were compared to 26 patients eligible for stem cell transplantation who received four induction cycles followed by a melphalan-based transplant. Complete remission rates were 57 % in the transplanted group compared to 24 % in the non-transplanted group ($p=0.02$). However, median time to progression and progression-free survival were not different between the two groups. Five-year overall survival was 49 % vs. 46 % in the two groups. This small study suggested that in elderly myeloma patients, the introduction of novel agents resulted in equivalent time to progression, progression-free, and overall survival, raising the question of the utility of stem cell transplantation in older patients [11].

Nonsecretory Disease

The benefit of stem cell transplantation does not appear to depend upon whether patients have secretory or nonsecretory disease. Treatment-related mortality, progression-free survival, and overall survival are comparable between the two groups [12]. It also does not appear that outcome after autologous stem cell transplantation depends on whether patients had an antecedent plasma cell proliferative disorder including MGUS, smoldering myeloma, or solitary plasmacytoma of bone. Patients with a preexisting plasma cell dyscrasia appear to do just as well; but patients with a preexisting MGUS appear to have a better outcome following high-dose therapy, likely reflecting more indolent disease and favorable biology compared with those patients presenting with de novo myeloma [13].

Response Status

The goal of stem cell transplantation is to increase the complete response (CR) rate, which is consistently associated with better outcomes. In one study after high-dose therapy, the complete response rate following induction increased from 8 to 37 %. Patients who achieved a CR had an event-free survival and overall survival that was statistically longer. This supports the use of stem cell transplantation in an effort to improve the complete response rate achievable with induction chemotherapy [14]. In a group receiving total therapy as defined at the University of Arkansas, the benefit of complete response was limited to the high-risk subgroup as identified by gene expression profile. This high-risk group, which compromised 13 % of patients, had lengthened survival only when achieving a complete response. The majority of patients with low-risk disease had similar survival expectations whether or not a CR was achieved [15]. In the era of novel agents, the achievement of a complete response remains significantly associated with event-free and overall survival prolongation. Patients achieving a CR had an event-free survival of 61 months compared to those who did not at 40 months. The benefit of achieving a complete response extended to older patients as well as younger patients. Quality of response is significantly associated with event-free and overall survival [16]. In a review of the IFM database, the benefit of complete response depended on the type of treatment and was not identical for all patients. In the elderly, treatment designed to induce a higher CR rate appeared to be more toxic. The achievement of complete response was deemed necessary in patients with poor-risk disease but was not as critical for long survival in more indolent multiple myeloma [17].

Remission status prior to stem cell transplantation was also an important prognostic factor. Patients who achieve a complete response before a stem cell transplantation have a better overall survival than those patients in partial response before autologous stem cell transplantation, suggesting that improving induction will result in an improved outcome post-transplant [18].

There are certain populations of patients that can be identified that do not appear to benefit from stem cell transplantation. The rate of early progression after transplantation is significantly higher among patients transplanted with progressive disease. Progression-free and overall survival from the first transplant is shorter in patients with progressive disease at 0.6 years and 1.1 year, respectively. Patients with progressive refractory myeloma do not benefit from autologous transplantation. Transplantation can be applied early after an initial induction therapy or can be used as salvage after the first relapse. In a retrospective analysis of 285 patients, those who received early stem cell mobilization and delayed stem cell transplantation had a similar overall survival compared to patients who had early stem cell transplantation. In both groups, the 4-year survival rate was >80 % [19]. Factors that predict for a good outcome using salvage stem cell transplantation include duration of remission of more than 12 months after first transplant. Patients who relapsed in less than 12 months do not appear to benefit from salvage stem cell transplantation.

Risk-Stratification

Cytogenetics appears to impact outcomes following stem cell transplantation. Patients who are considered high risk based on genetics by fluorescence in situ hybridization (FISH) t(4;14), t(14;16), t(14;20) del 17p13, or a high proliferation index have a median progression-free survival of less than 12 months; and in these 25 % of patients, the transient benefit may not justify intervention with high-dose therapy [20]. The application of genomics to identify high-risk patients has revealed that activation of one of the three cyclin-D genes predicts early treatment failure [21]. High-risk cytogenetics and persistent minimal residual disease predict unsustained complete response after autologous stem cell transplantation. Twelve percent of 241 patients showed unsustained complete response and a median overall survival of only 39 months. The presence of baseline high-risk cytogenetics by FISH had a hazard ratio of 17.3 and identified patients at risk of early progression following high-dose therapy, raising the question as to whether it is an appropriate intervention.

Choice of Induction Therapy

The only area in which investigators agree is that patients who are candidates for stem cell transplantation should not be exposed to stem cell toxic agents, which include melphalan and purine nucleoside analogs. In the era where vincristine, doxorubicin, dexamethasone (VAD), or dexamethasone alone was used as an induction agent, the outcome had very little impact on post-transplant results. In that era, complete responses occurred in less than 5 % of patients. Partial responses occurred in no greater than 50 % of patients, and stem cell transplantation was highly effective even in patients who failed to achieve a PR with induction therapy. In an analysis of patients largely before the introduction of novel agents, the median time to progression was 27.1 months with VAD and 24.7 months with single agent dexamethasone, suggesting that in the pre-novel agent era, the nature of initial treatment had no long-term impact on outcome [22]. However, it has been demonstrated that a level of residual myeloma at the completion of induction just prior to transplant was an independent predictor of outcome. When patients were analyzed for minimal residual disease in the novel agent era, the median event-free survival in those with a low amount of minimal residual disease was longer than patients with high minimal residual disease at 35 vs. 20 months. Moreover, survival was significantly better in patients who had the deeper response (70 vs. 45 months). A multivariable analysis found that the pre-transplant disease level was an independent prognostic factor [23]. Based on this and similar data, initiatives to try and maximize the number of complete responses and very good partial responses (VGPRs) at the completion of induction were introduced.

One of the first novel agent combinations was thalidomide and dexamethasone, and it was compared in a retrospective matched-case control analysis of 200 patients who received the VAD regimen. Thal-Dex resulted in a significantly higher response rate and a deeper reduction in myeloma cell mass, although the Thal-Dex arm had greater degree of deep vein thrombosis and was suggested in this retrospective analysis to be superior to VAD [24]. An induction regimen that included melphalan, dexamethasone, bortezomib, and thalidomide, before autologous hematopoietic stem cell infusions, was introduced in patients who were candidates for stem cell transplantation. This single-arm study showed significant anti-myeloma activity in patients with advanced-stage disease [25].

The Spanish Myeloma Group initiated a phase II trial studying bortezomib and dexamethasone. A PR or greater was seen in 65 % with an additional 17.5 % minor responses. Post stem cell transplantation, the response rate was 88 % with 33 % complete response and 22 % VGPR. This was an early demonstration of the efficacy of bortezomib as a pre-transplant conditioning regimen in newly diagnosed patients [26]. Clinical studies with bortezomib-based induction subsequently demonstrated no adverse impact on stem cell mobilization or the quality of the stem cells as defined by engraftment times [27].

The Nordic Myeloma Study Group conducted a prospective randomized trial of VAD vs. cyclophosphamide-dexamethasone. No novel agents were included and comparable response rates after stem cell transplantation resulted; and in both groups, the median event-free survival was 29 months; the 3-year survival was 75 %. This suggested that an alkylator-based regimen that does not contain a novel agent provides no benefit in terms of induction and that effective alternatives to VAD require a novel agent [28].

A single-arm study looking at bortezomib administered before stem cell transplantation followed by maintenance therapy post-transplant was reported in 40 patients. The overall response rate was 83 % with a CR + VGPR rate of 50 %. Disease-free and overall survival at 3 years was 38.2 % and 63.1 %, respectively [29]. In a prospective randomized trial, 135 patients received thalidomide from induction through tandem transplantation. These patients were analyzed in comparison with an equal number of patients who had double stem cell transplantation and did not have thalidomide as part of induction therapy. Stem cell transplantation resulted in a significant improvement in the response rate, 49–68 % reflecting the value of stem cell transplantation in the novel agent era. The thalidomide arm had a greater proportion of VGPR and longer progression-free survival. Overall survival at 5 years did not reach statistical significance (69 % vs. 53 %), presumably related to salvage use of novel agents. The benefits of thalidomide were an increase in the rate of VGPR or better response, time to progression, and progression-free survival. Seventeen percent of patients discontinued thalidomide related to toxicity. The addition of first-line thalidomide to a tandem transplant program improved clinical outcomes [30]. The same cooperative group did a prospective randomized study of bortezomib–thalidomide–dexamethasone (VTD) and compared it with thalidomide-dexamethasone (TD) as induction therapy before and consolidation therapy after tandem stem cell transplantation. Four hundred eighty patients were enrolled and randomly assigned to the VTD or TD arms. After induction therapy, a complete or near-complete response was achieved in 31 % of patients receiving VTD and 11 % on TD. Grade III or IV adverse events were significantly higher in the three-drug arm particularly peripheral neuropathy (10 % in VTD vs. 2 % in TD). VTD induction therapy significantly improved the rate of complete or near-complete response and is now widely considered the standard of induction therapy in continental Europe for those who are eligible for transplant [31].

One group combined the VTD described in the preceding paragraph with VAD and alternated them with each cycle. Combining both regimens the cumulative complete response rate after stem cell transplantation was 48 %. The 3-year overall and event-free survival were 75.1 % and 48.3 %, respectively. This approach of alternating VTD with VAD reduced the use of bortezomib without compromising the ultimate CR rate [32].

A single-arm study of bortezomib–dexamethasone followed by DCEP (dexamethasone, cyclophosphamide, etoposide, and cisplatin) resulted in an overall response rate of 86 %, which was independent of International Stage and FISH genetics. In patients who completed induction, consolidation, and transplant, the overall response rate was 96 %; and the bortezomib–dexamethasone was so active, it called into question whether the DCEP regimen was required [33].

Bortezomib plus dexamethasone was compared in a prospective randomized fashion to VAD as induction treatment prior to autologous transplantation by the French IFM Trial Collaborative. Bortezomib–dexamethasone produced a higher response rate when measured by CR, VGPR, and overall response rate compared with VAD. The CR rate was 14.8 % vs. 6.4 %, VGPR 37.7 % vs. 15.1 %, and overall response rate 78.5 % vs. 62.8 %. This is independent of International Stage or cytogenetic abnormalities. Hematologic toxicity and deaths related to toxicity were more frequent with VAD. Peripheral neuropathy was significantly higher with bortezomib and dexamethasone. Bortezomib plus dexamethasone improved CR and VGPR rates compared with VAD, and bortezomib plus dexamethasone is considered a standard induction therapy to which all other regimens are compared [34]. A study of bortezomib as induction therapy before transplant followed by lenalidomide as consolidation and maintenance in patients age 65–75 was initiated. After bortezomib-based induction, 58 % had a greater than VGPR or better, including 13 % complete response. After Mel-100, 82 % achieved VGPR or better, 38 % CR emphasizing the ability of transplant to upgrade and deepen the response, even with novel agent induction. Two-year overall survival is 86 %. Bortezomib as induction before autologous transplantation followed by lenalidomide is effective and well-tolerated [35].

In patients with renal insufficiency, the use of novel agents is not straightforward. Lenalidomide requires dose reduction in renal insufficiency, although thalidomide and bortezomib require minimal change. An exploratory study of 31 patients who had a creatinine clearance of <50 (seven on dialysis) was performed. Patients received 4 months of thalidomide-dexamethasone followed by peripheral blood stem cell collection and transplantation. PR or greater was achieved in 74 %, 26 % ≥ VGPR. Renal functional improvement in those achieving a PR was 82 %. Median event-free survival was 30 months. Thalidomide and dexamethasone was active, and it was felt that addition of bortezomib could deepen the responses even further [36].

A randomized trial to compare bortezomib–dexamethasone as induction to a combination of reduced-dose bortezomib and thalidomide plus dexamethasone vtD enrolled 199 patients. After four cycles, the complete response rate was the same in both the VD and the vtD arms, but the VGPR or better rate was significantly higher in the vtD arm (49 % vs. 36 %); and after transplant, increased to 74 % vs. 58 % with VD induction. Moreover, the reduced doses of bortezomib and thalidomide translated into a reduced incidence of peripheral neuropathy from 34 to 14 % in the vtD arm and can be considered a new triple combination before stem cell transplantation [37].

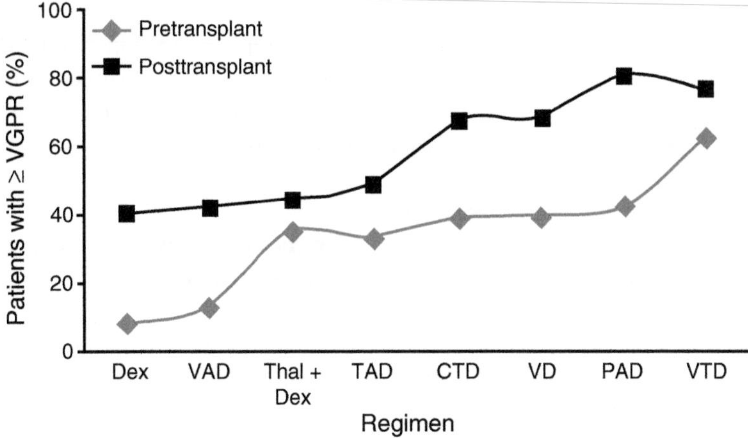

Fig. 10.1 Incremental response to SCT after induction therapy. Incremental response to stem cell transplant after induction therapy. *CTD* cyclophosphamide, thalidomide, dexamethasone; *DEX* dexamethasone; *PAD* bortezomid, Adriamycin, dexamethasone; *TAD* thalidomide, Adriamycin, dexamethasone; *Thal* thalidomide; *VAD* vincristine, Adriamycin, dexamethasone (dex); *VD* bortezomib, dexamethasone; *VGPR* very good partial response; *VTD* bortezomib, thalidomide, dexamethasone

In Great Britain, the use of cyclophosphamide, thalidomide, and dexamethasone as induction therapy was tested in the MRC Myeloma IX trial. Induction randomized transplant-eligible patients to cyclophosphamide, thalidomide, dexamethasone (CTD) vs. cyclophosphamide, vincristine, doxorubicin, and dexamethasone (C-VAD). CTD produced a higher overall response rate (82.5 % vs. 71.2 %), complete response rate (13.0 % vs. 8.1 %), and post-transplant CR (50 % vs. 37.2 %). There was a trend toward a late survival benefit with the CTD arm in responders. A trend toward a survival advantage for CTD was also observed in patients with favorable FISH. CTD produced more constipation and somnolence but a lower incidence of cytopenias. This all-oral regimen is an effective induction therapy for myeloma [38].

In conclusion, the most common regimens currently being used pre-stem cell transplantation are: in Europe, VTD; in Britain, CTD; in France, vtD. Although phase III studies of induction have not been completed in the United States, based on our referral practice, bortezomib and dexamethasone often with cyclophosphamide or lenalidomide as a third agent appear to be the most commonly used induction regimens; however, data regarding the depth of response post-transplant and the relapse-free survival are not yet mature. It does appear, however, that even in the era of novel agents, stem cell transplantation provides additional improvements in depth of response (Fig. 10.1) [39].

Mobilization

The total number of stem cells collectible determines which patients can safely undergo stem cell transplantation. Patients who fail to collect a requisite number of CD34 cells are not candidates for the procedure. In addition to ensuring engraftability, there is evidence that early lymphocyte recovery related to natural killer cells that are collected in the apheresis product actually improves survival in patients with multiple myeloma. Therefore, collecting CD34 cells as well as autologous NK-cells positively affects the recovery of absolute lymphocyte count [40].

Virtually all stem cell products are contaminated by multiple myeloma cells. By polymerase chain reaction (PCR) in one study, 69 % of harvests were contaminated demonstrating an immunoglobulin heavy chain rearrangement. Purging does not remove PCR-positive cells and does not alter response or survival rates [41]. In an EBMT registry study, the risk of relapse after autologous transplantation was not related to the infused tumor cell load, and the outcome did not improve with CD34 selection. CD34 selection can reduce tumor cells by 2.2 logs, but there is no significant difference in 5-year overall and event-free survival between purged and unpurged recipients. In fact, infections appear to be higher in those patients who have purged products. Therefore, attempts to reduce the number of reinfused tumor cells may not alter outcome [42]. Higher doses of CD34 peripheral blood stem cells shorten hematopoietic reconstitution and reduce hospitalization rates. Stable engraftment results from the transplantation of 2 to 3×10^6 CD34 cells/kg. Patients who receive $<3 \times 10^6$ CD34 cells/kg will engraft but do have a longer median time to leukocyte and platelet recovery. As a consequence, we have set our goal at $>3 \times 10^6$ CD34 cells/kg to reduce the transfusion requirement of platelets post-transplantation [43]. In another study, days to engraftment and the proportion of patients who reached blood count thresholds were compared across 3 CD34 cell dose levels (2–4, 4–6, and >6). Using those cutoffs, neutrophil and platelet engraftment times were similar regardless of cell dose [44].

The quality of stem cells does not appear to be an issue as long as the numbers reach predetermined thresholds. When comparing collections of <3, 3–5, and $>5 \times 10^6$ CD34/kg, days to platelet engraftment were significantly lower in patients with a collection of <3, but the quality of the stem cells from low mobilizers was comparable to those from high mobilizers [45].

The use of chemotherapy plus growth factor enhances the yield of stem cells but does not appear to improve outcomes for patients with multiple myeloma, and the concept of in vivo purging is not borne out by reported outcomes. There is no difference in outcomes or engraftment between those patients who receive cyclophosphamide at a dose of 2.4 g/m^2 vs. those who are treated with 7 g/m^2. The lower dose of cyclophosphamide results in excellent yields and significantly lowers utilization of filgrastim [46]. Although cyclophosphamide is the most common chemotherapy-mobilizing agent, other regimens have been attempted to improve on those outcomes. The addition of etoposide to cyclophosphamide resulted in increased toxicity in the etoposide-cyclophosphamide arm without significant improvement in CD34 cell yield or response rates [47].

Effects of Myeloma Therapy on Mobilization

When thalidomide is part of the induction regimen, there is a significant reduction in CD34 cells when compared with a non-thalidomide-containing regimen (9.8 vs. 10.9×10(6), $p=0.02$). However, engraftment after transplantation showed no difference. The number of total CD34 cells, although significantly lower, was sufficient for tandem transplantation [48]. When a regimen of low-dose cyclophosphamide for mobilization (1–2 g/m^2) was compared to intermediate-dose (3–4 g/m^2), the 3–4 g/m^2 cyclophosphamide dose resulted in 88 % success in collecting $>4 \times 10^6$ CD34 cells vs. 65 % in the low-dose cyclophosphamide group. Correlates of collection failure were prior melphalan or >12 months of prior therapy. Cyclophosphamide, 3–4 g/m^2, seems to be an optimal dosage.

Lenalidomide has been shown to reduce the yield of stem cell collection but does not prevent a successful harvest. This reduced yield can be overcome by using cyclophosphamide priming. Sufficient stem cells for two transplants were collected from all patients mobilized with cyclophosphamide 3 g/m^2 plus GCSF vs. 33 % mobilized with filgrastim alone [49]. Mobilization with cyclophosphamide is often required to obtain adequate numbers of stem cells in patients who receive lenalidomide induction therapy [50]. Although cyclophosphamide improves mobilization yields, it does not improve outcome in patients receiving stem cell transplantation. It does not increase overall complete response rates or improve time to progression for patients with myeloma undergoing stem cell transplantation [51].

Cyclophosphamide in doses exceeding 4 g/m^2 is potentially cardiotoxic to transplant patients. Echocardiographic measurements reveal a barely nonsignificant decrease in cardiac output after high-dose cyclophosphamide infusion. The precipitation of heart failure is manifest by an increase in BNP. Careful cardiac monitoring is required when high-dose cyclophosphamide is used in patients with myeloma [52].

Substituting intravenous melphalan for cyclophosphamide in an attempt to improve mobilization has been attempted. This strategy is feasible but frequently requires hospitalization and transfusion and is not widely used with the proposed melphalan dose of 60 mg/m^2. In less-developed nations where expenses are a prime consideration, one can collect stem cells and refrigerate them to allow for conditioning and reinfusion. Without cryopreservation and dimethyl sulfoxide, an apheresis product can be kept in a blood bank refrigerator at 4 °C for 2 days prior to infusion, resulting in an effective and safe method, which simplifies the procedure and does not require liquid nitrogen storage facilities [53].

Growth-Factor Mobilization

Prospective randomized studies looking at split doses of growth factor vs. once-daily administration of growth factor is not associated with superior clinical efficacy and does not have an impact on red cell or platelet requirement or hospitalization duration. Once-daily growth factor suffices [54].

Attempts to simplify the administration of growth factor by using pegylated filgrastim instead of standard filgrastim have been attempted. In fact, pegfilgrastim seems to be a reasonable substitute, with a single dose resulting in adequate mobilization. A comparative study of 6 vs. 12 mg of pegfilgrastim resulted in no benefit, suggesting that 6 mg of pegfilgrastim is sufficient for mobilization in myeloma patients [55]. Using chemotherapy with pegfilgrastim is safe, efficacious, and feasible. Again, 6 mg of pegfilgrastim is sufficient for adequate mobilization [56]. In a randomized phase II study of pegfilgrastim vs. filgrastim for lymphoma and myeloma, pegfilgrastim was found to be safe and effective and was a cost-effective alternative [57].

Plerixafor

The introduction of plerixafor has had a profound effect on the ability to safely mobilize patients with multiple myeloma. Plerixafor allowed successful collection of CD34 cells in 70 % of previously transplanted patients, overcoming the negative effect of poor prognostic factors that predict for poor mobilization [58]. In one study, plerixafor resulted in a median fourfold increase in the number of circulating CD34 cells from baseline. Fourteen of 17 myeloma patients predicted to be poor mobilizers achieved $>2 \times 10^6$ CD34 cells/kg within three apheresis procedures [59]. In a study of 20 patients with myeloma and 1 with light chain amyloidosis that had advanced renal failure, the use of plerixafor successfully mobilized 20 of 21. Five patients had mild to moderate GI symptoms that did not prevent apheresis. Plerixafor was found to be effective in mobilizing stem cells in patients with renal failure [60]. Plerixafor can also overcome the stem cell toxic effects of prior fludarabine and lenalidomide exposure. In fludarabine-exposed patients, 58 % achieve successful salvage mobilization. Salvage mobilization utilizing plerixafor is successful in the majority of patients previously treated with lenalidomide. In lenalidomide-exposed patients, the minimum required numbers of CD34 cells were collected from 69 % of patients in a median of 2 days [61]. The Mayo Clinic suggested protocol used for the collection of stem cells in patients with multiple myeloma is given in Table 10.2.

Stem Cell Transplantation Conditioning

The first regimen to be used for the conditioning of patients for autologous transplantation was melphalan with total body radiation, a regimen that was used because of its efficacy in allogeneic transplantation in multiple myeloma. However, a prospective randomized phase III study established melphalan 200 mg/m^2 (melphalan-200) as the standard of care for conditioning because it

Table 10.2 Mayo algorithm for stem cell mobilization

1. G-CSF 10 μg/kg daily for 4 days (a) If collecting for one transplant: Check CD34 level peripheral blood evening of d4 G-CSF, if <10/μL add plerixafor 240 μg/kg (160 μg/kg if creatinine clearance <50 mL/min); begin collection *d*+5 (b) If collecting for more than one transplant: Check CD34 level peripheral blood evening of d4 G-CSF, if <20/μL add plerixafor as outlined in 1(a)
2. If patient has relapsed or refractory myeloma at completion of induction or circulating plasma cells are detectable in the peripheral blood, give cyclophosphamide 1.5 g/m² for two consecutive days. Initiate G-CSF 10 μg/kg daily on *d*+3. Check CD34 level peripheral blood daily when recovery WBC>1.0. If <10/μL, continue measurement of CD34 for three consecutive days. If after 3 days CD34+ <10/μL begin plerixafor
3. Once apheresis begins: (a) If stem yield apheresis one <1.5×10^6 CD34/kg add plerixafor (b) If yield for apheresis after first falls below 0.5×10^5 CD34/kg add plerixafor (c) If after addition of plerixafor CD34 yield <0.5×10^6 CD34/kg for two consecutive days, collection failure stop mobilization procedure

was less toxic and at least as effective as melphalan 140 with 800 cGy of total body radiation therapy [62]. Thus melphalan-200 is considered the standard conditioning regimen for autologous transplantation in myeloma.

Radiation

Attempts to improve conditioning have involved combinations of chemotherapy and have also used radio-emitting pharmaceuticals in an attempt to improve myeloma cell kill without increasing toxicity. Studies on the use of holmium had to be abandoned because of an unacceptable incidence of thrombotic thrombocytopenic purpura due to radiation damage to the microvasculature of the kidney. Two studies have been published on the use of the radioisotope, samarium, as part of the conditioning regimen combined with melphalan for the treatment of multiple myeloma. Phase I studies have been performed to achieve doses where the target of absorbed radiation to the red marrow was 40 Gy. Using this isotope, no nephrotoxicity, hemorrhagic cystitis, or delayed radiation nephritis was observed as it had been with holmium. Median times to neutrophil and platelet engraftment were 12 and 11 days, respectively, with no graft failures and an overall response rate of 94 % [63]. When this data was updated [64], 59 % of the study patients achieved a VGPR or better with a median overall and progression-free survival from study entry of 6.2 and 1.5 years, respectively. Samarium-melphalan conditioning was safe and well-tolerated and has potential to be combined with novel agents.

In a phase I–II trial, patients with responding multiple myeloma received tandem stem cell transplantations with the first transplant at melphalan-200 and the second involving total marrow irradiation starting at 1,000 cGy. Dose-limiting toxicity was seen at 1,800 cGy. The toxicities included reversible enteritis and lower extremity deep venous thrombosis. At a median of 35 months, progression-free and overall survival for all patients was 49 % and 82 %, respectively. Total marrow radiation as part of tandem autologous stem cell transplantation produced an encouraging complete response rate. Late toxicities need to be reported. The appropriate dose for further trials was 1,600 cGy as the maximum tolerated dose for stem cell transplantation candidates [65].

New techniques to deliver total marrow radiation are currently under active exploration. Total body radiation is associated with significant toxicities, but targeted total body radiation using helical tomotherapy reduces the dose delivered to normal organs. The dose levels of total marrow irradiation in this study were 10, 12, 14, and 16 Gy delivered at 2 Gy daily/twice daily. Toxicities were primarily grade 1–2 and included mucositis, vomiting, fatigue, and diarrhea. Helical tomotherapy for total marrow irradiation is an ongoing therapeutic exploration [66].

Combinations with Melphalan

In a randomized trial, 56 patients were randomly assigned to melphalan-200 or Idarubicin, cyclophosphamide, and melphalan 200 mg/m². Infections were higher in the intensified treatment arm, with a treatment-related mortality of 20 % vs. 0 % with standard melphalan. The study was terminated early with no difference in response rates. Intensified conditioning with this specific triplet had intolerably high toxicity without improved outcomes, demonstrating that more is not necessarily better [67].

A study of patients receiving busulfan-melphalan conditioning with the monitoring of busulfan plasma concentrations was performed in 44 patients. There were four treatment-related deaths, which should be considered unacceptably high. No veno-occlusive disease was seen [68].

A single daily dose of intravenous busulfan and melphalan was used as a conditioning regimen for myeloma patients. Busulfan was given as a single daily dose day −5 through day −3, and melphalan 140 mg/m^2 was given on day −2. There was no veno-occlusive disease. There were two treatment-related deaths (3.6 %); 27 of 49 patients achieved a CR or NCR and 21 a PR. The 1-year overall and progression-free survival rates were 96 % and 87 %, respectively. In this study, busulfan-melphalan was associated with acceptable toxicity [69].

A prospective randomized study of busulfan 12 mg/kg plus melphalan 140 vs. melphalan 200/m^2 has been concluded. Conditioning with busulfan plus melphalan was associated with longer progression-free survival but equivalent survival to that achieved with melphalan-200. There was a higher frequency of veno-occlusive disease-related deaths. This study involved oral busulfan and whether an intravenous formulation would result in greater efficacy is unknown [70].

Carmustine has also been added to melphalan in a phase I–II trial [71]. Dose-limiting toxicity was pulmonary, presumably related to carmustine. Treatment-related mortality was 2 %, considered acceptable. The CR + nCR rate was 49 %. The progression-free and overall survival was 2.3 and 4.7 years, respectively. Carmustine can be combined with high-dose melphalan and produce a high response rate.

A phase I–II dose-finding trial combining bortezomib as part of the conditioning with high-dose melphalan has been reported. Patients were randomized to receive a single escalating dose of bortezomib (1, 1.3, or 1.6 mg/m^2) either 24 h before or 24 h after high-dose melphalan. The overall response rate for all patients was 87 % with 51 % VGPR or better. Pharmacodynamic studies showed greater plasma cell apoptosis among patients who received bortezomib following melphalan. A single dose of bortezomib administered after high-dose melphalan was recommended. Schedules for future clinical investigations are underway [72].

Infusion of mitoxantrone with bolus melphalan as a stem cell transplantation conditioning regimen for myeloma has been explored in a small number of patients. Mitoxantrone was infused on days −6, −5, with melphalan given on day −1. The median overall survival was 5.7 years with 37 % of patients alive >7 years. Myelosuppression and mucositis were the most frequent adverse events [73].

Arsenic trioxide, ascorbic acid, and melphalan have been combined to determine the safety and efficacy of this triplet as a preparative regimen in myeloma patients. Two doses of arsenic trioxide were used (0.15 mg/kg IV for 7 days and 0.25 mg/kg for 7 days). No dose-limiting toxicity, graft failure, or non-relapse mortality was seen through day 100. The CR rate was 25 %. The overall response rate was 85 %. Median progression-free survival was 25 months. No adverse effect of arsenic trioxide on melphalan pharmacokinetics was seen. The addition of arsenic-ascorbic acid to high-dose melphalan was safe and well-tolerated [74]. A phase II trial of high-dose topotecan, melphalan, and cyclophosphamide has been reported. The common adverse events were grade 1–3 mucositis, nausea, and diarrhea. Topotecan, melphalan, and cyclophosphamide were safe and active with an overall response and progression-free survival rate comparable to high-dose melphalan [75]. For allogeneic stem cell transplantation, there has been one retrospective study comparing melphalan TBI with cyclophosphamide TBI [76]. The overall complete remission rate in patients receiving melphalan TBI was greater than that for cyclophosphamide ($p = 0.085$). A higher proportion of patients with active disease at the time of transplant achieved CR with melphalan TBI compared with cyclophosphamide TBI (53 % vs. 33 %, $p = 0.009$). Relapsed and progression rates at 5 years were lower for the melphalan TBI arm compared with cyclophosphamide (36.7 % vs. 81 %). Five-year survival for the melphalan regimen was 44 and 28 % for cyclophosphamide. Melphalan TBI is generally considered the accepted conditioning regimen standard for sibling transplant for myeloma.

Melphalan-200

The studies discussed earlier are all phase II trials, and as discussed earlier, melphalan-200 still remains the standard non-study conditioning regimen for multiple myeloma. Melphalan conditioning, however, is not benign. In a study of 109 myeloma patients receiving melphalan-200, oral mucositis assessments were made through day 30, and severe oral mucositis occurred in 46 % of patients with multiple myeloma with a mean duration of 5.3 days. The time from initiation of conditioning to peak oral mucositis was 12 days and was significantly associated with higher chemotherapy dose per kilogram of body weight and poor performance status. Age was not a factor. This high rate of oral mucositis and subsequent hospitalization necessitates/justifies greater exploration into preventative measures for myeloma transplant patients [77].

Post-transplant Maintenance

Attempts to improve the progression-free survival and overall survival by adding consolidation and maintenance following stem cell transplantation have been ongoing since the onset of transplantation. Initially, attempts at using maintenance cytotoxic chemotherapy following transplantation were attempted. Cytotoxic consolidation chemotherapy given to 75 myeloma patients produced no event-free or overall survival advantage [78]. During the 1990s, α2 interferon given on a 3-times-per-week basis was a very popular post-transplant maintenance therapy for multiple myeloma. However, despite early positive results, a large meta-analysis encompassing over 750 patients in 12 trials showed that the difference in overall survival at 5 years was <3 %, and the use of interferon has largely been abandoned [79]. The tolerability of interferon, because of the flu-like symptoms, arthralgias, and reduced quality of life, impacted significantly.

Thalidomide

A total of seven published studies on the use of maintenance thalidomide after autologous stem cell transplantation have been published. Of the seven published studies, three demonstrated a clinical benefit for those patients and four did not. In an NCI Canada study, a randomized phase II trial showed a median progression-free survival post-transplant of 32.3 months. However, thalidomide was found to be very poorly tolerated; and because it could not be maintained for long periods of time, the ability to demonstrate benefit was limited [80]. In a trial of 668 patients, the 5-year progression-free survival between the thalidomide and non-thalidomide arms were 56 % and 44 %, respectively ($p = 0.01$), but there was no difference in overall survival [81]. Severe peripheral neuropathy and deep vein thrombosis occurred more frequently in the thalidomide group. Thalidomide increased the frequency of complete responses and extended event-free survival. A separate analysis showed that there was a survival advantage in those patients who had abnormal cytogenetics. In the IFM-9902 trial, patients post-transplant were randomized to one of three arms, which was: (1) no maintenance, (2) pamidronate maintenance, and (3) pamidronate and thalidomide maintenance [82]. In this study, both progression-free survival and overall survival favored the thalidomide-containing arm. With longer follow-up, the survival benefit of thalidomide was lost. In a study using maintenance thalidomide at 100 mg per day, 76 % had to discontinue the agent due to poor tolerance. The inability to take thalidomide for long periods of time is a strong disadvantage to its consideration as a maintenance agent because of the high toxicity [83].

In HOVON-50 trial, patients were randomized to maintenance interferon or thalidomide at 50 mg per day [84]. Event-free survival was superior in the thalidomide arm. Overall survival was not different.

Immunotherapy

Immunotherapy has been attempted for post-transplant myeloma patients. Idiotype-pulsed antigen-presenting cells can be prepared using the patient's serum monoclonal protein obtained at diagnosis as idiotype and then administered using autologous dendritic cells that have been presensitized to the monoclonal protein. This vaccine trial was associated with improved overall survival compared to historical controls, but no phase III data exists [85].

Lenalidomide

Two key trials have recently been published looking at lenalidomide maintenance at 10–15 mg per day until relapse. In the IFM-2005-02 study, following a transplant, patients were consolidated with lenalidomide for 2 months and then were randomized to lenalidomide or placebo. In this study, progression-free survival was improved, but overall survival was not. In this study, the possibility of an increased risk of second primary cancers was raised, leading to early termination of the study. Four years after randomization, no overall survival benefit was seen [86]. However, the chemotherapy trials network program and the Cancer and Leukemia Group B (CALGB) randomized patients to 10 mg of lenalidomide or placebo after a single stem cell transplantation. In this study, not only was time to progression improved from 21.9 to 42 months, but overall survival achieved statistical significance. A total of 35 patients who received lenalidomide (15 %) and 53 patients who received placebo (22 %) have died (p=0.03). Second primary cancers were seen in 8 % of lenalidomide patients and 3 % of placebo patients. Lenalidomide maintenance therapy initiated at day 100 was associated with more toxicity but a significantly longer time to disease progression and significantly improved overall survival among patients with myeloma [87].

Bortezomib-Based Combinations

A study of consolidation VTD in autografted myeloma, who had achieved a VGPR after transplant, administered four courses of therapy. Of 39 patients enrolled, the number of immunofixation-defined complete responses increased from 15 to 49 % after VTD. Molecular remissions were identified in 18 %. No patient in molecular response had relapsed with a median follow-up of 42 months. It was estimated that the VTD consolidation reduced the tumor burden by four logs. Persistent molecular response in autologous transplanted myeloma patients can lead to prolonged disease-free survival [88]. In a phase II open-label trial of bortezomib in patients who did not achieve a complete response after autologous stem cell transplantation, 48 evaluable patients were enrolled. Bortezomib monotherapy was feasible, safe, and well-tolerated with 8 % complete responses, 2 % unconfirmed complete responses, and 23 % partial responses [89]. A phase II study investigating prolonged weekly bortezomib and dexamethasone followed by thalidomide and dexamethasone as maintenance has recently been reported. Fifty-three percent achieved a complete response after bortezomib maintenance therapy, upgrading the response from 33 % pre-bortezomib. Prolonged sequential weekly bortezomib–dexamethasone–thalidomide maintenance therapy upgraded CR responses without grade III–IV neuropathy [90]. The administration of bortezomib appears to have value even in patients with unfavorable cytogenetics such as -17p. In one trial where bortezomib was administered before and after stem cell transplantation, the adverse impact of -17p on progression-free and overall survival was significantly reduced. The median progression-free survival in the non-bortezomib arm was 12 vs. 26.2 months in the bortezomib arm, a 3-year overall survival of 17 % vs. 69 % strongly commending the use of bortezomib with unfavorable cytogenetics [91]. In the HOVON-65 trial bortezomib given one dose every 2 weeks for 2 years as maintenance following either single or tandem transplant showed superior progression-free and overall survival compared to a non-bortezomib induction, transplant, and thalidomide maintenance. This trial also showed that bortezomib provided benefit in high-risk patients with del17p13 or creatinine >2 mg/dL [92].

The use of maintenance therapy has been widely adopted in many countries based on the survival advantage associated with lenalidomide. Bortezomib maintenance may also prove to be effective. Whether all subsets of patients benefit from maintenance and whether it should be the standard of care remains uncertain at this time. Finally, quality of life and potential toxicity of maintenance therapy should be taken into consideration for the individual patient.

Tandem Transplantation

Although tandem transplantation has been a standard since the inception of the myeloma transplant program in Little Rock, AR, it was not until 2003 that tandem transplant was shown to improve overall survival among patients with myeloma, particularly those who did not have a VGPR after the first transplant [93]. Although a second transplant did not deepen the response rate of patients, at 7 years, patients failing to achieve a VGPR after the first transplant had survival improved from 11 to 43 %. This study predates the introduction of novel agents but set a standard for which patients should be considered for tandem transplantation. Much of the benefit of second transplant has been attributed to its ability to produce a complete response for those patients who have not achieved a complete response after the first transplant. In the Spanish Myeloma Study Group, 30 % of patients achieved a complete response after first transplant. This was increased after transplant 2 for a final CR rate of 48 %. The complete response data suggested that the second transplant was the most important prognostic factor for overall survival. There was an improved overall and event-free survival for patients receiving a tandem transplant, which was 55 % at 5 years for the tandem group [94].

In a feasibility trial, 214 patients were seen in a group enrolled in a program modeled after Total Therapy 1; 13 % never made it to the first stem cell transplantation due to progression. An additional 16 % did not proceed with the second auto transplant related to complications seen after the first transplant. In other words, a third of patients with newly diagnosed symptomatic myeloma on an intention-to-treat basis never complete tandem transplantation. Those that do are, therefore, a selected group [95]. An IFM study of tandem transplant where the second transplant was conditioned with Mel-220 plus dexamethasone led to a median overall and event-free survival of 41 and 30 months, respectively. This was a selected patient population considered high-risk by virtue of high β2 microglobulin levels and metaphase chromosome 13 deletion [96]. Total Therapy 1 were the first trials exploring tandem transplantation; and in a report with a median follow-up of 12 years, survival was 17 % at 15 years and 7 % event-free survival at 15 years. Predictors of long-term survival were normal metaphase cytogenetics, normal LDH, and ability to complete the second transplant. The 10-year event-free and overall survivals were 15 % and 33 %, respectively, in this era prior to novel agent induction [97].

The Bologna-96 trial was a prospective randomized study of second compared with double autologous stem cell transplantation. In this trial, double stem cell transplantation produced a superior complete response rate, relapse-free survival, and event-free survival but did not prolong overall survival. The benefit offered by second stem cell transplantation was seen in patients who failed to achieve a near-complete response after the first auto transplant [98]. This prospective randomized study did not validate the concept of a second transplant in tandem since it did not prolong overall survival. In another feasibility study of tandem transplants in patients under the age of 65, the number of complete responses was 29 % after two transplants. The incremental response rate following the second transplant did not produce an advantage in event-free or overall survival. On an intention to treat basis, the first transplant was completed in 80 % of patients, but only 42 % received a second transplant. Inadequate numbers of stem cells, transplant-related toxicity of the first transplant, and early progression were all reasons why a second transplant could not be performed [99]. A feasibility study from Japan started with 40 patients, but only 28 completed the second transplant. The complete response rate was 28 %. The 5-year progression-free and overall survivals were 20.3 % and 66.5 %, respectively [100]. An attempt to improve on these outcomes resulted in an exploratory trial where the first transplant was actually submyeloablative; and then 6 months later, the patients received Mel-200. The median interval between the two transplant procedures was 239 days. Subsequent to the first transplant (Mel-100), 48 % achieved a complete response, 33 % a VGPR. The 1,000-day overall survival was 73 %. Mel-100 was tolerated in the outpatient setting [101]. In a review of the five trials comparing single vs. double transplant, an improved progression-free survival was seen in three of the five. Overall survival was significantly prolonged in only one, limited to those patients failing to achieve a VGPR [102]. In a meta-analysis of tandem vs. single autologous stem cell transplantation, the use of tandem transplant did not result in improved overall or event-free survival. The tandem transplant was associated with improved response rates but at a risk of a significant increase in treatment-related mortality. This protocol reviewed six randomized trials enrolling over 1,800 patients. The statistically significant increase in treatment-related mortality had a risk ratio of 1.71 [103].

A second transplant need not always be performed in tandem. Second transplants can be done at the time of progression and as such become a useful salvage strategy. In a group of 32 patients with relapsing multiple myeloma after a first auto transplant, a second salvage transplant was performed. The responses were: longer in 7, the same in 16, and shorter in 9. The second transplant resulted in a treatment-related mortality of 3 %. Median event-free survival after the first transplant was 15.7 months and was 12.9 months after the second transplant with a median overall survival of 79.1 months, again suggesting that a second auto stem cell transplantation can be considered a useful salvage tool [104]. Recently, the Princess Margaret Hospital reported on the role of a second autologous stem cell transplantation as salvage in 81 patients. The median time to progression after the second stem cell transplantation was 19 months. Treatment-related mortality was 2.6 %. The median overall survival following transplant was 28.5 months. The best outcome was observed in patients whose time to progression was >24 months after the first stem cell transplantation, as these patients had a progression-free survival of >1 year and an overall survival of 6 years [105]. Potential disadvantages of saving a second transplant for salvage at the time of relapse have been reported. Twenty-five consecutive patients who received a second transplant for relapsed disease were seen to experience more nephrotoxicity, delayed platelet engraftment, and an 8 % treatment-related mortality [106].

Both autologous and allogeneic stem cell transplantation have been used for salvage. When salvage auto and allotransplant were compared at MD Anderson Cancer Center, no difference in progression-free survival (6.8 vs. 7.3 months) or overall survival (29 vs. 13 months) was seen. The best predictor of overall survival was >1 year between the first and the salvage transplant. A relapse remained the major problem even for those patients receiving auto transplants [107]. In summary, tandem auto stem cell transplantation has only been demonstrated to improve survival in one study. A meta-analysis does not show benefit. However, collecting sufficient stem cells for two transplants is prudent. A second transplant at the time of progression (if the response to the first transplant was over 1 year) is a reasonable approach to management.

Allogeneic Stem Cell Transplantation

Allogeneic transplantation is discussed in detail in a separate chapter. A brief discussion is provided below to distinguish the benefits and risks compared with autologous transplantation.

The ability of allogeneic-reactive T-cells to cure multiple myeloma remains an ongoing question. The IFM-9903 trial compared autologous stem cell transplantation followed by a dose-reduced allograft with a tandem autologous transplant. Accrual was limited to patients defined as being high risk, which in that era was a β2 microglobulin level >3 mg/L and metaphase chromosome 13 deletion at diagnosis. Induction was vincristine-doxorubicin-dexamethasone, and randomization was biologic based on donor availability. On an intent-to-treat basis, overall and event-free survival was not different. The event-free survival of 166 patients receiving tandem autologous transplantation was similar to the event-free survival of the 46 patients who underwent allogeneic transplantation (35 vs. 31.7 months). Overall survival in the tandem transplant group was 47.2 vs. 35 months in the allogeneic transplant group ($p=0.07$). Allogeneic transplant did not add benefit [108].

The only reported positive trial indicating improved survival was reported by Bruno et al. In this trial of patients with newly diagnosed myeloma, the survival in recipients of an autograft followed by an HLA-identical sibling allograft was superior to those who received tandem stem cell transplantations with 80 vs. 54 months overall and 35 vs. 29 months relapse-free survival (both $p<0.05$) [109]. This trial launched a number of subsequent trials trying to confirm the survival advantage of an allogeneic transplant. A review from the European Myeloma Transplant Database for patients transplanted between 1994 and 2003 was performed in an attempt to determine the optimal source of stem cells for allografting. Peripheral blood stem cells have faster engraftment and more frequent chronic graft-versus-host, but overall survival and progression-free survival were similar to using bone marrow as the source. There was a lower response rate and a higher relapse rate for reduced-intensity conditioned transplants compared to myeloablative transplants [110]. When data was updated between 1998 and 2002, looking at 320 reduced-intensity grafts and 196 myeloablative grafts, non-relapse mortality was significantly lower for reduced-intensity conditioning, but overall survival was not significantly different. Reduced-intensity conditioning reduces non-relapse mortality, but it is offset by an increase in relapse risk. Therefore, it did not impact overall survival [111].

A review of 158 patients who had stem cell transplants (72 myeloablative, 86 autologous) showed the overall survival at 5 years in the allogeneic stem cell transplantation cohort was 48 % compared to 46 % in the autologous cohort. The 10-year survival was, likewise, not significantly different between the two groups. Risk of relapse was reduced in those patients who had acute graft-versus-host disease [112]. There have been attempts to reduce the chronic graft-versus-host disease risk by T-cell depleting the graft and then post-transplant add back of allogeneic-reactive T-cells. This technique requires further evaluation. Donor lymphocyte infusion has been used in Europe predominantly in an effort to manage relapsed disease [113]. A Spanish study of tandem autologous transplant vs. autograft followed by reduced-intensity allotransplant showed a higher complete response rate and a trend that did not achieve statistical significance for progression-free survival in favor of the auto-allo arm. However, transplant-related mortality was 16 % compared to 5 % with auto, and 66 % of patients at risk developed chronic graft-versus-host disease. There was no statistical difference in event-free and overall survival [114]. The Bruno trial comparing tandem auto with auto and reduced-intensity conditioning allogeneic was updated; and with a median follow-up of 5 years, complete remission was achieved in 53 % of the patients receiving allografting. Chronic graft-versus-host disease was not correlated with complete response or response duration [115].

A long-term follow-up of allogeneic transplant results in Seattle was performed on 102 myeloma patients with a median follow-up of 6.3 years. Seventy-four percent developed extensive chronic graft-versus-host disease. Five-year non-relapse mortality was 18 %. Among 95 patients with measurable disease, 59 achieved a complete remission. Median progression-free survival was 3 years. Five-year overall survival was 64 %. In a multivariate analysis, β2 microglobulin and delaying the allogeneic transplant to more than 10 months after the start of treatment correlated with shorter overall and progression-free survival [116]. Reduced-intensity conditioning allogeneic transplant results from MD Anderson was reported in 51 patients. Cumulative treatment-related mortality at 1 year was 25 %. The overall survival at 2 years was 32 % in a heavily pre-treated relapsed refractory group of patients. Fourteen percent of patients were in remission 6 years after allogeneic transplant. A fraction of patients can achieve durable remission when transplanted in relapse [117].

The German Myeloma Transplant Study Group reported an intensified myeloablative conditioning regimen with in vivo T-cell depletion using anti-thymocyte globulin followed by allografting. Treatment-related mortality was 17 %. A complete response was seen in 53 %. The median overall survival was estimated at 12 years with an event-free survival of 35 % at 10 years. Only patients who achieved a complete response achieved long-term disease-free survival [118]. The same group published results of allogeneic transplant using an unrelated donor after relapse following autologous transplantation. The incidence of relapse at 3 years was 55 %. The estimated 5-year progression-free and overall survival were 20 % and 26 %, respectively, suggesting that transplant after relapse using a matched unrelated donor is not expected to produce long-term benefit.

In a consensus statement by the International Myeloma Working Group, it was felt that convincing evidence was lacking that reduced-intensity transplantation improved survival compared with autologous transplantation and that reduced-intensity transplantation in myeloma should only be performed in the context of clinical trials [119]. Another long-term follow-up study of tandem autologous transplant vs. reduced-intensity allogeneic transplant reported a progression-free survival at 60 months, auto-allo vs. auto-auto at 35 % and 18 %, respectively. However, overall survival at 60 months was 65 % vs. 58 %. Non-relapse mortality at 24 months was 12 % in the auto-allo vs. 3 % in the auto-auto cohort. Graft-versus-host disease was seen acutely in 20 % and chronic graft-versus-host disease in 31 % [120].

A seminal study by the Chemotherapy Trials Network has recently been published; 710 patients of whom 625 had standard-risk disease received an autologous transplant; 156 of 189 patients with standard-risk disease in the auto-allo group and 366 of 436 of the auto-auto group went on to receive a second transplant. There was also an assignment to observation-vs.-maintenance therapy. Maintenance and no maintenance did not impact progression-free and overall survival. Three-year progression-free survival estimates were 43 and 46 % in the auto-allo and auto-auto group, respectively. Overall survival at 3 years was 77 % vs. 80 % (not significant). This important study showed that non-myeloablative allogeneic stem cell transplantation after an auto stem cell transplantation was not more effective than a tandem autologous transplant for standard-risk myeloma [121]. One important stratification factor is that patients receiving an allotransplant have the same outcome whether they lack or possess unfavorable cytogenetic features such as t(4;14) or deletion 17p. This suggests allotransplant overcomes unfavorable genetic features that lead to unfavorable outcomes in patients receiving conventional chemotherapy or auto stem cell transplantation. Therefore, the possibility that allogeneic stem cell transplantation could improve outcomes in patients with high-risk cytogenetics should be considered [122]. A statistical analysis of 148 patients demonstrated that a longer progression-free survival was seen when allotransplant was used for remission consolidation, and high-risk cytogenetics only affected progression-free survival and not overall survival [123].

A comparison of outcomes between related and unrelated donors showed no difference in acute graft-versus-host disease, chronic graft-versus-host disease, treatment-related mortality, and progression-free survival [124].

In conclusion, with the exception of the study by Bruno et al., no survival benefit has been demonstrated for allogeneic transplant. A small subset of patients has prolonged disease-free survival, suggesting a significant graft-versus-myeloma effect exists but is not as strong as that seen with chronic myelogenous or acute leukemia. A patient population that would derive benefit still has yet to be defined [125]. Consistent findings are that a lower relapse rate in patients who are receiving allotransplant is offset by non-relapse mortality associated with chronic graft-versus-host disease, eliminating any survival benefit. When transplantation is performed, outcomes are better when done earlier and while chemosensitivity is maintained. It is unclear that high-risk genetics have an unfavorable effect. Graft-versus-host disease reduces relapse rates [126].

References

1. Matsui W, Borrello I, Mitsiades C. Autologous stem cell transplantation and multiple myeloma cancer stem cells. Biol Blood Marrow Transplant. 2012;18:S27–32.
2. Child JA, Morgan GJ, Davies FE, et al. High-dose chemotherapy with hematopoietic stem-cell rescue for multiple myeloma. N Engl J Med. 2003;348: 1875–83.
3. Levy V, Katsahian S, Fermand JP, Mary JY, Chevret S. A meta-analysis on data from 575 patients with multiple myeloma randomly assigned to either high-dose therapy or conventional therapy. Medicine. 2005;84:250–60.
4. Ferrara F, Palmieri S, Viola A, et al. Outpatient-based peripheral blood stem cell transplantation for patients with multiple myeloma. Hematol J. 2004;5: 222–6.
5. Anderson KO, Giralt SA, Mendoza TR, et al. Symptom burden in patients undergoing autologous stem-cell transplantation. Bone Marrow Transplant. 2007;39:759–66.
6. Knudsen LM, Nielsen B, Gimsing P, Geisler C. Autologous stem cell transplantation in multiple myeloma: outcome in patients with renal failure. Eur J Haematol. 2005;75:27–33.
7. Bird JM, Fuge R, Sirohi B, et al. The clinical outcome and toxicity of high-dose chemotherapy and autologous stem cell transplantation in patients with myeloma or amyloid and severe renal impairment: a British Society of Blood and Marrow Transplantation study. Br J Haematol. 2006;134:385–90.
8. Raab MS, Breitkreutz I, Hundemer M, et al. The outcome of autologous stem cell transplantation in patients with plasma cell disorders and dialysis-dependent renal failure. Haematologica. 2006;91: 1555–8.
9. Parikh GC, Amjad AI, Saliba RM, et al. Autologous hematopoietic stem cell transplantation may reverse renal failure in patients with multiple myeloma. Biol Blood Marrow Transplant. 2009;15:812–6.
10. Qazilbash MH, Saliba RM, Hosing C, et al. Autologous stem cell transplantation is safe and feasible in elderly patients with multiple myeloma. Bone Marrow Transplant. 2007;39:279–83.
11. Offidani M, Leoni P, Corvatta L, et al. ThaDD plus high dose therapy and autologous stem cell transplantation does not appear superior to ThaDD plus maintenance in elderly patients with de novo multiple myeloma. Eur J Haematol. 2010;84:474–83.
12. Kumar S, Perez WS, Zhang M-J, et al. Comparable outcomes in nonsecretory and secretory multiple myeloma after autologous stem cell transplantation. Biol Blood Marrow Transplant. 2008;14:1134–40.
13. Kumar SK, Dingli D, Lacy MQ, et al. Outcome after autologous stem cell transplantation for multiple myeloma in patients with preceding plasma cell disorders. Br J Haematol. 2008;141:205–11.
14. Nadal E, Gine E, Blade J, et al. High-dose therapy/ autologous stem cell transplantation in patients with chemosensitive multiple myeloma: predictors of complete remission. Bone Marrow Transplant. 2004;33:61–4.
15. Haessler J, Shaughnessy Jr JD, Zhan F, et al. Benefit of complete response in multiple myeloma limited to high-risk subgroup identified by gene expression profiling. Clin Cancer Res. 2007;13:7073–9.
16. Lahuerta JJ, Mateos MV, Martinez-Lopez J, et al. Influence of pre- and post-transplantation responses on outcome of patients with multiple myeloma: sequential improvement of response and achievement of complete response are associated with longer survival. J Clin Oncol. 2008;26:5775–82.
17. Harousseau J-L, Attal M, Avet-Loiseau H. The role of complete response in multiple myeloma. Blood. 2009;114:3139–46.
18. Kim JS, Kim K, Cheong J-W, et al. Complete remission status before autologous stem cell transplantation is an important prognostic factor in patients with multiple myeloma undergoing upfront single autologous transplantation. Biol Blood Marrow Transplant. 2009;15:463–70.
19. Kumar SK, Lacy MQ, Dispenzieri A, et al. Early versus delayed autologous transplantation after immunomodulatory agents-based induction therapy in patients with newly diagnosed multiple myeloma. Cancer. 2012;118:1585–92.
20. Bergsagel PL. Individualizing therapy using molecular markers in multiple myeloma. Clin Lymphoma Myeloma. 2007;7 Suppl 4:S170–4.
21. Shaughnessy Jr JD, Barlogie B. Using genomics to identify high-risk myeloma after autologous stem cell transplantation. Biol Blood Marrow Transplant. 2006;12:77–80.
22. Kumar SK, Dingli D, Dispenzieri A, et al. Impact of pretransplant therapy in patients with newly diagnosed myeloma undergoing autologous SCT. Bone Marrow Transplant. 2008;41:1013–9.
23. Korthals M, Sehnke N, Kronenwett R, et al. The level of minimal residual disease in the bone marrow of patients with multiple myeloma before high-dose

therapy and autologous blood stem cell transplantation is an independent predictive parameter. Biol Blood Marrow Transplant. 2012;18:423–31.

24. Cavo M, Zamagni E, Tosi P, et al. Superiority of thalidomide and dexamethasone over vincristine-doxorubicindexamethasone (VAD) as primary therapy in preparation for autologous transplantation for multiple myeloma. Blood. 2005;106:35–9.
25. Palumbo A, Avonto I, Bruno B, et al. Intermediate-dose melphalan (100 mg/m^2)/bortezomib/thalidomide/dexamethasone and stem cell support in patients with refractory or relapsed myeloma. Clin Lymphoma Myeloma. 2006;6:475–7.
26. Rosinol L, Oriol A, Mateos MV, et al. Phase II PETHEMA trial of alternating bortezomib and dexamethasone as induction regimen before autologous stem-cell transplantation in younger patients with multiple myeloma: efficacy and clinical implications of tumor response kinetics. J Clin Oncol. 2007;25: 4452–8.
27. Oakervee H, Popat R, Cavenagh JD. Use of bortezomib as induction therapy prior to stem cell transplantation in frontline treatment of multiple myeloma: impact on stem cell harvesting and engraftment. Leuk Lymphoma. 2007;48:1910–21.
28. Mellqvist U-H, Lenhoff S, Johnsen HE, et al. Cyclophosphamide plus dexamethasone is an efficient initial treatment before high-dose melphalan and autologous stem cell transplantation in patients with newly diagnosed multiple myeloma: results of a randomized comparison with vincristine, doxorubicin, and dexamethasone. Cancer. 2008;112:129–35.
29. Uy GL, Goyal SD, Fisher NM, et al. Bortezomib administered pre-auto-SCT and as maintenance therapy post transplant for multiple myeloma: a single institution phase II study. Bone Marrow Transplant. 2009;43:793–800.
30. Cavo M, Di Raimondo F, Zamagni E, et al. Short-term thalidomide incorporated into double autologous stem-cell transplantation improves outcomes in comparison with double autotransplantation for multiple myeloma. J Clin Oncol. 2009;27:5001–7.
31. Cavo M, Tacchetti P, Patriarca F, et al. Bortezomib with thalidomide plus dexamethasone compared with thalidomide plus dexamethasone as induction therapy before, and consolidation therapy after, double autologous stem-cell transplantation in newly diagnosed multiple myeloma: a randomised phase 3 study. Lancet. 2010;376:2075–85.
32. Chim CS, Lie AKW, Chan EYT, et al. A staged approach with vincristine, adriamycin, and dexamethasone followed by bortezomib, thalidomide, and dexamethasone before autologous hematopoietic stem cell transplantation in the treatment of newly diagnosed multiple myeloma. Ann Hematol. 2010;89:1019–27.
33. Corso A, Barbarano L, Mangiacavalli S, et al. Bortezomib plus dexamethasone can improve stem cell collection and overcome the need for additional chemotherapy before autologous transplant in patients with myeloma. Leuk Lymphoma. 2010;51: 236–42.
34. Harousseau J-L, Attal M, Avet-Loiseau H, et al. Bortezomib plus dexamethasone is superior to vincristine plus doxorubicin plus dexamethasone as induction treatment prior to autologous stem-cell transplantation in newly diagnosed multiple myeloma: results of the IFM 2005–01 phase III trial. J Clin Oncol. 2010;28:4621–9.
35. Palumbo A, Gay F, Falco P, et al. Bortezomib as induction before autologous transplantation, followed by lenalidomide as consolidation-maintenance in untreated multiple myeloma patients. [Erratum appears in J Clin Oncol. 2010 May 1;28(13):2314]. J Clin Oncol. 2010;28:800–7.
36. Tosi P, Zamagni E, Tacchetti P, et al. Thalidomide-dexamethasone as induction therapy before autologous stem cell transplantation in patients with newly diagnosed multiple myeloma and renal insufficiency. Biol Blood Marrow Transplant. 2010;16:1115–21.
37. Moreau P, Avet-Loiseau H, Facon T, et al. Bortezomib plus dexamethasone versus reduced-dose bortezomib, thalidomide plus dexamethasone as induction treatment before autologous stem cell transplantation in newly diagnosed multiple myeloma. Blood. 2011;118:5752–8. quiz 5982.
38. Morgan GJ, Davies FE, Gregory WM, et al. Cyclophosphamide, thalidomide, and dexamethasone as induction therapy for newly diagnosed multiple myeloma patients destined for autologous stem-cell transplantation: MRC Myeloma IX randomized trial results. Haematologica. 2012;97: 442–50.
39. Kumar SK, Mikhael JR, Buadi FK, et al. Management of newly diagnosed symptomatic multiple myeloma: updated Mayo Stratification of Myeloma and Risk-Adapted Therapy (mSMART) consensus guidelines. Mayo Clin Proc. 2009;84(12):1095–110.
40. Porrata LF, Gastineau DA, Padley D, Bundy K, Markovic SN. Re-infused autologous graft natural killer cells correlates with absolute lymphocyte count recovery after autologous stem cell transplantation. Leuk Lymphoma. 2003;44:997–1000.
41. Galimberti S, Morabito F, Guerrini F, et al. Peripheral blood stem cell contamination evaluated by a highly sensitive molecular method fails to predict outcome of autotransplanted multiple myeloma patients. Br J Haematol. 2003;120:405–12.
42. Bourhis J-H, Bouko Y, Koscielny S, et al. Relapse risk after autologous transplantation in patients with newly diagnosed myeloma is not related with infused tumor cell load and the outcome is not improved by CD34+ cell selection: long term follow-up of an EBMT phase III randomized study. Haematologica. 2007;92:1083–90.
43. Klaus J, Herrmann D, Breitkreutz I, et al. Effect of CD34 cell dose on hematopoietic reconstitution and outcome in 508 patients with multiple myeloma undergoing autologous peripheral blood stem cell transplantation. Eur J Haematol. 2007;78:21–8.

44. Stiff PJ, Micallef I, Nademanee AP, et al. Transplanted CD34(+) cell dose is associated with long-term platelet count recovery following autologous peripheral blood stem cell transplant in patients with non-Hodgkin lymphoma or multiple myeloma. Biol Blood Marrow Transplant. 2011;17:1146–53.
45. Jiang L, Malik S, Litzow M, et al. Hematopoietic stem cells from poor and good mobilizers are qualitatively equivalent. Transfusion. 2012;52:542–8.
46. Petrucci MT, Avvisati G, La Verde G, et al. Intermediate-dose cyclophosphamide and granulocyte colony-stimulating factor is a valid alternative to high-dose cyclophosphamide for mobilizing peripheral blood CD34+ cells in patients with multiple myeloma. Acta Haematol. 2003;109:184–8.
47. Gojo I, Guo C, Sarkodee-Adoo C, et al. High-dose cyclophosphamide with or without etoposide for mobilization of peripheral blood progenitor cells in patients with multiple myeloma: efficacy and toxicity. Bone Marrow Transplant. 2004;34:69–76.
48. Breitkreutz I, Lokhorst HM, Raab MS, et al. Thalidomide in newly diagnosed multiple myeloma: influence of thalidomide treatment on peripheral blood stem cell collection yield. Leukemia. 2007;21:1294–9.
49. Mark T, Stern J, Furst JR, et al. Stem cell mobilization with cyclophosphamide overcomes the suppressive effect of lenalidomide therapy on stem cell collection in multiple myeloma. Biol Blood Marrow Transplant. 2008;14:795–8.
50. Nazha A, Cook R, Vogl DT, et al. Stem cell collection in patients with multiple myeloma: impact of induction therapy and mobilization regimen. Bone Marrow Transplant. 2011;46:59–63.
51. Dingli D, Nowakowski GS, Dispenzieri A, et al. Cyclophosphamide mobilization does not improve outcome in patients receiving stem cell transplantation for multiple myeloma. Clin Lymphoma Myeloma. 2006;6:384–8.
52. Zver S, Zadnik V, Bunc M, Rogel P, Cernelc P, Kozelj M. Cardiac toxicity of high-dose cyclophosphamide in patients with multiple myeloma undergoing autologous hematopoietic stem cell transplantation. Int J Hematol. 2007;85:408–14.
53. Ramzi M, Zakerinia M, Nourani H, Dehghani M, Vojdani R, Haghighinejad H. Non-cryopreserved hematopoietic stem cell transplantation in multiple myeloma, a single center experience. Clin Transplant. 2012;26:117–22.
54. Jang G, Ko OB, Kim S, Lee DH, Huh J, Suh C. Prospective randomized comparative observation of single- versus split-dose lenograstim to enhance engraftment after autologous stem cell transplantation in patients with multiple myeloma or non-Hodgkin's lymphoma. Transfusion. 2008;48(4):640–6.
55. Bruns I, Steidl U, Kronenwett R, et al. A single dose of 6 or 12 mg of pegfilgrastim for peripheral blood progenitor cell mobilization results in similar yields of CD34+ progenitors in patients with multiple myeloma. Transfusion. 2006;46:180–5.
56. Kroschinsky F, Holig K, Platzbecker U, et al. Efficacy of single-dose pegfilgrastim after chemotherapy for the mobilization of autologous peripheral blood stem cells in patients with malignant lymphoma or multiple myeloma. Transfusion. 2006;46:1417–23.
57. Sebban C, Lefranc A, Perrier L, et al. A randomised phase II study of the efficacy, safety and cost-effectiveness of pegfilgrastim and filgrastim after autologous stem cell transplant for lymphoma and myeloma (PALM study). Eur J Cancer. 2012;48:713–20.
58. Basak GW, Jaksic O, Koristek Z, et al. Haematopoietic stem cell mobilization with plerixafor and G-CSF in patients with multiple myeloma transplanted with autologous stem cells. Eur J Haematol. 2011;86:488–95.
59. Attolico I, Pavone V, Ostuni A, et al. Plerixafor added to chemotherapy plus G-CSF is safe and allows adequate PBSC collection in predicted poor mobilizer patients with multiple myeloma or lymphoma. Biol Blood Marrow Transplant. 2012;18:241–9.
60. Douglas KW, Parker AN, Hayden PJ, et al. Plerixafor for PBSC mobilisation in myeloma patients with advanced renal failure: safety and efficacy data in a series of 21 patients from Europe and the USA. Bone Marrow Transplant. 2012;47:18–23.
61. Malard F, Kroger N, Gabriel IH, et al. Plerixafor for autologous peripheral blood stem cell mobilization in patients previously treated with fludarabine or lenalidomide. Biol Blood Marrow Transplant. 2012;18:314–7.
62. Moreau P, Facon T, Attal M, et al. Comparison of 200 mg/m(2) melphalan and 8 Gy total body irradiation plus 140 mg/m(2) melphalan as conditioning regimens for peripheral blood stem cell transplantation in patients with newly diagnosed multiple myeloma: final analysis of the Intergroupe Francophone du Myelome 9502 randomized trial. Blood. 2002;99:731–5.
63. Dispenzieri A, Wiseman GA, Lacy MQ, et al. A phase I study of 153Sm-EDTMP with fixed high-dose melphalan as a peripheral blood stem cell conditioning regimen in patients with multiple myeloma. Leukemia. 2005;19:118–25.
64. Dispenzieri A, Wiseman GA, Lacy MQ, et al. A phase II study of (153)Sm-EDTMP and high-dose melphalan as a peripheral blood stem cell conditioning regimen in patients with multiple myeloma. Am J Hematol. 2010;85:409–13.
65. Somlo G, Spielberger R, Frankel P, et al. Total marrow irradiation: a new ablative regimen as part of tandem autologous stem cell transplantation for patients with multiple myeloma. Clin Cancer Res. 2011;17:174–82.
66. Wong JYC, Rosenthal J, Liu A, Schultheiss T, Forman S, Somlo G. Image-guided total-marrow irradiation using helical tomotherapy in patients with multiple myeloma and acute leukemia undergoing hematopoietic cell transplantation. Int J Radiat Oncol Biol Phys. 2009;73:273–9.

67. Fenk R, Schneider P, Kropff M, et al. High-dose idarubicin, cyclophosphamide and melphalan as conditioning for autologous stem cell transplantation increases treatment-related mortality in patients with multiple myeloma: results of a randomised study. Br J Haematol. 2005;130:588–94.
68. Clopes A, Sureda A, Sierra J, et al. Absence of veno-occlusive disease in a cohort of multiple myeloma patients undergoing autologous stem cell transplantation with targeted busulfan dosage. Eur J Haematol. 2006;77:1–6.
69. Blanes M, de la Rubia J, Lahuerta JJ, et al. Single daily dose of intravenous busulfan and melphalan as a conditioning regimen for patients with multiple myeloma undergoing autologous stem cell transplantation: a phase II trial. Leuk Lymphoma. 2009;50:216–22.
70. Lahuerta JJ, Mateos MV, Martinez-Lopez J, et al. Busulfan 12 mg/kg plus melphalan 140 mg/m^2 versus melphalan 200 mg/m^2 as conditioning regimens for autologous transplantation in newly diagnosed multiple myeloma patients included in the PETHEMA/GEM2000 study. Haematologica. 2010;95:1913–20.
71. Comenzo RL, Hassoun H, Kewalramani T, et al. Results of a phase I/II trial adding carmustine (300 mg/m^2) to melphalan (200 mg/m^2) in multiple myeloma patients undergoing autologous stem cell transplantation. Leukemia. 2005;20:345–9.
72. Lonial S, Kaufman J, Tighiouart M, et al. A phase I/II trial combining high-dose melphalan and autologous transplant with bortezomib for multiple myeloma: a dose- and schedule-finding study. Clin Cancer Res. 2010;16:5079–86.
73. Beaven AW, Moore DT, Sharf A, Serody JS, Shea TC, Gabriel DA. Infusional mitoxantrone plus bolus melphalan as a stem cell transplant conditioning regimen for multiple myeloma. Cancer Invest. 2011;29:214–9.
74. Qazilbash MH, Saliba RM, Nieto Y, et al. Arsenic trioxide with ascorbic acid and high-dose melphalan: results of a phase II randomized trial. Biol Blood Marrow Transplant. 2008;14:1401–7.
75. Kazmi SMA, Saliba RM, Donato M, et al. Phase II trial of high-dose topotecan, melphalan and CY with autologous stem cell support for multiple myeloma. Bone Marrow Transplant. 2011;46:510–5.
76. Hunter HM, Peggs K, Powles R, et al. Analysis of outcome following allogeneic haemopoietic stem cell transplantation for myeloma using myeloablative conditioning—evidence for a superior outcome using melphalan combined with total body irradiation. Br J Haematol. 2005;128:496–502.
77. Blijlevens N, Schwenkglenks M, Bacon P, et al. Prospective oral mucositis audit: oral mucositis in patients receiving high-dose melphalan or BEAM conditioning chemotherapy—European Blood and Marrow Transplantation Mucositis Advisory Group. J Clin Oncol. 2008;26:1519–25.
78. Fassas ABT, Spencer T, Desikan R, et al. Cytotoxic chemotherapy following tandem autotransplants in multiple myeloma patients. Br J Haematol. 2002; 119:164–8.
79. The Myeloma Trialists' Collaborative Group. Interferon as therapy for multiple myeloma: an individual patient data overview of 24 randomized trials and 4012 patients. Br J Haematol. 2001;113:1020–34.
80. Stewart AK, Chen CI, Howson-Jan K, et al. Results of a multicenter randomized phase II trial of thalidomide and prednisone maintenance therapy for multiple myeloma after autologous stem cell transplant. Clin Cancer Res. 2004;10:8170–6.
81. Barlogie B, Tricot G, Anaissie E, et al. Thalidomide and hematopoietic-cell transplantation for multiple myeloma. N Engl J Med. 2006;354:1021–30.
82. Attal M, Harousseau J-L, Leyvraz S, et al. Maintenance therapy with thalidomide improves survival in patients with multiple myeloma. Blood. 2006;108:3289–94.
83. Martino M, Console G, Callea V, et al. Low tolerance and high toxicity of thalidomide as maintenance therapy after double autologous stem cell transplant in multiple myeloma patients. Eur J Haematol. 2007;78:35–40.
84. Lokhorst H, van der Holt B, Zweegman S, et al. A randomized phase 3 study on the effect of thalidomide combined with adriamycin, dexamethasone, and high-dose melphalan, followed by thalidomide maintenance in patients with multiple myeloma. Blood. 2010;115:1113–20.
85. Lacy MQ, Mandrekar S, Dispenzieri A, et al. Idiotype-pulsed antigen-presenting cells following autologous transplantation for multiple myeloma may be associated with prolonged survival. Am J Hematol. 2009;84:799–802 [Erratum appears in Am J Hematol. 2010 Apr;85(4):309].
86. Attal M, Lauwers-Cances V, Marit G, et al. Lenalidomide maintenance after stem-cell transplantation for multiple myeloma. N Engl J Med. 2012;366:1782–91.
87. McCarthy PL, Owzar K, Hofmeister CC, et al. Lenalidomide after stem-cell transplantation for multiple myeloma. N Engl J Med. 2012;366:1770–81.
88. Ladetto M, Pagliano G, Ferrero S, et al. Major tumor shrinking and persistent molecular remissions after consolidation with bortezomib, thalidomide, and dexamethasone in patients with autografted myeloma. J Clin Oncol. 2010;28:2077–84.
89. Rifkin RM, Greenspan A, Schwerkoske JF, et al. A phase II open-label trial of bortezomib in patients with multiple myeloma who have undergone an autologous peripheral blood stem cell transplant and failed to achieve a complete response. Invest New Drugs. 2012;30:714–22.
90. Sahebi F, Frankel PH, Farol L, et al. Sequential bortezomib, dexamethasone, and thalidomide maintenance therapy after single autologous peripheral stem cell transplantation in patients with multiple myeloma. Biol Blood Marrow Transplant. 2012;18:486–92.
91. Neben K, Lokhorst HM, Jauch A, et al. Administration of bortezomib before and after autologous stem cell transplantation improves outcome in multiple myeloma patients with deletion 17p. Blood. 2012;119:940–8.

92. Sonneveld P, Schmidt-Wolf I, van der Holt B, et al. Bortezomib induction and maintenance treatment in patients with newly diagnosed multiple myeloma: Results of the randomized phase III HOVON-65/ GMMG-HD4 trial. J Clin Oncol. 2012;30:2946–55.
93. Attal M, Harousseau J-L, Facon T, et al. Single versus double autologous stem-cell transplantation for multiple myeloma. [Erratum appears in N Engl J Med. 2004 Jun17;350(25):2628]. N Engl J Med. 2003;349:2495–502.
94. Lahuerta JJ, Grande C, Martinez-Lopez J, et al. Tandem transplants with different high-dose regimens improve the complete remission rates in multiple myeloma. Results of a Grupo Espanol de Sindromes Linfoproliferativos/Trasplante Autologo de Medula Osea phase II trial. Br J Haematol. 2003;120:296–303.
95. Galli M, Nicolucci A, Valentini M, et al. Feasibility and outcome of tandem stem cell autotransplants in multiple myeloma. Haematologica. 2005;90:1643–9.
96. Moreau P, Hullin C, Garban F, et al. Tandem autologous stem cell transplantation in high-risk de novo multiple myeloma: final results of the prospective and randomized IFM 99-04 protocol. Blood. 2006;107:397–403.
97. Barlogie B, Tricot GJ, van Rhee F, et al. Long-term outcome results of the first tandem autotransplant trial for multiple myeloma. Br J Haematol. 2006;135:158–64.
98. Cavo M, Tosi P, Zamagni E, et al. Prospective, randomized study of single compared with double autologous stem-cell transplantation for multiple myeloma: Bologna 96 clinical study. J Clin Oncol. 2007;25(17):2434–41.
99. Corso A, Mangiacavalli S, Barbarano L, et al. Limited feasibility of double transplant in multiple myeloma: results of a multicenter study on 153 patients aged <65 years. Cancer. 2007;109:2273–8.
100. Sunami K, Shinagawa K, Sawamura M, et al. Phase I/II study of tandem high-dose chemotherapy with autologous peripheral blood stem cell transplantation for advanced multiple myeloma. Int J Hematol. 2009;90:635–42.
101. Novitzky N, Thomson J, Thomas V, du Toit C, Mohamed Z, McDonald A. Combined submyeloablative and myeloablative dose intense melphalan results in satisfactory responses with acceptable toxicity in patients with multiple myeloma. Biol Blood Marrow Transplant. 2010;16:1402–10.
102. Blade J, Rosinol L. Advances in therapy of multiple myeloma. Curr Opin Oncol. 2008;20:697–704.
103. Kumar A, Kharfan-Dabaja MA, Glasmacher A, Djulbegovic B. Tandem versus single autologous hematopoietic cell transplantation for the treatment of multiple myeloma: a systematic review and meta-analysis. J Natl Cancer Inst. 2009;101:100–6.
104. Krivanova A, Hajek R, Krejci M, et al. Second autologous transplantation for multiple myeloma patients relapsing after the first autograft—a pilot study for the evaluation of experimental maintenance therapies. Report of the prospective non-randomized pilot study of the Czech Myeloma Group. Onkologie. 2004;27: 275–9.
105. Jimenez-Zepeda VH, Mikhael J, Winter A, et al. Second autologous stem cell transplantation as salvage therapy for multiple myeloma: impact on progression-free and overall survival. Biol Blood Marrow Transplant. 2012;18:773–9.
106. Burzynski JA, Toro JJ, Patel RC, et al. Toxicity of a second autologous peripheral blood stem cell transplant in patients with relapsed or recurrent multiple myeloma. Leuk Lymphoma. 2009;50:1442–7.
107. Qazilbash MH, Saliba R, De Lima M, et al. Second autologous or allogeneic transplantation after the failure of first autograft in patients with multiple myeloma. Cancer. 2006;106:1084–9.
108. Garban F, Attal M, Michallet M, et al. Prospective comparison of autologous stem cell transplantation followed by dose-reduced allograft (IFM99-03 trial) with tandem autologous stem cell transplantation (IFM99-04 trial) in high-risk de novo multiple myeloma. Blood. 2006;107:3474–80.
109. Bruno B, Rotta M, Patriarca F, et al. A comparison of allografting with autografting for newly diagnosed myeloma. N Engl J Med. 2007;356:1110–20.
110. Gahrton G, Iacobelli S, Bandini G, et al. Peripheral blood or bone marrow cells in reduced-intensity or myeloablative conditioning allogeneic HLA identical sibling donor transplantation for multiple myeloma. Haematologica. 2007;92:1513–8.
111. Crawley C, Iacobelli S, Bjorkstrand B, Apperley JF, Niederwieser D, Gahrton G. Reduced-intensity conditioning for myeloma: lower nonrelapse mortality but higher relapse rates compared with myeloablative conditioning. Blood. 2007;109:3588–94.
112. Kuruvilla J, Shepherd JD, Sutherland HJ, et al. Long-term outcome of myeloablative allogeneic stem cell transplantation for multiple myeloma. Biol Blood Marrow Transplant. 2007;13:925–31.
113. Levenga H, Levison-Keating S, Schattenberg AV, Dolstra H, Schaap N, Raymakers RA. Multiple myeloma patients receiving pre-emptive donor lymphocyte infusion after partial T-cell-depleted allogeneic stem cell transplantation show a long progression-free survival. Bone Marrow Transplant. 2007;40:355–9.
114. Rosinol L, Perez-Simon JA, Sureda A, et al. A prospective PETHEMA study of tandem autologous transplantation versus autograft followed by reduced-intensity conditioning allogeneic transplantation in newly diagnosed multiple myeloma. Blood. 2008;112:3591–3.
115. Bruno B, Rotta M, Patriarca F, et al. Nonmyeloablative allografting for newly diagnosed multiple myeloma: the experience of the Gruppo Italiano Trapianti di Midollo. Blood. 2009;113:3375–82.
116. Rotta M, Storer BE, Sahebi F, et al. Long-term outcome of patients with multiple myeloma after autologous hematopoietic cell transplantation and nonmyeloablative allografting. Blood. 2009;113:3383–91.

117. Efebera YA, Qureshi SR, Cole SM, et al. Reduced-intensity allogeneic hematopoietic stem cell transplantation for relapsed multiple myeloma. Biol Blood Marrow Transplant. 2010;16:1122–9.
118. Kroger N, Einsele H, Derigs G, Wandt H, Krull A, Zander A. Long-term follow-up of an intensified myeloablative conditioning regimen with in vivo T cell depletion followed by allografting in patients with advanced multiple myeloma. Biol Blood Marrow Transplant. 2010;16:861–4.
119. Lokhorst H, Einsele H, Vesole D, et al. International Myeloma Working Group consensus statement regarding the current status of allogeneic stem-cell transplantation for multiple myeloma. J Clin Oncol. 2010;28:4521–30.
120. Bjorkstrand B, Iacobelli S, Hegenbart U, et al. Tandem autologous/reduced-intensity conditioning allogeneic stem-cell transplantation versus autologous transplantation in myeloma: long-term follow-up. [Erratum appears in J Clin Oncol. 2011 Sep 20;29(27):3721]. J Clin Oncol. 2011;29:3016–22.
121. Krishnan A, Pasquini MC, Logan B, et al. Autologous haemopoietic stem-cell transplantation followed by allogeneic or autologous haemopoietic stem-cell transplantation in patients with multiple myeloma (BMT CTN 0102): a phase 3 biological assignment trial. Lancet Oncol. 2011;12:1195–203.
122. Roos-Weil D, Moreau P, Avet-Loiseau H, et al. Impact of genetic abnormalities after allogeneic stem cell transplantation in multiple myeloma: a report of the Societe Francaise de Greffe de Moelle et de Therapie Cellulaire. Haematologica. 2011;96:1504–11.
123. Bashir Q, Khan H, Orlowski RZ, et al. Predictors of prolonged survival after allogeneic hematopoietic stem cell transplantation for multiple myeloma. Am J Hematol. 2012;87:272–6.
124. El-Cheikh J, Crocchiolo R, Boher JM, et al. Comparable outcomes between unrelated and related donors after reduced-intensity conditioning allogeneic hematopoietic stem cell transplantation in patients with high-risk multiple myeloma. Eur J Haematol. 2012;88:497–503.
125. Nishihori T, Kharfan-Dabaja MA, Ochoa-Bayona JL, Bazarbachi A, Pasquini M, Alsina M. Role of reduced intensity conditioning in allogeneic hematopoietic cell transplantation for patients with multiple myeloma. Hematol Oncol Stem Cell Ther. 2011;4:1–9.
126. Patriarca F, Einsele H, Spina F, et al. Allogeneic stem cell transplantation in multiple myeloma relapsed after autograft: a multicenter retrospective study based on donor availability. Biol Blood Marrow Transplant. 2012;18:617–26.

Allogeneic Stem Cell Transplantation

11

Martha Q. Lacy

Introduction

The survival of patients with multiple myeloma (MM) has improved over the past decade [1]. The most significant gains have been in patients without high-risk molecular markers. Despite these gains, multiple myeloma remains fatal and curative strategies are needed.

Allogeneic stem cell transplant (Allo-SCT) includes both myeloablative and nonmyeloablative or "reduced intensity conditioning" (RIC) transplants. Allogeneic transplant is appealing in theory because it avoids infusion of stem cells contaminated with myeloma cells and because there can be a beneficial graft vs. myeloma effect [2]. The role of Allo-SCT in myeloma, however, is debated due to the high mortality and morbidity. The high treatment-related mortality and significant toxicity from graft-versus-host disease (GVHD) have limited the role of this procedure in the treatment of myeloma.

Myeloablative AlloSCT

The earliest experience regarding myeloablative allo-SCT was reported by the transplant registries including the European Bone Marrow Transplantation (EBMT) and the Fred Hutchinson Cancer Center [3–5]. Early treatment-related mortality (TRM) ranged between 35 and 45 % [3–5] and complete remission rates varied between 36 [3] and 60 % [5]. Interpretations of these data are difficult because the reported patients were heterogeneous. They were not treated in prospective trials but were retrospective reports. Many patients had received several lines of previous chemotherapy and were chemotherapy-resistant at the time of transplant. In addition they received a variety of conditioning and GVHD prophylaxis regimens.

Subsequently, the EBMT compared 334 patients who received allogeneic transplants between 1983 and 1993 and 356 patients who received transplants between 1994 and 1998 [6]. The most important observation was a marked reduction in TRM from 46 to 30 % at 2 years between the two time periods. The median overall survival (OS) for the later transplants was 50 months. Nevertheless, the transplant-related mortality of 30 % was still deemed unacceptably high.

There are two prospective trials that tried to examine the role of myeloablative AlloSCT in myeloma [7, 8]. Neither was randomized but instead selection to the allogeneic arm was based on availability of an HLA-matched donor.

Patients enrolled in the US intergroup trial S9321 [7] were treated with four cycles of VAD. Patients were randomly assigned to either high-dose therapy with melphalan (MEL) plus total body irradiation (TBI) or to standard dose

M.Q. Lacy, M.D. (✉)
Division of Hematology, Mayo Clinic,
200 First Street, SW, Rochester, MN 55905, USA
e-mail: lacy.martha@mayo.edu

M.A. Gertz and S.V. Rajkumar (eds.), *Multiple Myeloma: Diagnosis and Treatment*,
DOI 10.1007/978-1-4614-8520-9_11, © Mayo Foundation for Medical Education and Research 2014

therapy with VBMCP. Patients who were <55 years of age with an HLA-compatible sibling donor were offered the option of allogeneic transplantation with MEL 140 mg/m^2 plus TBI. However, this arm was closed when an excessive first-year treatment-related mortality rate of 53 % was observed after enrollment of 36 eligible patients. With 7 years of follow-up the OS of the conventional chemotherapy, autologous, and allogeneic transplant groups were identical at 39 %. It was intriguing that AlloSCT group showed a survival plateau while the other two groups did not, suggesting long-term benefit.

The Haemato Oncology Foundation for Adults in the Netherlands (HOVON) 24 study was designed to compare AutoSCT with semi-intensive treatment; however, patients with an HLA-identical sibling donor could proceed to a partially T cell-depleted myeloablative AlloSCT using cyclophosphamide/TBI conditioning [8]. TRM among the AlloSCT patients exceeded 30 % while PFS and OS were inferior to the matched group of patients receiving only autologous SCT.

The EBMT performed a retrospective, case-matched comparison of AutoSCT and AlloSCT [9]. In their retrospective analysis of data compiled by the European Blood and Marrow Transplantation Group, there was inferior OS for myeloma patients treated with AlloSCT compared to case-matched controls treated with AutoSCT (18 vs. 36 months). This was due to a higher TRM of 41 % vs. 13 %, respectively. There was a trend, however, for better survival in the allogeneic patients surviving at 1 year.

Reduced Intensity Conditioning AlloSCT

Another strategy is to use ASCT to cytoreduce the myeloma followed by a reduced intensity conditioning AlloSCT (allo-RIC). After two large series reported encouraging results [10, 11] five prospective trials have looked at this approach [12–17] (Table 11.1). Only one of the five trials noted improved OS in patients undergoing tandem auto/allo transplants [13]. Graft vs. myeloma effect appears to be tightly linked to GVHD, which has the potential to significantly affect quality of life.

Bruno and colleagues [13, 15] enrolled 162 consecutive patients with newly diagnosed myeloma who were <65 years of age. All patients were initially treated with VAD, followed by high-dose melphalan and ASCT. Patients without an HLA-identical sibling received a second ASCT. Patients with an HLA-identical sibling then received nonmyeloablative TBI and stem cells from the sibling. The median OS was longer in the 80 patients with HLA-identical siblings than in the 82 patients without HLA-identical siblings (80 vs. 54 months, $P=0.01$).

The IFM enrolled 503 patients with high-risk MM (beta2-microglobulin level greater than 3 mg/L and chromosome 13 deletion at diagnosis) in two clinical trials [14]. In both protocols, the induction regimen consisted of VAD followed by first ASCT prepared by melphalan 200 mg/m^2. Patients with an HLA-identical sibling donor were subsequently treated with allo-RIC

Table 11.1 Tandem autologous SCT vs. Auto/allo SCT

	CR (%)	EFS/PFS	OS	cGVHD
	Auto/allo vs. Auto/auto			Auto/allo
Bruno	53 vs. 20	Median 35 vs. 29 months	Median 80 vs. 54 months	32 %
IFM	62 vs. 38	Median 25 vs. 30 months	Median 35 vs. 41 months	43 %
PETHEMA	40 vs. 11	41 % vs. 31 % at 5 years	62 % vs. 60 % at 5 years	66 %
Bjorkstrand	51 vs. 41	35 % vs. 18 % at 60 months	65 % vs. 58 % at 60 months	54 %
BMT-CTN	58 vs. 45	43 % vs. 46 % at 3 years	77 % vs. 80 % at 3 years	54 %

(IFM99-03 trial), and patients without an HLA-identical sibling donor were randomly assigned to undergo second ASCT prepared by melphalan 220 mg/m^2 and 160 mg dexamethasone with or without anti-IL-6 monoclonal antibody (IFM99-04 protocol). Two hundred and eighty-four patients in the IFM99-03 trial and 219 in the IFM99-04 trial were enrolled. There were no differences in OS or EFS.

The PETHEMA group enrolled 110 patients with MM who had failed to achieve at least near-complete remission (nCR) after a first ASCT [17]. They received a second ASCT (85 patients) or an allo-RIC (25 patients), depending on the availability of an HLA-identical sibling donor. Those who received the allo-RIC had higher rates of complete remission (40 % vs. 11 %, $P=0.001$) but no difference in EFS and OS. They noted a 66 % incidence of chronic GVHD.

The European Bone Marrow Transplant (EBMT), MM subcommittee enrolled 357 patients up to age 69 [12] from 23 participating centers. Patients with an HLA-identical sibling were allocated to the ASCT- allo-RIC arm and the remaining to a tandem ASCT arm. Complete response rates were higher in the ASCT- allo-RIC group as was PFS, but there was no difference in OS with a median follow-up of 61 months. Only 41 % of patients in the tandem ASCT arm actually got a second ASCT whereas 85 % of patients in the ASCT- allo-RIC group received their second transplant.

The Blood Marrow Transplant Clinical Trials Network (BMT CTN) enrolled 710 patients [16] and biologically randomized them to tandem ASCT or ASCT- allo-RIC. Compared with tandem autologous SCT, the auto-allo strategy did not improve progression-free survival (PFS) or overall survival and had more than double the treatment-related mortality. Additionally, there was no apparent overall survival or PFS benefit with the auto-allo approach in a subgroup of high-risk patients. More than half of patients in the auto-allo group had chronic GVHD.

Myeloablative vs. RIC Allogeneic Transplant

The EBMT has retrospectively compared RIC with standard ablative conditioning for AlloSCT in MM [18]. Between 1998 and 2002, 196 patients conditioned with myeloablative regimens were compared with 320 patients undergoing RIC. TRM was significantly lower for the reduced-intensity group, but there was no difference in OS between the two groups. Furthermore, PFS was inferior for patients receiving RIC due to a doubling of the relapse rate in the RIC group. The CIBMTR did a similar retrospective analysis in 1,211 patients undergoing AlloSCT for MM between 1989 and 2005 [19]. Although they did not specifically compare myeloablative regimens to RIC, they found over time the use of myeloablative regimens decreased over time while RIC increased. The TRM improved over time, the OS at 5 years was similar among the groups, primarily because of increased risk of relapse in the latest cohort.

Given the toxicity of this approach—rates of chronic GVHD of 50 %—and the lack of suitable donors, allogeneic transplant, whether myeloablative or RIC, should be considered experimental in patients with myeloma.

Syngeneic Transplant

The first syngeneic bone marrow transplant in MM was reported in 1982 [20]. Although only a small fraction of myeloma patients have a syngeneic donor, interest in this approach was fueled by the report from Bensinger and colleagues describing outcomes in 11 patients who underwent syngeneic bone marrow or stem cell or transplant [21]. Nine had relapsed or refractory disease. TRM was 18 %. Responses were seen in eight of nine evaluable patients including five who achieved a CR. Among the five patients who achieved a CR, three relapsed on days 539, 737, and 1,706 and died on days 1,759, 1,596, and 1,736, respectively; one patient died of myelodysplastic syndrome on day 1,407 without evidence of MM and one patient was still alive and disease-free 3,297 days after transplant. One of the two long-term survivors has a persistent monoclonal protein in the blood 15 years post-transplant.

The EBMT compared outcomes with syngeneic transplantation to allogeneic and autologous transplantation [22]. Twenty-five patients with MM received syngeneic transplants. The outcome was compared in a case-matched analysis to 125 patients who underwent autologous transplantation, and 125 who underwent allogeneic transplantation. Remission rates did not differ between the groups. The median overall and progression-free survival for the twins was 73 and 72 months, respectively. The overall survival tended to be better (73 vs. 44 months) and the progression-free survival was significantly better (72 vs. 25 months) than with autologous transplantation and both were significantly better than with allogeneic transplantation. Three of 17 patients who entered complete remission following transplantation had relapsed at follow-up. The relapse rate was significantly lower than following autologous transplantation and similar to the relapse rate with allogeneic transplantation.

Donor Lymphocyte Infusions

A graft vs. myeloma effect has been noted after the administration of donor peripheral blood mononuclear cells for relapse after allogeneic transplantation (567,568). DLI has been used in two ways in myeloma patients. Initially, it was used to treat relapsed or residual disease after full myeloablative AlloSCT (567,568). Subsequently, it was used to re-introduce T-cells into a patient who had received an allogeneic T cell-depleted graft (569,570). Most recently, it has been implemented in the context of allo-RIC programs to treat mixed chimerism, as well as for the older indications (571–573). In the largest DLI series for relapsed MM ($n = 54$), 52 % of patients responded (35 % with a partial response and 17 % with a complete response). The majority of patients received some chemotherapy before DLI. PFS and OS were 19 and 23 months, respectively. Rates of overall acute GVHD and of grade III–IV acute GVHD were 57 % and 20 %, respectively. Rates of overall chronic GVHD and of extensive GVHD were 47 % and 30 %, respectively. Acute and chronic GVHD following DLI were the strongest predictors for response (574).

References

1. Kumar SK, Rajkumar SV, Dispenzieri A, et al. Improved survival in multiple myeloma and the impact of novel therapies. Blood. 2008;111(5):2516–20.
2. Badros A, Barlogie B, Morris C, et al. High response rate in refractory and poor-risk multiple myeloma after allotransplantation using a nonmyeloablative conditioning regimen and donor lymphocyte infusions. Blood. 2001;97(9):2574–9 [Erratum appears in Blood 2001 Jul 15;98(2):271; Blood 2001 Sep 15;98(6):1653].
3. Bensinger WI, Buckner CD, Anasetti C, et al. Allogeneic marrow transplantation for multiple myeloma: an analysis of risk factors on outcome. Blood. 1996;88(7):2787–93.
4. Gahrton G, Tura S, Ljungman P, et al. Allogeneic bone marrow transplantation in multiple myeloma. European Group for Bone Marrow Transplantation. N Engl J Med. 1991;325(18):1267–73.
5. Gahrton G, Tura S, Ljungman P, et al. Prognostic factors in allogeneic bone marrow transplantation for multiple myeloma [see comments]. J Clin Oncol. 1995;13(6):1312–22.
6. Gahrton G, Svensson H, Cavo M, et al. Progress in allogenic bone marrow and peripheral blood stem cell transplantation for multiple myeloma: a comparison between transplants performed 1983–93 and 1994–8 at European Group for Blood and Marrow Transplantation centres. Br J Haematol. 2001;113(1):209–16.
7. Barlogie B, Kyle RA, Anderson KC, et al. Standard chemotherapy compared with high-dose chemoradiotherapy for multiple myeloma: final results of phase III US Intergroup Trial S9321. J Clin Oncol. 2006;24(6):929–36.
8. Lokhorst HM, Segeren CM, Verdonck LF, et al. Partially T-cell-depleted allogeneic stem-cell transplantation for first-line treatment of multiple myeloma: a prospective evaluation of patients treated in the phase III study HOVON 24 MM. J Clin Oncol. 2003;21(9):1728–33.
9. Bjorkstrand BB, Ljungman P, Svensson H, et al. Allogeneic bone marrow transplantation versus autologous stem cell transplantation in multiple myeloma: a retrospective case-matched study from the European

Group for Blood and Marrow Transplantation. Blood. 1996;88(12):4711–8.

10. Kroger N, Schwerdtfeger R, Kiehl M, et al. Autologous stem cell transplantation followed by a dose-reduced allograft induces high complete remission rate in multiple myeloma. Blood. 2002;100(3):755–60.
11. Maloney DG, Molina AJ, Sahebi F, et al. Allografting with nonmyeloablative conditioning following cytoreductive autografts for the treatment of patients with multiple myeloma. Blood. 2003;102(9):3447–54.
12. Bjorkstrand B, Iacobelli S, Hegenbart U, et al. Tandem autologous/reduced-intensity conditioning allogeneic stem-cell transplantation versus autologous transplantation in myeloma: long-term follow-up. J Clin Oncol. 2011;29(22):3016–22. Prepublished on 2011/07/07 as DOI JCO.2010.32.7312 [pii] 10.1200/JCO.2010.32.7312.
13. Bruno B, Rotta M, Patriarca F, et al. A comparison of allografting with autografting for newly diagnosed myeloma. N Engl J Med. 2007;356(11):1110–20.
14. Garban F, Attal M, Michallet M, et al. Prospective comparison of autologous stem cell transplantation followed by dose-reduced allograft (IFM99-03 trial) with tandem autologous stem cell transplantation (IFM99-04 trial) in high-risk de novo multiple myeloma. Blood. 2006;107(9):3474–80.
15. Giaccone L, Storer B, Patriarca F, et al. Long-term follow up of a comparison of non-myeloablative allografting with autografting for newly diagnosed myeloma. Blood. 2011;117(24):6721–7. Prepublished on 2011/04/15 as DOI blood-2011-03-339945 [pii] 10.1182/blood-2011-03-339945.
16. Krishnan A, Pasquini MC, Logan B, et al. Autologous haemopoietic stem-cell transplantation followed by allogeneic or autologous haemopoietic stem-cell transplantation in patients with multiple myeloma (BMT CTN 0102): a phase 3 biological assignment trial. Lancet Oncol. 2011;12(13):1195–203. doi:10.1016/s1470-2045(11)70243-1.
17. Rosinol L, Perez-Simon JA, Sureda A, et al. A prospective PETHEMA study of tandem autologous transplantation versus autograft followed by reduced-intensity conditioning allogeneic transplantation in newly diagnosed multiple myeloma. Blood. 2008;112(9):3591–3. Prepublished on 2008/07/10 as DOI blood-2008-02-141598 [pii] 10.1182/blood-2008-02-141598.
18. Crawley C, Iacobelli S, Bjorkstrand B, Apperley JF, Niederwieser D, Gahrton G. Reduced-intensity conditioning for myeloma: lower nonrelapse mortality but higher relapse rates compared with myeloablative conditioning. Blood. 2007;109(8):3588–94.
19. Kumar S, Zhang MJ, Li P, et al. Trends in allogeneic stem cell transplantation for multiple myeloma: a CIBMTR analysis. Blood. 2011;118(7):1979–88. Prepublished on 2011/06/22 as DOI 10.1182/blood-2011-02-337329.
20. Osserman EF, DiRe LB, DiRe J, Sherman WH, Hersman JA, Storb R. Identical twin marrow transplantation in multiple myeloma. Acta Haematol. 1982;68(3):215–23.
21. Bensinger WI, Demirer T, Buckner CD, et al. Syngeneic marrow transplantation in patients with multiple myeloma. Bone Marrow Transplant. 1996;18(3):527–31. Prepublished on 1996/09/01 as DOI.
22. Gahrton G, Svensson H, Bjorkstrand B, et al. Syngeneic transplantation in multiple myeloma—a case-matched comparison with autologous and allogeneic transplantation. European Group for Blood and Marrow Transplantation. Bone Marrow Transplant. 1999;24(7):741–5. Prepublished on 1999/10/12 as DOI 10.1038/sj.bmt.1701975.

New Agents for Multiple Myeloma

12

Shaji Kumar and Arleigh McCurdy

Introduction

The treatment paradigm for multiple myeloma has significantly shifted in the past decade, as a result of new treatment agents, a better refinement of the supportive care approaches, a deeper understanding of the disease biology, and risk stratification-based approaches to treatment of myeloma. However, a relatively small proportion of patients are able to obtain long-term disease control with any of these treatment approaches, with the majority relapsing after various treatments and eventually becoming refractory to all available options. Hence it is imperative, we continue to work on developing newer treatments that represent improved versions of available drug classes as well as newer classes of drugs. In addition, there has been significant focus on developing new combinations of existing as well as novel therapeutic agents. In the current chapter, we will examine the new drugs that have been recently approved as well as those that are currently in clinical trials. Broadly, these drugs can be classified into those belonging to currently used classes of drugs, and new drug classes.

S. Kumar, M.D. (✉) • A. McCurdy, M.D.
Division of Hematology, Mayo Clinic,
200 First Street, SW, Rochester, MN 55905, USA
e-mail: kumar.shaji@mayo.edu

Pomalidomide

Pomalidomide (CC-4047) is the most recent IMiD to be evaluated in clinical trials and was recently approved for treatment of relapsed myeloma. It is a thalidomide derivative with overlapping mechanisms of action with lenalidomide and thalidomide [1, 2]. The drug had shown potent anti-myeloma activity in the in vitro setting and set the stage for clinical evaluation. In terms of potential immune effects, in preclinical studies it significantly increases serum interleukin (IL)-2 receptor and IL-12 levels [3]. In vitro studies also have shown potent inhibitory effect on osteoclasts differentiation [4]. Pomalidomide also affects inflammation via transcriptional inhibition of cyclooxygenase-2 (COX-2) production, which is associated with increased prostaglandins in human lipopolysaccharide (LPS)-stimulated monocytes [5].

Efficacy results: Among patients with multiple myeloma, pomalidomide has been studied extensively in the setting of relapsed disease (Table 12.1). Initial phase I trials established pomalidomide as well tolerated in maximum tolerated dose (MTD) of 2 mg daily or 5 mg on alternate days [3, 6]. These studies using pomalidomide predominantly as monotherapy have shown an excellent activity with an overall response rate of 52 % [7].

M.A. Gertz and S.V. Rajkumar (eds.), *Multiple Myeloma: Diagnosis and Treatment*,
DOI 10.1007/978-1-4614-8520-9_12, © Mayo Foundation for Medical Education and Research 2014

Table 12.1 Results with pomalidomide

	IFM (21/28)	IFM (28/28)	Mayo (2 mg)	Mayo (4 mg)	MM02 (Ph 1)	MM02 (Ph 2)
N	43	41	35	35	28	120
CR	2	0	0	3	4	1
>VGPR	9	5	14	11	4	1
>PR	42	39	26	26	25	25
>MR	41	39	49	40	50	38
DOR	4 months	4 months	12 months	NA	NA	NA

In the first phase II trial conducted by Lacy and colleagues 60 patients with relapsed myeloma, who had 2–3 prior regimens, were treated with 2 mg pomalidomide daily, along with weekly 40 mg oral dexamethasone [8]. Thirty-eight patients (63 %) achieved confirmed response including complete response in 3 patients (5 %), very good partial response in 17 patients (28 %), and partial response in 18 patients (30 %). Responses were seen in 40 % of lenalidomide-refractory patients, 37 % of thalidomide-refractory patients, and 60 % of bortezomib-refractory patients. In addition, 74 % of patients with high-risk cytogenetic or molecular markers (hypodiploidy or karyotypic deletion of chromosome 13, FISH showing the presence of translocations t(4;14) or t(14;16) or deletion 17p, or plasma cell labeling index ≥3 %) had a response. Overall, the drug was well tolerated with the most common serious adverse effect being Grade 3 or 4 hematologic toxicity, which was seen in a third of the patients [8]. The median progression-free survival (PFS) time was 11.6 months and was not significantly different in patients with high-risk disease compared with patients with standard-risk disease. A series of patient cohorts with different resistance profiles were treated in this trial, such as bortezomib-refractory and dual refractory to bortezomib and lenalidomide, and also different dosing strategies such as increasing the dose to 4 mg for lack of response or starting therapy with 4 mg dose [9–11].

Richardson and colleagues in another phase I/II dose escalation study showed that 4 mg pomalidomide daily given for 3 of 4 weeks is the MTD for that dosing schema [12]. Overall response rate in this study was 25 %, and the phase II study is currently ongoing. The IFM group performed a randomized phase II trial looking at two dosing schedules, 21/28 or 28/28 days with pomalidomide administered at 4 mg daily with weekly dexamethasone. The overall response rate and the duration of response (DOR) were similar with the two strategies as was the overall toxicity [13].

Adverse effects: Myelosuppression was the most common as well as dose limiting toxicity in clinical trials. Grade 3/4 neutropenia has been seen in about 30–60 % of patients and is more common than thrombocytopenia or anemia. The risk of thromboembolic complications appears to be similar to that reported with other IMiDs, and similar anticoagulation strategies have been employed. New onset neuropathy is infrequent but worsening of pre-existing neuropathy has been seen. Other common side effects include orthostatic hypotension, skin rash, and constipation. Like thalidomide, pomalidomide may have the potential for severe birth defects requiring strict contraceptive requirements for its use.

Carfilzomib

Carfilzomib, also known as PR-171, targets the chymotrypsin-like activity of the 20S proteasome [14–18]. Carfilzomib is a selective inhibitor and binds most specifically to the chymotrypsin-like protease, with less activity against the other subunits. In addition, carfilzomib demonstrates less reactivity against non-proteasomal proteases when compared to bortezomib.

Efficacy results: Carfilzomib has been shown to have significant anti-myeloma activity in the

Table 12.2 Results with carfilzomib

Trial	N	Population	Number prior lines	Overall response rate (%)	MR/SD (%)	Median TTP (months)
003-A0	39	Refractory	5	18	8/41	5.1
003-A1	257	Refractory	5	24	13/32	3.7 (PFS)
004 (Bz exposed)	35	Relapsed	1–3	17	12/35	4.6
004 (Bz naïve)	126	Relapsed	1–3	47.6	14/18	54 % @ 9 months
006 (Combo with len/dex)	40	Relapsed	1–3	62.5	–/15	10.2 (PFS)

setting of relapsed myeloma both in bortezomib-naïve and bortezomib-refractory patients (Table 12.2). The toxicity pattern suggested that the drug is well tolerated, and in particular seemed to have very low rate of neuropathy. In the initial phase I study, carfilzomib was administered intravenously on 2 consecutive days for 3 weeks of a 4-week cycle at doses ranging from 1.2 to 27 mg/m^2 [19]. The dose escalation phase enrolled 37 patients followed by a dose-expansion phase with 11 patients. During dose expansion, carfilzomib was administered starting with 20 mg/m^2 during the first week (days 1 and 2) and then escalated to 27 mg/m^2 thereafter. A MTD was not reached. The main hematologic Grade 3 or higher adverse events were anemia and thrombocytopenia. Notably, there were no observations of Grade 3 or more peripheral neuropathy. Carfilzomib was cleared rapidly with an elimination half-life of less than 30 min but still induced dose-dependent inhibition of the 20S chymotrypsin-like proteasome activity. At doses of 15–27 mg/m^2, there was evidence of activity among patients with multiple myeloma and with non-Hodgkin lymphoma. In PX-171-003-A0 (20 mg/m^2 carfilzomib throughout), 46 patients with relapsed and refractory multiple myeloma were enrolled [20]. All patients had progressive disease on study entry and 100 % had received prior bortezomib alone or in combination with other agents; 70 % were refractory to prior bortezomib, and 22 % were removed from bortezomib therapy due to development of severe peripheral neuropathy. The response rate using IMWG criteria was 16.7 % (7 PRs) and there were an additional 3 (7 %) durable (>6 weeks) MRs; the DOR was similar for MRs and PRs at ~7.2 months. Study PX-171-003-A1 enrolled 266 relapsed and refractory patients at 20 mg/m^2 for cycle 1, and escalation to 27 mg/m^2 thereafter for patients who tolerate the drug [21]. In this trial, 82 % of the patients had at least four prior therapies, 84 % were refractory or intolerant to bortezomib, and 95 % were refractory to the last therapy. The responses included 6 % patients with VGPR or better, 18 % with a PR, and 13 % with an MR. In addition, stable disease was seen in 32 % of patients. The median PFS was 3.7 months and the median OS was 15.6 months. PX-171-004 was designed to assess the effect of carfilzomib on patients with MM who had 1–3 prior therapies, i.e., were less heavily pretreated than those in PX-171-003 [22, 23]. In the cohort of patients with at least one prior bortezomib-based therapy, the overall response rate was 17.1 % and the median DOR was over 10.6 months with the median time to progression of 4.6 months. The most common adverse events were fatigue (62.9 %), nausea (60.0 %), and vomiting (42.9 %). No exacerbation of baseline peripheral neuropathy was observed. In the cohort of patients with bortezomib-naïve disease (n=129), patients received either 20 mg/m^2 throughout (cohort 1) or only for cycle 1 followed by 27 mg/m^2 for the remaining cycles (cohort 2). The overall response rate was 42.4 % in cohort 1 and 52.2 % in cohort 2. Median DOR was 13.1 months and not reached, and median time to progression was 8.3 months and not reached, respectively.

Adverse effects: Toxicities have generally been manageable. In relapsed or refractory MM patients treated at 20–27 mg/m^2, the most common adverse events (AEs) are anemia, fatigue, nausea, diarrhea, and cyclic thrombocytopenia.

Peripheral neuropathy of any grade regardless of relationship to study drug is <15 % despite the majority of patients entering these studies with existing Grade 1 or 2 peripheral neuropathy. The most common Grade 3/4 AEs are anemia (14 %), thrombocytopenia (12 %), pneumonia (6 %), and fatigue (5 %). Importantly, Grade 3/4 neutropenia occurs in <5 % and Grade 3/4 peripheral neuropathy in <3 % (includes neuropathy, peripheral neuropathy, and neuropathic pain), despite the fact that nearly all of the patients have these conditions as a result of their prior drug therapies and disease. These results are consistent with the lack of myelosuppressive and neuropathic effects of carfilzomib in preclinical studies.

Ixazomib (MLN9708)

MLN9708 is the first oral proteasome inhibitor to enter clinical trials. It is an orally bioavailable, potent, reversible, specific inhibitor of the 20S proteasome. It is a citrate ester that immediately hydrolyzes to MLN2238, a dipeptidyl leucine boronic acid which represents the biologically active moiety. In comparison to bortezomib it has similar selectivity and potency, but faster dissociation from proteasome resulting in greater tissue penetration. The drug has demonstrated antitumor activity in solid tumor and hematologic malignancy xenograft models, including in vivo models of MM, leading to clinical trials.

Efficacy results: Two phase I trials with expansion cohorts have been conducted with single agent MLN9708 [24, 25]. The first trial administered MLN9708 twice weekly (days 1, 4, 8, 11) of a 21-day cycle and the other trial had the drug administered once weekly for 3 out of 4 weeks. The MTD for the drug has been determined and ongoing phase 3 trials are examining the efficacy of the drug in combination with lenalidomide or alkylating agents.

Adverse effects: The drug is reasonably well tolerated with gastrointestinal and hematologic adverse events being the most common. Skin rash has been seen, especially in combination with lenalidomide. Efficacy has been seen in both trials, especially at the higher doses with some patients achieving a VGPR to therapy. Unlike bortezomib, MLN9708 has not been associated with a significant peripheral neuropathy with mostly Grade 1 neuropathies observed in studies so far.

New Drug Classes

Monoclonal Antibodies

Monoclonal antibody therapy has been quite successful in lymphoid malignancies, but similar approaches in myeloma have been beset by the heterogeneous expression of surface proteins in myeloma.

Elotuzumab: More recently, early trials with the humanized monoclonal antibody, elotuzumab (HuLuc63), have shown encouraging results. It induces antibody-dependent cell cytotoxicity-mediated apoptosis in vitro and significantly reduced tumor growth in preclinical myeloma models [26]. In a phase I study in patients who had received 1–3 prior therapies for myeloma, escalating doses of elotuzumab (2.5, 5, 10, and 20 mg/kg IV) were administered on days 1 and 11 in combination with bortezomib (1.3 mg/m^2 IV) administered on days 1, 4, 8, and 11 of a 21-day cycle [27]. Dexamethasone 20 mg PO was added for patients with disease progression on days 1, 2, 4, 5, 8, 9, 11, and 12 of subsequent cycles. No DLTs were observed during cycle 1 and the MTD was not reached. The most frequent Grade 3/4 side effects were lymphopenia, fatigue, thrombocytopenia, neutropenia, hyperglycemia, peripheral neuropathy, pneumonia, and anemia. A partial response or better was observed in 13/27 (48 %) evaluable patients, including 7 % CR and 41 % PR. The results of the initial trials looking at the combination with lenalidomide were more promising [28]. The study enrolled three escalating dose cohorts of elotuzumab (5, 10, and 20 mg/kg IV), administered on days 1, 8, 15, and 22 of a 28-day cycle in the first two cycles, and then days 1 and 15 of each subsequent cycle, along with lenalidomide 25 mg PO daily on days 1–21 and dexamethasone 40 mg PO weekly. No DLTs were observed up to 20 mg/kg during the escalation phase and hence no MTD was established. The most frequent Grade 3/4 toxicities were neutropenia and thrombocytopenia, and two patients experienced serious infusion-related reactions. A partial response or better was seen in 82 % (23/28) of treated patients and 96 % (21/22) of lenalidomide-naïve patients.

Daratumumab: Daratumumab is a human CD38 monoclonal antibody directed against CD38-expressing myeloma tumor cells and kills via antibody-dependent cell-mediated cytotoxicity, complement-dependent cytotoxicity, and apoptosis [29–31]. In a phase I study, 32 patients with relapsed myeloma were treated with daratumumab over a 9-week period at doses ranging from 0.005 to 24 mg/kg. Initial data suggest potential clinical activity of this drug. Among patients getting ≤2 mg/kg, 4/20 achieved minimal reduction in paraprotein levels, but higher efficacy was seen in those receiving higher doses. Among those getting 4 mg/kg group, 3/3 had a reduction in paraprotein, while in the 8 mg/kg group, 2/3 had a reduction in paraprotein and in the 16 mg/kg cohort, 2/3 had a reduction in paraprotein of at least 25 %. The most common adverse events reported were infusion-related events, predominantly during the initial infusions.

The inflammatory cytokine interleukin (IL)-6 is a survival factor for malignant plasma cells and is secreted by myeloma cells. Preclinical data suggest that CNTO328, a novel human–mouse chimeric monoclonal antibody targeting IL-6, has an inhibitory effect on tumor burden and potentiates bortezomib-mediated apoptosis. Initial studies support the feasibility of combining the antibody with bortezomib in patients with relapsed myeloma [32].

HDAC Inhibitors

Inhibition of histone deacetylase (HDAC) provides a novel approach for cancer treatment. Histones are part of the core proteins of nucleosomes, and acetylation and deacetylation of these proteins play an important role in the regulation of gene expression. Deacetylated histones bind tightly to the DNA and limit access of transcription factors inhibiting transcription, while acetylation neutralizes the charge of histones and generates a more open DNA conformation, allowing gene expression. In normal cells, balanced activity of two groups of enzymes, histone acetyltransferase (HAT) and HDAC, control the amount of acetylation. Aberrant recruitment of HDAC and the resulting modification of chromatin structure has been implicated in malignant transformation of cells. HDAC inhibitors are thought to affect multiple pathways involved in MM and correct the deregulation of genes involved in apoptosis and cell cycle arrest, thus potentially sensitizing MM cells to apoptosis [33, 34].

Several HDAC inhibitors have been evaluated in the context of myeloma, including suberoylanilide hydroxamic acid (SAHA; vorinostat) [35], ITF2357 [36], LBH589 (panobinostat) [37], and romidepsin [38]. Results so far suggest limited single agent activity in patients with MM [34].

A phase I trial of oral vorinostat (200, 250, or 300 mg twice daily for 5 days/week/4-week cycle or 200, 300, or 400 mg twice daily for 14 days/3-week cycle) was conducted in patients with relapsed/refractory multiple myeloma [39]. Thirteen patients were enrolled; MTD was not reached. Drug-related adverse experiences included fatigue, anorexia, dehydration, diarrhea, and nausea. Of ten evaluable patients, one had a minimal response (MR) and nine had stable disease.

Romidepsin is an HDAC inhibitor that has demonstrated cytotoxicity against multiple myeloma cell lines in vitro. In a phase II trial, patients with multiple myeloma who were refractory to standard therapy were treated with romidepsin (13 mg/m^2) given as a 4-h intravenous infusion on days 1, 8, and 15 every 28 days [38]. No objective responses were seen among the 123 patients treated.

While this class of drugs does not seem to have significant single agent activity, combinations of HDACi with newer drugs, especially bortezomib, appear to be promising based on the initial phase II trials. A phase I trial evaluated escalating doses of bortezomib (1–1.3 mg/m^2 on days 1, 4, 8, and 11 and vorinostat at 100–500 mg orally daily for 8 days of each 21-day cycle) in patients with relapsed/refractory multiple myeloma [40]. The most common toxicities were myelosuppression, fatigue, and diarrhea. The overall response rate was 42 %, including three partial responses among nine bortezomib-refractory patients. In another phase I trial, patients with relapsed or refractory MM were randomized to oral vorinostat (200 mg twice daily or 400 mg once daily for 14 days) in combination with bortezomib (0.7 or 0.9 mg/m^2 on days 4, 8, 11, and 15 or 0.9, 1.1, or 1.3 mg/m^2 on days 1, 4, 8, and 11) [41]. The best responses observed in the 33 evaluable patients were PR (36.4 %), MR (18.2 %), and SD (39.4 %) including 18 % PR in patients with previous bortezomib therapy. Vorinostat 400 mg once daily plus bortezomib 1.3 mg/m^2 on days 1, 4, 8, and 11 was considered the MTD. However, a phase 3 trial of vorinostat and bortezomib failed to demonstrate any substantial improvement in PFS in patients with relapsed MM.

The combination of panobinostat and bortezomib also has been explored in early stage trials. In a phase Ib trial, 29 patients were treated with escalating doses of panobinostat and bortezomib [42]. Overall, hematologic adverse events were frequent. Non-hematologic side effects included diarrhea, fever, nausea, fatigue, and asthenia. Encouraging clinical efficacy was observed with 14 partial response or better (50 %) among 28 evaluable patients, including 4 with complete response (CR). The overall response rate was 64 % including minor responses, and activity was seen in patients refractory to bortezomib. Similar results have also been noted with combination of romidepsin with bortezomib.

Heat Shock Protein 90 Inhibitors

Heat shock protein 90 (Hsp90) is a molecular chaperone that is induced in response to cellular stress and leads to stabilization of various client proteins involved in cell cycle control and apoptotic signaling. Its overexpression can contribute to tumor cell survival by stabilizing aberrant signaling proteins leading to increased proliferation. Hsp90 inhibitors decrease MM proliferation and sensitize MM cells to other anticancer agents [43]. Several Hsp90 inhibitors have been evaluated in early stage clinical trials.

Tanespimycin was one of the early Hsp90 inhibitors to be tested in myeloma. In a phase I dose escalation study, tanespimycin (150–525 mg/m^2) was given on days 1, 4, 8, and 11 of each 3-week cycle for up to eight cycles to a group of heavily pretreated patients with relapsed/refractory myeloma. Common adverse events included diarrhea, back pain, fatigue, nausea, anemia, and thrombocytopenia. One patient (3 %) achieved minimal response (MR), with a PFS of 3 months. Fifteen patients (52 %) achieved SD with a median PFS of 2.1 months. Overall, tanespimycin monotherapy was well tolerated with limited evidence of activity [44]. In another phase I study, the safety and activity of the Hsp90 inhibitor, KOS-953 (a formulation of 17-AAG), was dose escalated from 150 to 340 mg/m^2 with manageable toxicity.

Based on the preclinical studies, Hsp90 inhibitors have been evaluated in combination with bortezomib. In a multicenter phase I/II trial tanespimycin (100–340 mg/m^2) was combined with bortezomib (0.7–1.3 mg/m^2) given on days 1, 4, 8, and 11 of each 21-day cycle [45]. The highest tested dose of tanespimycin at 340 mg/m^2 and bortezomib at 1.3 mg/m^2 was selected for a phase II portion. Seventy-two patients with relapsed or relapsed and refractory multiple myeloma (MM) were enrolled; 63 patients (89 %) completed the study. The combination was well tolerated and among 67 efficacy-evaluable patients, there were 2 (3 %) complete responses and 8 (12 %) partial responses, for an objective response rate (ORR) of 27 %, including 8 (12 %) minimal responses.

Inhibitors of the PI3K/Akt Pathway Including mTOR Inhibitors

This pathway, which consists of a series of kinases, including PI3K, Akt, mTOR, and p70S6K, as well as several intervening signaling molecules, plays an important role in the regulation of cell growth, proliferation, and survival [46–48]. The PI3K/Akt pathway is critical for proliferation and survival of the myeloma cell and mediates some of the anti-apoptotic and proliferative effects of IL6 [49], IGF-1 [49, 50], SDF-1α [51], and HGF.

Perifosine is the best-studied Akt inhibitor in the setting of myeloma [52]. Initial trials focused on perifosine as a single agent. In a phase II trial of perifosine, alone or with dexamethasone, 64 patients with relapsed myeloma and median of four lines of prior therapies were enrolled [53]. Among 48 patients evaluable for response, best response to single agent after two cycles was MR in 1 patient and stable disease in 22 patients (46 %). Addition of dexamethasone in 37 patients with disease progression led to a partial response in 13 %. Most common adverse events included nausea, vomiting, diarrhea, fatigue, increased creatinine, and anemia. Subsequent trials examined the combination of perifosine with lenalidomide or bortezomib [54, 55]. Other PI3K inhibitors in phase I studies include PI-103, BGT-226, BEZ-235, XL-765, XL-147, and the PDK-1 inhibitors derived from staurosporin and celecoxib [36].

The mTOR kinase, downstream in the PI3K/Akt pathway is a serine/threonine kinase that on activation, facilitates cell cycle progression from G1 into S-phase by phosphorylating p70S6 kinase (p70S6K) and 4E-BP1 [56, 57]. mTOR inhibitors include the macrolide rapamycin, and its analogues temsirolimus (CCI-779) and everolimus (RAD001) [58]. Preclinical studies confirm the anti-MM activity of rapamycin and its analogues [59, 60]. Both CCI779 and RAD001 have been studied in phase II trials in patients with relapsed disease with very little clinically relevant anti-myeloma activity. Better understanding of the reciprocal activity of TORC1 and TORC2 has shed light on potential mechanisms of action and has led to development of dual inhibitors. In addition, combined targeting of the PI3K/Akt/mTOR pathways may provide a way to enhance activity and several dual inhibitors are currently going through early phase trials [34].

Cell Cycle Agents

ARRY-520: ARRY-520 is a kinesin spindle protein inhibitor that arrests cells in mitosis and induces apoptosis due to degradation of the BCL2 family survival protein MCL-1 [61–63]. In the initial phase I study, 31 patients with relapsed or refractory MM with ≥2 prior lines of therapy [including both bortezomib (BTZ) and an immunomodulatory (IMiD) agent], were enrolled. The MTD was determined to be 1.25 mg/m^2/day without G-CSF and 1.5 mg/m^2/day with use of prophylactic G-CSF support. The most commonly reported treatment-related adverse events included anemia, leukopenia, neutropenia, thrombocytopenia, as well as anorexia, blurred vision, diarrhea, dizziness, fatigue, febrile neutropenia, mucositis, nausea, and rash. In this study, three confirmed partial responses (PR) and 1 confirmed minimal response (MR) were observed.

Given the synergy observed with dexamethasone in preclinical myeloma models, ARRY-520 was combined with dexamethasone in a subsequent study [64]. The study included 2 cohorts, cohort 1 receiving 1.5 mg/m^2/day ARRY-520 IV on days 1 and 2 every 2 weeks with prophylactic G-CSF support and cohort 2 receiving 40 mg dex weekly. The most common treatment-related adverse events in both cohorts included thrombocytopenia, anemia, neutropenia, and fatigue. Of 32 patients in cohort 1, confirmed responses (≥minor response (MR)) were observed in 6 patients (19 %) with 5 PR (16 %). Among the 18 evaluable patients in cohort 2, the ORR (≥MR) was 28 %, with four patients ≥PR (22 %).

Dinaciclib: Dinaciclib is a novel, potent, small molecule inhibitor of cyclin-dependent kinases (CDKs), with selective inhibition of CDK1, CDK2, CDK5, and CDK9. In a phase I/II study, 29 patients with relapsed MM and measurable disease were enrolled provided they had not more than four prior lines of therapy for MM [65]. The dose level of 50 mg/m^2 was determined to be the MTD for the phase II portion. The overall confirmed response rate was 3 of 27 (11 %); including two patients at 40 mg/m^2 dose (1 VGPR, 1 PR) and one patient at 50 mg/m^2 dose (1 VGPR) with a PR or better. In addition, two patients at 50 mg/mg^2 dose achieved an MR; translating to an overall response rate of 18.5 % (5 of 27). Leukopenia and thrombocytopenia were the most common hematological AEs, and gastrointestinal symptoms, alopecia, and fatigue were the most common non-hematological AEs seen in the study.

References

1. Verhelle D, Corral LG, Wong K, et al. Lenalidomide and CC-4047 inhibit the proliferation of malignant B cells while expanding normal CD34+ progenitor cells. Cancer Res. 2007;67(2):746–55.
2. Galustian C, Meyer B, Labarthe MC, et al. The anti-cancer agents lenalidomide and pomalidomide inhibit the proliferation and function of T regulatory cells. Cancer Immunol Immunother. 2009;58(7):1033–45.
3. Schey SA, Fields P, Bartlett JB, et al. Phase I study of an immunomodulatory thalidomide analog, CC-4047, in relapsed or refractory multiple myeloma. J Clin Oncol. 2004;22(16):3269–76.
4. Anderson G, Gries M, Kurihara N, et al. Thalidomide derivative CC-4047 inhibits osteoclast formation by down-regulation of PU.1. Blood. 2006;107(8):3098–105.
5. Ferguson GD, Jensen-Pergakes K, Wilkey C, et al. Immunomodulatory drug CC-4047 is a cell-type and stimulus-selective transcriptional inhibitor of cyclooxygenase 2. J Clin Immunol. 2007;27(2):210–20.
6. Streetly MJ, Gyertson K, Daniel Y, Zeldis JB, Kazmi M, Schey SA. Alternate day pomalidomide retains anti-myeloma effect with reduced adverse events and evidence of in vivo immunomodulation. Br J Haematol. 2008;141(1):41–51.
7. Streetly M, Stewart O, Gyertson K, Kazmi MA, Schey S. Pomalidomide monotherapy for relapsed myeloma is associated with excellent responses and prolonged progression free and overall survival. ASH Annu Meet Abstr. 2009;114(22):3878.
8. Lacy MQ, Hayman SR, Gertz MA, et al. Pomalidomide (CC4047) plus low-dose dexamethasone as therapy for relapsed multiple myeloma. J Clin Oncol. 2009;27(30):5008–14.
9. Lacy MQ, Hayman SR, Gertz MA, et al. Pomalidomide (CC4047) plus low dose dexamethasone (Pom/dex) is active and well tolerated in lenalidomide refractory multiple myeloma (MM). Leukemia. 2010;24(11):1934–9.
10. Short KD, Rajkumar SV, Larson D, et al. Incidence of extramedullary disease in patients with multiple myeloma in the era of novel therapy, and the activity of pomalidomide on extramedullary myeloma. Leukemia. 2011;25(6):906–8.
11. Lacy M, Mandrekar S, Gertz MAA, et al. Pomalidomide plus low-dose dexamethasone in myeloma refractory to both bortezomib and lenalidomide: comparison of two dosing strategies in dual-refractory disease. ASH Annu Meet Abstr. 2010;116(21):863.
12. Richardson PG, Siegel D, Baz R, et al. A phase I/II multi-center, randomized, open label dose escalation study to determine the maximum tolerated dose, safety, and efficacy of pomalidomide alone or in combination with low-dose dexamethasone in patients with relapsed and refractory multiple myeloma who have received prior treatment that includes lenalidomide and bortezomib. ASH Annu Meet Abstr. 2010;116(21):864.
13. Leleu X, Attal M, Moreau P, et al. Phase II study of 2 modalities of pomalidomide (CC4047) plus low-dose dexamethasone as therapy for relapsed multiple myeloma. IFM 2009-02. ASH Annu Meet Abstr. 2010;116(21):859.
14. Kuhn DJ, Chen Q, Voorhees PM, et al. Potent activity of carfilzomib, a novel, irreversible inhibitor of the ubiquitin-proteasome pathway, against preclinical models of multiple myeloma. Blood. 2007;110(9):3281–90.
15. Kuhn DJ, Orlowski RZ, Bjorklund CC. Second generation proteasome inhibitors: carfilzomib and immunoproteasome-specific inhibitors (IPSIs). Curr Cancer Drug Targets. 2011;11(3):285–95.
16. O'Connor OA, Stewart AK, Vallone M, et al. A phase I dose escalation study of the safety and pharmacokinetics of the novel proteasome inhibitor carfilzomib (PR-171) in patients with hematologic malignancies. Clin Cancer Res. 2009;15(22):7085–91.
17. Parlati F, Lee SJ, Aujay M, et al. Carfilzomib can induce tumor cell death through selective inhibition of the chymotrypsin-like activity of the proteasome. Blood. 2009;114(16):3439–47.
18. Sacco A, Aujay M, Morgan B, et al. Carfilzomib-dependent selective inhibition of the chymotrypsin-like activity of the proteasome leads to antitumor activity in Waldenstrom's macroglobulinemia. Clin Cancer Res. 2011;17(7):1753–64.
19. Alsina M, Trudel S, Furman RR, et al. A phase I single-agent study of twice-weekly consecutive-day dosing of the proteasome inhibitor carfilzomib in patients with relapsed or refractory multiple myeloma or lymphoma. Clin Cancer Res. 2012;18(17):4830–40.
20. Jagannath S, Vij R, Stewart AK, et al. An open-label single-arm pilot phase II study (PX-171-003-A0) of low-dose, single-agent carfilzomib in patients with relapsed and refractory multiple myeloma. Clin Lymphoma Myeloma Leuk. 2012;12(5):310–8.
21. Siegel DS, Martin T, Wang M, et al. A phase II study of single-agent carfilzomib (PX-171-003-A1) in patients with relapsed and refractory multiple myeloma. Blood. 2012;120(14):2817–25.
22. Vij R, Siegel DS, Jagannath S, et al. An open-label, single-arm, phase II study of single-agent carfilzomib in patients with relapsed and/or refractory multiple myeloma who have been previously treated with bortezomib. Br J Haematol. 2012;158(6):739–48.

23. Vij R, Wang M, Kaufman JL, et al. An open-label, single-arm, phase II (PX-171-004) study of single-agent carfilzomib in bortezomib-naive patients with relapsed and/or refractory multiple myeloma. Blood. 2012;119(24):5661–70.
24. Kumar S, Bensinger WI, Reeder CB, et al. Weekly dosing of the investigational oral proteasome inhibitor MLN9708 in patients with relapsed and/or refractory multiple myeloma: results from a phase I dose-escalation study. ASH Annu Meet Abstr. 2011;118(21):816.
25. Richardson PG, Baz R, Wang L, et al. Investigational agent MLN9708, an oral proteasome inhibitor, in patients (Pts) with relapsed and/or refractory multiple myeloma (MM): results from the expansion cohorts of a phase I dose-escalation study. ASH Annu Meet Abstr. 2011;118(21):301.
26. Tai YT, Dillon M, Song W, et al. Anti-CS1 humanized monoclonal antibody HuLuc63 inhibits myeloma cell adhesion and induces antibody-dependent cellular cytotoxicity in the bone marrow milieu. Blood. 2008;112(4):1329–37.
27. Jakubowiak AJ, Benson Jr DM, Bensinger W, et al. Elotuzumab in combination with bortezomib in patients with relapsed/refractory multiple myeloma: updated results of a phase I study. ASH Annu Meet Abstr. 2010;116(21):3023.
28. Lonial S, Vij R, Harousseau J-L, et al. Elotuzumab in combination with lenalidomide and low-dose dexamethasone in patients with relapsed/refractory multiple myeloma: interim results of a phase I study. ASH Annu Meet Abstr. 2010;116(21):1936.
29. Tai Y-T, de Weers M, Li X-F, et al. Daratumumab, a novel potent human anti-CD38 monoclonal antibody, induces significant killing of human multiple myeloma cells: therapeutic implication. ASH Annu Meet Abstr. 2009;114(22):608.
30. Groen RW, van der Veer M, Hofhuis FM, et al. In vitro and in vivo efficacy of cd38 directed therapy with daratumumab in the treatment of multiple myeloma. ASH Annu Meet Abstr. 2010;116(21):3058.
31. Plesner T, Lokhorst H, Gimsing P, Nahi H, Lisby S, Richardson PG. Daratumumab, a CD38 monoclonal antibody in patients with multiple myeloma—data from a dose-escalation phase I/II study. ASH Annu Meet Abstr. 2012;120(21):73.
32. Rossi J-F, Manges RF, Sutherland HJ, et al. Preliminary results of CNTO 328, an anti-interleukin-6 monoclonal antibody, in combination with bortezomib in the treatment of relapsed or refractory multiple myeloma. Blood. 2008;112(11):867.
33. Ocio EM, Mateos VM, Maiso P, Pandiella A, San-Miguel JF. New drugs in multiple myeloma: mechanism of action and phase I/II clinical findings. Lancet Oncol. 2008;9:1157–65.
34. Mahindra A, Cirstea D, Raje N. Novel therapeutic targets for multiple myeloma. Future Oncol. 2010;6(3): 407–18.
35. Richardson PG, Mitslades CS, Colson K, et al. Final results of a phase I trial of oral vorinostat (suberoylanilide hydroxamic acid, SAHA) in patients with advanced multiple myeloma. Blood. 2007;110:Abstract 1179.
36. Galli M, Salmoiraghi S, Golay J, et al. A phase II multiple dose clinical trial of histone deactylase inhibitor5 ITF2357 in patients with relapsed or progressive multiple myeloma: preliminary results. Blood. 2007; 2007(110):Abstract 1175.
37. Wolf JL, Siegel D, Matous J, et al. A phase II study of oral panobinostat (LBH589) in adult patients with advanced refractory multiple myeloma. Blood. 2008;112(11):2774.
38. Niesvizky R, Ely S, Mark T, et al. Phase II trial of the histone deacetylase inhibitor romidepsin for the treatment of refractory multiple myeloma. Cancer. 2011; 117(2):336–42.
39. Richardson P, Mitsiades C, Colson K, et al. Phase I trial of oral vorinostat (suberoylanilide hydroxamic acid, SAHA) in patients with advanced multiple myeloma. Leuk Lymphoma. 2008;49(3):502–7.
40. Badros A, Burger AM, Philip S, et al. Phase I study of vorinostat in combination with bortezomib for relapsed and refractory multiple myeloma. Clin Cancer Res. 2009;15(16):5250–7.
41. Weber D, Badros AZ, Jagannath S, et al. Vorinostat plus bortezomib for the treatment of relapsed/refractory multiple myeloma: early clinical experience. Blood. 2008;112(11):871.
42. San-Miguel JF, Sezer O, Siegel D, et al. A phase IB, multi-center, open-label dose-escalation study of oral panobinostat (LBH589) and I.V. bortezomib in patients with relapsed multiple myeloma. ASH Annu Meet Abstr. 2009;114(22):3852.
43. Mitsiades CS, Mitsiades N, McMullin CJ, et al. Antimyeloma activity of heat shock protein-90 inhibition. Blood. 2006;107(3):1092–100.
44. Richardson PG, Chanan-Khan AA, Alsina M, et al. Tanespimycin monotherapy in relapsed multiple myeloma: results of a phase I dose-escalation study. Br J Haematol. 2010;150(4):438–45.
45. Richardson PG, Chanan-Khan AA, Lonial S, et al. Tanespimycin and bortezomib combination treatment in patients with relapsed or relapsed and refractory multiple myeloma: results of a phase I/II study. Br J Haematol. 2011;153(6):729–40.
46. Bjornsti MA, Houghton PJ. The TOR pathway: a target for cancer therapy. Nat Rev Cancer. 2004;4(5): 335–48.
47. Sansal I, Sellers WR. The biology and clinical relevance of the PTEN tumor suppressor pathway. J Clin Oncol. 2004;22(14):2954–63.
48. Kharas MG, Fruman DA. ABL oncogenes and phosphoinositide 3-kinase: mechanism of activation and downstream effectors. Cancer Res. 2005;65(6):2047–53.
49. Tu Y, Gardner A, Lichtenstein A. The phosphatidylinositol 3-kinase/AKT kinase pathway in multiple myeloma plasma cells: roles in cytokine-dependent survival and proliferative responses. Cancer Res. 2000;60(23):6763–70.
50. Ge NL, Rudikoff S. Insulin-like growth factor I is a dual effector of multiple myeloma cell growth. Blood. 2000;96(8):2856–61.
51. Hideshima T, Chauhan D, Hayashi T, et al. The biological sequelae of stromal cell-derived factor-1alpha

in multiple myeloma. Mol Cancer Ther. 2002;1(7): 539–44.
52. Hideshima T, Catley L, Yasui H, et al. Perifosine, an oral bioactive novel alkylphospholipid, inhibits Akt and induces in vitro and in vivo cytotoxicity in human multiple myeloma cells. Blood. 2006;107(10): 4053–62.
53. Richardson P, Lonial S, Jakubowiak A, et al. Multicenter phase II study of perifosine (KRX-0401) alone and in combination with dexamethasone (dex) for patients with relapsed or relapsed/refractory multiple myeloma (MM): promising activity as combination therapy with manageable toxicity. ASH Annu Meet Abstr. 2007;110(11):1164.
54. Richardson P, Wolf J, Jakubowiak A, et al. Phase I/II results of a multicenter trial of perifosine (KRX-0401) + bortezomib in patients with relapsed or relapsed/ refractory multiple myeloma who were previously relapsed from or refractory to bortezomib. Blood. 2008;112(11):870.
55. Jakubowiak AJ, Richardson PG, Zimmerman TM, et al. Final phase I results of perifosine in combination with lenalidomide and dexamethasone in patients with relapsed or refractory multiple myeloma (MM). ASH Annu Meet Abstr. 2010;116(21):3064.
56. Brunn GJ, Hudson CC, Sekulic A, et al. Phosphorylation of the translational repressor PHAS-I by the mammalian target of rapamycin. Science. 1997;277(5322):99–101.
57. Burnett PE, Barrow RK, Cohen NA, Snyder SH, Sabatini DM. RAFT1 phosphorylation of the translational regulators p70 S6 kinase and 4E-BP1. Proc Natl Acad Sci U S A. 1998;95(4):1432–7.
58. Ma WW, Adjei AA. Novel agents on the horizon for cancer therapy. CA Cancer J Clin. 2009;59:111–37.
59. Frost P, Moatamed F, Hoang B, et al. In vivo antitumor effects of the mTOR inhibitor CCI-779 against human multiple myeloma cells in a xenograft model. Blood. 2004;104(13):4181–7.
60. Stromberg T, Dimberg A, Hammarberg A, et al. Rapamycin sensitizes multiple myeloma cells to apoptosis induced by dexamethasone. Blood. 2004; 103(8):3138–47.
61. Lonial S, Cohen A, Zonder J, et al. The novel KSP inhibitor ARRY-520 demonstrates single-agent activity in refractory myeloma: results from a phase II trial in patients with relapsed/refractory multiple myeloma (MM). ASH Annu Meet Abstr. 2011;118(21):2935.
62. Shah JJ, Cohen AD, Zonder JA, et al. Phase I trial of ARRY-520 in relapsed/refractory multiple myeloma (RR MM). J Clin Oncol. 2010;28(15_Suppl):8132.
63. Shah JJ, Zonder J, Cohen A, et al. ARRY-520 shows durable responses in patients with relapsed/refractory multiple myeloma in a phase I dose-escalation study. ASH Annu Meet Abstr. 2011;118(21):1860.
64. Shah JJ, Zonder JA, Cohen A, et al. The novel KSP inhibitor ARRY-520 is active both with and without low-dose dexamethasone in patients with multiple myeloma refractory to bortezomib and lenalidomide: results from a phase II study. ASH Annu Meet Abstr. 2012;120(21):449.
65. Kumar SK, LaPlant BR, Chng WJ, et al. Phase I/II trial of a novel CDK inhibitor dinaciclib (SCH727965) in patients with relapsed multiple myeloma demonstrates encouraging single agent activity. ASH Annu Meet Abstr. 2012;120(21):76.

Biological Therapy for Multiple Myeloma

13

Camilo Ayala-Breton, Stephen J. Russell, and Kah-Whye Peng

Introduction

The National Cancer Institute defines biological therapy as: "A form of treatment that implies the administration of substances which produce a biological reaction in the organism thus enhancing or restoring the host immune response, modifying the behavior of cancer cells, blocking the pathways of cell neoplastic transformation and tumor ability to metastasize, or facilitating the repair of cells damaged by aggressive forms of cancer treatment. It includes the use of sera, antitoxins, vaccines, genes, cells, tissues, and organs." In this chapter we will highlight different biological therapies that have been recently used against multiple myeloma (MM).

C. Ayala-Breton • K.-W. Peng
Department of Molecular Medicine, Mayo Clinic, 200 First Street SW, Rochester, MN 55905, USA
e-mail: peng.kah@mayo.edu

S.J. Russell, M.D. (✉)
Division of Hematology and Department of Molecular Medicine, Mayo Clinic, 200 First Street, SW, Rochester, MN 55905, USA
e-mail: sjr@mayo.edu

Monoclonal Antibodies

Monoclonal antibodies can kill or compromise targeted cancer cells directly by interfering with the signaling functions of key receptors, or indirectly by recruiting host effector functions including the complement cascade, NK cells, neutrophils, and macrophages, which interact with the antibody-coated cell via their Fc receptors [1, 2]. Alternatively, through various protein engineering strategies, antibody Fc fragments specifically recognizing a cancer cell surface antigen can be fused to a wide variety of foreign proteins or peptides that are capable of killing or compromising the targeted cells. Thus, immunotoxins consist of an Fc fragment fused to a ribosomal toxin and bispecific antibodies can be made by fusing two single chain antibodies tail to tail, to produce an engineered protein that cross-links tumor cells to host effector cells [3]. After a long period of preclinical development, monoclonal antibodies have emerged as extremely versatile and effective anticancer drugs, some of the most notable examples being anti-CD20 antibodies for B-cell lymphoma, anti-Her2 antibodies for breast cancer, anti-EGFR antibodies for lung cancer, and anti-VEGFR antibodies for a variety of malignancies [4–6]. Thus, there is enormous optimism that monoclonal antibodies will provide significant benefit to myeloma patients. Accordingly, numerous potentially suitable

M.A. Gertz and S.V. Rajkumar (eds.), *Multiple Myeloma: Diagnosis and Treatment*, DOI 10.1007/978-1-4614-8520-9_13, © Mayo Foundation for Medical Education and Research 2014 myeloma cell surface targets have been identified and there are many antibody-based antimyeloma therapies currently in preclinical development or in early phase clinical trials. The most notable examples are summarized below.

CD20

Rituximab, a human/mouse hybrid monoclonal antibody [7], was the first antibody tested as a therapy for multiple myeloma. Although successful for the treatment of non-Hodgkin lymphoma, this monoclonal antibody has limited efficacy for MM. In one study [8], 19 patients with multiple myeloma having variable levels of CD20 were treated with Rituximab for 4 weeks. Sixty four percent of the patients did not respond, and all the responders had CD20+ myeloma cells suggesting that patients could be selected for this therapy based on their CD20 levels, an observation that has been reported by other researchers [9]. Rituximab use in MM is therefore limited to those few patients expressing CD20 on their plasma cells [10].

Beta2-Microglobulin

Beta2-microglobulin (β_2M) is an 11.6 kDa polypeptide, a component of the major histocompatibility complex (MHC) class I molecule on the cell surface of nucleated cells. One of its main functions is to interact with and stabilize the structure of the MHC class I α chain. Monoclonal antibodies directed to β_2M have a pro-apoptotic effect on MM cells and have been shown to recruit MHC class I molecules to lipid rafts and triggering the caspase-9 cascade [11]. Anti-β_2M mAbs were nontoxic in mice expressing human HLA-A2 α-chain and were therapeutically effective against subcutaneous multiple myeloma [12]. Human testing has not been reported.

CD38

CD38 is a 46-kDa type II transmembrane glycoprotein expressed on lymphoid and myeloid cells but not in mature lymphocytes [13]. It is overexpressed on MM cells [14]. Daratumumab binds CD38 and kills MM cells by antibody-dependent cell-mediated cytotoxicity (ADCC) and complement-dependent cytotoxicity (CDC). Daratumumab controlled tumor growth in a mouse model of MM and is currently being evaluated alone or in combination with bortezomib, lenalidomide, and dexamethasone in four ongoing phase I/II clinical trials (http://www.clinicaltrials.gov) [15].

CD40

CD40 is highly expressed in MM. It is a transmembrane glycoprotein of the tumor necrosis factor receptor superfamily, involved in B-cell activation, differentiation, and the formation of germinal centers. Lucatumumab (HCD122, CHIR-12.12) is a fully human IgG1 monoclonal antibody that blocks the interaction of CD40 and its ligand. It also induces ADCC and binds to CD138+ cells from >80 % of MM patients [16]. In a phase I study in patients with relapsed/refractory MM, doses of lucatumumab in excess of 3 mg/kg resulted in only mild to moderate adverse effects, and almost half of the patients had disease stabilization [17]. Dacetuzumab (SGN-40) (Seattle Genetics, Inc., Bothell, WA, USA) is a humanized monoclonal antibody directed to CD40 that kills MM cells by ADCC and apoptosis induction. A phase I multi-dose study in relapsed/refractory MM patients showed good tolerability at doses up to 12 mg/kg with steroid pre-medication [18]. Best clinical response was stable disease in 9 of 44 treated patients.

CD47

CD47 is an *N*-glycosylated transmembrane protein expressed in all hematopoietic cells [19] but is highly expressed on myeloma cells [20]. An anti-CD47 monoclonal antibody did not induce ADCC or CDC but promoted phagocytosis of human MM cells by macrophages. Using the SCID-hu model in which primary myeloma cells were grown in human fetal bone, the anti-CD47 inhibited growth of the myeloma cells in vivo [21]. Human testing has not yet been reported.

CD54 (ICAM-1)

CD54 is a surface glycoprotein that binds leukocyte function-associated antigen 1 (CD11a/CD18) and is present at low levels in leukocytes and endothelial cells as well as on malignant plasma cells [22]. A murine IgG2a[kappa] monoclonal anti-human CD54 antibody (UV3) was generated against human myeloma cells but was further engineered into a mouse/human chimeric IgG1[kappa] antibody (cUV3) [23, 24]. This chimeric antibody is equally effective at binding to CD54+ cells and induces cell killing by ADCC and CDC in vitro. Furthermore, it significantly extended the survival of SCID mice bearing disseminated ARH-77 myeloma cells from 29 days (untreated controls) to 150 days (anti-CD54 treatment) [25].

CD56

An isoform of the neural cell adhesion molecule (NCAM) and NK cells marker and is a membrane glycoprotein of the immunoglobulin superfamily. CD56-positive plasma cells were found in 66 % of the tested MM patients, while normal plasma cells do not express CD56 [26, 27]. huN901-DM1, a humanized monoclonal antibody against CD56, conjugated to DM1, a potent cytotoxic agent, preferentially kills CD56+ MM cells. In SCID mice with OPM2 human MM xenografts, this conjugated antibody decreased the secretion of paraprotein, inhibited tumor growth, and increased mice survival [28].

CD74

CD74 is a cell surface-expressed epitope of the HLA class II-associated invariant chain and the monoclonal antibody LL1 binds to this protein. CD74 is expressed in association with HLA-DR and is involved in the maturation of B cells. CD74 expression was observed in 19 out of 22 MM patients. LL1 mAb inhibited the growth of an MM cell line expressing CD74 [29]. A humanized version of this antibody was tested in vitro and in vivo, showing a significant reduction in the tumor growth [30]. To increase potency, LL1 was conjugated to doxorubicin at a ratio of 8 molecules of drug to 1 mAb. The antibody-drug conjugate showed better efficacy in human tumor xenografts compared to either antibody alone or free antibody plus free drug [31].

CD138 (Syndecan-1)

CD138 is a member of the heparan sulfate proteoglycan family, expressed on plasma cells, and is a diagnostic marker of multiple myeloma [32]. Three antibodies anti-CD138 have been used to treat MM. An example is the nBT062 murine/human chimeric monoclonal antibody (CLB) conjugated with cytotoxic maytansinoid moieties. These conjugates were active against patient-derived primary MM cells, but are not toxic against CD138– cells from healthy donors. Also, in tumor xenografts, these three antibodies present activity against MM and can block the adhesion of MM to bone marrow stromal cells. The mechanism of action is by induction of G_2-M cell cycle arrest and apoptosis [33].

CS1 (CD2 Subset 1, CD319, CRACC, SLAMF7, 19A24)

CS1, a member of the signaling lymphocyte-activating molecule-related receptor family, is exclusively expressed on plasma cells and highly expressed on MM cells. A humanized monoclonal antibody against CS1 (HuLuc63) can mediate NK cell-mediated ADCC towards MM cells [34, 35]. Elotuzumab (HuLuc63) in combination with bortezomib can further reduce the tumor burden of patient-derived MM tumors established in SCID mice [36]. Due to its strong in vitro and in vivo anti-MM properties, elotuzumab in combination with bortezomib was used in a phase I clinical trial against MM. Patients received 2.5–20 mg/kg of elotuzumab without dose-limiting toxicities. Six cycles of elotuzumab in combination with bortezomib resulted in 48 % objective response rate with time to progression of 9.46 months of the patients [37].

Interleukin-6

Interleukin-6 (IL-6) is a cytokine whose functions include regulation of the immune response, acute-phase response, and bone metabolism. Increased levels of this cytokine have been observed in B-cells malignancies. Expression of IL-6 in the BM contribute to the growing of MM tumors [38]. Some anti-IL6 monoclonal antibodies have been tested against MM: mAb 1339 is a high-affinity fully human anti-IL-6 mAb (IgG1); it was able to inhibit MM growth in humanized mice [39]. The (CLB IL6/8; K_d 6.25×10^{-12} M) was used in a phase I dose escalating study, 12 patients received total doses of this antibody ranging from 140 to 1,120 mg. Importantly, it presented low toxicity, low immunogenicity, and a long half-life. Although the evaluation of the efficacy was not the aim of the study, a significant decrease in the C-reactive protein was observed in 11 out of 12 patients, indicating IL-6 blocking although no reduction in the M protein level (>50 %) was observed [40].

Myeloma Vaccines

While "complete remissions" are frequently achieved with modern myeloma therapy, the disease usually relapses. This has provided a strong impetus for the development of vaccination strategies that can eliminate residual unseen myeloma cells with the goal of converting complete remissions to cures. However, available evidence to support the optimistic view that this is an attainable goal remains relatively scant. For example, myeloma virtually never regresses spontaneously and virtually always relapses after successful therapy indicating that the immune system has minimal contribution to the control of the disease. However, occasional patients relapsing after allogeneic stem cell transplant have had remarkable disease responses when infused with T cells harvested from their original stem cell donors. Certain monoclonal antibodies have also been shown to mediate disease regression in some treated patients [41–44]. Thus, there is at least some clinical evidence that myeloma cells can be destroyed by humoral and/or cellular immune responses. In addition to these clinical observations, there have been several preclinical studies demonstrating that various vaccine formulations can provoke a protective or even therapeutic antimyeloma immune response [45, 46]

As to the question of which antigens to use in a myeloma vaccine formulation, a possibility is to use a single purified antigen such as the idiotypic immunoglobulin. But this protein is shed (secreted) so efficiently from the myeloma cells that it provides a poor target for a humoral response and contains very few unique peptides so may also be a poor target for T cell responses. At the other extreme, the entire repertoire of potential myeloma antigens can be harnessed by using the myeloma cell as the basis for a vaccine, either directly or indirectly, for example by vaccinating with dendritic cells that have somehow "sampled" the myeloma cells or have been transfected with their genetic material. Given the enormous appeal of myeloma vaccination, the wide range of possible vaccine formulations, and the generally promising results that are obtained in preclinical model systems, there have been a large number of early phase clinical trials of myeloma vaccination, briefly reviewed below. But to date there are no approved products.

Peptide-Based Vaccines

This therapy consists of introducing small peptides derived from MM biomarkers to induce the immune response against the tumor cells [45].

These therapies are based in T-cell maturation by dendritic cells. Several studies have tried to enhance the maturation of DC and create a strong immune response. In one study, NK cells and DCs were stimulated by IFN-α, poly(I:C), and IL-2, resulting in an induction of Th-1 responses and in a superior induction of CTL specific for myeloma-associated antigens compared to the stimulation by standard DC [47].

There are several Tumor-Associated Antigens (TAA) utilized for in vitro experiments and clinical trials.

Cancer-testis antigen NY-ESO-1. NY-ESO-1 was discovered while screening an esophageal squamous cell carcinoma cDNA library against sera from a patient [48, 49]. NY-ESO-1 mRNA was found only in testis and ovary and not in non-germ line tissues but showed expression in a wide array of human cancers including MM [50]. NY-ESO-1 expression both at the RNA and protein level is most prevalent in advanced MM cases and the expression of NY-ESO-1 is related to the clonal evolution of MM. Various peptide vaccination trials against NY-ESO-1 have been conducted against solid tumors and in MM [50, 51].

Wilms' tumor gene (WT1). This protein is an oncogene and is involved in cell growing and differentiation. Since WT1 expression seems to be involved in tumorigenesis, it is a good candidate to be used as a cancer antigen for immunotherapy [52]. The low levels of expression of WT1 in normal progenitors make it possible to differentiate normal from malignant cells. Wt1-specific CTLs attack cancer but not normal cells in vivo and in vitro [52]. Myeloma cells are killed by WT1-specific CTLs, despite expressing lower levels of mRNA for WT1 compared to lymphoma cells; however, the levels of IFN gamma produced for WT1-specific CTLs were similar when stimulated with lymphoma and multiple myeloma cells [53]. An WT1-based immunotherapy in one patient resulted in reduction of the M protein in urine and a decrease of myeloma cells in bone marrow [54]

Mucin-1 (MUC-1). MUC-1 is a type I transmembranal protein present on multiple myeloma cells. In a study it was found that almost half of the patients tested present MUC-1-specific CTLs with no difference between peripheral blood and bone marrow [55]. This protein is overexpressed in 92 % of the analyzed multiple myeloma patients. It was also found that CTLs specific for MUC-1 were able to lyse in an antigen-specific manner tumor cells from multiple myeloma patients [56].

Receptor for hyaluronic-acid-mediated motility (RHAMM). RHAMM is expressed in the tumor cells of 80 % of the patients with MM but not in PBMC or CD34+ bone marrow stem cells [57]. In a Phase 1/2 vaccination trial, 10 patients with residual or controlled disease (4 of them with MM) received 4 subcutaneous doses at a biweekly interval of RHAMM R3 peptide. No signs of toxicity were observed in the patients while 3 weeks after vaccinations, 2 of them presented a reduction in plasma cells and ß2-microglobulin in the bone marrow. Seven (70 %) of ten vaccinated patients showed an increase of RHAMM-R3-specific T cells [58].

Dickkopf-1 (DKK1). DKK1 is a secreted protein that interacts with Lrp-6 and inhibits Wnt/ß-catenin signaling. Interestingly, MM cells but not normal tissue express DKK1; antibody treatment against DKK1 reduced tumor burden in mouse models [59, 60]. CTLs specific for DKK1 present strong cytotoxicity for MM cells from patients but they did not kill DC, B cells, and PBMC. DKK1-specific CTLs can be generated by stimulating autologous T cells with DCs pulsed with DKK1 peptides, making DKK1 an excellent candidate for immunotherapy against MM [61].

Survivin. It is an apoptosis inhibitor family member; it is expressed only in thymus cells, CD34+ bone marrow-derived hematopoietic progenitor cells, basal colonic epithelial cells, and activated endothelial cells. It is overexpressed in cancer cells, including MM. Specific T-Cells for an HLA-A2-restricted survivin peptide were found in 39 % of the analyzed patients with MM. MM cells from BM specimens of 7 of 11 patients were found to express survivin [62, 63].

HM1-24 Antigen. It is a B cell-restricted antigen, a type-II transmembrane glycoprotein originally identified as a target of monoclonal antibodies raised against MM cell lines. This protein is not expressed in their peripheral blood, bone marrow, liver, spleen, kidney, or heart [64]. A study was performed to find human leukocyte antigen (HLA)-A22 restricted T-cell epitopes within the HM1.24 antigen. The peptide sequence was scanned and eight peptides with the highest probability of being immunogenic were analyzed; the HM1.24 aa22-30 peptide (LLLGIGILV) showed the most frequent activation of CD8(+) T cells. This newly identified HLA-A2-restricted T-cell epitope is processed and presented by MHC class I and the activated CD8(+) T cells are able to lyse MM cell lines [65].

Melan-A. It is a melanocyte lineage-specific antigen commonly expressed by melanoma tumor cells. Melan-A and melan-analog-specific CD8+ T-cells are able to recognize HM1.24 antigen, and Melan-specific T-cells from MM patients are able to lyse autologous MM cells [66].

P21-activated serin kinase 2 (PAK2) and cyclin-dependent kinase inhibitor 1A (CDKN1A). PAK2 is a protein expressed in malignant lymphatic cells. In a test to identify 120 genes that discriminate normal and malignant PCs, CDKN1A was one of the most significantly differentially expressed genes [46].

Cancer-testis antigens. Cancer-testis antigens are expressed almost exclusively in germ line and malignancies in advanced MM patients. Their expression is not decreased or lost during the course of the disease [67]. It was found that MAGEC1/CT7, LAGE-1, and MAGEA3/6 were frequently expressed (77 %, 49 %, and 41 %, respectively). MAGEC1/CT7 is an ideal candidate for MM immunotherapy, since plasma cells of patients with MGUS express MAGE-C1/CT-7 but no other CT antigens and MAGEC1/CT7 is absent in nonmalignant plasma cells [68].

Idiotypic Vaccines

The myeloma idiotype (Id) is a B-cell tumor antigen determinant of the variable region within the immunoglobulin; this is a true cancer antigen since they all come from a unique B-cell clone [69].

The use of idiotypes as vaccines was proposed more than 30 years ago; in that study the author showed that Balb/C mice immunized against MM idiotypes can suppress the formation of tumors from the corresponding cells [70].

Several studies have been done to determine the optimal conditions of the Id vaccines; this include the use of immunogenic molecules such as keyhole limpet hemocyanin (KLH), the co-injection of GM-CSF, or the use of dendritic cells [71].

There have been a substantial amount of trials for using Id vaccination against MM. Table 13.1 shows some of the vaccination trials done in the past 10 years.

Adoptive Cell Therapy

The best available evidence to support the notion that adoptive cell therapy might be of value in multiple myeloma comes from case reports of patients relapsing after allogeneic stem cell transplant who had remarkable disease responses when infused with T cells harvested from their original stem cell donors [84]. The concept of adoptive cell therapy is that autologous or allogeneic cells (usually T or NK cells) can be expanded outside the body and administered by intravenous infusion, whereupon they will traffic to sites of active disease, recognize the myeloma cells, and kill them [85, 86]. Various genes can be introduced into the immune cells outside the body to enhance their performance. For example, chimeric T cell receptors can be used to redirect the specificity of the effector cells, enhancing their ability to recognize the myeloma cells, and to proliferate in the tumor microenvironment [87, 88]. T cells expressing this type of chimeric receptor are called T bodies and have recently shown considerable promise in the treatment of chronic lymphocytic leukemia when targeted to CD20 or EBV-associated lymphomas when targeted to EBV antigens, providing a strong impetus to the development of myeloma-specific T bodies [89, 90]. "Suicide" genes can also be introduced into the adoptively transferred cells as a safety measure so that they can be destroyed by pro-drug administration if they ever cause unacceptable toxicities [91]. As more is learned of the ligand-receptor systems that govern the extravasation and migration of various recirculating cells, the potential for genetic modifications to enhance their antimyeloma activity is expected to increase further. However, despite the promising

Table 13.1 Results of selected vaccination trials done in the past 10 years in multiple myeloma

Pts. (age)	Stage disease	Previous treatment	Vaccine	Route	Dose schedule	Immune response	Clinical outcome	References
12 (44–60)	Stage II or III	HDT and PBSCT	DC/Id	IV (DC/Id)	Two doses, 15 days apart (DC/Id)		Id-specific T-cell proliferation (2/12 pts.) KLH-specific T cell proliferation (12/12 pts.)	[72]
			KLH/Id	SC (Id/KLH)	Five doses, 4 weeks after the last DC/Id injection (Id/KLH + GM-CSF)		Partial response (8/12 pts.) Six patients alive and well (24–37 months follow-up)	
6 (ND)	Stage I		Id + IL-12 (3/6 pts.) Id + IL-12 + GM-CSF (3/6 pts.)	IC (Id, GM-CSF) SC (IL-12)	Immunizations at weeks 0, 2, 4, 6, 8, 14, and 30	Id-specific T cell response (4/6)	No toxicity Complete molecular regression (1/6 pts.) Reduction of clonotypical B cells (3/6 pts.) No major tumor reduction in all patients	[73]
15 (ND)	Stage II–III	Chem. PBPC infusion	KLH/Id + GM-CSF	SC	Immunization at weeks 0, 2, 6, 10, 14, 24, and 28	Anti-KLH IgG and IgM (9/10 pts.). IgG up to 2 years Anti-GM-CSF antibodies (3/15 pts.) Anti-Id IgG (3/15 pts.) and IgE (5/15 pts.) TCR diversity increased (6 pts.)	Progression-free survival 40 months Overall survival 82 months	[74]
4 (45–52)	DP	Allo-SCT Chem.	KLH/Id	Id	Three cycles of three vaccinations (every 1, 2, or 3 months)	Anti-KLH T antibody response (4/4 pts.)	Well-tolerated vaccination Monoclonal component slight decrease (2/4 pts.)	[75]
			DC (CD14+) + Id + GM-CSF + IL-4	SC	DC/Id (Id) + KLH/Id (SC) + GM-CSF	Anti-KLH T-cell proliferation response (4/4 pts.) Ex vivo secretion of TNFα, IL-6, IFN gamma	Stable MC levels SD (1/4 pts.)	
18 (46–82)	Stage I–II		Id + IL-12	IC	Id (IC), and IL-12 (SC) or GM-CSF	Id-specific T-cell response (9/18 pts.)	No clinical response (after 32 weeks)	[76]
			Id + IL-12 + GM-CSF	SC	Immunization at weeks 0, 2, 4, 6, 8, and 14	Th1 polarized response (IL-12-treated group 4/5 pts.)		
10(50–83)	Stage I–III		Id + GM-CSF Id + IL-12	IC	Immunization at weeks 0, 2, 4, 6, 8, and 14 (induction phase)	Overall Id-response in blood (5/10 pts.) and BM (4/10 pts.)	Progressive disease (6/10 pts.) at late testing time	[77]
			Id + IL-12 + GM-CSF		Immunization at weeks 30, 46, 62, 78, 94, and 110 (maintenance)	ID-specific T cells in blood and/or BM (6/10 pts.)	Mixed Th1/Th2 response (3/10 pts.) or Th2 (3/10 pts.)	

(continued)

Table 13.1 (continued)

Pts. (age)	Stage disease	Previous treatment	Vaccine	Route	Dose schedule	Immune response	Clinical outcome	References
28 (46–82)	Stage I or II	Untreated (24/28) Chem. (4/28)	Id + IL-12 Id + IL-12 + GM-CSF		Immunization at weeks 0, 2, 4, 6, 8, and 14 (induction phase) Immunization at weeks 30, 46, 62, 78, 94, and 110 (maintenance)	Idiotypic-specific T-cell response (16/28) Idiotypic-specific DTH response (3/28)	Local sink reaction to vaccine (19/28) Reduction of M protein (1/28) Minor response 21 months after last Immunization (1/28) ID-specific T cell response (3/16 responder pts.)	[78]
15 (37–68)	Stage I–III	ASCT	DC (CD14+) + Id + KLH	SC	Three SC and two IV doses 2 weeks apart	KLH-specific antibody response (15/15 pts.)	No serious adverse effects during vaccinations	[79]
				IV		KLH-specific T-cell proliferation (10/15 pts.) Id-specific T-cell proliferation (8/15 pts.)	Stable disease (7/15) Partial response (1/15)	
			DC (CD14+) + Id (class I peptide) + KLH		Monthly SC injections thereafter in case of SD observed	Id-positive DTH test (4/15)		
11 (51–87)	Stage I–II	Untreated (10/11)	Id + GM-CSF Id + IL-12	IC (Id)	Immunization at weeks 0, 2, 4, 6, 8, and 14 (induction phase)	Id-specific T-cell response (6/11)	Th1 cell response (6/11) Reduction of CMC (4/11) Stable levels of CMC (2/11)	[80]
		Treated (CPA, IFN, betamethasone)	Id + IL-12 + GM-CSF		Immunization at weeks 30, 46, 62, 78, 94, and 110 (maintenance)		Complete molecular remission (2/11)	
27 (30–69)	Stage II or III	Allo-SCT	Id-loaded APC	IV	Immunizations at weeks 0, 2, 4, and 16	ND	Overall survival of 5.3 years of treated patients, 3.4 years survival for database control group	[81]
9 (42–72)	Smoldering (8/9) SD (1/9)		DC + Id	IN (9/9)	Four DC vaccines (at days 1, 14, 21, and 28) Low dose IL-2 subcutaneously for 5 days after each DC vaccination	T-cell response to KLH and increase anti-Id B cells (all pts.) Id-specific response of T cells (4/9 pts.) Positive skin DTH to Id or KLH-pulsed DC (7/8 pts.)	Progressive Disease (4/9 pts.) SD (4/9 pts.) PD/SD (after 1 year) (1/9 pts.)	[82]
9 (42–68)	Stage I		Id + KLH	IV (5), SC (4)	Five vaccinations every 4 weeks	T-cell response to Id 5/9	No signs of allergic reactions Decrease of M protein (3/9) Decrease in plasma cell infiltration 2/7	[83]

Pts. patients, *HDT* high-dose chemotherapy, *PBSCT* peripheral blood stem cell transplantation, *DC* dendritic cells, *Id* idiotype, *KLH* keyhole limpet hemocyanin, *IV* intravenous, *SC* subcutaneous, *GM-CSF* granulocyte-macrophage colony-stimulating factor, *ND* non-described, *DP* disease progression, *Allo-SCT* allogeneic stem cell transplantation, *Chem.* chemotherapy, *PBPC* peripheral blood progenitor cell, *TCR* t-cell receptor, *MC* monoclonal component, *IC* intracutaneous, *SD* stable disease, *CMC* circulating myeloma cells future, it must be acknowledged that there has to date been relatively little clinical experience of adoptive cell transfer for myeloma therapy. A brief overview is provided below.

Allogeneic transplantations have resulted in an increase in the survival of multiple myeloma patients, and this efficacy might be due to graft-versus-disease effect mediated by alloreactive donor T cells. In a study comprising 62 reports received by the European Group for Blood and Marrow Transplantation (EBMT) registry between 1983 and 1993, 42 % of the patients achieved complete remission following bone marrow transplantation. It was observed that grade III to IV graft-versus-host disease was related to low survival while subtype immunoglobulin A myeloma were a positive prognosis factor [92].

γδ T cells can recognize tumor antigens through a non-MHC mechanism; their cytotoxicity against MM was evaluated after their expansion ex vivo, as part as an anti-MM immunotherapy. The expansion of γδ T cells from patients with MM was achieved by incubation of γδ T cells with IL-2 and zoledronate, the cells specifically lyzed MM cells and were not toxic against healthy normal cells from the same patient [93].

Human T cells expressing NKG2D receptors fused to CD3ζ cytoplasmic domain can kill MM cells in vitro and in vivo. The injection of these T cells into mice leads to an activation of the host immune system as indicated by an increase in the expression of CD69 in NK cells, CD4+, and CD8+ T cells. The long-term survival of the mice was increased and, interestingly, the mice were resistant to tumor re-challenge, indicating that an antitumor immunity was developed [94]. In a continuation of this work, a phase II clinical trial was done to analyze the effect of ex vivo-expanded NKG2D+ CD3+ CD8+ T cells after autologous transplantation. After this immune therapy, there was an increase in tumor-specificity immunity as indicated by an increase in the cell killing of autologous MM cells [95].

Natural Killer Cells

Natural killer (NK) cells are cytotoxic CD16+ CD56+ and CD3– lymphocytes (~10 % of peripheral blood lymphocytes) with the ability to lyse tumor cells and virus-infected cells. They also express cytokines that further amplify the immune response. The biologic mechanism that transformed cells or virus-infected cells utilize to downregulate MHC class I molecules on the cell surface involves ligands of the NK-cell inhibitory KIR (Killer immunoglobulin-like receptor). The lack of MHC class I triggers cell lysis by NK cells [96].

The feasibility of transfusing haplo-identical, T-cell depleted, KIR-ligand mismatched NK cells was investigated in patients with MM treated first with melphalan and fludarabine, followed by autologous stem cells transplantation. The NK cells were able to kill U266 myeloma cells and MM cells from patients. The transplanted NK cells survived in the donor for around 14 days, and around 8 days post-transplantation a potent anti-donor immune response was observed. An anti-HLA antigen antibody enhanced the killing effect of the transplanted NK cells, and 50 % of the treated patients achieved complete or near-complete remission [97].

NK can be also activated by tumor-associated antigens (TaNK cells) and exhibit a powerful killing of NK-resistant cells. In a study, TaNK were generated by NK cells from 21 MM patients; the TaNK cells were able to kill CD138+ cells while leaving CD138– bone marrow cells unaffected. Interestingly, TaNK derived from patients treated with dexamethasone did not show any loss of activity, supporting combination of TaNK and dexamethasone therapies [98].

NK cells from killer immunoglobulin-like receptor ligand (KIR-L) mismatched donors can overcome inhibitory signals from MM cells and show a superior cytotoxicity against MM cells. To expand NK cells, they are co-cultured with K562 cells expressing IL15 and 4-1BBL [99]. This expanded NK cells (exp-NK) can home to the tumor sites and also have anti-growth activity against OMP2 and primary MM xenograft tumors. Based on these results, a phase II clinical trial has been initiated to investigate the effect of exp-NK cells for relapsed/refractory GEP-defined high-risk MM [85].

NK-92 is an NK cell line that has been tested on clinical trials and has shown safety in a phase I trial of patients with advanced renal cell cancer and melanoma [100]. Another NK cell line KHYG-1 showed preferential killing for MM cells, demonstrating higher cytotoxicity against MM than NK-92 cells. The in vivo efficacy of NK-92 cells was also tested; this cell line was distributed to the tumor sites and was able to reduce myeloma burden in the treated mice [101].

NK cells from MM patients can be expanded ex vivo and show enhanced cytotoxicity against MM cells. This effect requires the interaction of the NK cells with the target MM cells. Importantly, there was no toxicity against normal cells [102].

Cytokine-Induced Killer Cells

One of the pioneering works of cytokine-induced immune effector cells is the characterization of Lymphokine-Activated Killer (LAK) cells. These cells are generated by the incubation of normal lymphocytes with IL-2. The resulting cells are cytotoxic effector cells whose activity is not restricted by MHC and are able to kill NK-resistant tumor cells [103].

A more potent type of cytokine-induced cells are cytokine-induced killer (CIK); these are generated by the incubation with IFN-γ for 1 day (to increase the numbers of IL-2 receptors on the cells), and then a dose of anti-CD3 (to trigger proliferation of T-cells) and IL-2 (to increase cytotoxicity). After a period of 28 days of incubation CD3+ CD56+ cells can be expanded by up to 1,000-fold and present a better cytotoxicity against tumors compared to CD3+ CD56− cells. These cells had little toxicity against a subset of normal human hematopoietic precursor cells [104, 105].

CIK cells have been used against multiple myeloma as shown by Marten et al. [106]. They showed that CIK cells were able to lyse in vitro MM cells extracted from a patient; this effect can be importantly enhanced by co-culturing CIK cells with DC pulsed with MM-specific antigen. Interestingly, the cytotoxicity was only observed in the CD138+ but not in the CD138− fraction of the bone marrow cells [106].

In a case report study, the use of CIK cells was tested in a man with MM and lung cancer, and concomitant with paraneoplastic dermatoses. CIK were obtained from PBMCs from MM patients and infused into this patient. The treatment resulted in a stabilization of MM and lung cancer without detectable progression of the disease, and without evident side effects [107].

Oncolytic Viruses

Oncolytic viruses are viruses with evolved or engineered tropisms that render them capable of selectively destroying cancer cells [108, 109]. Multiple myeloma is an ideal target disease for systemic oncolytic virotherapy because it is incurable, disseminated from the outset, highly vascular, expresses minimal extracellular matrix, is metabolically active, and provides an excellent substrate for virus propagation [110, 111]. Also, myeloma patients have lower titers of both natural (IgM) and immune (IgG) antiviral antibodies, both because of disease-associated immune paresis and because of the immunosuppressive activity of the treatment regimens that are routinely used for myeloma therapy. For this reason, there are several different oncolytic viruses under development for multiple myeloma [112–118]. Several have shown promise in preclinical myeloma models, and a select few have already entered clinical trials. In addition to these modern studies, there is a single case report from a Japanese study published in 1987 in which a patient with IgA myeloma had a definite (but minor) disease response after a single intravenous administration of an attenuated vaccinia virus [119, 120]. Results to date are summarized below.

The oncolytic properties against MM have been investigated for six viruses: Measles virus, Vesicular Stomatitis virus, Reovirus, Coxsackievirus A21 (CVA21), Adenovirus (Ad), and Vaccinia virus [121].

Adenovirus

Non-enveloped viruses with a double-stranded DNA genome. This virus utilizes CAR as the attachment protein, while $\alpha v\beta 3$ and $\alpha v\beta 5$ are necessary for virus internalization [122].

Due to the presence of the adenovirus receptors (CAR and αvß5) expressed in MM but not in BM MNCs, Ad can be used to purge MM cells ex vivo. Treatment with adenovirus expressing the thymidine kinase gene (TK) under the DF3 promoter followed by a treatment with ganciclovir was able to reduce the number of MM cells by 6 logs while leaving normal BM mononuclear cells unaffected [123].

A loss of function of the p53 protein has been observed in MM cells in 50 % of the analyzed patients and is thought to be related to tumor progression [124]. In a preclinical study, treatment with an adenovirus expressing p53 resulted in a rapid induction of apoptosis in less than 24 h in MM cells expressing low levels of Bcl-2. Importantly, at doses necessary to kill up to 80 % of the myeloma cells, no toxicity was observed in purified CD34+ cells and lymphocytes [125].

The use of a selectively replicating adenovirus, named AdEHCD40L, has been tested as a treatment against MM. For this virus, the viral E1A and E4 genes were put under promoters containing the estrogen response element and hypoxia response, therefore this virus is able to replicate only in cells expressing HIF-1α, E2F-1, and estrogen receptors. Importantly MM cells do express these proteins [126, 127]. Moreover, adenovirus receptors are expressed in MM but not normal BM cells. When tested in murine models bearing MM xenografts, AdEHCD40L was able to reduce tumor growth by 50 % [128].

When tested in primary MM cell from patients, an adenovirus type 5 (Ad5) was shown to infect and kill MM cells with 70-fold reduced infectivity in CD138− cells. Since Ad5 has been approved as an oncolytic agent for solid tumors, using Ad5 as a treatment of MM seems plausible [129].

Coxsackievirus A21

This non-enveloped virus belongs to the picornaviridae family; its genome is a positive single-stranded RNA. Cell entry of this virus requires the expression of ICAM-1 and DAF proteins [130]; once internalized the virus kills the cell by different cellular mechanisms.

Since MM overexpress ICAM-1 and DAF on the cell surface, the ability of CVA21 to purge MM contaminated autographs was tested in samples from 10 MM patients. It was shown that the virus present a strong cytopathic effect specific for MM cells and a reduced toxicity for normal human PBMC cells [131].

One of the main concerns of using oncolytic viruses to treat patients with multiple myeloma is safety. It has been observed that immunocompromised mice, treated with CVA-21, present with damage in the skeletal muscle, indicative of myositis [132]. Although CVA-21 can promote rapid tumor regression, it is imperative to increase its safety. Therefore, CVA-21 was modified to include target elements of muscle-specific miRNAs. This modified virus was able to cause MM tumors regression in mice while preventing myositis and increasing mice survival [132].

Measles Virus

Measles virus belongs to the family Paramyxoviridae, genus Morbillivirus; its genome is negative-strand RNA that encodes for six structural proteins (N, P, M, F, H, and L) and two nonstructural accessory proteins (C and V). The Edmonston vaccine strain of this virus enters cells through two main receptors: CD46, a cell surface glycoprotein present in all the cells except red blood cells and it is overexpressed in most types of cancer, including multiple myeloma; and SLAM (signaling lymphocyte-activation molecule) present on some B and T-cells [133–136].

MV therapy against MM began with Peng et al. where SCID mice bearing subcutaneous tumors of different MM cell lines were given intravenous doses of MV Edmonston strain. Tumor regression was seen for all the different types of tumors analyzed [137]. To enhance MV therapy, this virus has been engineered to express the thyroidal iodide symporter (NIS) allowing the internalization of ^{131}I as a source of ionizing radiation. The outcome of this dual therapy against was significant since MV-NIS in combination with ^{131}I were able to eliminate virus-resistant tumors [118].

One of the main drawbacks of using MV as part of an oncolytic therapy is the presence of neutralizing antibodies in most of the population due to measles vaccination programs. To counter this, cells carriers have been proposed and tested as vehicles for virus delivery. Peng et al. showed that infected MM1 human myeloma cells, macrophages, T cells can home to the tumor sites and promote cell fusion by the expression MV proteins. The use of cell carrier prevents the neutralization of MV by preexisting antibodies [138–140].

MV-NIS, in combination with cyclophosphamide to suppress antiviral cell-mediated immunity, was used in preclinical pharmacology and toxicology studies to support a Phase I clinical trial against multiple myeloma. The results indicate that MV-NIS did not result in any toxicity at the maximum dose of 10^7 $TCID_{50}$/mouse and a single minimum effective dose of 4×10^6 $TCID_{50}$/Kg resulted in controlled tumor growth, and higher doses resulted in tumor regression [141]. MV-NIS is currently in Phase I clinical testing at Mayo Clinic for patients with relapsed myeloma in combination with cyclophosphamide.

Reovirus

Reovirus belongs to the *reoviridae* family, is a non-enveloped virus with a genome composed of ten segments of dsRNA. PKR antiviral response is not active in cells with an activated Ras pathway, a signaling pathway downstream of EGFR, therefore reovirus replication is able to continue in these cells. Since, it is not able to infect normal cells, and it has a low pathogenicity in humans, reovirus has been tested as an oncolytic virus for different types of malignancies such as: gliomas, prostate, and breast cancer [142–145].

In MM, the two pathways commonly affected are the serine/threonine kinase Akt (in 50 % of the MM patient samples) and the guanine nucleotide exchange factor RAS/MAPK pathways (in 30–50 %). Activation of these pathways independently contributes to the survival of MM cells [146].

In susceptible tumors, these activated pathways can be exploited by reovirus, rendering the cells susceptible to the infection. Reovirus was also tested for its ability to purge tumor burden and as an oncolytic therapy. Stem cell transplantation is part of standard therapy against multiple myeloma; however there is a significant effect of contaminating tumor cells in disease relapse. In an ex vivo assay, tumor cells were combined with normal cells and the cocktail was purged by infection with reovirus. It was possible to complete purge up to 1 % of tumor burden in multiple myeloma cell lines after 3 days post-infection with reovirus [147]. As part of a combinatory therapy with bortezomib, Reovirus type three Dearing (Reolysin, Oncolytics Biotech) was able to significantly decrease tumor burden in a xenograft and syngeneic MM model [148, 149].

The oncolytic activity of reovirus was assessed in a disseminated model of human MM in SCID/NOD mice. One dose of 1×10^7 PFU has an impact in the disease progression and MM cells were not observed in four out of six reovirus-treated mice. Importantly, reovirus did not affect human hematopoietic stem cell re-population/differentiation [112].

Vaccinia Virus

Using vaccinia virus (VV) as an oncolytic virus raises issues about its safety in humans, since vaccinia-associated encephalitis has been described in immunosuppressed individuals [150, 151]. To increase the safety of VV for cancer therapy, a double deleted vaccinia virus (VVDD) has been engineered to replicate and kill preferentially tumor cells. This virus presents a deletion in the Thymidine Kinase (TK) gene, which is useful for the production of TTP in non-replicating cells, without this gene, the virus can only use the TTP present in the cell pool. The second deletion was in the gene VGF. This is a secreted protein that induces mitosis in the surrounding cells, preparing them for the vaccinia infection. VVDD specifically killed MM cell lines and primary MM cells from patients, while showing low toxicity in PBMCs of normal donors. Its oncolytic activity was also assessed in murine models where VV inhibited tumor xenograft growth with a single dose of 10^9 PFU [117].

Vesicular Stomatitis Virus

Vesicular Stomatitis virus is part of the family Rabdoviridae; it has a single-stranded negative-sense RNA which encodes for five structural proteins: N, P, M, G, and L. VSV has a fast replication kinetics, is potently cytopathic, has a broad tropism but can be attenuated to specifically infect tumor cells. However, it is quite sensitive to the antiviral effects of type I interferon. However, since many cancer cells cannot mount an effective IFN antiviral response due to a dysregulated IFN response pathway, VSV is able to preferentially spread and replicate in many cancer cells. In samples from patients with MM, this virus was able to kill CD138+ cells while leaving CD138− cells unaffected [152].

VSV have been also engineered to include the NIS gene to increase the bystander killing effect by the incorporation of the radioisotope ^{131}I. Furthermore, M protein of VSV has been mutated in the 51st aminoacid (Δ51) of the matrix (M) protein. The VSVΔ51 virus is unable to block the interferon induction in normal responsive cells; however it will selectively spread in cancer cells with a disrupted IFN response [153]. Immunocompetent mice bearing syngeneic MM tumors, treated with VSVΔ51-NIS and ^{131}I, showed an increase in the survival; tumor regression was also enhanced. Importantly, VSVΔ51-NIS did not induce neurotoxicity at the doses tested [153].

Even though VSVΔ51-NIS showed good efficacy against MM, its replication was compromised. Therefore, new VSVs encoding the IFNß gene with and without NIS were produced. These viruses are not neurotoxic and their replication was not as compromised as VSVΔ51NIS. VSV-IFNß killed CD138+ MM cells while leaving CD138− cells unaffected. In immunocompetent animals, VSV- IFNß-NIS caused complete cure of large established myeloma 5TGM1 tumors in immunocompetent mice [111]. VSV virus is able to kill MM cells even in mice with disseminated MM disease, significantly improving the survival of these tumor bearing mice [113].

Conclusions

The past decade has been a time of tremendous progress in the development and approval of new biologically based therapeutics for cancer treatment. In particular, it is estimated that monoclonal antibodies constitute approximately 40 % of the biological products currently being developed, and many believe that the next generation of blockbuster drugs will belong to this class. Promising antitumor activities have been seen with engineered T cells which are retargeted to recognize tumor cell surface antigens using genetically encoded chimeric T cell receptors, an advance that builds upon significant scientific advances and improved understanding of formulations and methods to maintain T cell activity. Several oncolytic virotherapy products are now undergoing pivotal Phase II/III clinical evaluation and we envisage that these novel agents, which debulk tumors as well as elicit host immune responses to eradicate residual disease, hold much promise as biologics for myeloma therapy.

References

1. Baskar S, Muthusamy N. Antibody-based therapeutics for the treatment of human B cell malignancies. Curr Allergy Asthma Rep. 2012;13:33–43.
2. Dimitrov DS. Therapeutic proteins. Methods Mol Biol. 2012;899:1–26.
3. Kreitman RJ, Pastan I. Immunotoxins in the treatment of hematologic malignancies. Curr Drug Targets. 2006;7(10):1301–11.
4. Maloney DG. Anti-CD20 antibody therapy for B-cell lymphomas. N Engl J Med. 2012;366(21): 2008–16.
5. Jelovac D, Wolff AC. The adjuvant treatment of HER2-positive breast cancer. Curr Treat Options Oncol. 2012;13(2):230–9.
6. Vale CL, et al. Does anti-EGFR therapy improve outcome in advanced colorectal cancer? A systematic review and meta-analysis. Cancer Treat Rev. 2012;38(6):618–25.

7. Reff ME, et al. Depletion of B-cells in-vivo by a chimeric mouse-human monoclonal-antibody to Cd20. Blood. 1994;83(2):435–45.
8. Treon SP, et al. CD20-directed serotherapy in patients with multiple myeloma: biologic considerations and therapeutic applications. J Immunother. 2002;25(1):72–81.
9. Greipp PT, et al. Reply to 'Rituximab in CD20 positive multiple myeloma' by P Moreau et al. Leukemia. 2008;22(1):214–5.
10. Kapoor P, et al. Anti-CD20 monoclonal antibody therapy in multiple myeloma. Br J Haematol. 2008;141(2):135–48.
11. Yang J, et al. Targeting beta2-microglobulin for induction of tumor apoptosis in human hematological malignancies. Cancer Cell. 2006;10(4):295–307.
12. Yang J, et al. Human-like mouse models for testing the efficacy and safety of anti-beta2-microglobulin monoclonal antibodies to treat myeloma. Clin Cancer Res. 2009;15(3):951–9.
13. Malavasi F, et al. Human CD38: a glycoprotein in search of a function. Immunol Today. 1994;15(3): 95–7.
14. Lin P, et al. Flow cytometric immunophenotypic analysis of 306 cases of multiple myeloma. Am J Clin Pathol. 2004;121(4):482–8.
15. de Weers M, et al. Daratumumab, a novel therapeutic human CD38 monoclonal antibody, induces killing of multiple myeloma and other hematological tumors. J Immunol. 2011;186(3):1840–8.
16. Tai YT, et al. Human anti-CD40 antagonist antibody triggers significant antitumor activity against human multiple myeloma. Cancer Res. 2005;65(13): 5898–906.
17. Bensinger W, et al. A phase 1 study of lucatumumab, a fully human anti-CD40 antagonist monoclonal antibody administered intravenously to patients with relapsed or refractory multiple myeloma. Br J Haematol. 2012;159(1):58–66.
18. Hussein M, et al. A phase I multidose study of dacetuzumab (SGN-40; humanized anti-CD40 monoclonal antibody) in patients with multiple myeloma. Haematologica. 2010;95(5):845–8.
19. Mawby WJ, et al. Isolation and characterization of CD47 glycoprotein: a multispanning membrane protein which is the same as integrin-associated protein (IAP) and the ovarian tumour marker OA3. Biochem J. 1994;304(Pt 2):525–30.
20. Zhan F, et al. Global gene expression profiling of multiple myeloma, monoclonal gammopathy of undetermined significance, and normal bone marrow plasma cells. Blood. 2002;99(5):1745–57.
21. Kim D, et al. Anti-CD47 antibodies promote phagocytosis and inhibit the growth of human myeloma cells. Leukemia. 2012;26(12):2538–45.
22. Ahsmann EJ, et al. Lymphocyte function-associated antigen-1 expression on plasma cells correlates with tumor growth in multiple myeloma. Blood. 1992;79(8): 2068–75.
23. Huang YW, Burrows FJ, Vitetta ES. Cytotoxicity of a novel anti-ICAM-1 immunotoxin on human myeloma cell lines. Hybridoma. 1993;12(6):661–75.
24. Smallshaw JE, et al. The generation and antimyeloma activity of a chimeric anti-CD54 antibody, cUV3. J Immunother. 2004;27(6):419–24.
25. Huang YW, Richardson JA, Vitetta ES. Anti-CD54 (ICAM-1) has antitumor activity in SCID mice with human myeloma cells. Cancer Res. 1995;55(3): 610–6.
26. Kraj M, et al. Clinicopathological correlates of plasma cell CD56 (NCAM) expression in multiple myeloma. Leuk Lymphoma. 2008;49(2):298–305.
27. Harada H, et al. Phenotypic difference of normal plasma cells from mature myeloma cells. Blood. 1993;81(10):2658–63.
28. Tassone P, et al. In vitro and in vivo activity of the maytansinoid immunoconjugate huN901-N2′-deacetyl-N2′-(3-mercapto-1-oxopropyl)-maytansine against CD56+ multiple myeloma cells. Cancer Res. 2004;64(13):4629–36.
29. Burton JD, et al. CD74 is expressed by multiple myeloma and is a promising target for therapy. Clin Cancer Res. 2004;10(19):6606–11.
30. Stein R, et al. Antiproliferative activity of a humanized anti-CD74 monoclonal antibody, hLL1, on B-cell malignancies. Blood. 2004;104(12):3705–11.
31. Sapra P, et al. Anti-CD74 antibody-doxorubicin conjugate, IMMU-110, in a human multiple myeloma xenograft and in monkeys. Clin Cancer Res. 2005;11(14):5257–64.
32. Sanderson RD, Lalor P, Bernfield M. B lymphocytes express and lose syndecan at specific stages of differentiation. Cell Regul. 1989;1(1):27–35.
33. Ikeda H, et al. The monoclonal antibody nBT062 conjugated to cytotoxic Maytansinoids has selective cytotoxicity against CD138-positive multiple myeloma cells in vitro and in vivo. Clin Cancer Res. 2009;15(12):4028–37.
34. Hsi ED, et al. CS1, a potential new therapeutic antibody target for the treatment of multiple myeloma. Clin Cancer Res. 2008;14(9):2775–84.
35. Tai YT, et al. Anti-CS1 humanized monoclonal antibody HuLuc63 inhibits myeloma cell adhesion and induces antibody-dependent cellular cytotoxicity in the bone marrow milieu. Blood. 2008;112(4): 1329–37.
36. van Rhee F, et al. Combinatorial efficacy of anti-CS1 monoclonal antibody elotuzumab (HuLuc63) and bortezomib against multiple myeloma. Mol Cancer Ther. 2009;8(9):2616–24.
37. Benson Jr DM, Byrd JC. CS1-directed monoclonal antibody therapy for multiple myeloma. J Clin Oncol. 2012;30(16):2013–5.
38. Klein B, et al. Interleukin-6 in human multiple myeloma. Blood. 1995;85(4):863–72.
39. Fulciniti M, et al. A high-affinity fully human anti-IL-6 mAb, 1339, for the treatment of multiple myeloma. Clin Cancer Res. 2009;15(23):7144–52.

40. van Zaanen HC, et al. Chimaeric anti-interleukin 6 monoclonal antibodies in the treatment of advanced multiple myeloma: a phase I dose-escalating study. Br J Haematol. 1998;102(3):783–90.
41. Lonial S, et al. Elotuzumab in combination with lenalidomide and low-dose dexamethasone in relapsed or refractory multiple myeloma. J Clin Oncol. 2012;30(16):1953–9.
42. Allegra A, et al. Monoclonal antibodies: potential new therapeutic treatment against multiple myeloma. Eur J Haematol. 2013;90:441–68.
43. Jakubowiak AJ, et al. Phase I trial of anti-CS1 monoclonal antibody elotuzumab in combination with bortezomib in the treatment of relapsed/refractory multiple myeloma. J Clin Oncol. 2012;30(16):1960–5.
44. Moreau P, et al. A combination of anti-interleukin 6 murine monoclonal antibody with dexamethasone and high-dose melphalan induces high complete response rates in advanced multiple myeloma. Br J Haematol. 2000;109(3):661–4.
45. Zhou F-L, et al. Peptide-based immunotherapy for multiple myeloma: current approaches. Vaccine. 2010;28(37):5939–46.
46. Zhang L, et al. Immunogenic targets for specific immunotherapy in multiple myeloma. Clin Dev Immunol. 2012;2012:820394.
47. Nguyen-Pham TN, et al. Induction of myeloma-specific cytotoxic T lymphocytes responses by natural killer cells stimulated-dendritic cells in patients with multiple myeloma. Leuk Res. 2011;35(9): 1241–7.
48. Chen YT, et al. A testicular antigen aberrantly expressed in human cancers detected by autologous antibody screening. Proc Natl Acad Sci U S A. 1997;94(5):1914–8.
49. Gnjatic S, et al. NY-ESO-1: review of an immunogenic tumor antigen. Adv Cancer Res. 2006;95: 1–30.
50. Szmania S, Tricot G, van Rhee F. NY-ESO-1 immunotherapy for multiple myeloma. Leuk Lymphoma. 2006;47(10):2037–48.
51. van Rhee F, et al. NY-ESO-1 is highly expressed in poor-prognosis multiple myeloma and induces spontaneous humoral and cellular immune responses. Blood. 2005;105(10):3939–44.
52. Oka Y, et al. WT1 peptide vaccine for the treatment of cancer. Curr Opin Immunol. 2008;20(2):211–20.
53. Azuma T, et al. Myeloma cells are highly sensitive to the granule exocytosis pathway mediated by WT1-specific cytotoxic T lymphocytes. Clin Cancer Res. 2004;10(21):7402–12.
54. Tsuboi A, et al. Wilms tumor gene WT1 peptide-based immunotherapy induced a minimal response in a patient with advanced therapy-resistant multiple myeloma. Int J Hematol. 2007;86(5):414–7.
55. Choi C, et al. Enrichment of functional CD8 memory T cells specific for MUC1 in bone marrow of patients with multiple myeloma. Blood. 2005;105(5): 2132–4.
56. Brossart P, et al. The epithelial tumor antigen MUC1 is expressed in hematological malignancies and is recognized by MUC1-specific cytotoxic T-lymphocytes. Cancer Res. 2001;61(18):6846–50.
57. Giannopoulos K, et al. Expression of RHAMM/CD168 and other tumor-associated antigens in patients with B-cell chronic lymphocytic leukemia. Int J Oncol. 2006;29(1):95–103.
58. Schmitt M, et al. RHAMM-R3 peptide vaccination in patients with acute myeloid leukemia, myelodysplastic syndrome, and multiple myeloma elicits immunologic and clinical responses. Blood. 2008;111(3): 1357–65.
59. Tian E, et al. The role of the Wnt-signaling antagonist DKK1 in the development of osteolytic lesions in multiple myeloma. N Engl J Med. 2003;349(26):2483–94.
60. Yaccoby S, et al. Antibody-based inhibition of DKK1 suppresses tumor-induced bone resorption and multiple myeloma growth in vivo. Blood. 2007;109(5):2106–11.
61. Qian J, et al. Dickkopf-1 (DKK1) is a widely expressed and potent tumor-associated antigen in multiple myeloma. Blood. 2007;110(5):1587–94.
62. Grube M, et al. CD8+ T cells reactive to survivin antigen in patients with multiple myeloma. Clin Cancer Res. 2007;13(3):1053–60.
63. Schmidt SM, et al. Survivin is a shared tumor-associated antigen expressed in a broad variety of malignancies and recognized by specific cytotoxic T cells. Blood. 2003;102(2):571–6.
64. Goto T, et al. A novel membrane antigen selectively expressed on terminally differentiated human B cells. Blood. 1994;84(6):1922–30.
65. Hundemer M, et al. Identification of a new HLA-A2-restricted T-cell epitope within HM1.24 as immunotherapy target for multiple myeloma. Exp Hematol. 2006;34(4):486–96.
66. Christensen O, et al. Melan-A/MART1 analog peptide triggers anti-myeloma T-cells through crossreactivity with HM1.24. J Immunother. 2009;32(6):613–21.
67. Atanackovic D, et al. Longitudinal analysis and prognostic effect of cancer-testis antigen expression in multiple myeloma. Clin Cancer Res. 2009;15(4): 1343–52.
68. Andrade VC, et al. Prognostic impact of cancer/testis antigen expression in advanced stage multiple myeloma patients. Cancer Immun. 2008;8:2.
69. Ruffini PA, et al. Idiotypic vaccination for B-cell malignancies as a model for therapeutic cancer vaccines: from prototype protein to second generation vaccines. Haematologica. 2002;87(9):989–1001.
70. Lynch RG, et al. Myeloma proteins as tumor-specific transplantation antigens. Proc Natl Acad Sci U S A. 1972;69(6):1540–4.
71. Houet L, Veelken H. Active immunotherapy of multiple myeloma. Eur J Cancer. 2006;42(11):1653–60.
72. Reichardt VL, et al. Idiotype vaccination of multiple myeloma patients using monocyte-derived dendritic cells. Haematologica. 2003;88(10):1139–49.

73. Rasmussen T, et al. Idiotype vaccination in multiple myeloma induced a reduction of circulating clonal tumor B cells. Blood. 2003;101(11):4607–10.
74. Coscia M, et al. Long-term follow-up of idiotype vaccination in human myeloma as a maintenance therapy after high-dose chemotherapy. Leukemia. 2004;18(1):139–45.
75. Bendandi M, et al. Combined vaccination with idiotype-pulsed allogeneic dendritic cells and soluble protein idiotype for multiple myeloma patients relapsing after reduced-intensity conditioning allogeneic stem cell transplantation. Leuk Lymphoma. 2006;47(1):29–37.
76. Abdalla AO, et al. Idiotype protein vaccination in combination with adjuvant cytokines in patients with multiple myeloma—evaluation of T-cell responses by different read-out systems. Haematologica. 2007;92(1):110–4.
77. Abdalla AO, et al. Long-term effects of idiotype vaccination on the specific T-cell response in peripheral blood and bone marrow of multiple myeloma patients. Eur J Haematol. 2007;79(5):371–81.
78. Hansson L, et al. Long-term idiotype vaccination combined with interleukin-12 (IL-12), or IL-12 and granulocyte macrophage colony-stimulating factor, in early-stage multiple myeloma patients. Clin Cancer Res. 2007;13(5):1503–10.
79. Curti A, et al. Phase I/II clinical trial of sequential subcutaneous and intravenous delivery of dendritic cell vaccination for refractory multiple myeloma using patient-specific tumour idiotype protein or idiotype (VDJ)-derived class I-restricted peptides. Br J Haematol. 2007;139(3):415–24.
80. Abdalla AO, et al. Idiotype vaccination in patients with myeloma reduced circulating myeloma cells (CMC). Ann Oncol. 2008;19(6):1172–9.
81. Lacy MQ, et al. Idiotype-pulsed antigen-presenting cells following autologous transplantation for multiple myeloma may be associated with prolonged survival. Am J Hematol. 2009;84(12):799–802.
82. Yi Q, et al. Optimizing dendritic cell-based immunotherapy in multiple myeloma: intranodal injections of idiotype-pulsed CD40 ligand-matured vaccines led to induction of type-1 and cytotoxic T-cell immune responses in patients. Br J Haematol. 2010;150(5):554–64.
83. Rollig C, et al. Induction of cellular immune responses in patients with stage-I multiple myeloma after vaccination with autologous idiotype-pulsed dendritic cells. J Immunother. 2011;34(1):100–6.
84. Rosenblatt J, Avigan D. Cellular immunotherapy for multiple myeloma. Best Pract Res Clin Haematol. 2008;21(3):559–77.
85. Garg TK, et al. Highly activated and expanded natural killer cells for multiple myeloma immunotherapy. Haematologica. 2012;97(9):1348–56.
86. Ramos CA, Dotti G. Chimeric antigen receptor (CAR)-engineered lymphocytes for cancer therapy. Expert Opin Biol Ther. 2011;11(7):855–73.
87. Rosenberg SA. Raising the bar: the curative potential of human cancer immunotherapy. Sci Transl Med. 2012;4(127):127ps8.
88. Sadelain M, Brentjens R, Riviere I. The promise and potential pitfalls of chimeric antigen receptors. Curr Opin Immunol. 2009;21(2):215–23.
89. Till BG, Press OW. Treatment of lymphoma with adoptively transferred T cells. Expert Opin Biol Ther. 2009;9(11):1407–25.
90. Biagi E, et al. Chimeric T-cell receptors: new challenges for targeted immunotherapy in hematologic malignancies. Haematologica. 2007;92(3):381–8.
91. Di Stasi A, et al. Inducible apoptosis as a safety switch for adoptive cell therapy. N Engl J Med. 2011;365(18):1673–83.
92. Gahrton G, et al. Prognostic factors in allogeneic bone marrow transplantation for multiple myeloma. J Clin Oncol. 1995;13(6):1312–22.
93. Saitoh A, et al. Anti-tumor cytotoxicity of gammadelta T cells expanded from peripheral blood cells of patients with myeloma and lymphoma. Med Oncol. 2008;25(2):137–47.
94. Barber A, Meehan KR, Sentman CL. Treatment of multiple myeloma with adoptively transferred chimeric NKG2D receptor-expressing T cells. Gene Ther. 2011;18(5):509–16.
95. Meehan KR, et al. Adoptive cellular therapy using cells enriched for NKG2D(+)CD3(+)CD8(+)T cells after autologous transplantation for myeloma. Biol Blood Marrow Transplant. 2012;19:129–37.
96. Patil S, Schwarer T. Natural killer cells—new understanding of basic biology may lead to more effective allogeneic haematopoietic stem cell transplantation. Intern Med J. 2009;39(10):639–47.
97. Shi J, et al. Infusion of haplo-identical killer immunoglobulin-like receptor ligand mismatched NK cells for relapsed myeloma in the setting of autologous stem cell transplantation. Br J Haematol. 2008;143(5):641–53.
98. Katodritou E, et al. Tumor-primed natural killer cells from patients with multiple myeloma lyse autologous, NK-resistant, bone marrow-derived malignant plasma cells. Am J Hematol. 2011;86(12):967–73.
99. Fujisaki H, et al. Expansion of highly cytotoxic human natural killer cells for cancer cell therapy. Cancer Res. 2009;69(9):4010–7.
100. Arai S, et al. Infusion of the allogeneic cell line NK-92 in patients with advanced renal cell cancer or melanoma: a phase I trial. Cytotherapy. 2008;10(6):625–32.
101. Swift BE, et al. Natural killer cell lines preferentially kill clonogenic multiple myeloma cells and decrease myeloma engraftment in a bioluminescent xenograft mouse model. Haematologica. 2012;97(7):1020–8.
102. Alici E, et al. Autologous antitumor activity by NK cells expanded from myeloma patients using GMP-compliant components. Blood. 2008;111(6):3155–62.
103. Grimm EA, et al. Lymphokine-activated killer cell phenomenon. Lysis of natural killer-resistant fresh

solid tumor cells by interleukin 2-activated autologous human peripheral blood lymphocytes. J Exp Med. 1982;155(6):1823–41.
104. Schmidt-Wolf IG, et al. Use of a SCID mouse/human lymphoma model to evaluate cytokine-induced killer cells with potent antitumor cell activity. J Exp Med. 1991;174(1):139–49.
105. Linn YC, Hui KM. Cytokine-induced NK-like T cells: from bench to bedside. J Biomed Biotechnol. 2010;2010:435745.
106. Marten A, et al. Enhanced lytic activity of cytokine-induced killer cells against multiple myeloma cells after co-culture with idiotype-pulsed dendritic cells. Haematologica. 2001;86(10):1029–37.
107. Lin J, et al. Autologous cytokine-induced killer cells in the treatment of multiple myeloma concomitant with lung cancer and paraneoplastic dermatoses. Intern Med. 2010;49(21):2341–6.
108. Kelly E, Russell SJ. History of oncolytic viruses: genesis to genetic engineering. Mol Ther. 2007; 15(4):651–9.
109. Russell SJ, Peng KW, Bell JC. Oncolytic virotherapy. Nat Biotechnol. 2012;30(7):658–70.
110. Stief AE, McCart JA. Oncolytic virotherapy for multiple myeloma. Expert Opin Biol Ther. 2008;8(4): 463–73.
111. Naik S, et al. Curative one-shot systemic virotherapy in murine myeloma. Leukemia. 2012;26(8):1870–8.
112. Thirukkumaran CM, et al. Reovirus as a viable therapeutic option for the treatment of multiple myeloma. Clin Cancer Res. 2012;18:4962–72.
113. Naik S, et al. Potent systemic therapy of multiple myeloma utilizing oncolytic vesicular stomatitis virus coding for interferon-beta. Cancer Gene Ther. 2012;19(7):443–50.
114. Bartee E, et al. Selective purging of human multiple myeloma cells from autologous stem cell transplantation grafts using oncolytic myxoma virus. Biol Blood Marrow Transplant. 2012;18(10):1540–51.
115. Chen CY, et al. Species D adenoviruses as oncolytics against B-cell cancers. Clin Cancer Res. 2011;17(21): 6712–22.
116. Hadac EM, Kelly EJ, Russell SJ. Myeloma xenograft destruction by a nonviral vector delivering oncolytic infectious nucleic acid. Mol Ther. 2011;19(6):1041–7.
117. Deng H, et al. Oncolytic virotherapy for multiple myeloma using a tumour-specific double-deleted vaccinia virus. Leukemia. 2008;22(12):2261–4.
118. Dingli D, et al. Image-guided radiovirotherapy for multiple myeloma using a recombinant measles virus expressing the thyroidal sodium iodide symporter. Blood. 2004;103(5):1641–6.
119. Kawa A, Arakawa S. The effect of attenuated vaccinia virus AS strain on multiple myeloma; a case report. Jpn J Exp Med. 1987;57(1):79–81.
120. Munguia A, et al. Cell carriers to deliver oncolytic viruses to sites of myeloma tumor growth. Gene Ther. 2008;15(10):797–806.
121. Thirukkumaran CM, Morris DG. Oncolytic virotherapy for multiple myeloma: past, present, and future. Bone Marrow Res. 2011;2011:632948.
122. Wickham TJ, et al. Integrins ±v^{2}3 and ±v^{2}5 promote adenovirus internalization but not virus attachment. Cell. 1993;73(2):309–19.
123. Teoh G, et al. Adenovirus vector-based purging of multiple myeloma cells. Blood. 1998;92(12):4591–601.
124. Neri A, et al. p53 gene mutations in multiple myeloma are associated with advanced forms of malignancy. Blood. 1993;81(1):128–35.
125. Liu Q, Gazitt Y. Adenovirus-mediated delivery of p53 results in substantial apoptosis to myeloma cells and is not cytotoxic to flow-sorted CD34(+) hematopoietic progenitor cells and normal lymphocytes. Exp Hematol. 2000;28(12):1354–62.
126. Otsuki T, et al. Estrogen receptors in human myeloma cells. Cancer Res. 2000;60(5):1434–41.
127. Wilson CS, et al. Cyclin D1 and E2F-1 immunoreactivity in bone marrow biopsy specimens of multiple myeloma: relationship to proliferative activity, cytogenetic abnormalities and DNA ploidy. Br J Haematol. 2001;112(3):776–82.
128. Fernandes MS, et al. Growth inhibition of human multiple myeloma cells by an oncolytic adenovirus carrying the CD40 ligand transgene. Clin Cancer Res. 2009;15(15):4847–56.
129. Senac JS, et al. Infection and killing of multiple myeloma by adenoviruses. Hum Gene Ther. 2010;21(2):179–90.
130. Shafren DR, et al. Coxsackievirus A21 binds to decay-accelerating factor but requires intercellular adhesion molecule 1 for cell entry. J Virol. 1997; 71(6):4736–43.
131. Au GG, et al. Oncolytic Coxsackievirus A21 as a novel therapy for multiple myeloma. Br J Haematol. 2007;137(2):133–41.
132. Kelly EJ, et al. Engineering microRNA responsiveness to decrease virus pathogenicity. Nat Med. 2008;14(11):1278–83.
133. Naniche D, et al. Human membrane cofactor protein (CD46) acts as a cellular receptor for measles virus. J Virol. 1993;67(10):6025–32.
134. Tatsuo H, et al. SLAM (CDw150) is a cellular receptor for measles virus. Nature. 2000;406(6798):893–7.
135. Ong HT, et al. Oncolytic measles virus targets high CD46 expression on multiple myeloma cells. Exp Hematol. 2006;34(6):713–20.
136. Msaouel P, Dispenzieri A, Galanis E. Clinical testing of engineered oncolytic measles virus strains in the treatment of cancer: an overview. Curr Opin Mol Ther. 2009;11(1):43–53.
137. Peng KW, et al. Systemic therapy of myeloma xenografts by an attenuated measles virus. Blood. 2001;98(7):2002–7.
138. Liu C, Russell SJ, Peng KW. Systemic therapy of disseminated myeloma in passively immunized mice using measles virus-infected cell carriers. Mol Ther. 2010;18(6):1155–64.

139. Peng KW, et al. Tumor-associated macrophages infiltrate plasmacytomas and can serve as cell carriers for oncolytic measles virotherapy of disseminated myeloma. Am J Hematol. 2009;84(7):401–7.
140. Ong HT, et al. Evaluation of T cells as carriers for systemic measles virotherapy in the presence of antiviral antibodies. Gene Ther. 2007;14(4):324–33.
141. Myers RM, et al. Preclinical pharmacology and toxicology of intravenous MV-NIS, an oncolytic measles virus administered with or without cyclophosphamide. Clin Pharmacol Ther. 2007;82(6):700–10.
142. Wilcox ME, et al. Reovirus as an oncolytic agent against experimental human malignant gliomas. J Natl Cancer Inst. 2001;93(12):903–12.
143. Thirukkumaran CM, et al. Oncolytic viral therapy for prostate cancer: efficacy of reovirus as a biological therapeutic. Cancer Res. 2010;70(6):2435–44.
144. Norman KL, et al. Reovirus oncolysis of human breast cancer. Hum Gene Ther. 2002;13(5):641–52.
145. Comins C, et al. Reovirus: viral therapy for cancer 'as nature intended'. Clin Oncol. 2008;20(7):548–54.
146. Steinbrunn T, et al. Mutated RAS and constitutively activated Akt delineate distinct oncogenic pathways, which independently contribute to multiple myeloma cell survival. Blood. 2011;117(6):1998–2004.
147. Thirukkumaran CM, et al. Reovirus oncolysis as a novel purging strategy for autologous stem cell transplantation. Blood. 2003;102(1):377–87.
148. Kelly KR, et al. Reovirus therapy stimulates endoplasmic reticular stress, NOXA induction, and augments bortezomib-mediated apoptosis in multiple myeloma. Oncogene. 2012;31(25):3023–38.
149. Vidal L, et al. A phase I study of intravenous oncolytic reovirus type 3 Dearing in patients with advanced cancer. Clin Cancer Res. 2008;14(21): 7127–37.
150. Gurvich EB, Vilesova IS. Vaccinia virus in postvaccinal encephalitis. Acta Virol. 1983;27(2):154–9.
151. Turkel SB, Overturf GD. Vaccinia necrosum complicating immunoblastic sarcoma. Cancer. 1977;40(1): 226–33.
152. Lichty BD, et al. Vesicular stomatitis virus: a potential therapeutic virus for the treatment of hematologic malignancy. Hum Gene Ther. 2004;15(9): 821–31.
153. Goel A, et al. Radioiodide imaging and radiovirotherapy of multiple myeloma using VSV(Delta51)-NIS, an attenuated vesicular stomatitis virus encoding the sodium iodide symporter gene. Blood. 2007;110(7):2342–50.

Management of Treatment Complications and Supportive Care

14

Francis Buadi and Asher Chanan Khan

Introduction

Multiple myeloma patients usually present with complications related to the proliferation of clonal plasma cells or the toxic effect of monoclonal proteins [1]. Therapy is indicated when complications referred to as the CRAB criteria is present [2, 3]. These include hypercalcemia (C), renal insufficiency (R), anemia (A), and lytic bone lesions or osteoporosis (B), as defined by the myeloma working group [4]. In a study at the Mayo clinic, anemia was the presenting sign in 73 % of the patients, lytic bone lesions 66 %, hypercalcemia 13 %, and renal insufficiency 19 % [5]. Although the definitive therapy for multiple myeloma is directed at the plasma cell malignancy, appropriate immediate intervention for these complications is essentially for the long-term outcome of these patients. The major cause of death in multiple myeloma patients is infection and renal failure and failure to reverse acute renal failure will significantly impact long-term survival [6]. Failure also to recognize and appropriately treat pathologic bone fractures and cord compression will have significant effect on quality of life, even with effective treatment of the multiple myeloma. The current armamentarium of drugs for the management of multiple myeloma is extensive and these have changed significantly over the last decade. The traditional agents such as alkylators, anthracyclines, and platinum [7–10] have given way to immunomodulatory drugs (Thalidomide, Lenalidomide, Pomalidomide) and the proteosome inhibitors Bortezomib and Carfilzomib [11–20]. In addition to the primary complications of multiple myeloma, all these drugs also do come with their own peculiar side effects which will have to be effectively monitored and managed during their use. Multiple myeloma patients are leaving longer and therefore their quality of life as they live with this disease should be optimized by effectively preventing, reducing, and managing complications associated with this disease [21]. This chapter will review complications associated with multiple myeloma and its management.

Bone Disease and Hypercalcemia

Hypercalcemia

Hypercalcemia is seen in about 13 % of multiple myeloma cases at the time of initial presentation [5]. These patients may present with nausea, vomiting, polyuria, confusion, and in severe

F. Buadi, M.B., Ch.B. (✉)
Division of Hematology, Mayo Clinic,
200 First Street, SW, Rochester, MN 55905, USA
e-mail: buadi.francis@mayo.edu

A.C. Khan, M.D.
Division of Hematology and Medical Oncology,
Mayo Clinic Florida, Jacksonville, FL, USA
e-mail: chanan-khan.asher@mayo.edu

M.A. Gertz and S.V. Rajkumar (eds.), *Multiple Myeloma: Diagnosis and Treatment*,
DOI 10.1007/978-1-4614-8520-9_14, © Mayo Foundation for Medical Education and Research 2014

cases coma. The hypercalcemia may be the cause or contribute to acute renal failure in these patients. Osteoclastic activity in the absence of osteoblastic activity thought to be driven by cytokines such as interleukin (IL)-6, IL-3, osteoprotegerin, and receptor activator of nuclear factor-k ligand (RANK-L) has been implicated as the cause of hypercalcemia in multiple myeloma [22, 23]. These patients should be treated aggressively with hydration and forced diuresis [24, 25]. Although it is recommended to infuse isotonic saline at a rate of about 200 mL/h to generate urine out of 100 mL/h at the minimum, one will have to be careful in multiple myeloma patients, since the median age at diagnosis is in the seventh decade and most patients may have comorbid conditions precluding rapid hydration. Bisphosphonate use has become an integral part of the management of hypercalcemia. They are very effective and can result in sustained control of calcium level while definitive therapy for the myeloma is administered. Both pamidronate and zoledronic acid (ZA) are effective; however, dose adjustment is needed for zoledronic acid in the setting of acute renal failure [26–30]. Calcitonin alone or in combination with glucocorticoids is also effective and may be beneficial especially in cases refractory to bisphosphonates [31–33]. Denosumab a monoclonal antibody that binds RANK-L is also effective in the management of hypercalcemia [34–36]. Although not the current standard of care, it may become a major treatment for refractory hypercalcemia in myeloma patients and also those with simultaneous renal function impairment in whom bisphosphonate may not be ideal.

Imaging

Bone destruction presenting in the form of osteolytic lesion, osteopenia, osteoporosis, and pathologic fractures is common in multiple myeloma and in a significant number of cases is the initial presenting feature [5]. The bone destruction is due to increased bone resorption as a result of osteoclast activity without reciprocal osteoblastic activity maintained by the effect of cytokines such as IL-1, IL-6, and TNF secreted by myeloma cells and bone marrow stromal cells [37–39]. Detailed radiologic evaluation of all bones should be performed in all patients. Metastatic bone survey is considered the standard of care. Magnetic resonance imaging (MRI) and whole body computerized tomography scanning with positron emission tomography (CT/PET) may be required for better evaluation of abnormal bony lesions or any areas of concern [40–42]. These skeletal complications are associated with significant morbidity.

Treatment of Bone Pain

Bone pain is usually the initial symptom and should be treated with analgesics or radiation treatment. Adequate analgesic therapy including nonsteroidal anti-inflammatory drugs (NSAID) and narcotics may be required to control pain. One must be cautious with the use of NSAID since 20 % of multiple myeloma patients may present with some degree of renal insufficiency. Palliative radiation is associated with rapid pain and disease control [43]. The recommended dose of local radiotherapy for control of bone pain in myeloma is 10–20 Gy given in 5–10 fractions [44–46]. Radiation therapy should be used judiciously, to prevent exposing significant amount of bone marrow to radiation, since this may affect hematopoietic reserve.

Vertebral Augmentation

The services of orthopedic surgeon may be needed for evaluation and management of pathologic fractures or areas at risk for pathologic fractures especially weight bearing long bones. Vertebral compression fractures (VCF) have been treated with vertebroplasty, balloon kyphoplasty, or radiation therapy [47–50]. In the VERTOS study, short-term clinical outcome of patients with subacute or chronic painful osteoporotic VCF treated with percutaneous vertebroplasty (PV) was compared with optimal pain medication (OPM) [51]. Thirty four patients were enrolled in the study. Eighteen patients were randomized to be treated by PV and 16 patients by OPM. Pain relief and improvement of mobility, function, and stature after PV was immediate and significantly better in the short term compared with OPM treatment. A larger multicenter study randomized 300 patients to kyphoplasty treatment ($n=149$) or nonsurgical care ($n=151$) [52]. At 1 month, the mean physical component score (36 physical component summary score on a 0–100 scale) improved by 7.2 points (95 % CI 5.7–8.8) in the kyphoplasty group and by 2.0 points (0.4–3.6) in the nonsurgical group ($P<0.0001$). The benefit of these vertebral procedures in controlling pain has, however, not been confirmed in all studies. One of such studies looked at 78 patients randomized to vertebroplasty ($n=38$) and placebo ($n=40$) with a 6-month follow-up [53]. Vertebroplasty did not result in a significant advantage in any measured outcome at any time point. At 3 months, the mean (±SD) reductions in the score for pain in the vertebroplasty and control groups were 2.6±2.9 and 1.9±3.3, respectively. Similar improvements were seen in both groups with respect to pain at night and at rest, physical functioning, quality of life, and perceived improvement.

In the INvestigational Vertebroplasty Efficacy and Safety Trial (INVEST) study, patients with osteoporotic VCF were randomized to undergo vertebroplasty or a control procedure [54]. After 1 month, patients were allowed to cross over and undergo the alternate procedure. Co-primary outcomes were patient-reported function, measured with the modified Roland-Morris Disability Questionnaire (RDQ), and pain (on a scale of 1–10) at 1 year [55]. One hundred thirty-one participants (68 in the vertebroplasty group and 63 in the control group) were included in the analyses. Patients in both groups showed improvements in pain and function at 1 year. In Intention-to-treat analyses, patients randomized to vertebroplasty did not differ from control subjects in terms of RDQ results (difference, 1.37 points; 95 % confidence interval [CI]: −0.88, 3.62; ($P=0.231$)), but reported lower levels of pain (difference, 1.02 points; 95 % CI: 0.04, 2.01; ($P=0.042$)). Eleven of 68 patients who underwent vertebroplasty (16 %) and 38 of 63 control subjects (60 %) crossed over and elected to undergo the alternate procedure ($P<0.001$). In the as-treated analyses, patients treated with vertebroplasty did not differ from control subjects in terms of RDQ results (difference, 0.66 points; 95 % CI: −1.98, 3.30; $P=0.625$) or pain (difference, 0.85 points; 95 % CI: −0.35, 2.05; $P=0.166$). They concluded that vertebroplasty may provide a modest reduction in pain at 1 year compared with a control procedure; however, no difference in functional disability was observed.

Bisphosphonates

The benefit of bisphosphonate therapy, pamidronate or zoledronic acid in reducing skeletal events in multiple myeloma has been shown in multiple clinical studies [56–59]. In a randomized study by Berenson el al, 392 patients with stage III myeloma and at least one lytic lesion received either placebo (179) or pamidronate 90 mg intravenously administered as a 4-h infusion monthly (198). After 21 cycles, the proportion of patients who developed any skeletal event was lower in the pamidronate-group ($P=0.015$). The mean number of skeletal events per year was less in the pamidronate-group (1.3) than in placebo-treated patients (2.2; $P=0.008$) [60].

In the MRC Myeloma IX study 1,960 patients were randomized to zoledronic acid (981) and clodronic acid (979). Zoledronic acid reduced mortality by 16 % (95 % CI 4–26) versus clodronic acid (hazard ratio [HR] 0.84, 95 % CI 0.74–0.96; $P=0.0118$) and extended median overall survival by 5.5 months (50.0 versus 44.5 months; $P=0.04$). Zoledronic acid also significantly improved progression-free survival by 12 % (95 % CI 2–20) versus clodronic acid (HR 0.88, 95 % CI 0.80–0.98; $P=0.0179$), and increased median progression-free survival by 2.0 months (19.5 versus 17.5 months; $P=0.07$) [61]. Pamidronate is given intravenously over 2 h at a dose of 90 mg every 4 weeks. No dosage adjustment is recommended in renal impairment when given monthly. Zoledronic acid is administered as an intravenous infusion over 15 min at a dose of 4 mg every 4 weeks. Dose adjustment is however required for patients with renal impairment. Zoledronic acid or pamidronate are equally effective. Rosen et al. compared zoledronic acid to pamidronate in patients with breast cancer and myeloma and concluded that zoledronic acid

(4 mg) via 15-min intravenous infusion was as effective and well tolerated as 90 mg of pamidronate in the treatment of osteolytic and mixed bone metastases/lesions in patients with advanced breast cancer or multiple myeloma [57]. Oral calcium and vitamin D supplements should be recommended for all patients on bisphosphonate therapy. The duration of therapy is not clearly defined. Long-term use has been associated with stress fractures [62–64]. Treatment is therefore recommended for a total of 2 years and frequency of administration can be reduced to every 3 months in the second year for those who achieve complete response and/or plateau phase [65]. For patients whose disease is active, or who have threatening bone disease beyond 2 years, therapy can be continued at a reduced frequency.

The enthusiasm for routine and continuous use of bisphosphonates has been affected by the risk of osteonecrosis of the jaw (ONJ) [66–69]. This risk may be reduced by good dental hygiene and referral of patients with chronic periodontal problems to a dentist for treatment and dental extraction prior to starting bisphosphonate therapy [70–72]. Antibiotic prophylaxis before dental procedures may be helpful in patients on bisphosphonates [73]. Patients should be continuously evaluated for the development of osteonecrosis of the mandible.

Denosumab

Denosumab, a monoclonal antibody that binds RANK-L, has been used for bone disease prevention in myeloma patients. In a large study Denosumab was superior to zoledronic acid in delaying time to first on-study skeletal related events (SRE) by a median of 8.21 months, reducing the risk of a first SRE by 17 % (hazard ratio, 0.83 [95 % confidence interval (CI): 0.76–0.90]; $P<0.001$). This study included 180 multiple myeloma patients, 87 received Denosumab and 93 received Zoledronic acid. Efficacy was demonstrated for first and multiple events and across patient subgroups. Disease progression and overall survival were similar between the treatments. ONJ occurred at a similar rate 1.8 % with Denosumab and 1.3 % with zoledronic acid ($P=0.13$) [74]. A combined analysis of three phase III trials in patients with metastatic bone disease receiving antiresorptive therapies also confirmed the same risk of ONJ. Another study randomly assigned patients with advanced cancer and multiple myeloma in a double-blind, double-dummy design to receive monthly subcutaneous Denosumab 120 mg ($n=886$) or intravenous ZA 4 mg (dose adjusted for renal impairment; $n=890$). Daily supplemental calcium and vitamin D were strongly recommended. Denosumab was non-inferior to ZA in delaying time to first on-study SRE (hazard ratio, 0.84; 95 % CI, 0.71–0.98; $P=0.0007$). Denosumab was not statistically superior to ZA in delaying time to first on-study SRE ($P=0.06$ adjusted for multiplicity) or time to first-and-subsequent (multiple) SRE (rate ratio, 0.90; 95 % CI, 0.77–1.04; $P=0.14$) [75]. It is possible that denosumab is going to be increasingly used for myeloma bone disease.

Renal Complications

Approximately 20 % of multiple myeloma patients will present with some degree of renal insufficiency and up to 50 % during the course of the disease [5, 76]. The Spanish cohort of 423 multiple myeloma patients reported renal insufficiency in 22.2 % of the patients similar to the 19 % reported in the Mayo clinic series [5, 77]. This is usually due to light chain cast nephropathy, hypercalcemia, dehydration, renal tubular dysfunction, nephrotoxic medications, and intravenous contrast dye. In a small percentage this may be related to the simultaneous presence of renal diseases associated with monoclonal gammopathy such as light chain deposition disease, membranoproliferative glomerulonephritis, and amyloidosis [78].

Prognosis

Long-term survival can be improved if one can achieve rapid reversal of the renal failure. In the Blade series the median survival of the 94 patients with renal failure was 8.6 months, whereas that of the 329 patients with normal renal function was 34.5 months ($P<0.001$). The median survival was 28.3 months in those who recovered their renal function not significantly different from those with normal renal function at presentation ($P=0.97$). Analysis of data from 1,435 elderly patients enrolled in four European phase III trials showed that after a median follow-up of 33 months, the 3-year OS was 66 % in patients without renal failure and 38 % in those with renal failure (HR 2.02, 95 % CI 1.5–2.70, $P<0.001$) [79]. The Greek myeloma study group evaluation of 756 newly diagnosed patients showed that the presence of renal failure at diagnosis was associated with inferior survival 19.5 versus 40.4 months for patients without renal failure ($P<0.001$) [76]. In the Nordic myeloma study group evaluation of 775 multiple myeloma patients, renal failure was observed in 29 % of the cases at the time of diagnosis [80]. Normalization of renal function was seen in 58 % by the end of the first year of diagnosis with most occurring within the first 3 months. Reversibility of renal failure was more frequently observed in patients with moderate renal failure, hypercalcemia, and low Bence Jones protein excretion. Patients who needed dialysis had a poor prognosis, with a median survival of 3.5 months. A 12-months landmark analysis showed that reversibility of renal failure was an important prognostic factor and that reversibility of renal failure improves long-term survival similar to the finding by Blade. Renal failure with need for dialysis is generally irreversible; however, some patients may benefit from intensive management and survive for a longer period with good quality of life.

Treatment of Cast Nephropathy

Effective management of acute renal failure and rapid reversal of renal damage is not only essential for the ability to allow adequate dosing and to use all known effective medications, but data suggest that lack of improvement in renal function has a significant effect on long-term survival [80]. Approximately 20–70 % of patients will recover their renal function with aggressive management of the renal failure and effective multiple myeloma therapy. The use of novel agents has had a significant effect in these patients. In a study of 41 newly diagnosed patients treated with high-dose dexamethasone containing regimens with or without Thalidomide and Bortezomib, renal failure was reversed in 73 % of all patients within a median of 1.9 months. Those treated with thalidomide and/or bortezomib had a reversibility rate of 80 % within a median of 0.8 months. Patients who responded to treatment had a better rate of reversal of renal failure 85 % versus 56 %, $P=0.046$, confirming the importance of effective myeloma therapy [81].

Plasma Exchange

The role of plasma exchange (PLEX) in the management of acute renal failure in multiple myeloma patients remains controversial. This is probably so because not all renal failure in multiple myeloma patients is related to light chain cast nephropathy. Review of 190 multiple myeloma patients with kidney biopsy at the Mayo clinic showed that paraprotein-associated lesions were seen in 73 % of patients and 25 % had non-paraprotein-associated lesions. Myeloma cast nephropathy was seen in 33 %, monoclonal immunoglobulin deposition disease in 22 %, and amyloidosis in 21 %. Non-paraprotein-associated lesions were acute tubular necrosis (9 %), hypertensive arteriosclerosis (6 %), and diabetic nephropathy (5 %) [82]. The largest randomized study evaluating the role of PLEX is from the Canadian apheresis group. In this study 104 patients were randomized to conventional chemotherapy therapy in addition to PLEX ($n=61$) or conventional chemotherapy alone ($n=43$) [83]. The primary outcome was a composite measure of death, dialysis dependence, or glomerular filtration rate less than 30 mL/min per 1.73 m^2. This occurred in 33 of 57 (57.9 %) patients in the PLEX group and in 27 of 39 (69.2 %) patients in the control group (difference between groups, 11.3 % [95 % CI, −8.3–29.1 %]; $P=0.36$). Concluding that, there was no benefit in the use of PLEX. Kidney biopsies were not performed in this study and therefore other causes of renal failure not responsive to PLEX may have been included.

Two other small randomized studies have also looked at the role of PLEX in multiple myeloma-associated acute renal failure. In 1990, Johnson and colleagues published a study of 21 patients who were randomly assigned either to PLEX and chemotherapy or to chemotherapy alone [84]. There was no significant difference in renal recovery or patient survival; however in the PLEX group, 3/7 dialysis-dependent patients were able to come of dialysis, compared with none in the control group (43 % versus 0 %). This difference was not statistically significant, probably, because of the small sample size.

The second study by Zucchelli and colleagues, however, reported a positive outcome with the use of PLEX in addition to chemotherapy [85]. This study randomized 29 patients to PLEX ($n=15$) in addition chemotherapy and hemodialysis when needed or to chemotherapy ($n=14$) in addition to preemptive intermittent peritoneal dialysis. At 2 months 11/13 (85 %) in the PLEX group had recovered sufficient renal function to stop dialysis, compared with 2/11 (18 %) in the control group ($P<0.01$). Patient survival at 1 year was also superior in the PLEX group 66 % compared with 28 % in the control group. A Mayo clinic retrospective review of 14 patients who received bortezomib and median of 8 PLEXs (range, 3–14) starting within 7 days after the diagnosis of cast nephropathy showed that 6 patients (43 %) had a complete renal response, which was defined as normalization of the serum creatinine level within 6 months. An additional six patients had a partial renal response, which was defined as a reduction in the serum creatinine level of more than 50 % from the maximum value or freedom from hemodialysis within 6 months among patients who were initially undergoing hemodialysis [86]. In view of the fact that improvement in renal function is associated with improved survival, PLEX should be considered in selected cases of myeloma-related acute renal failure. Patients who most probably will benefit are those with high circulating immunoglobulin light chain and light chain cast nephropathy on a kidney biopsy. Leung et al. reviewed data on 40 patients with myeloma and renal insufficiency looking at PLEX in relation to kidney biopsy finding and immunoglobulin-free light change reduction. They found that 18 of 40 (45 %) patients achieved a renal response after PLEX. Twenty-eight patients had serum immunoglobulin-free light measured before and after PLEX, serum FLC was reduced by >50 % in 11 of 14 renal responders, but in only 6 of 14 nonresponders ($P=0.05$). Three quarters of the patients with biopsy-proven cast nephropathy resolved their renal disease when the free light chains present in the serum were reduced by half or more, but there was no significant response when the reduction was less. The median time to a response was about 2 months [78]. Therefore, where possible a kidney biopsy should be considered, to determine if PLEX will be beneficial.

Drug Therapy

The primary goal in these situations should be rapid reduction of tumor burden using effective chemotherapy. Response rates in the range of 60–90 % have been seen with the current chemotherapy regimen available for multiple myeloma [12, 14, 87–89]. Most of these drugs have been used in myeloma patients with acute renal failure [81, 90–95]. Thalidomide in combination with dexamethasone was given to 20 patients with refractory multiple myeloma and renal insufficiency, 45 % achieved a partial response and 25 % minor response [92]. Recovery to a normal renal function was observed in 12 of 15 responsive patients. Bortezomib has been well studied in myeloma patients with renal failure. The safety and efficacy of Bortezomib was detailed in a study of 10 patients with CrCl <30 mL/min, by Jagannath et al. [96]. Seven patients completed 8 cycles of treatment; 4 patients received the full dose of 1.3 mg/m^2, and 3 patients received 1.0 mg/m^2. Responses were seen in these heavily pretreated patients, with no increased toxicity compared to those with normal renal function. Renal function did not appear to affect the 1-h post dose proteasome inhibition or its recovery. Ludwig reported on 8 patients with myeloma-associated renal failure with a median creatinine of 9.05 (5.2–12.0) mg/mL treated with Bortezomib 1.0 or 1.3 mg/m^2 on day 1, 4, 8, and 11 on a 3-week cycle [97]. Five out of the 8 patients experienced reversal of renal failure with their median creatinine level decreasing from 9.05 (5.2–12.0 mg/dL) to 2.1 mg/dL (0.8–2.4 mg/dL). All of the improvement was seen in two and a half months after starting therapy and was associated with disease response to chemotherapy. A multicenter retrospective study of 24 patients with renal failure all requiring dialysis except one, treated with Bortezomib-based chemotherapy regimen, showed an overall hematologic response rate of 75 %. One patient was spared dialysis and 3 others were able to discontinue dialysis [98]. In view of all these studies, myeloma patients with renal insufficiency should be treated with Bortezomib-based chemotherapy regimen.

A phase II study of Carfilzomib, a new proteasome inhibitor in patients with multiple myeloma and varying degrees of renal impairment, including patients on chronic hemodialysis, showed no differences in carfilzomib clearance or exposure among patients with normal renal function and renal impairment. Adverse events (AEs) were similar among groups. Although nearly 50 % of patients were refractory to bortezomib and lenalidomide, end of study overall response rate was 25.5 % with 7.9 months median duration of response. In conclusion, the pharmacokinetics and safety of carfilzomib were not influenced by the degree of baseline renal impairment, including patients on dialysis, and carfilzomib was well tolerated and demonstrated promising efficacy [95].

Stem Cell Transplantation

For those patients who are well enough to proceed to an autologous stem cell transplant as part of their myeloma therapy, further recovery in renal function may occur [99, 100]. The benefit of autologous stem cell transplant in myeloma patients with renal failure was published by Badros et al. [100]. They reviewed 81 multiple myeloma patients with renal failure (creatinine >176.8 μmol/L) at the time of autologous stem cell transplantation (auto-SCT), including 38 patients on dialysis. Conditioning regimen was melphalan 200 mg/m^2 in 60 patients (27 on dialysis). The remaining 21 patients (11 on dialysis) received melphalan 140 mg/m^2 because of excessive toxicity with the 200 mg/2 dosing. Thirty-one patients (38 %) completed tandem auto-SCT, including 11 on dialysis. Complete hematologic remission (CR) was achieved in 21 patients (26 %) after first auto-SCT and 31 patients (38 %) after tandem auto-SCT. Two patients discontinued dialysis after auto-SCT. Probabilities of event-free survival (EFS) and OS at 3 years were 48 % and 55 %, respectively. The same group also looked at 59 patients on dialysis at the time of autologous stem cell transplant [101]. A total of 37 patients had been on dialysis for more than 6 months. Of 54 patients evaluable for renal function improvement, 13 (24 %) became dialysis-independent at a median of 4 months after auto-SCT (range: 1–16). Dialysis duration ≤6 months prior to first auto-SCT and pre-transplant creatinine clearance >10 mL/min were significant for renal function recovery. This treatment option should be offered to myeloma patients with renal failure who are otherwise eligible for autologous stem cell transplant and early in the disease course because of the potential benefit.

Anemia

Most patients with multiple myeloma have anemia at the time of diagnosis and almost all will develop anemia as a result of disease progression or therapy. A review of initial presenting features of 1,027 patients at the Mayo clinic showed that anemia (hemoglobin concentration ≤12 g/dL) was present initially in 73 % of patients, 35 % had hemoglobulin ≤10 g/dL, and severe anemia requiring transfusion support was seen in 8 % [5]. The anemia is typically normocytic normochromic and the usual symptom is fatigue. Almost all patients with progressive disease do develop anemia. Bone marrow failure as a result of replacement by plasma cells is the usual cause of the anemia, although decreased erythropoiesis mediated by cytokines such as TNFa, IL-1, and IL-6 may also occur [38, 102]. Anemia of chronic disease with its various mechanisms such as ineffective erythropoiesis, decreased red cell survival, dysfunctional iron metabolism, and impaired erythropoietin response is well known. Other factors such vitamin deficiency, chronic renal failure, and iron deficiency may play a role. Case reports of hemolytic anemia in patients with multiple myeloma have been reported [103–105].

Although development of anemia has been reported in about 4–20 % of patients treated with current novel agents, it usually should improve or resolve with treatment [87, 106, 107]. Persistent anemia during therapy may be related to the effect of chemotherapy or disease progression. Lack of improvement in anemia should prompt evaluation for other causes of anemia such as vitamin and erythropoietin deficiency. If anemia persists, despite adequate response to therapy, other causes such as iron, vitamin B12, and folates deficiencies should be considered. Vitamin B12 deficiency has been reported in patients with multiple myeloma [108–111]. Appropriate vitamin replacement therapy should be instituted and is usually associated with improvement in hemoglobin. A small percentage of multiple myeloma patients may have simultaneous amyloidosis with malabsorption syndrome leading to folate deficiency.

Treatment of Anemia

Those presenting with severe symptomatic anemia should receive red cell transfusion. This usually results in improvement of symptoms such as fatigue and general weakness. The need for transfusion support should decrease with disease response to therapy.

Renal insufficiency with relative erythropoietin deficiency is common in this population. These patients may benefit from erythropoietin replacement therapy. The use of erythropoietin-stimulating factors (ESA) in multiple myeloma, however, should not be routine. Most patients will maintain a reasonable hemoglobulin on initiation of therapy for their multiple myeloma and will not require ESA. The goal of therapy should be to improve quality of life and reduce or eliminate the need for red cell transfusion. The role and benefit of appropriate use of ESA has been shown in multiple studies [102, 112–116]. The use of ESA has been associated with improvement in hemoglobulin in about 60–75 % of patients and also a better quality of life. Although the use of ESA is accepted by all societies (NCCN, EORTC, and ASCO-ASH) involved in the use of these agents, the threshold for initiation varies [117–120]. Most recommend starting ESA for hemoglobulin of less than 10 g/dL with a target hemoglobulin of 11–12 g/dL. The ESA available include erythropoietin alpha, beta, and darbepoetin and they are of equivalent efficacy. The recommended starting dose of erythropoietin alpha or beta is 150 Units/kg three times a week or 40,000 Units weekly given subcutaneously. Darbepoetin is given at a dose of 2.25 μg/kg weekly or 500 μg subcutaneously every 3 weeks. In our practice at the Mayo clinic we do recommend initiating ESA for hemoglobulin <9 g/dL and prefer darbepoetin 200 μg every 2 weeks. Responses are usually seen in about 6–8 weeks and dose adjustments may be needed. Adequate iron stores are required for effective response to erythropoietin. A ferritin and iron saturation level should be checked and should be greater than 100 ng/dL and 20 %, respectively. Iron replacement should be given if levels are inadequate. Treatment should be discontinued if there is no improvement in red cell transfusion requirement or improvement in hemoglobulin. If desired hemoglobulin is achieved adjusting dose down by 25–40 % may be required to maintain acceptable hemoglobulin level. Treatment should be discontinued if hemoglobulin exceeds 12 g/dL. The use of ESA is associated with complications such as thromboembolism 3–7 %, hypertension 4–30 %, and renal failure 12 % [121–124]. These complications are also common in multiple myeloma, especially thromboembolism, which may be exacerbated in the setting of immunomodulatory drugs such as Thalidomide, Lenalidomide, and Pomalidomide [125, 126].

Infections

Infections are one of the major causes of mortality and morbidity in multiple myeloma [6, 127–129]. The increased risk of infection is due to multiple factors including immunodeficiency (Polyclonal hypogammaglobulinemia) and neutropenia as a result of disease and chemotherapy [130–133]. In a study of 3,107 newly diagnosed cases of multiple myeloma by the MRC of UK, 299 died within the first 60 days of diagnosis and out of this 135 (45 %) were attributed to infections [6]. Specifically pneumonia occurred in 89 (66 %) of 135 bacterial infections. Most of the patients did not have severe neutropenia at the time of diagnosis, and only 11 of the 135 deaths from infection were classified as having neutropenia-associated. The most common organisms cultured were streptococcus pneumoniae, *Staphylococcus aureus*, and *Escherichia coli*. The risk and type of infection in multiple myeloma vary depending on whether the individual is newly diagnosed, receiving induction chemotherapy, in plateau phase, or at relapse [134–137]. Hargreaves et al. followed 102 patients in plateau phase and found that the risk of infection increased four times at the time of active disease [134]. In Perri's study the incidence of infection per patient years in the first 2 months was 4.68 compared to 1.04 for subsequent months [135]. The pattern of infection has changed over the years especially in the era of early diagnosis, more use of effective novel therapy, and the use of lower doses of corticosteroids [12, 129, 138]. Although there is less neutropenia with these new agents, the risk of bacterial infections ranges between 10 and 40 % [11, 139]. These novel therapies do also bring their own peculiar increased risk of certain infection, for example high risk of herpes zoster with Bortezomib [140–142]. The reported incidence is about 13 % in this population [143]. It is unclear if this high incidence will be seen with carfilzomib. Most of the carfilzomib studies did require herpes zoster prophylaxis [19, 144, 145].

Role of Prophylactic Therapy

The use of prophylaxis has therefore become an integral part of the management of multiple myeloma. Although there are no large randomized studies available, the few published literature suggest a benefit. This is even more important during periods of neutropenia and the first few months of therapy [146]. In a study conducted by Oken and colleagues, 54 patients with newly diagnosed multiple myeloma were randomized to receive prophylaxis with Trimethoprim-Sulfamethoxazole (TMP-SMX) 160/800 mg twice a day ($n=28$) versus placebo ($n=26$) for 2 months and followed for 3 months [147]. The incidence of bacterial infection was significantly lower in the prophylaxis group ($n=2$) compared to placebo ($n=11$). Most clinical trials using combination chemotherapy associated with increased risk of neutropenia recommend antibiotic prophylaxis [148, 149]. Bacterial prophylaxis using TMP-SMX 80/400 daily is therefore recommended. A quinolone or penicillin can be substituted for patients allergic to sulfa. [147]. The need for long-term bacterial prophylaxis should be reassessed after completion of induction therapy. Although uncommon, Pneumocystis jiroveci pneumonia (PJP) is associated with a high mortality [150–153]. If patients are to remain on long-term corticosteroid therapy, TMP-SMX for PJP prophylaxis is recommended especially those on high doses of corticosteroids [152, 154, 155]. Antiviral prophylaxis for herpes zoster is recommended for all patients receiving Bortezomib-based chemotherapy because of the high incidence of herpes Zoster [156, 157].

Vaccination

The value of vaccination against pneumococcus and influenza in multiple myeloma patients is not clearly defined and some studies suggest no benefit [158]. Most studies however have shown some immune response even in myeloma patients [159–162]. In view of the low risk associated with this vaccination, Pneumovax and influenza vaccination should be offered to all newly diagnosed patients.

Immune Globulin

Intravenous immunoglobulin (IVIG) has been available for several decades and has been frequently used in patients with multiple myeloma. However, randomized studies on the use of IVIG in multiple myeloma are limited [163–165]. In a randomized, double-blind, placebo-controlled, multicentre trial, 82 patients with stable multiple myeloma received monthly infusions of IVIG at 0.4 g/kg body weight or an equivalent volume of placebo (0.4 % albumin) intravenously for 1 year [166]. There were no episodes of septicemia or pneumonia in patients receiving IVIG compared with 10 in placebo patients ($P = 0.002$). IVIG also protected against recurrent infections in 60 patients who completed a year of treatment ($P = 0.021$). Before treatment, 54 of the patients who were immunized with Pneumovax had specific IgG responses measured. A poor pneumococcal IgG antibody response (less than twofold increase) identified patients who had maximum benefit from IVIG. No clear survival benefit, however, has been shown with the prophylactic use of IVIG. Although its use is not routinely recommended, it may be beneficial in reducing recurrent infection in a limited population.

Neuropathy

Patients with myeloma may also have neuropathy as a complication of their disease [167, 168]. In such cases it is necessary to rule out an associated primary amyloidosis, POEMS syndrome (Osteosclerotic myeloma), or cryoglobulinemia [169–173]. In patients who present with neurologic deficit, a detail neurologic evaluation should be done to rule out spinal cord compression due to tumor invasion of the spinal canal. Peripheral neuropathy may also occur from direct toxicity of the monoclonal proteins to peripheral nerve. However, in a larger number of cases the primary mechanism is not well understood [174]. Neurologic complications associated with the therapeutic interventions for controlling the multiple myeloma have become a major issue with the novel therapies. Although this has always been a major problem even with traditional chemotherapy agents used in the treatment of multiple myeloma such as vincristine and cisplatin [175–177], the incidence has significantly increased in the era of immunomodulatory drugs and proteasome inhibitors. Thalidomide, the first approved immunomodulatory drug for the management of myeloma, is associated with a 25–80 % incidence of neuropathy [178, 179]. This is related to dose and duration of therapy as seen in a study by Mileshkin and colleagues in which neuropathy increased from 38 % at 6 months to 73 % at 12 months, with 81 % of responding patients developing this complication [178]. Lenalidomide, however, has a significantly lower incidence of neuropathy with most studies reporting about 3–23 % incidence and only 3 % with greater than grade 3 neuropathy [107, 180–183]. The first-generation proteasome inhibitor Bortezomib is associated with a 35–80 % incidence of neuropathy [88, 184, 185]. The incidence of neuropathy is, however, significantly lower when administered by subcutaneous injection. In a phase III study comparing subcutaneous to intravenous delivery of bortezomib, peripheral neuropathy of any grade was 38 % versus 53 % ($P = 0.044$), grade 2 or worse 24 % versus 41 % ($P = 0.012$), and grade 3 or worse 6 % versus 16 % ($P = 0.026$) in favor of subcutaneous administration [186].

In a phase II study of Bortezomib in 64 newly diagnosed multiple myeloma patients, sensory polyneuropathy developed during treatment in 64 % of patients (grade 3 in 3 %) but this resolved in 85 % within a median of 98 days [183]. Underlying neuropathy, route of administration, frequency and duration of therapy, in addition to dose are risk factors for the development of neuropathy [168, 183, 186].

The new proteasome inhibitor carfilzomib has a lower incidence of peripheral neuropathy, with most studies reporting about 12–23 % peripheral neuropathy, primarily limited to grades 1 or 2

[19, 89, 144]. Grade 2 neuropathy can be very debilitating and significantly affect the quality of life of these patients, therefore neuropathy must be proactively looked for at every visit, and appropriate intervention such as discontinuation of drug or dose adjustment instituted [185, 187].

Treatment of Neuropathy

Preemptive evaluation and early management of neuropathy must be incorporated in the management of all multiple myeloma patients. Prior to starting therapy patients should be evaluated for signs and symptoms of peripheral neuropathy and educated about the symptoms and the importance of reporting them. There should be continuing evaluation during treatment so that appropriate interventions can be employed if necessary. This should begin with exclusion of other treatable causes of neuropathy such as vitamin B12 deficiency [109–111]. Specific management strategies are based on the severity of the peripheral neuropathy. In mild cases modification of dose, route of administration, and schedule may prevent progression. In the case of Bortezomib, weekly dosing and subcutaneous administration has been associated with less neuropathy [186, 188, 189]. In severe cases treatment will initially have to be discontinued and resume at lower doses after resolution of symptoms.

Therapeutic interventions include analgesic and antiepileptic agents and these may improve mood, sleep disturbance, and quality of life. Tricyclic antidepressants (amitriptyline) and anticonvulsants (gabapentin and pregabalin) have become the primary treatment for chemotherapy-induced peripheral neuropathy. The antiepileptic agent, gabapentin, has shown benefit in managing peripheral neuropathy. The starting dose should be 300 mg daily and this can be escalated to 2,700 mg depending on response. In diabetic-associated peripheral neuropathy pregabalin was found to be safe and effective in decreasing pain [190, 191]. The literature on its use in cancer and chemotherapy-associated neuropathy is limited. In a study of 30 children (median age 13.5 year) with chemotherapy-induced neuropathic pain, pregabalin was given at a daily dose of 150–300 mg for 8 weeks [192]. A significant and long-lasting pain relief was noted in 86 % of these patients. If pharmacologic therapy is required we do recommend gabapentin 300–2,700 mg daily or pregabalin 150–300 mg daily. In severe cases narcotic analgesics or the monoaminergic drug tramadol have been shown to be beneficial [193]. In our practice a topical formulation containing ketamine 0.5 %, lidocaine 2 %, and amitriptyline 2 % has been used with good symptomatic pain control. Other measures that may reduce pain and also reduce injury include wearing soft loose fit shoes and minimal bedding over feet at night.

Thrombosis

Cancers are associated with an increased risk of venous thromboembolic (VTE) disease [194–196]. The risk of thrombosis in multiple myeloma is estimated at about 3 % [125, 197]. Prior to the era of immunomodulatory drugs thrombosis in myeloma was attributed to the disease, immobilization as a result of bone pain, fractures, and dexamethasone therapy. It is also known that procoagulant factors may be upregulated in myeloma, while endogenous anticoagulants may be downregulated resulting in the increased risk of thrombosis [198]. Immunomodulatory drugs have been shown to increase cellular adhesion molecules, which may impair the function of endogenous anticoagulation [199, 200]. The immunomodulatory drugs thalidomide, lenalidomide, and Pomalidomide have become an integral part of myeloma therapy. Thalidomide and Lenalidomide in combination with dexamethasone have been associated with about 10–30 % risk of thrombosis [201–205]. Preemptive intervention is therefore recommended in all patients receiving immunomodulatory drugs [206]. The new immunomodulatory drug Pomalidomde is also associated with about 1.6–12.5 % risk of thrombosis [15, 16, 18, 207, 208]. Although the incidence reported in these studies are low, all these studies had thromboprophylaxis with aspirin or full anticoagulation. All patients on immunomodulatory drugs should be monitored closely for the development of VTE.

Prevention

Preventive therapies have included aspirin, low-molecular-weight heparin (LMWH), and warfarin [107, 209–213]. In a phase III study, 667 patients with previously untreated myeloma receiving thalidomide-containing regimens were randomized to aspirin (ASA 100 mg/day), warfarin (WAR 1.25 mg/day), or Enoxaparin (LMWH 40 mg/day) as thromboprophylaxis. ASA and WAR showed similar efficacy in reducing serious thromboembolic events, acute cardiovascular events, and sudden deaths compared with LMWH, except in elderly patients where WAR showed less efficacy than LMWH [214]. A prospective, open-label, randomized phase III trial compared the efficacy and safety of thromboprophylaxis with low-dose aspirin (ASA) or LMWH in patients with newly diagnosed MM, treated with lenalidomide-based chemotherapy. Overall 342 patients were randomly assigned to receive ASA 100 mg/day ($n=176$) or LMWH enoxaparin 40 mg/day ($n=166$). The incidence of VTE was 2.27 % in the ASA group and 1.20 % in the LMWH group. Compared with LMWH, the absolute difference in the proportion of VTE was 1.07 % (95 % confidence interval, −1.69–3.83; $P=0.452$) in the ASA group. ASA was an effective and less-expensive alternative to LMWH thromboprophylaxis [215]. LMWH and warfarin, however, do come with an increased risk of bleeding and since they have not been shown to be superior to aspirin, we do recommend aspirin as the initial thrombosis prophylaxis. Patients with prior history of thrombosis or other risk of thrombosis should be treated with full anticoagulation with LMWH or warfarin [216]. Those on immunomodulatory drugs who develop thrombosis while on aspirin should have their drug held and started on full anticoagulation. This can be resumed after they are well-anticoagulated [210].

References

1. Kyle RA, et al. Clinical course and prognosis of smoldering (asymptomatic) multiple myeloma. N Engl J Med. 2007;356(25):2582–90.
2. Blade J, Rosinol L. Complications of multiple myeloma. Hematol Oncol Clin North Am. 2007;21(6):1231–46.
3. Conte LG, et al. Clinical features and survival of Chilean patients with multiple myeloma. Rev Med Chil. 2007;135(9):1111–7.
4. International Myeloma Working Group. Criteria for the classification of monoclonal gammopathies, multiple myeloma and related disorders: a report of the International Myeloma Working Group. Br J Haematol. 2003;121(5):749–57.
5. Kyle RA, et al. Review of 1027 patients with newly diagnosed multiple myeloma. Mayo Clin Proc. 2003;78(1):21–33.
6. Augustson BM, et al. Early mortality after diagnosis of multiple myeloma: analysis of patients entered onto the United kingdom Medical Research Council trials between 1980 and 2002—Medical Research Council Adult Leukaemia Working Party. J Clin Oncol. 2005;23(36):9219–26.
7. Barlogie B, Smith L, Alexanian R. Effective treatment of advanced multiple myeloma refractory to alkylating agents. N Engl J Med. 1984;310(21):1353–6.
8. Alexanian R, Barlogie B, Tucker S. VAD-based regimens as primary treatment for multiple myeloma. Am J Hematol. 1990;33(2):86–9.
9. Dimopoulos MA, Kastritis E. Is there still place for VAD as primary treatment for patients with multiple myeloma who are candidates for high-dose therapy? Leuk Lymphoma. 2006;47(11):2271–2.
10. Kyle RA, Rajkumar SV. Treatment of multiple myeloma: a comprehensive review. Clin Lymphoma Myeloma. 2009;9(4):278–88.
11. Rajkumar SV, et al. Phase III clinical trial of thalidomide plus dexamethasone compared with dexamethasone alone in newly diagnosed multiple myeloma: a clinical trial coordinated by the Eastern Cooperative Oncology Group. J Clin Oncol. 2006;24(3):431–6.
12. Rajkumar SV, et al. Lenalidomide plus high-dose dexamethasone versus lenalidomide plus low-dose dexamethasone as initial therapy for newly diagnosed multiple myeloma: an open-label randomised controlled trial. Lancet Oncol. 2010;11(1):29–37.
13. Richardson PG, et al. Extended follow-up of a phase 3 trial in relapsed multiple myeloma: final time-to-event results of the APEX trial. Blood. 2007;110(10):3557–60.
14. Harousseau JL, et al. Bortezomib plus dexamethasone as induction treatment prior to autologous stem cell transplantation in patients with newly diagnosed multiple myeloma: results of an IFM phase II study. Haematologica. 2006;91(11):1498–505.
15. Leleu X, et al. Pomalidomide plus low-dose dexamethasone is active and well tolerated in bortezomib and lenalidomide-refractory multiple myeloma: Intergroupe Francophone du Myelome 2009-02. Blood. 2013;121(11):1968–75.
16. Lacy MQ, et al. Pomalidomide (CC4047) plus low-dose dexamethasone as therapy for relapsed multiple myeloma. J Clin Oncol. 2009;27(30):5008–14.

17. Lacy MQ, et al. Pomalidomide (CC4047) plus low dose dexamethasone (Pom/dex) is active and well tolerated in lenalidomide refractory multiple myeloma (MM). Leukemia. 2010;24(11):1934–9.
18. Lacy MQ, et al. Pomalidomide plus low-dose dexamethasone in myeloma refractory to both bortezomib and lenalidomide: comparison of 2 dosing strategies in dual-refractory disease. Blood. 2011; 118(11):2970–5.
19. Siegel DS, et al. A phase 2 study of single-agent carfilzomib (PX-171-003-A1) in patients with relapsed and refractory multiple myeloma. Blood. 2012;120(14):2817–25.
20. Vij R, et al. An open-label, single-arm, phase 2 (PX-171-004) study of single-agent carfilzomib in bortezomib-naive patients with relapsed and/or refractory multiple myeloma. Blood. 2012;119(24): 5661–70.
21. Kumar SK, et al. Improved survival in multiple myeloma and the impact of novel therapies. Blood. 2008;111(5):2516–20.
22. Roodman GD. Mechanisms of bone metastasis. N Engl J Med. 2004;350(16):1655–64.
23. Castellano D, et al. The role of RANK-ligand inhibition in cancer: the story of denosumab. Oncologist. 2011;16(2):136–45.
24. Elliott GT, McKenzie MW. Treatment of hypercalcemia. Drug Intell Clin Pharm. 1983;17(1):12–22.
25. Singer FR, et al. Treatment of hypercalcemia of malignancy with intravenous etidronate. A controlled, multicenter study. The Hypercalcemia Study Group. Arch Intern Med. 1991;151(3):471–6.
26. Davenport A, Goel S, Mackenzie JC. Treatment of hypercalcaemia with pamidronate in patients with end stage renal failure. Scand J Urol Nephrol. 1993;27(4):447–51.
27. Machado CE, Flombaum CD. Safety of pamidronate in patients with renal failure and hypercalcemia. Clin Nephrol. 1996;45(3):175–9.
28. Gucalp R, et al. Treatment of cancer-associated hypercalcemia. Double-blind comparison of rapid and slow intravenous infusion regimens of pamidronate disodium and saline alone. Arch Intern Med. 1994;154(17):1935–44.
29. Nussbaum SR, et al. Single-dose intravenous therapy with pamidronate for the treatment of hypercalcemia of malignancy: comparison of 30-, 60-, and 90-mg dosages. Am J Med. 1993;95(3):297–304.
30. Major PP, Coleman RE. Zoledronic acid in the treatment of hypercalcemia of malignancy: results of the international clinical development program. Semin Oncol. 2001;28(2 Suppl 6):17–24.
31. Sekine M, Takami H. Combination of calcitonin and pamidronate for emergency treatment of malignant hypercalcemia. Oncol Rep. 1998;5(1):197–9.
32. Binstock ML, Mundy GR. Effect of calcitonin and glutocorticoids in combination on the hypercalcemia of malignancy. Ann Intern Med. 1980;93(2): 269–72.
33. Wisneski LA, et al. Salmon calcitonin in hypercalcemia. Clin Pharmacol Ther. 1978;24(2):219–22.
34. Boikos SA, Hammers HJ. Denosumab for the treatment of bisphosphonate-refractory hypercalcemia. J Clin Oncol. 2012;30(29):e299.
35. Bech A, de Boer H. Denosumab for tumor-induced hypercalcemia complicated by renal failure. Ann Intern Med. 2012;156(12):906–7.
36. Body JJ, et al. Effects of denosumab in patients with bone metastases with and without previous bisphosphonate exposure. J Bone Miner Res. 2010;25(3):440–6.
37. Abildgaard N, et al. Biochemical markers of bone metabolism reflect osteoclastic and osteoblastic activity in multiple myeloma. Eur J Haematol. 2000;64(2):121–9.
38. Carter A, et al. The role of interleukin-1 and tumour necrosis factor-alpha in human multiple myeloma. Br J Haematol. 1990;74(4):424–31.
39. Merico F, et al. Cytokines involved in the progression of multiple myeloma. Clin Exp Immunol. 1993;92(1):27–31.
40. Walker R, et al. Magnetic resonance imaging in multiple myeloma: diagnostic and clinical implications. J Clin Oncol. 2007;25(9):1121–8.
41. Waheed S, et al. Standard and novel imaging methods for multiple myeloma: correlates with prognostic laboratory variables including gene expression profiling data. Haematologica. 2013;98(1):71–8.
42. Bartel TB, et al. F18-fluorodeoxyglucose positron emission tomography in the context of other imaging techniques and prognostic factors in multiple myeloma. Blood. 2009;114(10):2068–76.
43. Yaneva MP, Goranova-Marinova V, Goranov S. Palliative radiotherapy in patients with multiple myeloma. J BUON. 2006;11(1):43–8.
44. Adamietz IA, et al. Palliative radiotherapy in plasma cell myeloma. Radiother Oncol. 1991;20(2):111–6.
45. Leigh BR, et al. Radiation therapy for the palliation of multiple myeloma. Int J Radiat Oncol Biol Phys. 1993;25(5):801–4.
46. Mill WB, Griffith R. The role of radiation therapy in the management of plasma cell tumors. Cancer. 1980;45(4):647–52.
47. Saliou G, et al. Percutaneous vertebroplasty for pain management in malignant fractures of the spine with epidural involvement. Radiology. 2010;254(3): 882–90.
48. Lim BS, Chang UK, Youn SM. Clinical outcomes after percutaneous vertebroplasty for pathologic compression fractures in osteolytic metastatic spinal disease. J Korean Neurosurg Soc. 2009;45(6):369–74.
49. Bartolozzi B, et al. Percutaneous vertebroplasty and kyphoplasty in patients with multiple myeloma. Eur J Haematol. 2006;76(2):180–1.
50. Diamond TH, et al. Percutaneous vertebroplasty for acute vertebral body fracture and deformity in multiple myeloma: a short report. Br J Haematol. 2004;124(4):485–7.
51. Voormolen MH, et al. Percutaneous vertebroplasty compared with optimal pain medication treatment: short-term clinical outcome of patients with subacute or chronic painful osteoporotic vertebral compression

fractures. The VERTOS study. AJNR Am J Neuroradiol. 2007;28(3):555–60.
52. Wardlaw D, et al. Efficacy and safety of balloon kyphoplasty compared with non-surgical care for vertebral compression fracture (FREE): a randomised controlled trial. Lancet. 2009;373(9668):1016–24.
53. Buchbinder R, et al. A randomized trial of vertebroplasty for painful osteoporotic vertebral fractures. N Engl J Med. 2009;361(6):557–68.
54. Gray LA, et al. INvestigational Vertebroplasty Efficacy and Safety Trial (INVEST): a randomized controlled trial of percutaneous vertebroplasty. BMC Musculoskelet Disord. 2007;8:126.
55. Comstock BA, et al. *Investigational Vertebroplasty Safety and Efficacy Trial (INVEST): Patient-reported Outcomes through 1 Year*. Radiology, 2013 May 21. [Epub ahead of print].
56. Berenson JR, et al. Efficacy of pamidronate in reducing skeletal events in patients with advanced multiple myeloma. Myeloma Aredia Study Group. N Engl J Med. 1996;334(8):488–93.
57. Rosen LS, et al. Zoledronic acid versus pamidronate in the treatment of skeletal metastases in patients with breast cancer or osteolytic lesions of multiple myeloma: a phase III, double-blind, comparative trial. Cancer J. 2001;7(5):377–87.
58. Kraj M, et al. Comparative evaluation of safety and efficacy of pamidronate and zoledronic acid in multiple myeloma patients (single center experience). Acta Pol Pharm. 2002;59(6):478–82.
59. Ibrahim A, et al. Approval summary for zoledronic acid for treatment of multiple myeloma and cancer bone metastases. Clin Cancer Res. 2003;9(7):2394–9.
60. Berenson JR, et al. Long-term pamidronate treatment of advanced multiple myeloma patients reduces skeletal events. Myeloma Aredia Study Group. J Clin Oncol. 1998;16(2):593–602.
61. Morgan GJ, et al. First-line treatment with zoledronic acid as compared with clodronic acid in multiple myeloma (MRC Myeloma IX): a randomised controlled trial. Lancet. 2010;376(9757):1989–99.
62. Odvina CV, et al. Unusual mid-shaft fractures during long term bisphosphonate therapy. Clin Endocrinol (Oxf). 2009;72(2):161–8.
63. Napoli N, Novack D, Armamento-Villareal R. Bisphosphonate-associated femoral fracture: implications for management in patients with malignancies. Osteoporos Int. 2010;21(4):705–8.
64. Koh JS, et al. Femoral cortical stress lesions in long-term bisphosphonate therapy: a herald of impending fracture? J Orthop Trauma. 2010;24(2):75–81.
65. Lacy MQ, et al. Mayo clinic consensus statement for the use of bisphosphonates in multiple myeloma. Mayo Clin Proc. 2006;81(8):1047–53.
66. Ruggiero SL, et al. Osteonecrosis of the jaws associated with the use of bisphosphonates: a review of 63 cases. J Oral Maxillofac Surg. 2004;62(5):527–34.
67. Durie BG, Katz M, Crowley J. Osteonecrosis of the jaw and bisphosphonates. N Engl J Med. 2005;353(1):99–102; discussion 99–102.
68. Badros A, et al. Natural history of osteonecrosis of the jaw in patients with multiple myeloma. J Clin Oncol. 2008;26(36):5904–9.
69. Pozzi S, et al. Bisphosphonates-associated osteonecrosis of the jaw: a long-term follow-up of a series of 35 cases observed by GISL and evaluation of its frequency over time. Am J Hematol. 2009;84(12): 850–2.
70. Bagan J, et al. Recommendations for the prevention, diagnosis, and treatment of osteonecrosis of the jaw (ONJ) in cancer patients treated with bisphosphonates. Med Oral Patol Oral Cir Bucal. 2007;12(4): E336–40.
71. Chu V. Management of patients on bisphosphonates and prevention of bisphosphonate-related osteonecrosis of the jaw. Hawaii Dent J. 2008;39(5):9–12; quiz 17.
72. Landis BN, et al. Osteonecrosis of the jaw after treatment with bisphosphonates: is irreversible, so the focus must be on prevention. BMJ. 2006;333(7576): 982–3.
73. Montefusco V, et al. Antibiotic prophylaxis before dental procedures may reduce the incidence of osteonecrosis of the jaw in patients with multiple myeloma treated with bisphosphonates. Leuk Lymphoma. 2008;49(11):2156–62.
74. Lipton A, et al. Superiority of denosumab to zoledronic acid for prevention of skeletal-related events: a combined analysis of 3 pivotal, randomised, phase 3 trials. Eur J Cancer. 2012;48(16):3082–92.
75. Henry DH, et al. Randomized, double-blind study of denosumab versus zoledronic acid in the treatment of bone metastases in patients with advanced cancer (excluding breast and prostate cancer) or multiple myeloma. J Clin Oncol. 2011;29(9):1125–32.
76. Eleutherakis-Papaiakovou V, et al. Renal failure in multiple myeloma: incidence, correlations, and prognostic significance. Leuk Lymphoma. 2007; 48(2):337–41.
77. Blade J, et al. Renal failure in multiple myeloma: presenting features and predictors of outcome in 94 patients from a single institution. Arch Intern Med. 1998;158(17):1889–93.
78. Leung N, et al. Improvement of cast nephropathy with plasma exchange depends on the diagnosis and on reduction of serum free light chains. Kidney Int. 2008;73(11):1282–8.
79. Bringhen S, et al. Age and organ damage correlate with poor survival in myeloma patients: meta-analysis of 1435 individual patient data from 4 randomized trials. Haematologica. 2013;98(6):980–7.
80. Knudsen LM, Hjorth M, Hippe E. Renal failure in multiple myeloma: reversibility and impact on the prognosis. Nordic Myeloma Study Group. Eur J Haematol. 2000;65(3):175–81.
81. Kastritis E, et al. Reversibility of renal failure in newly diagnosed multiple myeloma patients treated with high dose dexamethasone-containing regimens and the impact of novel agents. Haematologica. 2007;92(4):546–9.

82. Nasr SH, et al. Clinicopathologic correlations in multiple myeloma: a case series of 190 patients with kidney biopsies. Am J Kidney Dis. 2012;59(6): 786–94.
83. Clark WF, et al. Plasma exchange when myeloma presents as acute renal failure: a randomized, controlled trial. Ann Intern Med. 2005;143(11):777–84.
84. Johnson WJ, et al. Treatment of renal failure associated with multiple myeloma. Plasmapheresis, hemodialysis, and chemotherapy. Arch Intern Med. 1990;150(4):863–9.
85. Zucchelli P, et al. Controlled plasma exchange trial in acute renal failure due to multiple myeloma. Kidney Int. 1988;33(6):1175–80.
86. Burnette BL, Leung N, Rajkumar SV. Renal improvement in myeloma with bortezomib plus plasma exchange. N Engl J Med. 2011;364(24):2365–6.
87. Rajkumar SV, et al. Multicenter, randomized, double-blind, placebo-controlled study of thalidomide plus dexamethasone compared with dexamethasone as initial therapy for newly diagnosed multiple myeloma. J Clin Oncol. 2008;26(13): 2171–7.
88. Jagannath S, et al. Bortezomib therapy alone and in combination with dexamethasone for previously untreated symptomatic multiple myeloma. Br J Haematol. 2005;129(6):776–83.
89. Jakubowiak AJ, et al. A phase 1/2 study of carfilzomib in combination with lenalidomide and low-dose dexamethasone as a frontline treatment for multiple myeloma. Blood. 2012;120(9):1801–9.
90. Ludwig H, Zojer N. Renal recovery with lenalidomide in a patient with bortezomib-resistant multiple myeloma. Nat Rev Clin Oncol. 2010;7(5): 289–94.
91. Dimopoulos MA, et al. Lenalidomide and dexamethasone for the treatment of refractory/relapsed multiple myeloma: dosing of lenalidomide according to renal function and effect on renal impairment. Eur J Haematol. 2010;85(1):1–5.
92. Tosi P, et al. Thalidomide alone or in combination with dexamethasone in patients with advanced, relapsed or refractory multiple myeloma and renal failure. Eur J Haematol. 2004;73(2):98–103.
93. Roussou M, et al. Treatment of patients with multiple myeloma complicated by renal failure with bortezomib-based regimens. Leuk Lymphoma. 2008;49(5):890–5.
94. Carlson K, Hjorth M, Knudsen LM. Toxicity in standard melphalan-prednisone therapy among myeloma patients with renal failure—a retrospective analysis and recommendations for dose adjustment. Br J Haematol. 2005;128(5):631–5.
95. Badros AZ, et al. *Carfilzomib in multiple myeloma patients with renal impairment: pharmacokinetics and safety*. Leukemia, 2013;27(8):1707–14.
96. Jagannath S, et al. Bortezomib in recurrent and/or refractory multiple myeloma. Initial clinical experience in patients with impared renal function. Cancer. 2005;103(6):1195–200.
97. Ludwig H, et al. Reversal of acute renal failure by bortezomib-based chemotherapy in patients with multiple myeloma. Haematologica. 2007;92(10):1411–4.
98. Chanan-Khan AA, et al. Activity and safety of bortezomib in multiple myeloma patients with advanced renal failure: a multicenter retrospective study. Blood. 2007;109(6):2604–6.
99. Tauro S, et al. Recovery of renal function after autologous stem cell transplantation in myeloma patients with end-stage renal failure. Bone Marrow Transplant. 2002;30(7):471–3.
100. Badros A, et al. Results of autologous stem cell transplant in multiple myeloma patients with renal failure. Br J Haematol. 2001;114(4):822–9.
101. Lee CK, et al. Dialysis-dependent renal failure in patients with myeloma can be reversed by high-dose myeloablative therapy and autotransplant. Bone Marrow Transplant. 2004;33(8):823–8.
102. Musto P, et al. Clinical results of recombinant erythropoietin in transfusion-dependent patients with refractory multiple myeloma: role of cytokines and monitoring of erythropoiesis. Eur J Haematol. 1997;58(5):314–9.
103. Vaiopoulos G, et al. Multiple myeloma associated with autoimmune hemolytic anemia. Haematologica. 1994;79(3):262–4.
104. Friedland M, Schaefer P. Myelomatosis and hemolytic anemia. Hemolytic anemia, a rare complication of multiple myeloma, is successfully managed by splenectomy. R I Med J. 1979;62(12):469–71.
105. Wada H, et al. Multiple myeloma complicated by autoimmune hemolytic anemia. Intern Med. 2004;43(7):595–8.
106. Kumar S, et al. Randomized, multicenter, phase 2 study (EVOLUTION) of combinations of bortezomib, dexamethasone, cyclophosphamide, and lenalidomide in previously untreated multiple myeloma. Blood. 2012;119(19):4375–82.
107. Gay F, et al. Lenalidomide plus dexamethasone versus thalidomide plus dexamethasone in newly diagnosed multiple myeloma: a comparative analysis of 411 patients. Blood. 2010;115(7): 1343–50.
108. Vlasveld LT. Low cobalamin (vitamin B12) levels in multiple myeloma: a retrospective study. Neth J Med. 2003;61(8):249–52.
109. Heyerdahl F, Kildahl-Andersen O. Myelomatosis and low level of vitamin B12. Tidsskr Nor Laegeforen. 1999;119(29):4321–2.
110. Perillie PE. Myeloma and pernicious anemia. Am J Med Sci. 1978;275(1):93–8.
111. Hansen OP, et al. Interrelationships between Vitamin B12 and folic acid in myelomatosis: cobalamin coenzyme and tetrahydrofolic acid function. Scand J Haematol. 1978;20(4):360–70.
112. Ludwig H, et al. Erythropoietin treatment of anemia associated with multiple myeloma. N Engl J Med. 1990;322(24):1693–9.
113. Osterborg A, et al. Randomized, double-blind, placebo-controlled trial of recombinant human

erythropoietin, epoetin beta, in hematologic malignancies. J Clin Oncol. 2002;20(10):2486–94.
114. Dammacco F, Castoldi G, Rodjer S. Efficacy of epoetin alfa in the treatment of anaemia of multiple myeloma. Br J Haematol. 2001;113(1):172–9.
115. Garton JP, et al. Epoetin alfa for the treatment of the anemia of multiple myeloma. A prospective, randomized, placebo-controlled, double-blind trial. Arch Intern Med. 1995;155(19):2069–74.
116. Cazzola M, et al. Recombinant human erythropoietin in the anemia associated with multiple myeloma or non-Hodgkin's lymphoma: dose finding and identification of predictors of response. Blood. 1995; 86(12):4446–53.
117. Rizzo JD, et al. Use of epoetin and darbepoetin in patients with cancer: 2007 American Society of Clinical Oncology/American Society of Hematology clinical practice guideline update. J Clin Oncol. 2008;26(1):132–49.
118. Straus DJ, et al. Quality-of-life and health benefits of early treatment of mild anemia: a randomized trial of epoetin alfa in patients receiving chemotherapy for hematologic malignancies. Cancer. 2006;107(8): 1909–17.
119. Charu V, et al. A randomized, open-label, multicenter trial of immediate versus delayed intervention with darbepoetin alfa for chemotherapy-induced anemia. Oncologist. 2007;12(10):1253–63.
120. Osterborg A, et al. Recombinant human erythropoietin in transfusion-dependent anemic patients with multiple myeloma and non-Hodgkin's lymphoma—a randomized multicenter study. The European Study Group of Erythropoietin (Epoetin Beta) Treatment in Multiple Myeloma and Non-Hodgkin's Lymphoma. Blood. 1996;87(7):2675–82.
121. Bennett CL, et al. Venous thromboembolism and mortality associated with recombinant erythropoietin and darbepoetin administration for the treatment of cancer-associated anemia. JAMA. 2008;299(8): 914–24.
122. Vanrenterghem Y, et al. Randomized trial of darbepoetin alfa for treatment of renal anemia at a reduced dose frequency compared with rHuEPO in dialysis patients. Kidney Int. 2002;62(6):2167–75.
123. Steurer M, et al. Thromboembolic events in patients with myelodysplastic syndrome receiving thalidomide in combination with darbepoietin-alpha. Br J Haematol. 2003;121(1):101–3.
124. Singh AK, et al. Correction of anemia with epoetin alfa in chronic kidney disease. N Engl J Med. 2006;355(20):2085–98.
125. Catovsky D, et al. Thromboembolic complications in myelomatosis. Br Med J. 1970;3(5720):438–9.
126. Galli M, et al. Recombinant human erythropoietin and the risk of thrombosis in patients receiving thalidomide for multiple myeloma. Haematologica. 2004;89(9):1141–2.
127. Doughney KB, Williams DM, Penn RL. Multiple myeloma: infectious complications. South Med J. 1988;81(7):855–8.
128. Paradisi F, Corti G, Cinelli R. Infections in multiple myeloma. Infect Dis Clin North Am. 2001;15(2): 373–84; vii–viii.
129. Espersen F, et al. Current patterns of bacterial infection in myelomatosis. Scand J Infect Dis. 1984;16(2):169–73.
130. Hopen G, et al. Granulocyte function in malignant monoclonal gammopathy. Scand J Haematol. 1983;31(2):133–43.
131. Jacobson DR, Zolla-Pazner S. Immunosuppression and infection in multiple myeloma. Semin Oncol. 1986;13(3):282–90.
132. Cesana C, et al. Risk factors for the development of bacterial infections in multiple myeloma treated with two different vincristine-adriamycin-dexamethasone schedules. Haematologica. 2003;88(9):1022–8.
133. Cheson BD, Plass RR, Rothstein G. Defective opsonization in multiple myeloma. Blood. 1980;55(4): 602–6.
134. Hargreaves RM, et al. Immunological factors and risk of infection in plateau phase myeloma. J Clin Pathol. 1995;48(3):260–6.
135. Perri RT, Hebbel RP, Oken MM. Influence of treatment and response status on infection risk in multiple myeloma. Am J Med. 1981;71(6):935–40.
136. Goranov S. Clinical problems of infectious complications in patients with multiple myeloma. Folia Med (Plovdiv). 1994;36(1):41–6.
137. Savage DG, Lindenbaum J, Garrett TJ. Biphasic pattern of bacterial infection in multiple myeloma. Ann Intern Med. 1982;96(1):47–50.
138. Shaikh BS, et al. Changing patterns of infections in patients with multiple myeloma. Oncology. 1982;39(2):78–82.
139. Weber D, et al. Thalidomide alone or with dexamethasone for previously untreated multiple myeloma. J Clin Oncol. 2003;21(1):16–9.
140. Kim SJ, et al. Bortezomib and the increased incidence of herpes zoster in patients with multiple myeloma. Clin Lymphoma Myeloma. 2008;8(4): 237–40.
141. Hasegawa Y, et al. Prophylaxis with acyclovir for herpes zoster infection during bortezomib-dexamethasone combination therapy. Rinsho Ketsueki. 2009;50(6):488–94.
142. Basler M, et al. The proteasome inhibitor bortezomib enhances the susceptibility to viral infection. J Immunol. 2009;183(10):6145–50.
143. Chanan-Khan A, et al. Analysis of herpes zoster events among bortezomib-treated patients in the phase III APEX study. J Clin Oncol. 2008;26(29): 4784–90.
144. Jagannath S, et al. An open-label single-arm pilot phase II study (PX-171-003-A0) of low-dose, single-agent carfilzomib in patients with relapsed and refractory multiple myeloma. Clin Lymphoma Myeloma Leuk. 2012;12(5):310–8.
145. Vij R, et al. An open-label, single-arm, phase 2 study of single-agent carfilzomib in patients with relapsed and/or refractory multiple myeloma who have been

previously treated with bortezomib. Br J Haematol. 2012;158(6):739–48.

146. Reuter S, et al. Impact of fluoroquinolone prophylaxis on reduced infection-related mortality among patients with neutropenia and hematologic malignancies. Clin Infect Dis. 2005;40(8):1087–93.
147. Oken MM, et al. Prophylactic antibiotics for the prevention of early infection in multiple myeloma. Am J Med. 1996;100(6):624–8.
148. Lee CK, et al. DTPACE: an effective, novel combination chemotherapy with thalidomide for previously treated patients with myeloma. J Clin Oncol. 2003;21(14):2732–9.
149. Reeder CB, et al. Cyclophosphamide, bortezomib and dexamethasone induction for newly diagnosed multiple myeloma: high response rates in a phase II clinical trial. Leukemia. 2009;23(7):1337–41.
150. van der Lelie J, et al. Pneumocystis carinii pneumonia in HIV-negative patients with haematologic disease. Infection. 1997;25(2):78–81.
151. Worth LJ, et al. An analysis of the utilisation of chemoprophylaxis against Pneumocystis jirovecii pneumonia in patients with malignancy receiving corticosteroid therapy at a cancer hospital. Br J Cancer. 2005;92(5):867–72.
152. Pagano L, et al. Pneumocystis carinii pneumonia in patients with malignant haematological diseases: 10 years' experience of infection in GIMEMA centres. Br J Haematol. 2002;117(2):379–86.
153. Peters SG, Prakash UB. Pneumocystis carinii pneumonia. Review of 53 cases. Am J Med. 1987;82(1):73–8.
154. Roblot F, et al. Pneumocystis carinii pneumonia in patients with hematologic malignancies: a descriptive study. J Infect. 2003;47(1):19–27.
155. Yale SH, Limper AH. Pneumocystis carinii pneumonia in patients without acquired immunodeficiency syndrome: associated illness and prior corticosteroid therapy. Mayo Clin Proc. 1996;71(1):5–13.
156. Vickrey E, et al. Acyclovir to prevent reactivation of varicella zoster virus (herpes zoster) in multiple myeloma patients receiving bortezomib therapy. Cancer. 2009;115(1):229–32.
157. Pour L, et al. Varicella-zoster virus prophylaxis with low-dose acyclovir in patients with multiple myeloma treated with bortezomib. Clin Lymphoma Myeloma. 2009;9(2):151–3.
158. Robertson JD, et al. Immunogenicity of vaccination against influenza, Streptococcus pneumoniae and Haemophilus influenzae type B in patients with multiple myeloma. Br J Cancer. 2000;82(7):1261–5.
159. Einarsdottir HM, et al. Nationwide study of recurrent invasive pneumococcal infections in a population with a low prevalence of human immunodeficiency virus infection. Clin Microbiol Infect. 2005;11(9): 744–9.
160. Shildt RA, et al. Polyvalent pneumococcal immunization of patients with plasma cell dyscrasias. Cancer. 1981;48(6):1377–80.
161. Landesman SH, Schiffman G. Assessment of the antibody response to pneumococcal vaccine in high-risk populations. Rev Infect Dis. 1981;3(Suppl): S184–97.
162. Lazarus HM, et al. Pneumococcal vaccination: the response of patients with multiple myeloma. Am J Med. 1980;69(3):419–23.
163. Gordon DS, et al. Phase I study of intravenous gamma globulin in multiple myeloma. Am J Med. 1984;76(3A):111–6.
164. Musto P, Brugiatelli M, Carotenuto M. Prophylaxis against infections with intravenous immunoglobulins in multiple myeloma. Br J Haematol. 1995;89(4):945–6.
165. Raanani P, et al. Immunoglobulin prophylaxis in chronic lymphocytic leukemia and multiple myeloma: systematic review and meta-analysis. Leuk Lymphoma. 2009;50(5):764–72.
166. Chapel HM, et al. Randomised trial of intravenous immunoglobulin as prophylaxis against infection in plateau-phase multiple myeloma. The UK Group for Immunoglobulin Replacement Therapy in Multiple Myeloma. Lancet. 1994;343(8905):1059–63.
167. Kelly Jr JJ, et al. The spectrum of peripheral neuropathy in myeloma. Neurology. 1981;31(1):24–31.
168. Richardson PG, et al. Single-agent bortezomib in previously untreated multiple myeloma: efficacy, characterization of peripheral neuropathy, and molecular correlations with response and neuropathy. J Clin Oncol. 2009;27(21):3518–25.
169. Kelly Jr JJ, et al. Osteosclerotic myeloma and peripheral neuropathy. Neurology. 1983;33(2):202–10.
170. Dispenzieri A, et al. POEMS syndrome: definitions and long-term outcome. Blood. 2003;101(7): 2496–506.
171. Wilson JR, Stittsworth Jr JD, Fisher MA. Electrodiagnostic patterns in MGUS neuropathy. Electromyogr Clin Neurophysiol. 2001;41(7): 409–18.
172. Noring L, et al. Peripheral neuropathy in patients with benign monoclonal gammopathy—a pilot study. J Neurol. 1982;228(3):185–94.
173. Nobile-Orazio E, et al. Peripheral neuropathy in monoclonal gammopathy of undetermined significance: prevalence and immunopathogenetic studies. Acta Neurol Scand. 1992;85(6):383–90.
174. Besinger UA, et al. Myeloma neuropathy: passive transfer from man to mouse. Science. 1981; 213(4511):1027–30.
175. Roelofs RI, et al. Peripheral sensory neuropathy and cisplatin chemotherapy. Neurology. 1984;34(7):934–8.
176. van der Hoop RG, et al. Incidence of neuropathy in 395 patients with ovarian cancer treated with or without cisplatin. Cancer. 1990;66(8):1697–702.
177. Windebank AJ, Grisold W. Chemotherapy-induced neuropathy. J Peripher Nerv Syst. 2008;13(1):27–46.
178. Mileshkin L, et al. Development of neuropathy in patients with myeloma treated with thalidomide: patterns of occurrence and the role of electrophysiologic monitoring. J Clin Oncol. 2006;24(27): 4507–14.
179. Plasmati R, et al. Neuropathy in multiple myeloma treated with thalidomide: a prospective study. Neurology. 2007;69(6):573–81.

180. Argyriou AA, Iconomou G, Kalofonos HP. Bortezomib-induced peripheral neuropathy in multiple myeloma: a comprehensive review of the literature. Blood. 2008;112(5):1593–9.
181. Dahut WL, et al. Phase I study of oral lenalidomide in patients with refractory metastatic cancer. J Clin Pharmacol. 2009;49(6):650–60.
182. Richardson PG, et al. A randomized phase 2 study of lenalidomide therapy for patients with relapsed or relapsed and refractory multiple myeloma. Blood. 2006;108(10):3458–64.
183. Richardson PG, et al. Frequency, characteristics, and reversibility of peripheral neuropathy during treatment of advanced multiple myeloma with bortezomib. J Clin Oncol. 2006;24(19):3113–20.
184. Richardson PG, et al. Bortezomib or high-dose dexamethasone for relapsed multiple myeloma. N Engl J Med. 2005;352(24):2487–98.
185. Richardson PG, et al. Reversibility of symptomatic peripheral neuropathy with bortezomib in the phase III APEX trial in relapsed multiple myeloma: impact of a dose-modification guideline. Br J Haematol. 2009;144(6):895–903.
186. Moreau P, et al. Subcutaneous versus intravenous administration of bortezomib in patients with relapsed multiple myeloma: a randomised, phase 3, non-inferiority study. Lancet Oncol. 2011;12(5):431–40.
187. El-Cheikh J, et al. Features and risk factors of peripheral neuropathy during treatment with bortezomib for advanced multiple myeloma. Clin Lymphoma Myeloma. 2008;8(3):146–52.
188. Hainsworth JD, et al. Weekly treatment with bortezomib for patients with recurrent or refractory multiple myeloma: a phase 2 trial of the Minnie Pearl Cancer Research Network. Cancer. 2008;113(4):765–71.
189. Suvannasankha A, et al. Weekly bortezomib/methylprednisolone is effective and well tolerated in relapsed multiple myeloma. Clin Lymphoma Myeloma. 2006;7(2):131–4.
190. Rosenstock J, et al. Pregabalin for the treatment of painful diabetic peripheral neuropathy: a double-blind, placebo-controlled trial. Pain. 2004;110(3):628–38.
191. Tolle T, et al. Pregabalin for relief of neuropathic pain associated with diabetic neuropathy: a randomized, double-blind study. Eur J Pain. 2008;12(2):203–13.
192. Vondracek P, et al. Efficacy of pregabalin in neuropathic pain in paediatric oncological patients. Eur J Paediatr Neurol. 2009;13(4):332–6.
193. Sindrup SH, et al. Tramadol relieves pain and allodynia in polyneuropathy: a randomised, double-blind, controlled trial. Pain. 1999;83(1):85–90.
194. Nordstrom M, et al. Deep venous thrombosis and occult malignancy: an epidemiological study. BMJ. 1994;308(6933):891–4.
195. Falanga A, Donati MB. Pathogenesis of thrombosis in patients with malignancy. Int J Hematol. 2001;73(2):137–44.
196. Hettiarachchi RJ, et al. Undiagnosed malignancy in patients with deep vein thrombosis: incidence, risk indicators, and diagnosis. Cancer. 1998;83(1):180–5.
197. Kristinsson SY, et al. Deep vein thrombosis after monoclonal gammopathy of undetermined significance and multiple myeloma. Blood. 2008;112(9):3582–6.
198. Uaprasert N, et al. Venous thromboembolism in multiple myeloma: current perspectives in pathogenesis. Eur J Cancer. 2010;46(10):1790–9.
199. Corso A, et al. Modification of thrombomodulin plasma levels in refractory myeloma patients during treatment with thalidomide and dexamethasone. Ann Hematol. 2004;83(9):588–91.
200. Elice F, et al. Thrombosis associated with angiogenesis inhibitors. Best Pract Res Clin Haematol. 2009;22(1):115–28.
201. Cavo M, et al. Deep-vein thrombosis in patients with multiple myeloma receiving first-line thalidomide-dexamethasone therapy. Blood. 2002;100(6):2272–3.
202. Camba L, et al. Thalidomide and thrombosis in patients with multiple myeloma. Haematologica. 2001;86(10):1108–9.
203. Menon SP, et al. Thromboembolic events with lenalidomide-based therapy for multiple myeloma. Cancer. 2008;112(7):1522–8.
204. Rus C, et al. Thalidomide in front line treatment in multiple myeloma: serious risk of venous thromboembolism and evidence for thromboprophylaxis. J Thromb Haemost. 2004;2(11):2063–5.
205. Carrier M, et al. Rates of venous thromboembolism in multiple myeloma patients undergoing immunomodulatory therapy with thalidomide or lenalidomide: a systematic review and meta-analysis. J Thromb Haemost. 2011;9(4):653–63.
206. Palumbo A, et al. Prevention of thalidomide- and lenalidomide-associated thrombosis in myeloma. Leukemia. 2008;22(2):414–23.
207. Richardson PG, et al. Phase 1 study of pomalidomide MTD, safety, and efficacy in patients with refractory multiple myeloma who have received lenalidomide and bortezomib. Blood. 2013;121(11):1961–7.
208. Schey SA, et al. Phase I study of an immunomodulatory thalidomide analog, CC-4047, in relapsed or refractory multiple myeloma. J Clin Oncol. 2004;22(16):3269–76.
209. Miller KC, et al. Prospective evaluation of low-dose warfarin for prevention of thalidomide associated venous thromboembolism. Leuk Lymphoma. 2006;47(11):2339–43.
210. Zangari M, et al. Deep vein thrombosis in patients with multiple myeloma treated with thalidomide and chemotherapy: effects of prophylactic and therapeutic anticoagulation. Br J Haematol. 2004;126(5):715–21.
211. Baz R, et al. The role of aspirin in the prevention of thrombotic complications of thalidomide and

anthracycline-based chemotherapy for multiple myeloma. Mayo Clin Proc. 2005;80(12):1568–74.
212. Zonder JA, et al. Thrombotic complications in patients with newly diagnosed multiple myeloma treated with lenalidomide and dexamethasone: benefit of aspirin prophylaxis. Blood. 2006;108(1):403; author reply 404.
213. Minnema MC, et al. Prevention of venous thromboembolism with low molecular-weight heparin in patients with multiple myeloma treated with thalidomide and chemotherapy. Leukemia. 2004;18(12):2044–6.
214. Palumbo A, et al. Aspirin, warfarin, or enoxaparin thromboprophylaxis in patients with multiple myeloma treated with thalidomide: a phase III, open-label, randomized trial. J Clin Oncol. 2011;29(8):986–93.
215. Larocca A, et al. Aspirin or enoxaparin thromboprophylaxis for patients with newly diagnosed multiple myeloma treated with lenalidomide. Blood. 2012;119(4):933–9; quiz 1093.
216. Jimenez-Zepeda VH, Dominguez-Martinez VJ. Acquired activated protein C resistance and thrombosis in multiple myeloma patients. Thromb J. 2006;4:11.

POEMS Syndrome (Takatsuki Syndrome)

15

Angela Dispenzieri

Introduction

POEMS syndrome [1], also known as osteosclerotic myeloma, Takatsuki syndrome [2], and Crow–Fukase syndrome [3, 4], is a rare paraneoplastic syndrome due to an underlying plasma cell disorder. The acronym POEMS refers to several, but not all, of the features of the syndrome: polyradiculoneuropathy, organomegaly, endocrinopathy, monoclonal plasma cell disorder, and skin changes. Not all of the features within the acronym are required to make the diagnosis. There are other important features not included in the POEMS acronym, including *p*apilledema, *e*xtravascular volume overload, *s*clerotic bone lesions, *t*hrombocytosis/erythrocytosis (P.E.S.T.), elevated VEGF levels, abnormal pulmonary function tests, and a predisposition towards thrombosis. Lastly, there is a Castleman's disease variant of POEMS syndrome that may not be associated with a clonal plasma cell disorder [5, 6]. Table 15.1 outlines the range of expected frequencies of each of the features based on the largest published series [2, 7–11].

VEGF is the cytokine that correlates best with disease activity [12–20], although it may not be the driving force of the disease based on the mixed results seen with anti-VEGF therapy [5, 21–29]. The pathogenesis of the syndrome is not well understood. VEGF, which is expressed by osteoblasts, macrophages, tumor cells [30] (including plasma cells) [31, 32], and megakaryocytes/platelets [33], is known to target endothelial cells, induce a rapid and reversible increase in vascular permeability, and be important in angiogenesis. Both IL-1β and IL-6 have been shown to stimulate VEGF production [30]. Interleukin 12 has also shown to be quite elevated in patients with POEMS syndrome [34]. Little is known about the plasma cells in POEMS syndrome except that more than 95 % of the time they are lambda light chain-restricted with restricted immunoglobulin light chain variable gene usage (IGLV1) [5].

Diagnosis

The constellation of an ascending peripheral neuropathy—especially demyelinating—and any of the following should elicit an in-depth search for POEMS syndrome: monoclonal protein (especially when lambda-restricted); thrombocytosis; anasarca; or papilledema. Making the diagnosis can be a challenge, but a good history and physical examination followed by appropriate testing—most notably radiographic assessment of bones [35], measurement of VEGF [14, 18, 36, 37], and careful analysis of a bone marrow biopsy [38]—can differentiate this syndrome

A. Dispenzieri, M.D. (✉)
Division of Hematology, Mayo Clinic,
200 First Street, SW, Rochester, MN 55905, USA
e-mail: dispenzieri.angela@mayo.edu

M.A. Gertz and S.V. Rajkumar (eds.), *Multiple Myeloma: Diagnosis and Treatment*,
DOI 10.1007/978-1-4614-8520-9_15, © Mayo Foundation for Medical Education and Research 2014

Table 15.1 Criteria for the diagnosis of POEMS syndrome[a]

		% Affected[b]
Mandatory major criteria (both required)	1. Polyradiculoneuropathy (typically demyelinating)	100
	2. Monoclonal plasma cell disorder (almost always λ)	100[c]
Other major criteria (one required)	3. Castleman's disease[d]	11–25
	4. Sclerotic bone lesions	27–97
	5. Vascular endothelial growth factor elevation[e]	
Minor criteria (one required)	6. Organomegaly (splenomegaly, hepatomegaly, or lymphadenopathy)	45–85
	7. Extravascular volume overload (edema, pleural effusion, or ascites)	29–87
	8. Endocrinopathy (adrenal, thyroid[f], pituitary, gonadal, parathyroid, pancreatic[f])	67–84
	9. Skin changes (hyperpigmentation, hypertrichosis, glomeruloid hemangiomata, plethora, acrocyanosis, flushing, white nails)	68–89
	10. Papilledema	29–64
	11. Thrombocytosis/polycythemia[g]	54–88
Other symptoms and signs	Clubbing, weight loss, hyperhidrosis, pulmonary hypertension/restrictive lung disease, thrombotic diatheses, diarrhea, low vitamin B_{12} values	

Taken with permission from Dispenzieri, A. (2012). "How I treat POEMS syndrome." Blood **119**(24): 5650–5658
POEMS, polyneuropathy, organomegaly, endocrinopathy, M-protein, skin changes
[a]The diagnosis of POEMS syndrome is confirmed when both of the mandatory major criteria, one of the three other major criteria, and one of the six minor criteria are present
[b]Summary of frequencies of POEMS syndrome features based on largest retrospective series [2, 7–11]
[c]Takasuki and Nakanishi series are included even though only 75 % of patients had a documented plasma cell disorder. Since these are among the earliest series describing the syndrome, they are included
[d]There is a Castleman's disease variant of POEMS syndrome that occurs *without* evidence of a clonal plasma cell disorder that is not accounted for in this table. This entity should be considered separately
[e]A plasma VEGF level of 200 pg/mL is 95 % specific and has 68 % sensitivity for a POEMS syndrome [28]
[f]Because of the high prevalence of diabetes mellitus and thyroid abnormalities, this diagnosis alone is not sufficient to meet this minor criterion
[g]Approximately 50 % of patients will have bone marrow changes that distinguish it from a typical MGUS or myeloma bone marrow [38]

from other conditions like chronic inflammatory polyradiculoneuropathy (CIDP), monoclonal gammopathy of undetermined significance (MGUS) neuropathy, and immunoglobulin light chain amyloid neuropathy. Other important baseline tests include CBC, creatinine, creatinine clearance, serum and urine protein electrophoresis with immunofixation, serum immunoglobulin free light chains, TSH, prolactin, parathyroid hormone, testosterone (or estradiol), luteinizing hormone, follicle stimulating hormone, plasma VEGF, bone marrow aspirate and biopsy with immunohistochemical stains to document lambda-restricted plasma cells, pulmonary function tests, electromyelogram with nerve conduction studies, and PET/CT—with special attention to the bone windows of the CT. A biopsy of a sclerotic lesion is not imperative in the proper clinical context.

Therapy

Treatment of the POEMS syndrome can be broken down into two major categories: targeting the underlying clone and targeting the rest of the syndrome. Both are important to achieve the best outcomes. An algorithm for choosing therapy is shown in Fig. 15.1. Monitoring for hematologic response is a challenge since the serum M-protein is typically small making standard multiple myeloma response criteria inapplicable in most cases. In addition, patients can derive substantial clinical benefit even in the absence of an M-protein response [39, 40]. In addition, despite the fact that the immunoglobulin free light chains are elevated in 90 % of POEMS patients, the ratio is normal in all but 18 % [41], making the test of limited value for patients with POEMS syndrome.

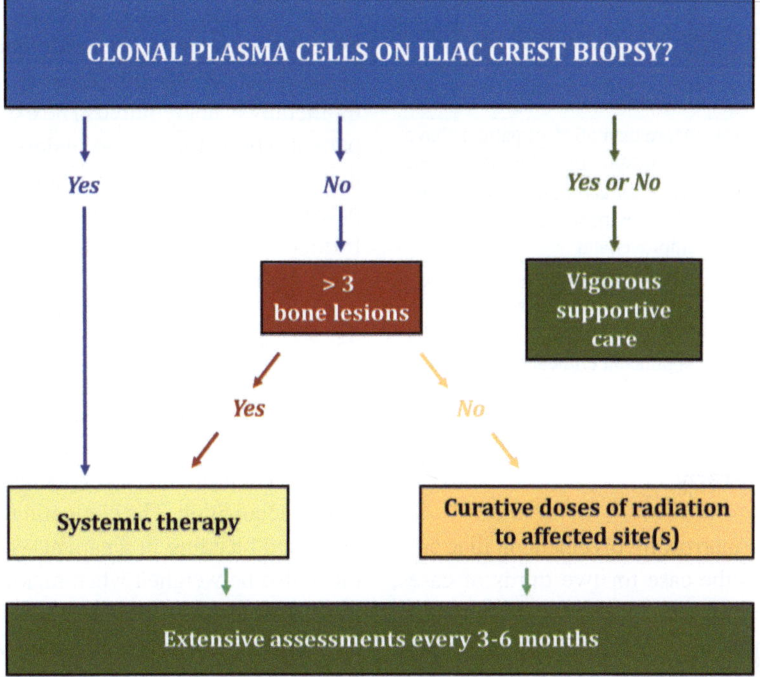

Fig. 15.1 Algorithm for the treatment of POEMS syndrome

Following VEGF is rather straight-forward, but spurious VEGF levels do occur. Following the other features of the syndrome is also challenging since there are more than two-dozen parameters that could be assessed in a given patient with POEMS syndrome [42]. Focusing on features present at baseline at each visit or at every other visit is the most effective approach to follow-up.

Radiation

If there is no involvement of the bone marrow on iliac crest biopsy as documented with immunohistochemical stains, but only one to three bone lesions, radiation is the preferred strategy. One-third of patients do not have clonal plasma cells on their iliac crest biopsy. These are the patients who present with a solitary or "multiple solitary plasmacytomas." The other two thirds of patients have a low burden of clonal plasma cells in their bone marrow, often akin to a "plasmacytoma plus [43]." For this first group, radiation doses of 40 Gy are most standard, since the goal for this group is potential cure [9, 44–47]. If a patient is rapidly deteriorating, simultaneous use of corticosteroids—e.g., dexamethasone 40 mg, days 1–4 every 2 weeks or daily prednisone at approximately 1 mg/kg—is reasonable as adjuvant therapy. The corticosteroids can be tapered over the ensuing months, but if decreased adrenal reserve at diagnosis adrenal insufficiency may be unmasked. It is important to note that assessing the bone marrow for clonality using flow cytometry alone is *insufficient* given the architecture of the small lambda clones characteristic of patients with POEMS. These small clones in an increased polyclonal background can be missed by flow cytometry. Using kappa and lambda immunohistochemistry, these small clones are seen in the bone marrow both in the interstitium and more importantly rimming lymphoid aggregates the latter of which is a pathognomonic finding [38]. Not only does radiation to an isolated (or even two or three) lesion(s) improve the symptoms of POEMS syndrome over the course of 3–36 months, but it can be curative.

Table 15.2 Activity of radiation, alkylator-based, and corticosteroid therapies for the treatment of POEMS syndrome

Regimen	Outcome
Radiation [9, 44–47]	More than 50 % of patients have significant clinical improvement
Mel-Dex [39]	81 % hematologic response rate; 100 % with some neurologic improvement
Corticosteroids [5]	≥15 % of patients have significant clinical improvement
ASCT [5]	100 % of surviving patients have significant clinical improvement

Systemic Therapy

If there is bone marrow involvement on iliac crest sampling, as is the case for two thirds of cases, 91 % of which are clonal lambda with a median plasma cell infiltrate of less than 5 % [38], radiation alone is less effective. These patients who have disseminated bone marrow disease by iliac crest biopsy or by innumerable sclerotic or mixed sclerotic and lytic lesions require systemic therapy. The sooner this plasma cell neoplasm is addressed with systemic chemotherapy, the better will be the recovery of the patient's peripheral neuropathy. Since there are no randomized clinical trials among patients with POEMS syndrome, recommendations for systemic therapy are based on case series and anecdotes. Therapeutic strategies are borrowed from other plasma cell disorders, most notably multiple myeloma and light chain amyloidosis. Corticosteroids may provide symptomatic improvement, but response duration is limited [5]. The most experience has been with alkylator-based therapy, either high dose with peripheral blood stem cell transplant or low dose with corticosteroids (Table 15.2).

Transplantation

For those patients well enough to tolerate high-dose melphalan (140–200 mg/m^2) as conditioning for autologous peripheral blood stem cell transplantation (ASCT), ASCT is my first choice based on our own experience and reports from others [19, 40, 48–60]. Because these patients have low-tumor burden and their plasma cell clone is not rapidly proliferating, induction chemotherapy is not required. The exceptions are the patient who is too sick to undergo ASCT immediately and the patient for whom there are anticipated delays to bring him/her to ASCT. In the former instance, cyclical cyclophosphamide (750 mg/m^2 intravenously every 3 weeks) with 4–5 days of corticosteroid or lenalidomide (15–25 mg orally, days 1–21 every 28 days) with weekly dexamethasone is an excellent option. Cyclophosphamide is often more expedient because there is no associated wait period or insurance hurdles that are associated with lenalidomide acquisition. The competing risks of thrombosis and bleeding in a patient who is at fall risk must also be weighed when making the decision about using the lenalidomide–dexamethasone combination and when choosing whether to use either aspirin or full anticoagulation with the lenalidomide–dexamethasone combination.

With ASCT, responses are durable, but relapses have been reported [27, 61]. We recently reviewed our series of 59 patients with POEMS syndrome who were treated with ASCT [62]. With a median follow-up of 45 months, 14 patients had relapsed or progressed. The progression-free survival was 98 % and 75 % at 1 and 5 years, respectively. Overall survival was 98 and 94 % at 1 and 5 years. Risk factors for progression included an immunoglobulin G-lambda monoclonal component and FDG-avid lesions on baseline PET scan. Tandem ASCT has been used to treat patients with POEMS [55, 63], but it is unclear if this approach is warranted given the excellent results with a single ASCT. Treatment-related morbidity and mortality can be minimized by recognizing and promptly treating an engraftment-type syndrome characterized by fevers, rash, diarrhea, weight gain, and respiratory symptoms and signs that occur anytime between days 7 and 15 post-stem cell infusion [40]. A starting dose of prednisone ranging between 20 and 1,500 mg/day has been used, but personal experience would place the daily starting dose anywhere between 1 and 2 mg/kg to 500 mg. The taper can typically start within 2 days and should be completed no sooner than 10 days.

Table 15.3 Activity of immune modulatory drug therapies for the treatment of POEMS syndrome

Thal after MP [68]	No hematological response but improved ascites; stabilized PN, splenomegaly, pulmonary hypertension
Thal + Dex after CAD [69]	CD/POEMS: improved ascites, effusions, pulmonary hypertension, peripheral neuropathy, renal function, IL-6 level
Thal + Dex [70]	*Nine patients*. VEGF improved in all; PN improved in 66 %; stable in 33 %; improved edema; no HCR
Thal after VAD, CTX, Bev [25]	Improved cardiopulmonary status, but no improved PN and rising VEGF
Len + Dex [64]	Improved ascites, PS, peripheral neuropathy, VEGF, testosterone, pulmonary function tests
Len + Dex [65]	*Nine patients*. All had hematologic response; clinical responses in all evaluable patients including PS, neurological syndrome, edema, and VEGF
Len ± Dex [66]	*Ten patients*. All had prior therapy a median of 4 months (range 1–36 months) prior to starting len. For 7, only Pred and IVIG were used as prior therapy, making it improbable that the salutatory effect was related to anything other than len. After a median of 7.5 cycles of len, all had clinical improvement despite the fact that only half achieved CR. Five were consolidated with ASCT
Len + CTX + Dex [67]	After 4 cycles of therapy, patient was able to walk without support, and, after 6 cycles, papilledema and IgA disappeared. One year after 9 cycles, she remains in remission

Bev bevacizumab, *CTX* cyclophosphamide, *Dex* dexamethasone, *HCR* hematological complete response, *HTN* hypertension, *Len* lenalidomide, *Mel* melphalan, *Pred* prednisone, *PS* performance status, *Thal* thalidomide, *VAD* vincristine, doxorubicin, dexamethasone, *VEGF* vascular endothelial growth factor

Table 15.4 Activity of proteosome inhibitors for the treatment of POEMS syndrome

Bortez + AD after VAD, CTX, Mel-Pred, +AD [71]	Improved M-protein, VEGF, paresthesias, splenomegaly, effusions, muscle strength, gynecomastia, and skin changes
Bortez + Dex [72]	Improved M-protein, polyneuropathy, hepatomegaly, testosterone; no change in electromyelography
Bortez × 5 cycles + Thali added at cycle 6 (prior Dex and Mel-Pred) [73]	Improvement of anasarca, peripheral neuropathy, VEGF, and PET scan with Bortez alone, but thali added because of persistent symptoms and signs. With thali, disappearance of pleural effusion, ascites, and M-protein and normalization of VEGF
Bortez Dex[a] [74]	Improvement by 3 cycles, but continued for 6. Complete remission 4 years after completing therapy. Improvement in adenopathy, pleural effusion and ascites, hepatosplenomegaly, and IL-6
Bortez, CTX, Dex [75]	Clinical response of anasarca within 6 weeks and tolerated therapy for 18 months achieving an nCR and a VEGF response. Peripheral neuropathy, hyperpigmentation, pulmonary hypertension improved significantly

Bortez bortezomib, *CS* corticosteroids, *CTX* cyclophosphamide, *Dex* dexamethasone, *HCR* hematological complete response, *HTN* hypertension, *Len* lenalidomide, *Mel* melphalan, *Pred* prednisone, *PS* performance status, *Thali* thalidomide, *VAD* vincristine, doxorubicin, dexamethasone, *VEGF* vascular endothelial growth factor

[a]Castleman's variant of POEMS syndrome

Splenomegaly was the baseline factor that best predicted for a complicated peri-transplant course [40]. Patients with POEMS typically have a higher than expected transfusion need with median numbers of platelet and erythrocyte transfusions being 5 apheresis units and 6 units, respectively, and delayed neutrophil engraftment.

Chemotherapy and Novel Agents

In the first reported prospective clinical trial to treat POEMS syndrome [39], 31 patients were treated with 12 cycles of low dose oral melphalan and dexamethasone and found that 81 % of patients had hematologic response, 100 % had VEGF response, and 100 % with at least some improvement in neurologic status. A limitation of this study is that follow-up was only 21 months.

Other promising treatments include lenalidomide (Table 15.3) [64–67], thalidomide [25, 68–70], and bortezomib (Table 15.4) [71–75], drugs all of which can have a direct anti-plasma cell effect as well as anti-VEGF and anti-TNF effects. Enthusiasm for the latter two therapies should be tempered by the high risk of peripheral neuropathy

Table 15.5 Activity of VEGF inhibition for the treatment of POEMS syndrome

Bev alone [21]	Death within 6 weeks
Bev+mycophenolate+ Dex [98]	One month after starting therapy, patient deteriorated further with worsening ascites and shortness of breath. Bev and Dex were discontinued. Mel and Pred were begun. Patient died 1 month later
Bev alone [22]	Worsening peripheral neuropathy, anasarca, multiorgan failure; died of pneumonia 5 weeks after therapy
Bev alone [23]	Improved pain, breathing, and walking
Bev+Mel-Dex [24]	Improved effusions/ascites
Prior VAD/CTX [25]	Improved edema, pain, weakness, and VEGF
Bev+CTX-Dex [26]	Initial worsening; repeat with Bev → improved pulmonary HTN, anasarca, skin changes
Bev+CTX-CS [27]	Initial improvement, but multiorgan failure and death
Bev+CTX-radiation [29]	*Two patients*. First patient treated with radiation and CTX and then Bev. Clinical improvement started before Bev. At radiological relapse, Bev no use, so lenalidomide plus Dex used with benefit. Second patient treated with same sequence, but course complicated by sepsis. Biochemical and early neurologic response before Bev started
Bev+CTX [28]	Clinical and biochemical relapse. No response to CTX, so bevacizumab added. Death

Bev bevacizumab, *CS* corticosteroids, *CTX* cyclophosphamide, *Dex* dexamethasone, *HCR* hematological complete response, *HTN* hypertension, *Len* lenalidomide, *Mel* melphalan, *Pred* prednisone, *PS* performance status, *VAD* vincristine, doxorubicin, dexamethasone, *VEGF* vascular endothelial growth factor

induced by these drugs. As mentioned above, the limited experience with lenalidomide so far has been positive. Our group observed dramatic improvements in a patient treated with the lenalidomide–dexamethasone combination [64]. In France, nine patients, one of whom was newly diagnosed, were treated with lenalidomide and dexamethasone [65]. Serious side effects were noted in three patients with two hematologic toxicities and a cutaneous allergy. All evaluable for hematologic response had at least a partial hematologic response, and clinical responses—including improvement in performance status and neurologic symptoms—were documented among the eight who had sufficient follow-up. One patient relapsed 5 months after discontinuing therapy, but responded to reintroduction of the drug. In a retrospective review of ten patients with previously treated POEMS syndrome who were treated with lenalidomide ± dexamethasone in Spain, all patients improved [66]. Median time from last therapy to lenalidomide was 4 months (range 1–36). Because the prior therapy in seven patients was intravenous immunoglobulin (IVIG) ± prednisone, which is a relatively ineffective regimen, the benefit observed in these patients most certainly would have been due to the lenalidomide ± dexamethasone. Yet another case report combining lenalidomide with cyclophosphamide and dexamethasone produced dramatic improvements lasting more than 1 year after completing therapy [67]. Thalidomide with dexamethasone has been reported to be effective in 12 patients [25, 68–70], but the risk of introducing thalidomide-induced small fiber neuropathy on top of the demyelinating peripheral neuropathy that is the dominant symptom of the POEMS syndrome cannot be disregarded.

Bortezomib use has been reported in three patients (Table 15.4) [71, 72, 75]. The first report is difficult to interpret since the patient had a number of chemotherapies prior to receiving a bortezomib, doxorubicin, and dexamethasone combination [71]. There was early evidence of improvement even before starting the bortezomib regimen. The second report, using 7 cycles of bortezomib and dexamethasone resulted in patient improvement, was more convincing [72]. We recently reported an astounding clinical and biochemical response in a patient with relapsed POEMS syndrome using the combination of cyclophosphamide, bortezomib, and dexamethasone [75]. Whether that response might have been achieved with cyclophosphamide and dexamethasone alone is unknown, but the patient was progressing on dexamethasone, and his anasarca began to resolve within weeks of initiating the combination.

Although an anti-VEGF strategy is theoretically appealing, the results with bevacizumab have been mixed (Table 15.5) [22–29]. Five patients who had also received alkylator during and/or predating the bevacizumab had benefit [24–26, 29], including one who had improvement, but was then consolidated with high-dose chemotherapy with autologous stem cell transplant [25], and another two who were treated with radiation and cyclophosphamide with initial clinical and VEGF response within approximately 6 months of therapy, but were given bevacizumab, and had "impressive improvement of neurologic symptoms [29]." These data are difficult to interpret since dramatic neurologic improvement does not typically occur in this syndrome until about 6–12 months after definitive treatment, which is precisely the time after radiation and cyclophosphamide that the bevacizumab was given in most of these cases. In four other case reports, patients receiving bevacizumab died very shortly thereafter [21, 22, 27, 28].

Other Treatments

Although IVIG and plasmapheresis are very effective for CIDP, neither of these therapies is helpful for patients with POEMS syndrome [76]. A recent report, however, describes reduction in serum VEGF and clinical improvement with single agent IVIG. The response was not durable, which prompted another course of IVIG with radiation to a solitary plasmacytoma [77]. Other treatments like interferon-alpha, tamoxifen, trans-retinoic acid, ticlopidine, argatroban, and strontium-89 have been reported as having activity mostly as single case reports [76].

Treatment of Neuropathy

The neuropathy is usually the dominant characteristic of the disease. The quality and extent of the neuropathy, which is typically peripheral, ascending, symmetrical, and affecting both sensation and motor function, should be elicited. Pain may be a dominant feature in about 10–15 % of patients, seemly more common in reports from Japan with reported rates of hyperesthesia or pain in 50–79 % of their subjects [78, 79]. The most common misdiagnosis made in patients with POEMS syndrome before the correct diagnosis is established is CIDP since both disorders are predominantly demyelinating neuropathies. In a series comparing 51 patients with POEMS and 46 patients with CIDP, patients with POEMS syndrome were significantly more likely to have muscle atrophy and distal dominant muscle weakness and to report severe leg pain [79]. Electrophysiologically, there is growing evidence that demyelination is predominant in the nerve trunk rather than in the distal nerve terminals. Axonal loss is also often seen in the lower limb nerves [79, 80].

The two best ways to approach the peripheral neuropathy are to target the clone (see above) and to direct the patient to work intensively with physical therapy and occupational therapy, and encourage stretching, strengthening, and balance exercises. Ankle braces, canes, walkers, and wheelchair should be used as needed. The painful peripheral neuropathy if present can be palliated with drugs like gabapentin, pregabalin, amitriptyline, nortriptyline, duloxetine, topical lidocaine patches, and topical ketamine, lidocaine, amitriptyline compounds.

Targeting Vascular Endothelial Growth Factor

Plasma and serum levels of vascular endothelial growth factor (VEGF) are markedly elevated in patients with POEMS [12, 30, 81] and correlate with the activity of the disease even better than the serum M-spike [14, 18, 28, 30]. We found that a plasma VEGF level of 200 pg/mL has a specificity of 95 % and a sensitivity of 68 % for POEMS syndrome [28]. Although VEGF is the best measure of disease activity for the majority of patients, reduction of levels using bevacizumab is not clearly effective therapy see section "Targeting

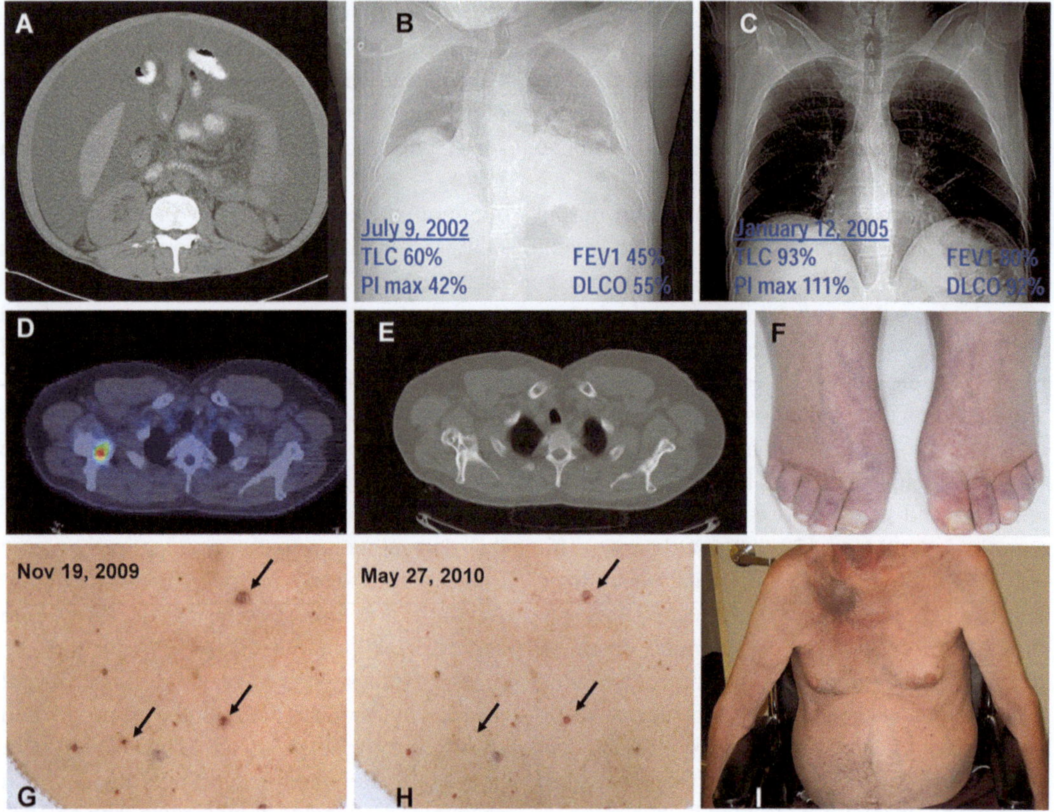

Fig. 15.2 Classic findings of POEMS syndromes taken with permission from Dispenzieri, A. (2012). "How I treat POEMS syndrome." Blood **119**(24): 5650–5658. (**a**) Massive ascites and lipodystrophy. (**b**) Chest radiograph and pulmonary function test results demonstrating reduced lung volumes due to neuromuscular weakness, small effusions, and reduced diffusing capacity of carbon monoxide. (**c**) Improved chest radiograph and pulmonary function tests 2.5 years after ASCT (same patient as (**b**)). (**d**) Fusion CT/PET of mixed lytic/sclerotic lesion in right scapula. (**e**) Bone windows of CT of mixed lytic/sclerotic lesion in right scapula. (**f**) Hyperemia of extremities and white nails. (**g**) Outcropping of cherry angiomata at diagnosis. (**h**) Shrinkage and disappearance of cherry angiomata after radiation to solitary osteosclerotic lesion right femur. (**i**) Plasmacytoma right scapula with overlying erythema as well as gynecomastia, muscle wasting, and ascites. Also present but unrelated is florid tinea corpis due to chronic steroid used for the incorrect diagnosis of CIDP

Plasma Cell Clone" even though it drops VEGF levels to undetectable levels. This paradox would suggest that VEGF is not the primary driver of the disease, but rather a surrogate. There are clinical assays available to measure both serum and plasma VEGF; the former levels are 10–50 times higher than the latter [82]. There is a debate as to which test is better, but it is imperative that one selects a laboratory assay and continues to use throughout the course of the patient's disease. I prefer the plasma VEGF since the higher level observed in serum is attributable to the release of VEGF from platelets in vitro during serum processing. I measure levels every 3–6 months to track a patient's progress. A rise in a patient's VEGF without any evidence of clinical deterioration should not be acted on but rather repeated in 1–3 months before considering a new therapy.

Signs of volume overload are present in the majority of patients in the form of peripheral edema; however, ascites, pleural effusions, and pericardial effusions may be present in as many as 50 % of patients depending on the series [2, 7–11]. After the peripheral neuropathy, refractory ascites and anasarca cause the most morbidity (Fig. 15.2a). The mechanism of this feature of the syndrome is not well understood, but it has been speculated that VEGF contributes to the capillary leak. Although this manifestation may be present at presentation or at relapse, it is one of the most common preterminal events. In extreme cases, the third spacing is not controllable with diuretics and patients become prerenal and even develop renal failure through this mechanism. Serial paracenteses and albumin-forced diuresis may provide benefit, but results can also be disappointing. In a recent personal case, neither bevacizumab nor cyclophosphamide–dexamethasone alleviated the third spacing, and the patient died about 4.5 years after his original diagnosis [28]. In another recent personal case, the combination of cyclophosphamide, bortezomib, and dexamethasone brought a patient from paracentesis dependence (Fig. 15.2a) to a diuretic-independent normal dry weight [75].

Treatment of Complications

Renal

Serum creatinine levels are normal in most cases, but serum cystatin C, a surrogate marker for renal function, is high in 71 % of patients [41]. In our experience, at presentation, fewer than 10 % of patients have proteinuria exceeding 0.5 g/24 h, and only 6 % have a serum creatinine greater than or equal to 1.5 mg/dL [9]. In another series from China, at diagnosis 37 % of patients had a creatinine clearance of less than 60 mL/min, and 9 % had a creatinine clearance of less than 30 mL/min and 15 % had microhematuria [10]. Overt renal disease appears to be more likely to occur in patients who have co-existing Castleman's disease. It may also occur as part of a preterminal event in association with uncontrollable ascites and anasarca. In the rare cases where there is significant kidney pathology warranting biopsy, the renal histologic findings are diverse with membranoproliferative features and evidence of endothelial injury being most common [49]. There is no known specific therapy to treat these instances of renal disease other than targeting the underlying plasma cell clone.

Pulmonary

Respiratory complaints are usually limited given patients' neurologic status impairing their ability to induce cardiovascular challenges, but abnormal pulmonary function tests are present in the majority [51, 83]. The pulmonary manifestations include pulmonary hypertension, restrictive lung disease, impaired neuromuscular respiratory function, and impaired diffusion capacity of carbon monoxide [83, 84]. Patients with significant neuromuscular weakness should be screened for sleep apnea so either CPAP or BiPAP can be prescribed as necessary. All of these abnormalities can improve with effective therapy targeting the plasma cell clone (Fig. 15.2b, c) [76, 83, 84].

Organomegaly

The hepatosplenomegaly and lymphadenopathy do not require specific therapy. The enlargement is typically not sufficient to cause localized discomfort. These tissues are often biopsied during the course of establishing a diagnosis. Except when there is co-existing Castleman's disease, biopsies of these tissues are uninformative. The organomegaly and adenopathy resolve with effective treatment of the underlying plasma cell disorder. When a patient has POEMS with co-existing Castleman's disease as is the case in up to 30 % of cases [5], the approach is not different except in these cases the interleukin 6 (IL-6) should also be followed. In contrast, if the patient has the POEMS variant of Castleman's disease, i.e., no plasma cell clone documented and potentially a less apparent or even absent peripheral neuropathy, but many of the other features of POEMS syndrome, the treatment strategy is different [6]. In these patients anti-IL-6 antibodies, anti-IL-6 receptor antibodies, and rituximab are therapies that should be considered in addition to alkylator and steroid-based therapy [85, 86]. Patients with Castleman's variant of POEMS should also be tested for HIV and HHV-8.

Endocrinopathy

Endocrinopathy is a central but poorly understood feature of POEMS. In a recent series [11], approximately 84 % of patients had a recognized endocrinopathy, with hypogonadism as the most common endocrine abnormality, followed by thyroid abnormalities, glucose metabolism abnormalities, and lastly by adrenal insufficiency. Endocrine abnormalities can improve after chemotherapy including successful tapering off of thyroid replacement, androgen replacement, and corticosteroid replacement in at least a third of patients. The clinically silent, but biochemically evident, rises in prolactin typically improve within the first year as well.

Papilledema

Papilledema (optic disc edema) is present in at least one-third of patients and may be associated with increased intracranial pressure. Of the 33 patients at our institution referred for a formal ophthalmologic examination during a 10-year period, 67 % had ocular signs and symptoms, the most common of which was papilledema in 52 % of those examined [87]. In most cases the optic disc edema is asymptomatic, but when it is not and when pressures are high, treatment with acetazolamide and corticosteroids may control symptoms until definitive chemo- or radiation-therapy directed at the underlying clone can control the disease. In rare cases, serial therapeutic lumbar puncture may be required. Ventriculoperitoneal shunts are typically not required. Response of the optic disc edema is typically rapid with clinical improvements noted within 3 months after ASCT.

Osteosclerotic Lesions

Osteosclerotic lesions occur in approximately 95 % of patients, and can be confused with benign bone islands, aneurysmal bone cysts, nonossifying fibromas, and fibrous dysplasia [7, 9, 88, 89]. Some lesions are densely sclerotic, while others are lytic with a sclerotic rim (Fig. 15.2d), while still others have a mixed soap-bubble appearance. FDG-PET/CT is a useful tool for screening for POEMS syndrome [35] as is (99m) Tc-HMDP bone scintigraphy [90]. Bone windows of CT body images (Fig. 15.2e) are often more informative than the scintigraphy at diagnosis especially if there is no lytic component to the bone lesion, but after treatment FDG-uptake is a useful tool to monitor response [91]. Bone lesions in POEMS syndrome do not typically cause bone pain or threaten skeletal integrity and therefore do not require any specific therapy other than using radiation to target the underlying clone. Radiating these lesions as primary therapy among those patients without bone marrow involvement is appropriate. Applying adjuvant radiation 12 months after ASCT to those FDG-avid lesions, which have not had reduction in their SUV, may also be appropriate on a case-to-case basis. Pathologic fractures are rare, but may occur.

Cutaneous

A whole skin examination should be performed looking for hyperpigmentation, hypertrichosis, acrocyanosis, dependent rubor (Fig. 15.2f), white nails, a recent outcropping of hemangioma (Fig. 15.2g), and sclerodermoid changes, flushing or clubbing. Also seen is facial lipoatrophy [59] and very rarely calciphylaxis [92]. Even more rarely can a violaceous skin patch overlying a solitary plasmacytoma of bone (Fig. 15.2i), associated with enlarged regional lymph node, be seen [93]. With the exception of calciphylaxis, none of the skin changes require any specific therapy and they all gradually improve after definitive therapy. In contrast, calciphylaxis can be devastating. There are four reports in the literature [92, 94–96], and I have seen two additional cases. Of these six, three patients died, two had resolution, and one did not have outcome described. Yoshikawa et al. treated their patient with etidronate with improvement in skin, but sudden death within 3 months of calciphylaxis.

Of the two cases I have seen, one died. Skin lesions, including hemangiomata, improve with therapy (Fig. 15.2h).

Hematologic

Approximately 50 % of patients with POEMS have thrombocytosis. Unlike multiple myeloma, anemia is rare unless there is co-existing Castleman's disease or renal insufficiency. Many patients are thought to have a JAK2 negative myeloproliferative disorder before the diagnosis of POEMS syndrome is made since megakaryocyte hyperplasia and megakaryocyte clustering are seen in 54 % and 93 % of cases, respectively [38]. The question of whether to treat these patients with hydroxyurea to lower their platelet count arises not infrequently. There are no data to guide whether lowering the platelet count is necessary with the exception of indirect data from our series on cerebrovascular events among patients with POEMS syndrome [97]. A high platelet count was a risk factor for developing a cerebral infarction. With these data in mind, hydroxyurea can be used in those patients with significant thrombocytosis who presented with a cerebral event if there is to be a delay in instituting therapy directed at the underlying clone. Lenalidomide–dexamethasone is less appealing in this same high-risk patient population unless full anticoagulation is being used. Once plasma cell-directed therapy has been commenced, hydroxyurea is not likely required. The erythrocytosis observed in approximately 10–15 % of patients is typically modest and treating the underlying plasma cell disorder is sufficient. Both thrombocytosis and erythrocytosis improve after therapy.

Summary

Patients with POEMS syndrome present with a complex conglomerate of symptoms, signs, and objective abnormalities, making the diagnosis, management, and follow-up a challenge. Early diagnosis and a prompt multidisciplinary approach increase the likelihood of reduced long-term irreversible morbidity. Parameters associated with the poorest outcomes include finger nail clubbing, respiratory symptoms, and extravascular volume overload [5]. The number of POEMS-specific features is not prognostic. The best choice of therapy has not been derived through clinical trials, but rather through case series. ASCT has become a favored therapy. Other therapies that are effective in myeloma also appear to be effective in patients with POEMS syndrome. Both therapies directed at other features of the disease as well as emotional support should be a major part of the care plan. Follow-up and measurement of response is difficult since no one measurement is reliable enough to direct therapy. VEGF response appears to correlate with disease activity better than serum M-spike or PET scan as long as anti-VEGF antibodies have not been used. Plasma cell-directed therapy can be deemed to have been effective as long as the VEGF normalizes even if there is a residual M-spike. If there is still FDG avidity on PET scan 1 year after completing therapy, adjuvant radiation can also be considered. If the primary therapy was radiation, and at 1 year there is still FDG avidity on PET scan but the VEGF is normal and the patient is otherwise continuing to improve clinically, observation is quite reasonable. Serial assessments of clinical stigmata (peripheral neuropathy, volume status, eyes, skin, and organomegaly) of blood (M-spike, VEGF, affected endocrine parameters) should be done every 3 months for at least the first several years. Pulmonary function tests and bone assessments should be done annually. Follow-up at least once or twice a year indefinitely is recommended since patients do relapse and these patients can be salvaged. Once the underlying pathogenesis of the disease is better understood, more targeted therapy will be possible.

Acknowledgment AD and this work are supported in part by NIH grants CA125614, CA107476, and CA111345 and the Predolin Foundation and the JABBS Foundation.

References

1. Bardwick PA, Zvaifler NJ, Gill GN, Newman D, Greenway GD, Resnick DL. Plasma cell dyscrasia with polyneuropathy, organomegaly, endocrinopathy, M protein, and skin changes: the POEMS syndrome.

Report on two cases and a review of the literature. Medicine. 1980;59(4):311–22.
2. Takatsuki K, Sanada I. Plasma cell dyscrasia with polyneuropathy and endocrine disorder: clinical and laboratory features of 109 reported cases. Jpn J Clin Oncol. 1983;13(3):543–55.
3. Crow R. Peripheral neuritis in myelomatosis. Br Med J. 1956;2:802–4.
4. Fukase M, Kakimatsu T, Nishitani H, et al. Report of a case of solitary plasmacytoma in the abdomen presenting polyneuropathy and endocrinological disorders. (Abstr.). Clin Neurol (Tokyo). 1969;9:657.
5. Dispenzieri A. POEMS syndrome: 2011 update on diagnosis, risk-stratification, and management. Am J Hematol. 2011;86(7):591–601. Prepublished on 2011/06/18 as DOI 10.1002/ajh.22050.
6. Dispenzieri A. Castleman disease. Cancer Treat Res. 2008;142:293–330.
7. Nakanishi T, Sobue I, Toyokura Y, et al. The Crow-Fukase syndrome: a study of 102 cases in Japan. Neurology. 1984;34(6):712–20.
8. Soubrier MJ, Dubost JJ, Sauvezie BJ. POEMS syndrome: a study of 25 cases and a review of the literature. French Study Group on POEMS Syndrome. Am J Med. 1994;97(6):543–53.
9. Dispenzieri A, Kyle RA, Lacy MQ, et al. POEMS syndrome: definitions and long-term outcome. Blood. 2003;101(7):2496–506.
10. Li J, Zhou DB, Huang Z, et al. Clinical characteristics and long-term outcome of patients with POEMS syndrome in China. Ann Hematol. 2011;90(7):819–26. Prepublished on 2011/01/12 as DOI 10.1007/s00277-010-1149-0.
11. Ghandi GY, Basu R, Dispenzieri A, Basu A, Montori V, Brennan MD. Endocrinopathy in POEMS syndrome: the Mayo Clinic experience. Mayo Clin Proc. 2007;82(7):836–42.
12. Watanabe O, Arimura K, Kitajima I, Osame M, Maruyama I. Greatly raised vascular endothelial growth factor (VEGF) in POEMS syndrome [Letter]. Lancet. 1996;347(9002):702.
13. Soubrier M, Guillon R, Dubost JJ, et al. Arterial obliteration in POEMS syndrome: possible role of vascular endothelial growth factor. J Rheumatol. 1998; 25(4):813–5.
14. Watanabe O, Maruyama I, Arimura K, et al. Overproduction of vascular endothelial growth factor/vascular permeability factor is causative in Crow-Fukase (POEMS) syndrome. Muscle Nerve. 1998; 21(11):1390–7.
15. Nishi J, Arimura K, Utsunomiya A, et al. Expression of vascular endothelial growth factor in sera and lymph nodes of the plasma cell type of Castleman's disease. Br J Haematol. 1999;104(3):482–5.
16. Soubrier M, Sauron C, Souweine B, et al. Growth factors and proinflammatory cytokines in the renal involvement of POEMS syndrome. Am J Kidney Dis. 1999;34(4):633–8.
17. Niimi H, Arimura K, Jonosono M, et al. VEGF is causative for pulmonary hypertension in a patient with Crow-Fukase (POEMS) syndrome. Intern Med. 2000;39(12):1101–4.
18. Scarlato M, Previtali SC, Carpo M, et al. Polyneuropathy in POEMS syndrome: role of angiogenic factors in the pathogenesis. Brain. 2005;128 (Pt 8):1911–20.
19. Kuwabara S, Misawa S, Kanai K, et al. Autologous peripheral blood stem cell transplantation for POEMS syndrome. Neurology. 2006;66(1):105–7.
20. Mineta M, Hatori M, Sano H, et al. Recurrent Crow-Fukase syndrome associated with increased serum levels of vascular endothelial growth factor: a case report and review of the literature. Tohoku J Exp Med. 2006;210(3):269–77.
21. Kanai K, Kuwabara S, Misawa S, Hattori T. Failure of treatment with anti-VEGF monoclonal antibody for long-standing POEMS syndrome. Intern Med. 2007; 46(6):311–3.
22. Straume O, Bergheim J, Ernst P. Bevacizumab therapy for POEMS syndrome. Blood. 2006;107(12): 4972–3; author reply 4973–4.
23. Dietrich PY, Duchosal MA. Bevacizumab therapy before autologous stem-cell transplantation for POEMS syndrome. Ann Oncol. 2008;19(3):595.
24. Badros A, Porter N, Zimrin A. Bevacizumab therapy for POEMS syndrome. Blood. 2005;106(3):1135.
25. Ohwada C, Nakaseko C, Sakai S, et al. Successful combination treatment with bevacizumab, thalidomide and autologous PBSC for severe POEMS syndrome. Bone Marrow Transplant. 2009;43(9): 739–40.
26. Badros A. Bevacizumab therapy for POEMS syndrome. Blood. 2006;107(12):author reply 4973–74.
27. Samaras P, Bauer S, Stenner-Liewen F, et al. Treatment of POEMS syndrome with bevacizumab. Haematologica. 2007;92(10):1438–9.
28. D'Souza A, Hayman SR, Buadi F, et al. The utility of plasma vascular endothelial growth factor levels in the diagnosis and follow-up of patients with POEMS syndrome. Blood. 2011;118(17):4663–5. Prepublished on 2011/09/02 as DOI 10.1182/blood-2011-06-362392.
29. Buxhofer-Ausch V, Gisslinger B, Stangl G, Rauschka H, Gisslinger H. Successful treatment sequence incorporating bevacizumab for therapy of polyneuropathy in two patients with POEMS syndrome. Leuk Res. 2012;36:e98–100. Prepublished on 2012/03/01 as DOI 10.1016/j.leukres.2012.01.018.
30. Soubrier M, Dubost JJ, Serre AF, et al. Growth factors in POEMS syndrome: evidence for a marked increase in circulating vascular endothelial growth factor. Arthritis Rheum. 1997;40(4):786–7.
31. Endo I, Mitsui T, Nishino M, Oshima Y, Matsumoto T. Diurnal fluctuation of edema synchronized with plasma VEGF concentration in a patient with POEMS syndrome. Intern Med. 2002;41(12):1196–8.
32. Nakano A, Mitsui T, Endo I, Takeda Y, Ozaki S, Matsumoto T. Solitary plasmacytoma with VEGF overproduction: report of a patient with polyneuropathy. Neurology. 2001;56(6):818–9.

33. Koga H, Tokunaga Y, Hisamoto T, et al. Ratio of serum vascular endothelial growth factor to platelet count correlates with disease activity in a patient with POEMS syndrome. Eur J Intern Med. 2002;13(1):70–4.
34. Kanai K, Sawai S, Sogawa K, et al. Markedly upregulated serum interleukin-12 as a novel biomarker in POEMS syndrome. Neurology. 2012;79(6):575–82. Prepublished on 2012/07/31 as DOI 10.1212/WNL.0b013e318263c42b.
35. Alberti MA, Martinez-Yelamos S, Fernandez A, et al. 18F-FDG PET/CT in the evaluation of POEMS syndrome. Eur J Radiol. 2010;76(2):180–2.
36. Nobile-Orazio E, Terenghi F, Giannotta C, Gallia F, Nozza A. Serum VEGF levels in POEMS syndrome and in immune-mediated neuropathies. Neurology. 2009;72(11):1024–6.
37. Briani C, Fabrizi GM, Ruggero S, et al. Vascular endothelial growth factor helps differentiate neuropathies in rare plasma cell dyscrasias. Muscle Nerve. 2010;43(2):164–7.
38. Dao LN, Hanson CA, Dispenzieri A, Morice WG, Kurtin PJ, Hoyer JD. Bone marrow histopathology in POEMS syndrome: a distinctive combination of plasma cell, lymphoid and myeloid findings in 87 patients. Blood. 2011;117(24):6438–44. Prepublished on 2011/03/10 as DOI 10.1182/blood-2010-11-316935.
39. Li J, Zhang W, Jiao L, et al. Combination of melphalan and dexamethasone for patients with newly diagnosed POEMS syndrome. Blood. 2011;117(24): 6445–9. Prepublished on 2011/03/12 as DOI 10.1182/blood-2010-12-328112.
40. Dispenzieri A, Lacy MQ, Hayman SR, et al. Peripheral blood stem cell transplant for POEMS syndrome is associated with high rates of engraftment syndrome. Eur J Haematol. 2008;80(5):397–406.
41. Stankowski-Drengler T, Gertz MA, Katzmann JA, et al. Serum immunoglobulin free light chain measurements and heavy chain isotype usage provide insight into disease biology in patients with POEMS syndrome. Am J Hematol. 2010;85(6):431–4.
42. Dispenzieri A. Ushering in a new era for POEMS. Blood. 2011;117(24):6405–6. Prepublished on 2011/06/18 as DOI 10.1182/blood-2011-03-342675.
43. Warsame R, Gertz MA, Lacy MQ, et al. Trends and outcomes of modern staging of solitary plasmacytoma of bone. Am J Hematol. 2012;87(7):647–51.
44. Morley JB, Schwieger AC. The relation between chronic polyneuropathy and osteosclerotic myeloma. J Neurol Neurosurg Psychiatry. 1967;30(5):432–42.
45. Davis L, Drachman D. Myeloma neuropathy. Arch Neurol. 1972;27:507–11.
46. Iwashita H, Ohnishi A, Asada M, Kanazawa Y, Kuroiwa Y. Polyneuropathy, skin hyperpigmentation, edema, and hypertrichosis in localized osteosclerotic myeloma. Neurology. 1977;27(7):675–81.
47. Reitan JB, Pape E, Fossa SD, Julsrud OJ, Slettnes ON, Solheim OP. Osteosclerotic myeloma with polyneuropathy. Acta Med Scand. 1980;208(1–2):137–44.
48. Giglia F, Chiapparini L, Fariselli L, et al. POEMS syndrome: relapse after successful autologous peripheral blood stem cell transplantation. Neuromuscul Disord. 2007;17(11–12):980–2.
49. Sanada S, Ookawara S, Karube H, et al. Marked recovery of severe renal lesions in POEMS syndrome with high-dose melphalan therapy supported by autologous blood stem cell transplantation. Am J Kidney Dis. 2006;47(4):672–9.
50. Ganti AK, Pipinos I, Culcea E, Armitage JO, Tarantolo S. Successful hematopoietic stem-cell transplantation in multicentric Castleman disease complicated by POEMS syndrome. Am J Hematol. 2005;79(3):206–10.
51. Dispenzieri A, Moreno-Aspitia A, Suarez GA, et al. Peripheral blood stem cell transplantation in 16 patients with POEMS syndrome, and a review of the literature. Blood. 2004;104(10):3400–7.
52. Schliamser LM, Hardan I, Sharif D, Zukerman E, Avshovich N, Attias D. Significant improvement of POEMS syndrome with pulmonary hypertension following autologous peripheral blood stem cell transplant. Blood. 2003;102(11(2 of 2)):5664 abstract.
53. Soubrier M, Ruivard M, Dubost JJ, Sauvezie B, Philippe P. Successful use of autologous bone marrow transplantation in treating a patient with POEMS syndrome. Bone Marrow Transplant. 2002;30(1):61–2.
54. Peggs KS, Paneesha S, Kottaridis PD, et al. Peripheral blood stem cell transplantation for POEMS syndrome. Bone Marrow Transplant. 2002;30(6):401–4.
55. Jaccard A, Royer B, Bordessoule D, Brouet JC, Fermand JP. High-dose therapy and autologous blood stem cell transplantation in POEMS syndrome. Blood. 2002;99(8):3057–9.
56. Rovira M, Carreras E, Blade J, et al. Dramatic improvement of POEMS syndrome following autologous haematopoietic cell transplantation. Br J Haematol. 2001;115(2):373–5.
57. Hogan WJ, Lacy MQ, Wiseman GA, Fealey RD, Dispenzieri A, Gertz MA. Successful treatment of POEMS syndrome with autologous hematopoietic progenitor cell transplantation. Bone Marrow Transplant. 2001;28(3):305–9.
58. Kuwabara S, Misawa S, Kanai K, et al. Neurologic improvement after peripheral blood stem cell transplantation in POEMS syndrome. Neurology. 2008; 71(21):1691–5.
59. Barete S, Mouawad R, Choquet S, et al. Skin manifestations and vascular endothelial growth factor levels in POEMS syndrome: impact of autologous hematopoietic stem cell transplantation. Arch Dermatol. 2010;146(6):615–23.
60. Laurenti L, De Matteis S, Sabatelli M, et al. Early diagnosis followed by front-line autologous peripheral blood stem cell transplantation for patients affected by POEMS syndrome. Leuk Res. 2008; 32(8):1309–12.
61. Imai N, Taguchi J, Yagi N, Konishi T, Serizawa M, Kobari M. Relapse of polyneuropathy, organomegaly, endocrinopathy, M-protein, and skin changes (POEMS) syndrome without increased level of vascular endothelial growth factor following successful

autologous peripheral blood stem cell transplantation. Neuromuscul Disord. 2009;19(5):363–5.
62. D'Souza A, Lacy M, et al. "Long-term outcomes after autologous stem cell transplantation for patients with POEMS syndrome (osteosclerotic myeloma): a single-center experience." Blood. 2012;120(1):56–62.
63. Kojima H, Katsuoka Y, Katsura Y, et al. Successful treatment of a patient with POEMS syndrome by tandem high-dose chemotherapy with autologous CD34+ purged stem cell rescue. Int J Hematol. 2006;84(2):182–5.
64. Dispenzieri A, Klein CJ, Mauermann ML. Lenalidomide therapy in a patient with POEMS syndrome. Blood. 2007;110(3):1075–6.
65. Jaccard A, Abraham J, Recher C, et al. Lenalidomide therapy in nine patients with POEMS syndrome. ASH Annu Meet Abstr. 2009;114(22):3872.
66. Tomas JF, Giraldo P, Lecumberri R, Nistal S. POEMS syndrome with severe neurological damage clinically recovered with lenalidomide. Haematologica. 2012;97(2):320–2. Prepublished on 2011/11/08 as DOI 10.3324/haematol.2011.041897.
67. Suyani E, Yagci M, Sucak GT. Complete remission with a combination of lenalidomide, cyclophosphamide and prednisolone in a patient with incomplete POEMS syndrome. Acta Haematol. 2011;126(4):199–201. Prepublished on 2011/08/19 as DOI 10.1159/000329896.
68. Sinisalo M, Hietaharju A, Sauranen J, Wirta O. Thalidomide in POEMS syndrome: case report. Am J Hematol. 2004;76(1):66–8.
69. Kim SY, Lee SA, Ryoo HM, Lee KH, Hyun MS, Bae SH. Thalidomide for POEMS syndrome. Ann Hematol. 2006;85(8):545–6.
70. Kuwabara S, Misawa S, Kanai K, et al. Thalidomide reduces serum VEGF levels and improves peripheral neuropathy in POEMS syndrome. J Neurol Neurosurg Psychiatry. 2008;79(11):1255–7. Prepublished on 2008/05/13 as DOI jnnp.2008.150177 [pii] 10.1136/jnnp.2008.150177.
71. Tang X, Shi X, Sun A, et al. Successful bortezomib-based treatment in POEMS syndrome. Eur J Haematol. 2009;83(6):609–10.
72. Kaygusuz I, Tezcan H, Cetiner M, Kocakaya O, Uzay A, Bayik M. Bortezomib: a new therapeutic option for POEMS syndrome. Eur J Haematol. 2010;84(2):175–7.
73. Ohguchi H, Ohba R, Onishi Y, et al. Successful treatment with bortezomib and thalidomide for POEMS syndrome. Ann Hematol. 2011;90(9):1113–4. Prepublished on 2010/12/15 as DOI 10.1007/s00277-010-1133-8.
74. Sobas MA, Alonso Vence N, Diaz Arias J, Bendana Lopez A, Fraga Rodriguez M, Bello Lopez JL. Efficacy of bortezomib in refractory form of multicentric Castleman disease associated to poems syndrome (MCD-POEMS variant). Ann Hematol. 2010;89(2):217–9.
75. Warsame R, Kohl I, Dispenzieri A. Successful use of cyclophosphamide, bortezomib and dexamethasone to treat a case of multiply relapsed POEMS syndrome. Eur J Haematol. 2012;88(6):549–50.
76. Dispenzieri A. POEMS syndrome. Blood Rev. 2007;21(6):285–99.
77. Terracciano C, Fiore S, Doldo E, et al. Inverse correlation between VEGF and soluble VEGF receptor 2 in POEMS with AIDP responsive to intravenous immunoglobulin. Muscle Nerve. 2010;42(3):445–8.
78. Koike H, Iijima M, Mori K, et al. Neuropathic pain correlates with myelinated fibre loss and cytokine profile in POEMS syndrome. J Neurol Neurosurg Psychiatry. 2008;79(10):1171–9.
79. Nasu S, Misawa S, Sekiguchi Y, et al. Different neurological and physiological profiles in POEMS syndrome and chronic inflammatory demyelinating polyneuropathy. J Neurol Neurosurg Psychiatry. 2012;83(5):476–9. Prepublished on 2012/02/18 as DOI 10.1136/jnnp-2011-301706.
80. Mauermann ML, Sorenson EJ, Dispenzieri A, et al. Uniform demyelination and more severe axonal loss distinguish POEMS syndrome from CIDP. J Neurol Neurosurg Psychiatry. 2012;83(5):480–6.
81. Hashiguchi T, Arimura K, Matsumuro K, et al. Highly concentrated vascular endothelial growth factor in platelets in Crow-Fukase syndrome. Muscle Nerve. 2000;23(7):1051–6.
82. Tokashiki T, Hashiguchi T, Arimura K, Eiraku N, Maruyama I, Osame M. Predictive value of serial platelet count and VEGF determination for the management of DIC in the Crow-Fukase (POEMS) syndrome. Intern Med. 2003;42(12):1240–3.
83. Allam JS, Kennedy CC, Aksamit TR, Dispenzieri A. Pulmonary manifestations in patients with POEMS syndrome: a retrospective review of 137 patients. Chest. 2008;133(4):969–74.
84. Lesprit P, Godeau B, Authier FJ, et al. Pulmonary hypertension in POEMS syndrome: a new feature mediated by cytokines. Am J Respir Crit Care Med. 1998;157(3 Pt 1):907–11.
85. van Rhee F, Fayad L, Voorhees P, et al. Siltuximab, a novel anti-interleukin-6 monoclonal antibody, for Castleman's disease. J Clin Oncol. 2010;28(23):3701–8. Prepublished on 2010/07/14 as DOI JCO.2009.27.2377 [pii] 10.1200/JCO.2009.27.2377.
86. Nishimoto N, Kanakura Y, Aozasa K, et al. Humanized anti-interleukin-6 receptor antibody treatment of multicentric Castleman disease. Blood. 2005;106(8):2627–32.
87. Kaushik M, Pulido JS, Abreu R, Amselem L, Dispenzieri A. Ocular findings in patients with polyneuropathy, organomegaly, endocrinopathy, monoclonal gammopathy, and skin changes syndrome. Ophthalmology. 2011;118(4):778–82.
88. Tanaka O, Ohsawa T. The POEMS syndrome: report of three cases with radiographic abnormalities. Radiologe. 1984;24(10):472–4.

89. Chong ST, Beasley HS, Daffner RH. POEMS syndrome: radiographic appearance with MRI correlation. Skeletal Radiol. 2006;35(9):690–5.
90. Shibuya K, Misawa S, Horikoshi T, et al. Detection of bone lesions by CT in POEMS syndrome. Intern Med. 2011;50(13):1393–6. Prepublished on 2011/07/02 as DOI.
91. Stefanelli A, Treglia G, Leccisotti L, et al. Usefulness of F-18 FDG PET/CT in the follow-up of POEMS syndrome after autologous peripheral blood stem cell transplantation. Clin Nucl Med. 2012;37(2):181–3. Prepublished on 2012/01/10 as DOI 10.1097/RLU.0b013e31823ea154.
92. Yoshikawa M, Uhara H, Arakura F, et al. Calciphylaxis in POEMS syndrome: a case treated with etidronate. Acta Derm Venereol. 2011;91(1):98–9. Prepublished on 2010/10/12 as DOI 10.2340/00015555-0968.
93. Lipsker D, Rondeau M, Massard G, Grosshans E. The AESOP (adenopathy and extensive skin patch overlying a plasmacytoma) syndrome: report of 4 cases of a new syndrome revealing POEMS (polyneuropathy, organomegaly, endocrinopathy, monoclonal protein, and skin changes) syndrome at a curable stage. Medicine. 2003;82(1):51–9. Prepublished on 2003/01/25 as DOI.
94. Lee FY, Chiu HC. POEMS syndrome with calciphylaxis: a case report. Acta Derm Venereol. 2011;91(1):96–7. Prepublished on 2010/10/30 as DOI 10.2340/00015555-0969.
95. Hineno A, Kinoshita T, Kinoshita M, et al. Calciphylaxis as a catastrophic complication in a patient with POEMS syndrome. Case Rep Neurol. 2009;1(1):47–53. Prepublished on 2009/01/01 as DOI 10.1159/000259906.
96. De Roma I, Filotico R, Cea M, Procaccio P, Perosa F. Calciphylaxis in a patient with POEMS syndrome without renal failure and/or hyperparathyroidism. A case report. Ann Ital Med Int. 2004;19(4):283–7.
97. Dupont SA, Dispenzieri A, Mauermann ML, Rabinstein AA, Brown Jr RD. Cerebral infarction in POEMS syndrome: incidence, risk factors, and imaging characteristics. Neurology. 2009;73(16): 1308–12.
98. Chong DY, Comer GM, Trobe JD. Optic disc edema, cystoid macular edema, and elevated vascular endothelial growth factor in a patient with POEMS syndrome. J Neuroophthalmol. 2007;27(3):180–3.

Solitary Plasmacytoma

16

David Dingli and Prashant Kapoor

Definition

Solitary plasmacytoma (SP) is the clinical condition characterized by the localized proliferation of clonal plasma cells. The definition of SP has been evolving as a result of improvement in imaging technology as well as the availability of more sensitive techniques that can detect small populations of clonal plasma cells in the bone marrow. Patients with SP do not have other lytic or sclerotic bone lesions or soft tissue masses, hypercalcemia, renal insufficiency, or anemia and no involvement of the bone marrow by clonal plasma cells (Table 16.1) [1–3]. Some series have included patients with two bone lesions and less than 5 or 10 % clonal plasma cells in the bone marrow [4–10]. The presence of a monoclonal protein in the serum or urine or the presence of elevated immunoglobulin free light chain (FLC) does not exclude the diagnosis. On the contrary, such biomarkers may provide important prognostic information and may guide management. SP is further divided into two entities: solitary plasmacytoma of bone (SPB) and extramedullary plasmacytoma (EMP) where the plasma cell clone generally arises from lymphoid tissues away from the bone marrow microenvironment that normally hosts these cells. SP is quite uncommon and constitutes less than 5 % of all plasma cell neoplasms [11]. Out of 45,366 patients with a plasma cell proliferative disorder seen at Mayo Clinic, Rochester, MN, between 1960 and 2011, 883 patients were diagnosed with SP (2 %). SPB is more common than EMP by a ratio of at least 2:1 [2, 12], although the comprehensive literature review by Alexiou et al. suggests a ratio closer to 5:1 [13]. SP is more common in males (~70 %) and the median age at diagnosis varies from 55 to 60 years, depending on the study [2, 5, 7, 8, 14, 15]. Almost a third of patients are below 50 years of age at the time of diagnosis. Thus, patients diagnosed with SP are significantly younger than those diagnosed with multiple myeloma.

Tissue Distribution

Virtually any organ in the body that has associated lymphoid tissue can be affected by a plasmacytoma. SPB can affect any bone but most commonly affects the vertebrae (42–61 %), followed by the pelvis (15 %), ribs (12 %), and long bones of the lower (12 %) and upper (10 %) extremity [2, 5, 16]. The most comprehensive analysis of the literature regarding the distribution of EMP was performed by Alexiou et al. [13]. EMP is found in the head and neck in up to 85 % of reported cases [2, 13, 14]. The paranasal sinuses are affected in circa 40 % of cases,

D. Dingli, M.D., Ph.D. (✉) • P. Kapoor, M.D.
Division of Hematology, Department of Internal Medicine, Mayo Clinic, 200 First St SW, Rochester, MN 55905, USA
e-mail: dingli.david@mayo.edu; kapoor.prashant@mayo.edu

M.A. Gertz and S.V. Rajkumar (eds.), *Multiple Myeloma: Diagnosis and Treatment*,
DOI 10.1007/978-1-4614-8520-9_16, © Mayo Foundation for Medical Education and Research 2014

Table 16.1 Diagnostic criteria for solitary plasmacytoma[a]

Solitary plasmacytoma of bone	Extramedullary plasmacytoma
Single area of bone destruction	Extramedullary plasma cell tumor
No clonal plasma cells in bone marrow	No clonal plasma cells in bone marrow
Normal skeletal survey and MRI[b]	Normal skeletal survey and MRI
No M-protein in serum and/or urine[c]	No M-protein in serum and/or urine[c]
No related organ or tissue impairment	No related organ or tissue impairment

[a]Adapted from [3]
[b]Excluding the single involved area
[c]A small M-component may be present in the serum and/or urine

followed by the nasopharynx (~12 %), oropharynx, and larynx (4 % each) [2, 14]. Other sites that have been reportedly affected by EMP include the gastrointestinal (GI) tract, urogenital tract, the skin, lung and pleura, central nervous system, the breast, and thyroid although no tissue seems free of the risk of developing EMP [13]. The most common sites afflicted in the GI tract are the stomach (11 %), colon (6.5 %), and the pancreas (3.9 %) while the small intestine is rarely affected. Regional lymph nodes are involved in less than 10 % of cases of EMP [13] although this seems to be higher in the case of GI plasmacytomas [15].

Biology

Given the relative rarity of SP, it is not surprising that there is very limited information about the etiology and mechanisms of progression in this disorder. The variable propensity of SP to progress to multiple myeloma would suggest that SP is a localized form of myeloma, and that similar mechanisms are responsible for disease pathogenesis. Metaphase cytogenetics and interphase fluorescent in situ hybridization (FISH) studies have identified the presence of recurrent chromosomal abnormalities in multiple myeloma that may play a role in pathogenesis and disease progression [17–22]. However, more importantly, these abnormalities have a major impact on prognosis and are used to risk stratify patients for the purpose of therapy [22–24]. These abnormalities are often also present in monoclonal gammopathy of undetermined significance (MGUS) [25] and in AL amyloidosis [26].

In a study of 38 cases of EMP, Bink et al. found recurrent chromosomal abnormalities in virtually all plasmacytomas [27]. The most common abnormalities were gains of the odd numbered chromosomes, present in 82 % of samples. Hyperdiploidy was seen in 54 % of tumors while breaks in 14q32 were observed in 37 % of cases. Loss of 13q14 was observed in 15 patients (40 %) with 9 of them also having a translocation involving the immunoglobulin heavy chain (*IGH*). The t(4;14)(p16;q32) representing the fusion of *IGH* with *FGFR3* was found in 6 patients (16 %). No cases with the t(11;14)(q13;q32), t(14;16)(q32;q23), or t(8;14)(q24;q32) were found in this series. Only one case had a break in *C-MYC* but this breakpoint did not bring the oncogene next to the *IGH* locus and was negative for the t(8;14). No translocation involving *MALT1*, *BCL6*, or *FOXP1* was identified. The study did not report testing for loss of *TP53* which is found in about 5 % of patients with myeloma [28]. In another study, cyclin D1 was expressed in 17 % of plasmacytomas [29]. In summary, the incidence of chromosomal abnormalities in SP appears to be quite similar to what is observed in multiple myeloma and MGUS [30]. To date, it is not known whether these recurrent chromosomal abnormalities are causal and what impact they have on the risk of progression from EMP to multiple myeloma. Clearly, more work is required in this field.

Clinical Presentation

The clinical presentations of SP are protean and depend on the location of the lesion. Both SPB and EMP can be associated with localized

AL amyloid deposition, presumably due to local production of the amyloidogenic immunoglobulin fragments. SPB often presents with pain due to bone destruction or a pathological fracture. In some older series, the time from symptom onset to diagnosis was 6 months [5]. Symptoms of a radiculopathy from pressure on nerve roots or cord compression can also be present. Sometimes, the tumor may be palpable due to soft tissue extension. Rarely, a patient with SPB can present with symptoms and signs of a demyelinating peripheral neuropathy and, in such a scenario, the possibility of the POEMS syndrome (polyneuropathy, organomegaly, endocrinopathy, monoclonal protein, and skin changes) needs to be considered [31, 32]. Some patients are asymptomatic and identified serendipitously after imaging studies for an unrelated purpose identify a lytic bone lesion.

Symptoms from EMP vary depending on the site of origin. The most common symptoms from EMP affecting the upper aerodigestive tract include nasal obstruction, epistaxis, pain, hoarseness, and hearing loss. A 4 cm EMP affecting the tonsillar fossa that was asymptomatic has been reported [33]. On endoscopy, the lesions appear as soft, gray, sessile, or pedunculated masses that may rarely ulcerate [34, 35]. EMP arising from the GI tract most commonly presents with abdominal pain and frequently leads to intestinal obstruction with nausea, vomiting, abdominal distention, and constipation. Malabsorption syndrome with associated weight loss is frequent, and EMP that affects the stomach can present with upper gastrointestinal bleeding. Rarely, the plasmacytoma can cause obstructive jaundice, intestinal perforation, and enteroenteric fistula [15]. There are myriad other presenting symptoms related to the location of the EMP, including hematuria (urinary tract), cough and/or dyspnea due to either airway obstruction or pleural effusion [36], and a midline neck mass (thyroid gland) that can rarely be misdiagnosed as medullary carcinoma [37]. The size of plasmacytomas varies: in one series, 66 % were below 5 cm in diameter, with 8 % being greater than 10 cm in diameter and 26 % with a diameter in between [2].

Diagnostic Testing

The diagnosis of SP is based on an adequate tissue specimen obtained either by a fine needle aspiration, a core biopsy, or by pathologic examination of tissue removed at the time of surgery. Apart from the obvious exclusion of multiple myeloma, it is critical for the clinician to rule out reactive plasmacytosis, granulomatous inflammation, mucosal-associated lymphoid tissue (MALT) lymphoma with plasmacytic differentiation, immunoblastic lymphoma, lymphoplasmacytic lymphoma, and undifferentiated carcinoma. Malignant plasma cells typically express CD138 and/or CD38, and clonality is proven by kappa and lambda light chain restriction. Immunohistochemical staining for IgG, IgA, and IgM is also required. The suggested diagnostic work-up is presented in Table 16.2. Multiple myeloma is excluded based on the results of the bone marrow biopsy, imaging studies, and the absence of end organ damage. It appears that EMP cells often express CD19, a marker that is normally not expressed in multiple myeloma cells and therefore may be a good marker to differentiate EMP from myeloma [38].

Laboratory Studies

Laboratory studies should include a complete blood count, chemistry panel with serum calcium, creatinine, lactate dehydrogenase, C-reactive

Table 16.2 Diagnostic work-up for solitary plasmacytoma

Laboratory
Complete blood count
Serum calcium
Serum creatinine
Serum and urine protein electrophoresis and immunofixation
Quantitative immunoglobulins (IgG, IgA, IgM)
Serum immunoglobulin free light chains
Lactate dehydrogenase
Beta-2 microglobulin
Bone marrow aspirate and biopsy with flow cytometry and/or immunofixation
Imaging
Skeletal survey
Magnetic resonance imaging of the axial skeleton and proximal long bones (marrow)
PET/CT (whole body)

protein, beta-2 microglobulin, and urinalysis. Monoclonal protein studies of the serum and urine are essential as are quantitative immunoglobulins and immunoglobulin FLC. The frequency of detection of a monoclonal protein in patients with SPB varies from 19 to 72 % [2, 5, 7, 16, 39–45]. In a study from the Mayo Clinic of 116 patients with SPB, we found a monoclonal protein in the serum and/or urine in 72 % of patients with 64 % of patients having a detectable serum monoclonal protein [7]. An abnormal serum FLC ratio may be found in 50 % of patients. An abnormal urine monoclonal protein is less common—in our series, 36 of 90 patients (40 %) who were tested had Bence Jones proteinuria, more often kappa than lambda (by a ratio of 3:1) [7]. When a serum monoclonal protein is present, this is less than 1.0 g/dL in up to 64 % of patients and greater than 2.0 g/dL in only 10 %. The median size of the serum M-spike was 0.5 g/dL (range 0–3.0 g/dL). The concentration of monoclonal protein in the urine is normally quite low: in our series, none of the patients had more than 0.2 g/24 h. In another series from MD Anderson Cancer Center, the median size of the serum M-spike was 0.7 g/dL with a range of 0.2–4.2 g/dL, while the median 24 h urine protein excretion was 44.8 mg (range 3–384 mg) [2]. A monoclonal protein is less common in EMP and is found in less than 25 % of cases [13, 33, 46]. Immunofixation studies of the serum and urine are essential to detect such low concentrations of the protein: in our series, 11 out of 63 patient samples had the monoclonal protein detected only by immunofixation. This is important since it appears that it is the *presence* and not the size of the urine M-spike in the urine that is linked with the risk of progression to multiple myeloma [7]. The levels of uninvolved immunoglobulins are usually in the normal range and compatible with a low tumor burden [1, 47]. If they are abnormal, systemic disease should be suspected and patients observed closely since they have a high risk of progression to active multiple myeloma [44].

A bone marrow aspirate and biopsy are also essential to rule out multiple myeloma [3].

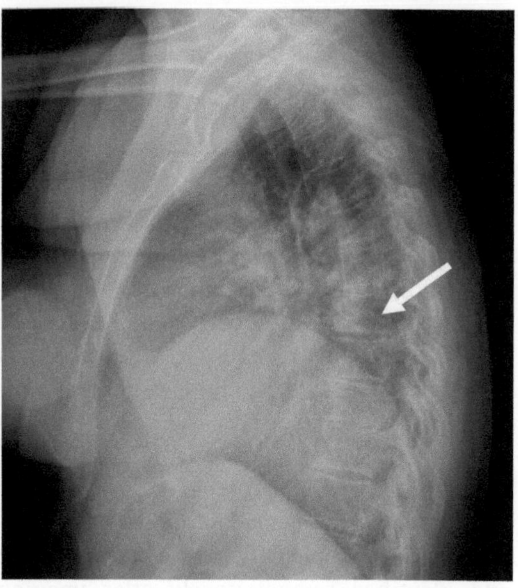

Fig. 16.1 Plain radiograph of a solitary plasmacytoma of bone affecting a thoracic vertebra. There is bone destruction without any sclerosis

Various case series in the past included patients with less than 5 or 10 % clonal plasma cells in the absence of other bone lesions on imaging [2, 5, 16, 40]. However, a more modern definition of SP would require the absence of clonal plasma cells in the bone marrow that includes immunophenotyping and multiparameter flow cytometry [3, 48].

Imaging

Once a clonal population of plasma cells is identified, proper staging of the disease is essential to determine whether the tumor is localized (SP) or disseminated, i.e., multiple myeloma. In the past, imaging studies were limited to metastatic skeletal surveys [2, 5, 6, 16, 40]. On plain X-rays, SPB typically appears as a purely lytic lesion with a clear margin without surrounding sclerosis (Fig. 16.1). The presence of diffuse osteoporosis without alternative explanation suggests that the patient either is at high risk of progression or has systemic rather than localized disease [49].

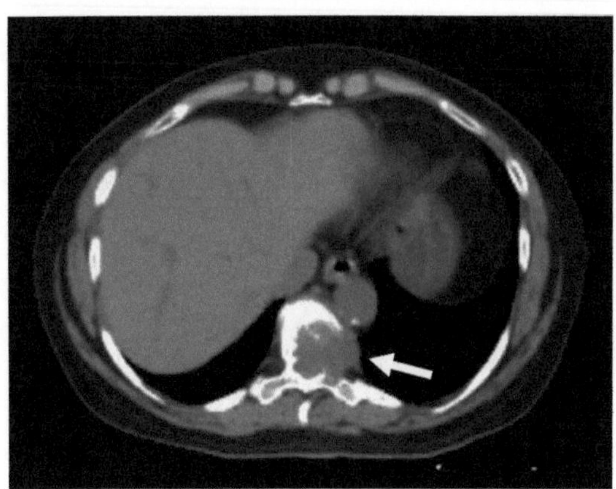

Fig. 16.2 Computerized tomography (CT) often shows the presence of soft tissue extension of the tumor that may or may not impinge on associated structures. CT is critical for proper planning of radiation therapy

However, the skeletal survey lacks sensitivity and a substantial number of patients would have evidence of additional sites of disease with more sensitive techniques such as magnetic resonance imaging (MRI) or combined computerized tomography and positron emission tomography (PET/CT). Computerized tomography (CT) is more sensitive and can detect smaller lesions that otherwise would be missed by plain radiography and often shows the soft tissue extension of such lesions that may be present in up to 37 % of cases (Fig. 16.2). CT is essential for the diagnosis of EMP as well as staging by providing information about the extent of local disease as well as regional lymph node involvement.

With MRI, SPB appears as an area of abnormal bone marrow signal due to marrow replacement with signal intensity similar to muscle on T1-weighted images (Fig.16.3a). The lesion appears hyperintense on T2-weighted images (Fig. 16.3b) and it enhances with gadolinium (Fig. 16.3c). There is often an extraosseous component that may impinge on the adjacent structures such as the spinal cord or nerve roots. In a series of 12 patients with suspected SPB, Moulopoulos et al. found MRI evidence of additional lesions in 4 of 12 patients [50]. In another series from the MD Anderson Cancer Center, Liebross et al. found that in patients with a plasmacytoma restricted to the thoracolumbar spine, only 1 of 7 patients with a negative MRI of the spine progressed to multiple myeloma compared to 7 out of 8 patients who were staged with a negative skeletal survey alone [40]. Limited MRI of the axial skeleton and proximal long bones can miss up to 10 % of lesions in patients with multiple myeloma and therefore under-stage the disease [51].

Whole body PET/CT imaging provides a number of advantages compared to other modalities: it is able to image most of the body in one session, can detect medullary and extramedullary disease in one examination, and distinguish between active tumor versus necrotic tissue. For these reasons, PET/CT (Fig. 16.4) is also indicated in the work-up of suspected solitary plasmacytoma [52–55]. In one study of 15 patients, PET/CT identified additional lesions (in bone and/or soft tissues) in 5 of these patients, upstaging the disease in almost 30 % and had a direct impact on therapy [52]. In another small series PET/CT identified additional, biopsy-proven plasmacytomas in 6 of 14 patients (43 %) [55]. Salaun et al. prospectively studied PET/CT and marrow MRI in 24 patients with SP. Both PET/CT and MRI missed some lesions, but overall, PET/CT was superior with a sensitivity of 98 % compared to 93 % (MRI) and a specificity of 99 % versus 94 %, respectively. The positive predictive value of PET/CT was 93 % compared to 84 % for MRI while the respective negative predictive values were 99 and 98 % [54].

From these studies, it can be concluded that PET/CT and MRI are complementary approaches and required for the proper staging of patients with suspected SP since they provide information on the local as well as potentially systemic disease burden. In the series reviewed here, no lesion was missed in any patient who underwent both imaging approaches. The recommended work-up for SP is presented in Table 16.2. Although staging systems for EMP have been proposed [56, 57], the value of these systems has not been validated. At present it appears that the pragmatic approach of localized versus disseminated disease is sufficient.

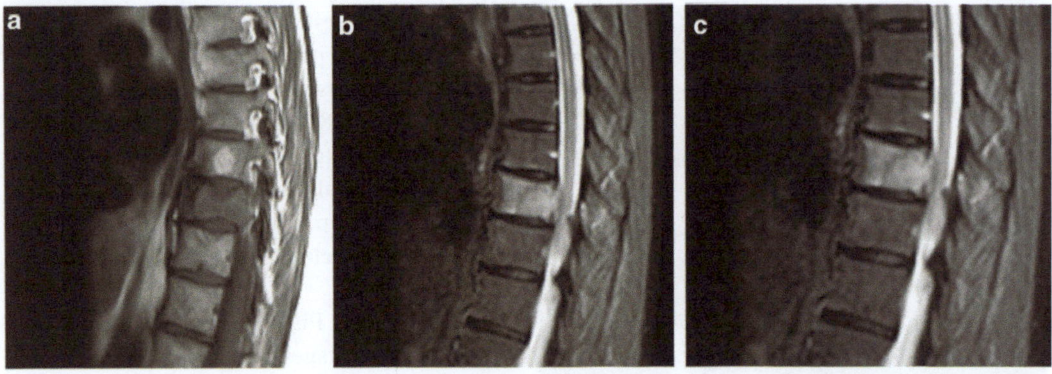

Fig. 16.3 Magnetic resonance imaging of SPB. In the absence of contrast (**a**), the plasmacytoma has the same tissue density as muscle but it enhances on STIR imaging (**b**) and with gadolinium (**c**). In the illustrated case, extension beyond the vertebra is also evident

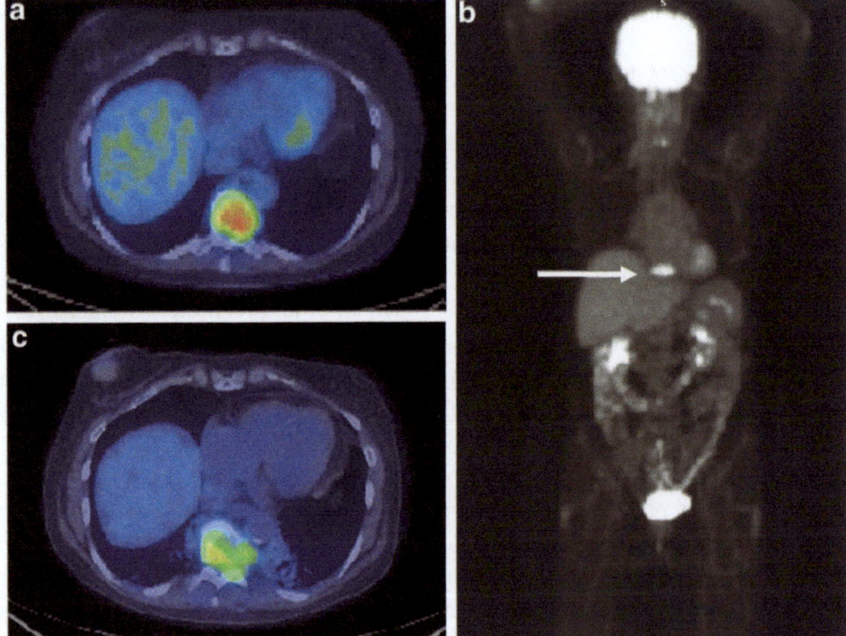

Fig. 16.4 Combined positron emission tomography and computerized tomography (PET/CT) shows the FDG avid lesion (**a**) and provides excellent staging of the disease by showing uptake only in the involved vertebra (**b**). PET/CT can be used for follow-up studies and show recurrence at the local site, including residual tumor tissue at the rim after radiation therapy (**c**)

Therapy

Malignant plasma cells are very sensitive to radiation, and therefore, the initial therapy of choice for SP is often local radiation therapy (RT) which can lead to local disease control in more than 80 % of patients. For the purpose of this discussion, therapy of SPB and EMP will be considered separately.

Solitary Plasmacytoma of Bone

Most patients are initially treated with RT and/or surgery with curative intent depending on the site of disease. In an analysis of the SEER database, spanning 1973–2005, Jawad and Scully identified 1,164 patients with skeletal plasmacytoma. They did not find any difference in survival between patients who were treated by radiation

Table 16.3 Radiation therapy for solitary plasmacytoma of bone

Series	*N*	Radiation (Gy)	Local failure (%)	Risk of prog. (%)	TTP (MM) (months)	Survival (months)
Knowling et al. [39]	25	35.0 (20–50)	0	50	17	84
McLain and Weinstein [6]	12	38.25 (24–50)	N.A.	50	N.A.	92
Frassica et al. [16]	46	39.75 (20–70)	11	57	18	111
Brinch et al. [42]	25	40.0 (28–60)	0	40	59	>120
Mayr et al. [61]	17	44.0 (21–54)	12	53	36	49
Holland et al.[45]	32	46.1 (16–62)	6	40	31	
Bolek et al. [41]	27	42.4 (28–60)	4	40	120	120
Liebross et al. [40]	57	50.0 (30–70)	4	N.A.	21	120
Tsang et al. [10]	32	35.0 (30–50)	13	60	24	120
Wilder et al. [47]	60	46.0 (30–70)	7	60	50	121
Knobel et al. [9]	206	40.0 (20–64)	12	51	21	120
Dagan et al. [76]	22	42.7 (15–54)	12	42	25	>120
Reed et al. [2]	59	45.0 (36–54)	8	56	60	>60

Risk of progression is reported at 5 years
TTP is median time in months to progression to multiple myeloma
N.A. refers to studies where this parameter could not be determined

versus surgery (60 % at 5 years and 40 % at 10 years for both treatment approaches) [58]. Several series have reported on the outcome of local RT and these are summarized in Table 16.3. Although the studies have been conducted in different eras, using different treatment technologies and with varying inclusion criteria, there is a certain consistency in the results: RT at a dose of around 40 Gy is associated with a high rate of local disease control (>85 %). Therapy is generally given daily at a rate of 1.8–2.0 Gy per fraction. The treatment field should include all the involved tissues identified by imaging as well as a margin of healthy tissue (at least 2 cm) [59]. In the case of SPB affecting vertebrae, the margin should include at least one uninvolved vertebra on either side [1]. Radiologic evidence of response is seen in approximately one-half of the patients using planar X-rays that show bone sclerosis and remineralization. Evidence of healing by CT and MRI is significantly less common [40].

The relationship between radiation dose and tumor size on the rate of tumor control is controversial. Mendelhall et al. reported a local failure rate of 31 % if the RT dose was <40 Gy and only a 6 % failure rate for a higher dose [60]. Frassica et al. did not observe any local failure rates when the dose of RT was 45 Gy or higher [16]. Tsang et al. reported that for bulky tumors (defined as a diameter >5 cm), a RT dose of ≤35 Gy was associated with a local failure rate of 83 %, while a radiation dose of >40 Gy was associated with a failure rate of 33 % in such tumors [10]. Similar observations had been reported by Mayr et al. [61] and Holland et al. [45]. Based on these results, the United Kingdom Myeloma Forum recommended that SPB less than 5 cm in diameter should be treated with 40 Gy in 20 fractions while tumors larger than 5 cm should receive up to 50 Gy [59]. Subsequently, however, a significantly larger analysis of 206 patients with SPB, performed by the Rare Cancer Network, did not find any evidence for such a relationship between dose, tumor size, and the risk of local treatment failure [9, 62]. Indeed, local failures even with RT doses greater than 50 Gy have been reported. Reed et al. also could not establish a clear relationship between the tumor size and the risk of local failure [2]. However, it is the general practice to give 45 Gy to plasmacytomas affecting the vertebrae [1, 9]. Local failure occurs in approximately 12 % of cases (Table 16.3). SPB may recur at the margin due to tumor extension outside the initial radiation portal (Fig. 16.4c), in-field, or rarely, within the draining lymph nodes [9, 40]. Therefore, in most series, no prophylactic radiation is given to the local draining lymph nodes [47, 62].

Surgery is normally reserved for patients with structural instability or neurological compromise. However, referral to an orthopedic or neurological surgeon is highly recommended for patients with spinal involvement. If a decompressive laminectomy is necessary, an anterior approach is generally recommended since this allows optimal access to the tumor and may interfere less with the subsequent RT that would be required [59, 63]. Reconstruction of the spine may require the use of expandable spacers or structural allografts. The role of vertebroplasty in the management of SPB has not been investigated.

It is not clear whether there is any role for adjuvant chemotherapy in the management of SPB. Although in principle chemotherapy may improve local tumor control when combined with RT, the evidence for this is mixed and the size of the studies small, making it difficult to provide any definite recommendation. One randomized controlled study showed that melphalan and prednisone (MP) therapy given for 3 years after RT reduced the incidence of progression to myeloma from 54 to 12 % after a median follow-up of 8.9 years [64]. However, this was a small trial ($N=25$ per arm) and given the young age of this patient population and the significant risk of myelodysplasia or leukemia with long-term melphalan therapy [65], it is difficult to recommend 3 years of therapy with this agent. Indeed, most experts would not recommend continuous MP therapy for longer than a year and perhaps restricted to ten cycles [66]. Currently, we do not recommend chemotherapy post-RT for this disease [59]. Although the combination of thalidomide and zoledronic acid delays the progression from smoldering to active myeloma [67], there are no data on the role of these agents in SPB. It may be reasonable to treat patients who have a single symptomatic plasmacytoma with imaging studies showing subtle bone disease with RT alone followed by close observation. If there is clear evidence of progression to myeloma, they should be treated as recommended by various groups [66, 68]. The role of autologous stem cell transplantation in the management of SPB is unclear since only a small number of patients with "high-risk disease" have been treated [69, 70].

With successful therapy, the monoclonal protein in the blood and/or urine generally decreases but it disappears completely less often. The decrease in the paraprotein may be quite slow and therefore may take a long time [71]. It is unusual for the serum M-protein to resolve completely if it is greater than 1.0 g/dL at the time of diagnosis [40]. In one study, the presence/absence of an M-protein at diagnosis or resolution of the M-protein after definitive RT did not have any impact on the risk of progression to multiple myeloma [16]. However, Liebross et al. reported that when the M-protein resolved, only 2 of 11 patients progressed to myeloma compared to 17 of 30 patients with a persistent M-protein [40]. Wilder et al. suggested that persistence of an M-protein for more than a year after RT is the single most important determinant of the risk of progression to myeloma, and such patients almost invariably progress to myeloma within 2 years [47]. These results suggest that patients with SPB need to be followed up closely after RT since there is considerable risk of progression to myeloma.

In a study that included 116 patients seen at the Mayo Clinic, we found that the main determinants of risk are: (1) Persistence of the serum M-protein 1–2 years after the diagnosis (HR 3.0, $p=0.02$), in agreement with Wilder et al. [47]. (2) Persistence of the urine M-protein (HR=3.6, $p=0.002$). (3) The size of the serum M-protein as a continuous variable (HR=2.0, $p<0.001$). Patients with a serum M-protein level of 0.5 g/dL or more 1–2 years after RT had a 50 % risk of progression to myeloma at 5 years, compared to patients with a serum M-protein <0.5 g/dL who had a progression risk of 13 % in the same time interval ($p<0.001$). (4) Patients with an abnormal serum FLC ratio at the time of diagnosis (<0.26 or >1.65) have a higher risk of progression compared with patients who have a normal ratio ($p=0.039$). The risk of progression to myeloma for patients with an abnormal ratio was 44 % at 5 years, 51 % at 10 years, and 51 % at 15 years while the risk for patients with a normal ratio was 26 %, 32 %, and 36 % for the same time intervals, respectively (Fig. 16.5a) [7]. In addition, an

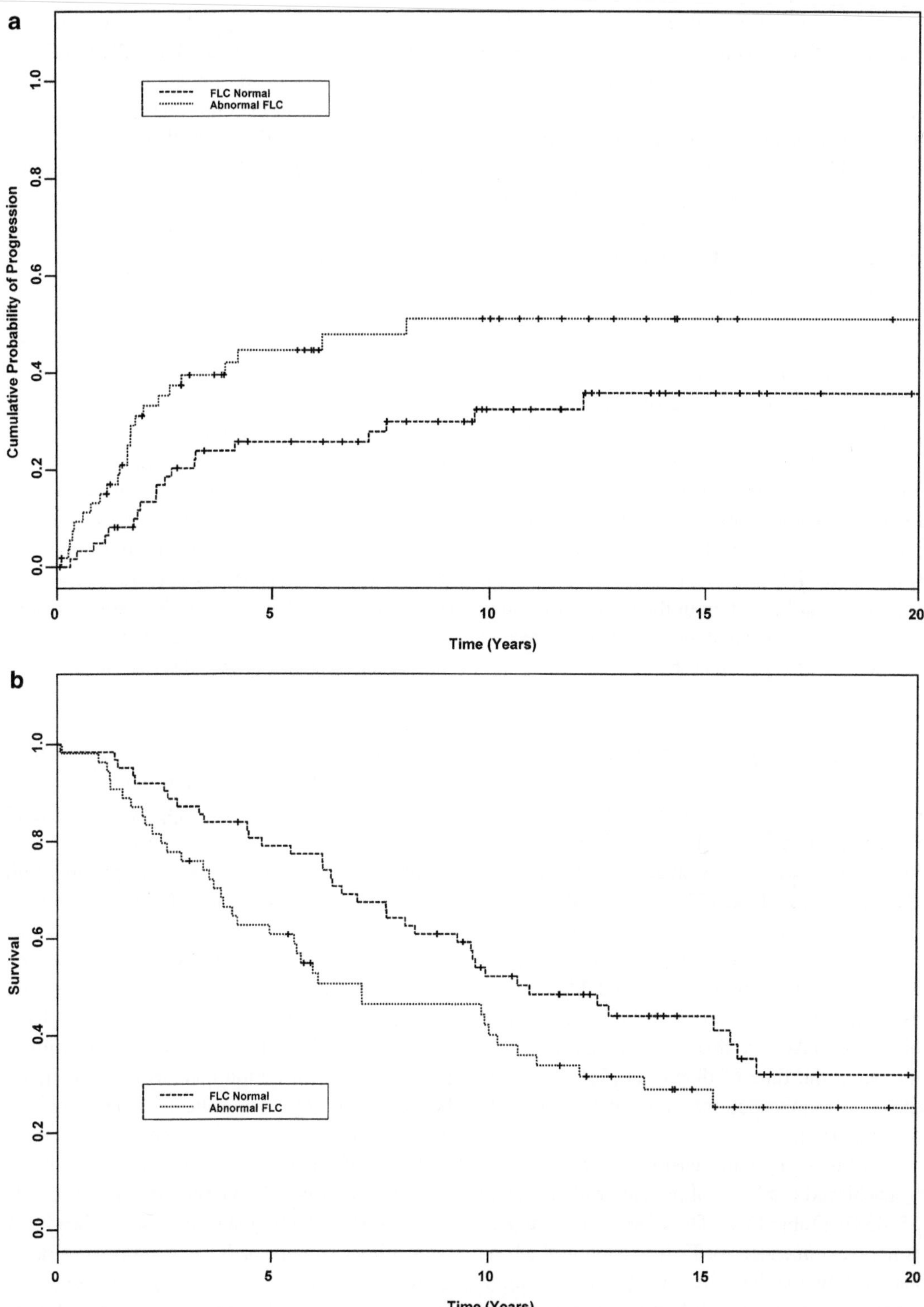

Fig. 16.5 The serum immunoglobulin free light chain (FLC) assay at diagnosis provides important prognostic information. An abnormal ratio at the time of diagnosis predicts the probability of progression to myeloma (**a**) as well as overall survival (**b**) [7]

abnormal FLC ratio (defined as <0.25 or >4.0) was associated with an adverse impact on overall survival (Fig. 16.5b). We developed a stratification model for risk of progression to multiple myeloma based on the FLC ratio at diagnosis and a serum M-protein concentration below 0.5 g/dL 1–2 years after diagnosis: patients with a normal FLC ratio and an M-protein below 0.5 g/dL were at the lowest risk of progression—13 % at 5 years, patients with either an abnormal FLC ratio or an M-protein >0.5 g/dL were at an intermediate risk (26 % at 5 years), while patients with both an abnormal FLC ratio and an elevated M-protein had the highest risk of progression (62 % at 5 years) (Fig. 16.6a) [7]. A persistently abnormal FLC ratio 1–2 years after diagnosis combined with the presence or absence of an M-protein below or above 0.5 g/dL was similarly prognostic for the risk of progression to myeloma (Fig. 16.6b). It is important to emphasize that the absence of an M-protein in the serum or urine at the time of diagnosis does not alter the risk of progression to myeloma [16].

Extramedullary Plasmacytoma

Once an EMP is found, it is currently not clear to what extent imaging studies should be performed to determine the proper staging of the disease. CT, PET/CT, or MRI [72] is essential to determine the extent of the disease and enable planning of therapy. We and others generally perform either a skeletal survey or limited MRI of the axial skeleton together with a bone marrow biopsy to make sure that systemic disease is not missed at the time of diagnosis [63]. However, these recommendations are not uniformly accepted [59].

EMP is highly radiosensitive, with local control achieved in >80 % of patients with a dose of 35–45 Gy (Table 16.4). Therefore, radical surgery is not recommended for EMP arising in the head and neck region, but care must be taken to minimize the risk of early and late side effects from the radiation while maximizing the chances of long-term disease control. Moreover, in a recent series with 68 patients who had EMP of the head and neck, the risk of progression to myeloma was higher with surgery compared to radiation (50 % versus 17 %) [14]. The impact of the radiation dose on the chances of control has been evaluated in a number of studies, but all included a small number of patients. The risk of local failure appears higher for tumors greater than 5 cm in diameter [10, 45], and therefore, some recommend a dose of up to 50 Gy for such bulky tumors [59, 73]. However, in the largest series reported to date, that included 52 patients with EMP, no dose–response relationship was found for tumors smaller or greater than 4 cm in diameter [62].

The optimal target volume for radiation is unclear. The United Kingdom Myeloma Forum recommends that a margin of at least 2 cm should be included in the radiation field [59]. More controversial is whether the associated draining lymph nodes should receive prophylactic RT, given the propensity of EMP to relapse within such nodes [10, 39, 41, 74–76]. Some groups include only clinically involved lymph nodes in the radiation field [10], whereas others have treated the local lymph nodes routinely [41]. In one series with 25 patients, only 4 received prophylactic RT to lymph nodes and yet no patient subsequently developed lymph node metastasis [2]. Other small series also support the view that RT to draining lymph nodes is generally not necessary [77, 78]. In an analysis of 128 patients with EMP who were treated with RT to the primary tumor bed alone, the overall recurrence rate was 7 % [72]. These observations, together with the considerable increase in toxicity associated with more extensive radiation, suggest that RT of the EMP itself may be enough in the vast majority of patients. Cervical lymph node irradiation should be reserved only for patients with clinically involved nodes or for those considered to have high risk of relapse, i.e., bulky disease, or if the primary tumor is in Waldeyer's ring [39, 46, 79].

For EMP affecting sites outside the head and neck, either surgery or RT is appropriate. Based on retrospective reviews, surgery seems to be the preferred form of therapy for patients with gut-associated EMP [13, 15]. In some series, patients have been treated both with surgery and RT [13, 62, 80]. There is no clear evidence that any one of

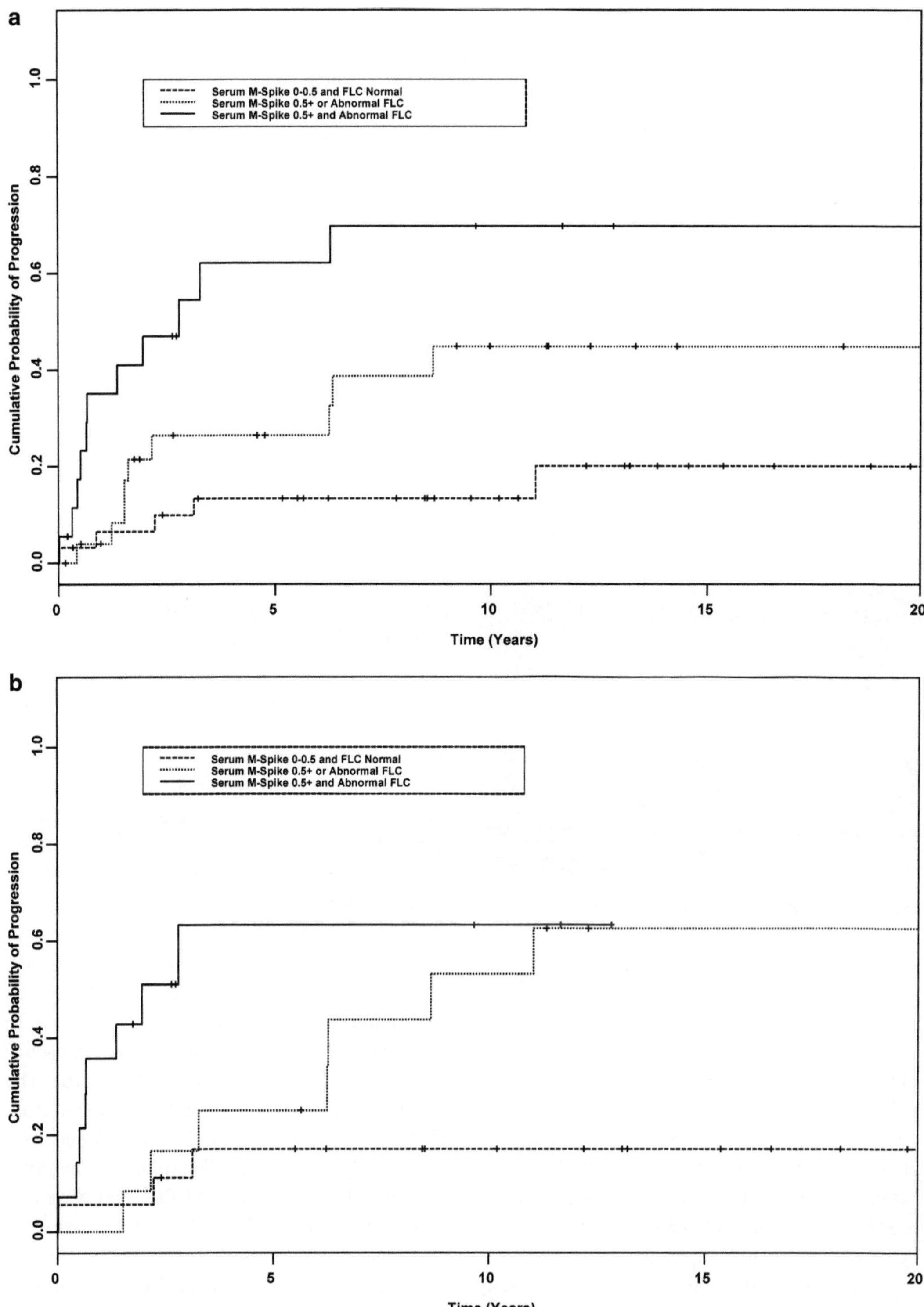

Fig. 16.6 Predictive value of the serum monoclonal proteins on the risk of progression to myeloma. The risk of progression of SPB to myeloma was stratified based on the presence/absence of an abnormal FLC ratio at diagnosis as well the size of the monoclonal protein at 1–2 years after diagnosis (**a**). The presence of one or two of these abnormalities incrementally increases the risk of progression (**a**). The presence of an abnormal FLC 1–2 years after diagnosis, combined with an M-protein abnormality, also is predictive of the progression risk (**b**) [7]

Table 16.4 Radiation therapy for extramedullary plasmacytoma

Series	*N*	Radiation (Gy)	Local failure (%)	Risk of prog. (%)	TTP (MM) (months)	Survival (months)
Knowling et al. [39]	25	35.0 (10–50)	16	30	23.4	100
Bolek et al. [41]	10	45.0 (9–50)	0	11	N.A.	180
Mayr et al. [61]	13	50.4 (40–60)	8	23	13	69
Holland et al. [45]	14	46.1 (16–62)	7	30	13	
Alexiou et al. [13]	7	40.0 (40–60)	22	N.A.	N.A.	300
Galieni et al. [80]	46	46.0 (30–60)	7	15	N.A.	>120
Tsang et al. [10]	14	35.0 (≤30–35)	7	17	24	120
Chao et al. [79]	16	45.0 (40–50.4)	0	25	13	>120
Ozsahin et al. [62]	52	40.0 (20–66)	26	26	36	>120
Bachar et al. [14]	68	35.0 (10–50)	13	23	34	>120
Dagan et al. [76]	10	43.0 (15–54)	0	10	144	>120
Reed et al. [2]	25	45.0 (36–53.4)	20	30	24	>120

Risk of progression is reported at 5 years
TTP is median time in months to progression to multiple myeloma
N.A. refers to studies where this parameter could not be determined

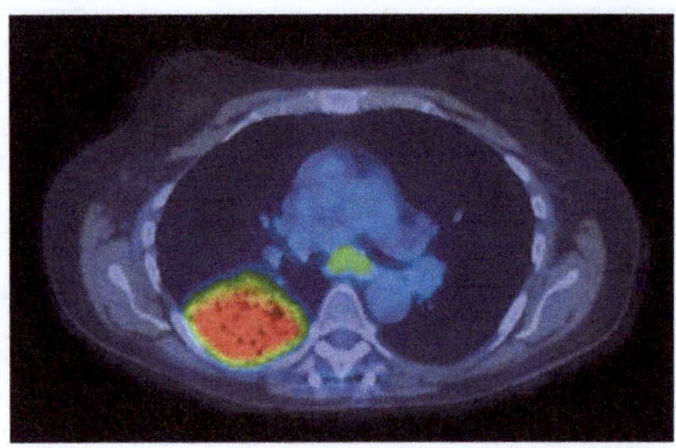

Fig. 16.7 PET/CT imaging showing delayed radiation pneumonitis after definitive therapy of SPB affecting a thoracic vertebra. Infectious and neoplastic disorders were excluded by biopsy and cultures and the patient responded rapidly to a course of glucocorticosteroids

these approaches is superior with respect to the risk of local recurrence or progression [13, 14, 62]. To date, there is no evidence that adjuvant chemotherapy is of value in EMP [80, 81]. Similarly, no data exist on the role of immunomodulatory agents, proteasome inhibitors, or bisphosphonates in the management of EMP.

Patients with SP should be followed closely during and after RT for detection and treatment of early or delayed adverse effects of RT including xerostomia, as well as radiation pneumonitis (Fig. 16.7) [82].

Relapse and Progression to Multiple Myeloma

Failure of local therapy in SP may manifest either by recurrence in the treated radiation field, in the rim outside the prior radiation field (Fig. 16.4c) or in the draining lymph nodes. Some patients may present with another isolated plasmacytoma although the majority progress to multiple myeloma. With modern therapy, the risk of local failure is low and should be less than 15 % (Tables 16.3 and 16.4). The risk of progression to myeloma is higher with SPB compared to EMP (~50 % compared to ~21 % at 5 years) [62]. It has to be emphasized that the risk of progression to myeloma is not related to the presence/absence of M-protein at the time of diagnosis [16]. The median time to progression to myeloma from SPB is circa 24 months although this can vary significantly (Table 16.3). The value of monitoring the monoclonal proteins and FLC has been discussed previously. The risk of progression to myeloma increases with time from 51 % at 5 years to 72 % at 10 years [9]. In the largest series of patients with SPB, the only determinant of the risk of progression to myeloma was age [9]. For patients younger than 60 years at the time of diagnosis, the risk of progression to myeloma at 10 years was 67 % versus 76 % for older patients ($p = 0.007$) [9]. The risk of local failure is least for disease affecting a vertebra.

In one series, that included 68 patients with EMP of the head and neck, the risk of progression to multiple myeloma was not the same for all sites and highest for the sinonasal tract (37 %) followed by the oropharynx (18 %) [14]. The risk of progression to multiple myeloma appeared to be lowest for patients treated with RT compared to those treated with surgery alone (17 % versus 50 %). Additional studies are needed to confirm these observations. The median time to progression to multiple myeloma from EMP taking all series into consideration is 24 months (Table 16.4). Similar to SPB, the presence/absence of an M-protein at the time of diagnosis has no impact on the risk of progression [42].

These observations suggest that patients with SP need careful observation. Although the risk of progression to myeloma is highest within the first few years after diagnosis, they require lifelong follow-up. Patients with local relapse may be treated with surgery or radiation depending on the site and prior radiation dose and tissue tolerance, taking the potential toxicities into consideration. If there is evidence of progression to multiple myeloma, they should be treated according to established guidelines or enrolled in clinical trials [66, 83, 84].

Prognosis

Most of the reported series, usually from major centers treating patients with these disorders, have reported excellent overall survival rates for both SPB and EMP with a median greater than 10 years (Tables 16.3 and 16.4). The multicenter Rare Cancer Treatment Network study reported a median overall survival of 74 % at 5 years and 54 % at 10 years [62]. However, analysis of the SEER database suggests that overall survival in the general population may be inferior and only 57 % at 5 years and 37 % at 10 years [58]. There are various potential explanations for these discrepancies including incomplete reporting and the inclusion of a significant number of patients who may have had myeloma in the SEER analysis. The only determinant of overall survival appears to be age at the time of diagnosis, with patients older than 60 years having an inferior overall survival [58, 62]. On a more optimistic note, there appears to be a trend for an improvement in prognosis for patients with SP treated between 1973 and 2005, perhaps due to better disease definition and referral to centers with expertise in the management of this disorder [58]. The main causes of death in patients who do not progress to multiple myeloma are cardiovascular and cerebrovascular in nature.

References

1. Dimopoulos MA, Moulopoulos LA, Maniatis A, Alexanian R. Solitary plasmacytoma of bone and asymptomatic multiple myeloma. Blood. 2000;96(6):2037–44.
2. Reed V, Shah J, Medeiros LJ, et al. Solitary plasmacytomas: outcome and prognostic factors after definitive radiation therapy. Cancer. 2011;117(19):4468–74.
3. Group IMW. Criteria for the classification of monoclonal gammopathies, multiple myeloma and related disorders: a report of the International Myeloma Working Group. Br J Haematol. 2003;121(5):749–57.
4. Corwin J, Lindberg RD. Solitary plasmacytoma of bone vs. extramedullary plasmacytoma and their relationship to multiple myeloma. Cancer. 1979;43(3):1007–13.
5. Bataille R, Sany J. Solitary myeloma: clinical and prognostic features of a review of 114 cases. Cancer. 1981;48(3):845–51.
6. McLain RF, Weinstein JN. Solitary plasmacytomas of the spine: a review of 84 cases. J Spinal Disord. 1989;2(2):69–74.
7. Dingli D, Kyle RA, Rajkumar SV, et al. Immunoglobulin free light chains and solitary plasmacytoma of bone. Blood. 2006;108(6):1979–83.
8. Warsame R, Gertz MA, Lacy MQ, et al. Trends and outcomes of modern staging of solitary plasmacytoma of bone. Am J Hematol. 2012;87(7):647–51.
9. Knobel D, Zouhair A, Tsang RW, et al. Prognostic factors in solitary plasmacytoma of the bone: a multicenter Rare Cancer Network study. BMC Cancer. 2006;6:118.
10. Tsang RW, Gospodarowicz MK, Pintilie M, et al. Solitary plasmacytoma treated with radiotherapy: impact of tumor size on outcome. Int J Radiat Oncol Biol Phys. 2001;50(1):113–20.
11. Dimopoulos MA, Goldstein J, Fuller L, Delasalle K, Alexanian R. Curability of solitary bone plasmacytoma. J Clin Oncol. 1992;10(4):587–90.

12. Dimopoulos MA, Hamilos G. Solitary bone plasmacytoma and extramedullary plasmacytoma. Curr Treat Options Oncol. 2002;3(3):255–9.
13. Alexiou C, Kau RJ, Dietzfelbinger H, et al. Extramedullary plasmacytoma: tumor occurrence and therapeutic concepts. Cancer. 1999;85(11):2305–14.
14. Bachar G, Goldstein D, Brown D, et al. Solitary extramedullary plasmacytoma of the head and neck—long-term outcome analysis of 68 cases. Head Neck. 2008;30(8):1012–9.
15. Lopes da Silva R. Extramedullary plasmacytoma of the small intestine: clinical features, diagnosis and treatment. J Dig Dis. 2012;13(1):10–8.
16. Frassica DA, Frassica FJ, Schray MF, Sim FH, Kyle RA. Solitary plasmacytoma of bone: Mayo Clinic experience. Int J Radiat Oncol Biol Phys. 1989;16(1): 43–8.
17. Fonseca R, Barlogie B, Bataille R, et al. Genetics and cytogenetics of multiple myeloma: a workshop report. Cancer Res. 2004;64(4):1546–58.
18. Bergsagel PL, Kuehl WM. Molecular pathogenesis and a consequent classification of multiple myeloma. J Clin Oncol. 2005;23(26):6333–8.
19. Chng WJ, Santana-Davila R, Van Wier SA, et al. Prognostic factors for hyperdiploid-myeloma: effects of chromosome 13 deletions and IgH translocations. Leukemia. 2006;20(5):807–13.
20. Zhan F, Huang Y, Colla S, et al. The molecular classification of multiple myeloma. Blood. 2006;108(6): 2020–8.
21. Chng WJ, Kuehl WM, Bergsagel PL, Fonseca R. Translocation t(4;14) retains prognostic significance even in the setting of high-risk molecular signature. Leukemia. 2008;22(2):459–61.
22. Avet-Loiseau H, Attal M, Campion L, et al. Long-term analysis of the IFM 99 trials for myeloma: cytogenetic abnormalities [t(4;14), del(17p), 1q gains] play a major role in defining long-term survival. J Clin Oncol. 2012;30(16):1949–52.
23. Stewart AK, Bergsagel PL, Greipp PR, et al. A practical guide to defining high-risk myeloma for clinical trials, patient counseling and choice of therapy. Leukemia. 2007;21(3):529–34.
24. Kapoor P, Kumar S, Fonseca R, et al. Impact of risk stratification on outcome among patients with multiple myeloma receiving initial therapy with lenalidomide and dexamethasone. Blood. 2009;114(3):518–21.
25. Avet-Loiseau H, Facon T, Daviet A, et al. 14q32 translocations and monosomy 13 observed in monoclonal gammopathy of undetermined significance delineate a multistep process for the oncogenesis of multiple myeloma. Intergroupe Francophone du Myelome. Cancer Res. 1999;59(18):4546–50.
26. Fonseca R, Ahmann GJ, Jalal SM, et al. Chromosomal abnormalities in systemic amyloidosis. Br J Haematol. 1998;103(3):704–10.
27. Bink K, Haralambieva E, Kremer M, et al. Primary extramedullary plasmacytoma: similarities with and differences from multiple myeloma revealed by interphase cytogenetics. Haematologica. 2008;93(4):623–6.
28. Chng WJ, Price-Troska T, Gonzalez-Paz N, et al. Clinical significance of TP53 mutation in myeloma. Leukemia. 2007;21(3):582–4.
29. Vasef MA, Medeiros LJ, Yospur LS, Sun NC, McCourty A, Brynes RK. Cyclin D1 protein in multiple myeloma and plasmacytoma: an immunohistochemical study using fixed, paraffin-embedded tissue sections. Mod Pathol. 1997;10(9):927–32.
30. Kumar S, Fonseca R, Ketterling RP, et al. Trisomies in multiple myeloma: impact on survival in patients with high-risk cytogenetics. Blood. 2012;119(9): 2100–5.
31. Dispenzieri A. POEMS syndrome: update on diagnosis, risk-stratification, and management. Am J Hematol. 2012;87(8):804–14.
32. Dispenzieri A, Kyle RA, Lacy MQ, et al. POEMS syndrome: definitions and long-term outcome. Blood. 2003;101(7):2496–506.
33. Medini E, Rao Y, Levitt SH. Solitary extramedullary plasmacytoma of the upper respiratory and digestive tracts. Cancer. 1980;45(11):2893–6.
34. Kapadia SB, Desai U, Cheng VS. Extramedullary plasmacytoma of the head and neck. A clinicopathologic study of 20 cases. Medicine. 1982;61(5):317–29.
35. Manganaris A, Conn B, Connor S, Simo R. Uncommon presentation of nasopharyngeal extramedullary plasmacytoma: a case report and literature review. B-ENT. 2010;6(2):143–6.
36. Nagai K, Ando K, Yoshida H, et al. Response of the extramedullary lung plasmacytoma with pleural effusion to chemotherapy. Ann Hematol. 1997;74(6): 279–81.
37. Bourtsos EP, Bedrossian CW, De Frias DV, Nayar R. Thyroid plasmacytoma mimicking medullary carcinoma: a potential pitfall in aspiration cytology. Diagn Cytopathol. 2000;23(5):354–8.
38. Yu SC, Chen SU, Lu W, Liu TY, Lin CW. Expression of CD19 and lack of miR-223 distinguish extramedullary plasmacytoma from multiple myeloma. Histopathology. 2011;58(6):896–905.
39. Knowling MA, Harwood AR, Bergsagel DE. Comparison of extramedullary plasmacytomas with solitary and multiple plasma cell tumors of bone. J Clin Oncol. 1983;1(4):255–62.
40. Liebross RH, Ha CS, Cox JD, Weber D, Delasalle K, Alexanian R. Solitary bone plasmacytoma: outcome and prognostic factors following radiotherapy. Int J Radiat Oncol Biol Phys. 1998;41(5):1063–7.
41. Bolek TW, Marcus Jr RB, Mendenhall NP. Solitary plasmacytoma of bone and soft tissue. Int J Radiat Oncol Biol Phys. 1996;36(2):329–33.
42. Brinch L, Hannisdal E, Abrahamsen AF, Kvaloy S, Langholm R. Extramedullary plasmacytomas and solitary plasma cell tumours of bone. Eur J Haematol. 1990;44(2):132–5.
43. Galieni P, Cavo M, Avvisati G, et al. Solitary plasmacytoma of bone and extramedullary plasmacytoma: two different entities? Ann Oncol. 1995;6(7):687–91.
44. Jackson A, Scarffe JH. Prognostic significance of osteopenia and immunoparesis at presentation in

patients with solitary myeloma of bone. Eur J Cancer. 1990;26(3):363–71.
45. Holland J, Trenkner DA, Wasserman TH, Fineberg B. Plasmacytoma. Treatment results and conversion to myeloma. Cancer. 1992;69(6):1513–7.
46. Liebross RH, Ha CS, Cox JD, Weber D, Delasalle K, Alexanian R. Clinical course of solitary extramedullary plasmacytoma. Radiother Oncol. 1999;52(3): 245–9.
47. Wilder RB, Ha CS, Cox JD, Weber D, Delasalle K, Alexanian R. Persistence of myeloma protein for more than one year after radiotherapy is an adverse prognostic factor in solitary plasmacytoma of bone. Cancer. 2002;94(5):1532–7.
48. San Miguel JF, Gutierrez NC, Mateo G, Orfao A. Conventional diagnostics in multiple myeloma. Eur J Cancer. 2006;42(11):1510–9.
49. Jackson A, Scarffe JH. Upper humeral cortical thickness as an indicator of osteopenia: diagnostic significance in solitary myeloma of bone. Skeletal Radiol. 1991;20(5):363–7.
50. Moulopoulos LA, Dimopoulos MA, Weber D, Fuller L, Libshitz HI, Alexanian R. Magnetic resonance imaging in the staging of solitary plasmacytoma of bone. J Clin Oncol. 1993;11(7):1311–5.
51. Lecouvet FE, Malghem J, Michaux L, et al. Skeletal survey in advanced multiple myeloma: radiographic versus MR imaging survey. Br J Haematol. 1999; 106(1):35–9.
52. Schirrmeister H, Buck AK, Bergmann L, Reske SN, Bommer M. Positron emission tomography (PET) for staging of solitary plasmacytoma. Cancer Biother Radiopharm. 2003;18(5):841–5.
53. Mulligan ME, Badros AZ. PET/CT and MR imaging in myeloma. Skeletal Radiol. 2007;36(1):5–16.
54. Salaun PY, Gastinne T, Frampas E, Bodet-Milin C, Moreau P, Bodere-Kraeber F. FDG-positron-emission tomography for staging and therapeutic assessment in patients with plasmacytoma. Haematologica. 2008;93(8):1269–71.
55. Nanni C, Rubello D, Zamagni E, et al. 18F-FDG PET/CT in myeloma with presumed solitary plasmocytoma of bone. In Vivo. 2008;22(4):513–7.
56. Wiltshaw E. The natural history of extramedullary plasmacytoma and its relation to solitary myeloma of bone and myelomatosis. Medicine. 1976;55(3): 217–38.
57. Woodruff RK, Whittle JM, Malpas JS. Solitary plasmacytoma. I: extramedullary soft tissue plasmacytoma. Cancer. 1979;43(6):2340–3.
58. Jawad MU, Scully SP. Skeletal plasmacytoma: progression of disease and impact of local treatment; an analysis of SEER database. J Hematol Oncol. 2009;2:41.
59. Soutar R, Lucraft H, Jackson G, et al. Guidelines on the diagnosis and management of solitary plasmacytoma of bone and solitary extramedullary plasmacytoma. Br J Haematol. 2004;124(6):717–26.
60. Mendenhall CM, Thar TL, Million RR. Solitary plasmacytoma of bone and soft tissue. Int J Radiat Oncol Biol Phys. 1980;6(11):1497–501.
61. Mayr NA, Wen BC, Hussey DH, et al. The role of radiation therapy in the treatment of solitary plasmacytomas. Radiother Oncol. 1990;17(4):293–303.
62. Ozsahin M, Tsang RW, Poortmans P, et al. Outcomes and patterns of failure in solitary plasmacytoma: a multicenter Rare Cancer Network study of 258 patients. Int J Radiat Oncol Biol Phys. 2006;64(1): 210–7.
63. Weber DM. Solitary bone and extramedullary plasmacytoma. Hematology Am Soc Hematol Educ Program. 2005:373–6, PMID is 16304406.
64. Aviles A, Huerta-Guzman J, Delgado S, Fernandez A, Diaz-Maqueo JC. Improved outcome in solitary bone plasmacytomata with combined therapy. Hematol Oncol. 1996;14(3):111–7.
65. Delauche-Cavallier MC, Laredo JD, Wybier M, et al. Solitary plasmacytoma of the spine. Long-term clinical course. Cancer. 1988;61(8):1707–14.
66. Kumar SK, Mikhael JR, Buadi FK, et al. Management of newly diagnosed symptomatic multiple myeloma: updated Mayo Stratification of Myeloma and Risk-Adapted Therapy (mSMART) consensus guidelines. Mayo Clin Proc. 2009;84(12):1095–110.
67. Witzig TE, Laumann KM, Lacy MQ, et al. A phase III randomized trial of thalidomide plus zoledronic acid versus zoledronic acid alone in patients with asymptomatic multiple myeloma. Leukemia. 2012;27(1):220–5.
68. Anderson KC, Alsina M, Bensinger W, et al. Multiple myeloma. J Natl Compr Canc Netw. 2011;9(10): 1146–83.
69. Dimopoulos MA, Papadimitriou C, Anagnostopoulos A, Mitsibounas D, Fermand JP. High dose therapy with autologous stem cell transplantation for solitary bone plasmacytoma complicated by local relapse or isolated distant recurrence. Leuk Lymphoma. 2003;44(1):153–5.
70. Jantunen E, Koivunen E, Putkonen M, Siitonen T, Juvonen E, Nousiainen T. Autologous stem cell transplantation in patients with high-risk plasmacytoma. Eur J Haematol. 2005;74(5):402–6.
71. Alexanian R. Localized and indolent myeloma. Blood. 1980;56(3):521–5.
72. Dimopoulos MA, Kiamouris C, Moulopoulos LA. Solitary plasmacytoma of bone and extramedullary plasmacytoma. Hematol Oncol Clin North Am. 1999;13(6):1249–57.
73. Mill WB, Griffith R. The role of radiation therapy in the management of plasma cell tumors. Cancer. 1980;45(4):647–52.
74. Hu K, Yahalom J. Radiotherapy in the management of plasma cell tumors. Oncology (Williston Park). 2000;14(1):101–8; 11; discussion 11–2; 15.
75. Susnerwala SS, Shanks JH, Banerjee SS, Scarffe JH, Farrington WT, Slevin NJ. Extramedullary plasmacytoma of the head and neck region: clinicopathological correlation in 25 cases. Br J Cancer. 1997;75(6): 921–7.
76. Dagan R, Morris CG, Kirwan J, Mendenhall WM. Solitary plasmacytoma. Am J Clin Oncol. 2009;32(6): 612–7.

77. Jyothirmayi R, Gangadharan VP, Nair MK, Rajan B. Radiotherapy in the treatment of solitary plasmacytoma. Br J Radiol. 1997;70(833):511–6.
78. Strojan P, Soba E, Lamovec J, Munda A. Extramedullary plasmacytoma: clinical and histopathologic study. Int J Radiat Oncol Biol Phys. 2002;53(3):692–701.
79. Chao MW, Gibbs P, Wirth A, Quong G, Guiney MJ, Liew KH. Radiotherapy in the management of solitary extramedullary plasmacytoma. Intern Med J. 2005; 35(4):211–5.
80. Galieni P, Cavo M, Pulsoni A, et al. Clinical outcome of extramedullary plasmacytoma. Haematologica. 2000;85(1):47–51.
81. Shih LY, Dunn P, Leung WM, Chen WJ, Wang PN. Localised plasmacytomas in Taiwan: comparison between extramedullary plasmacytoma and solitary plasmacytoma of bone. Br J Cancer. 1995;71(1): 128–33.
82. Arbetter KR, Prakash UB, Tazelaar HD, Douglas WW. Radiation-induced pneumonitis in the "nonirradiated" lung. Mayo Clin Proc. 1999;74(1):27–36.
83. Anderson KC, Alsina M, Bensinger W, et al. NCCN clinical practice guidelines in oncology: multiple myeloma. J Natl Compr Canc Netw. 2009;7(9):908–42.
84. Smith A, Wisloff F, Samson D. Guidelines on the diagnosis and management of multiple myeloma 2005. Br J Haematol. 2006;132(4):410–51.

Myeloma Bone Disease

17

Matthew T. Drake

Introduction

Skeletal complications are a major problem for patients affected by cancers which metastasize to or grow primarily within bone [1]. As advancements in chemotherapeutic regimens have led to progressive lifespan extension in patients with malignancies, efforts to limit both cancer-associated and treatment-associated skeletal complications have become increasingly important for the provision of optimal patient care.

Multiple Myeloma: The Skeletal Impact

Within the United States, nearly 22,000 patients are diagnosed with multiple myeloma (MM) each year, and nearly 11,000 MM-associated deaths occur annually [2]. Importantly, the last decade has witnessed continued improvement in the median survival of MM patients from diagnosis, as novel chemotherapeutic agents including immunomodulatory drugs (IMiDs) and proteasome inhibitors have become widely available, resulting in increased numbers of patients with prolonged periods of survival [3], including some with survival of greater than 10 years [4]. Accordingly, improving quality of life by limiting disease-associated complications has become an increasingly important aspect of caring for all patients with MM.

Unlike other malignancies in which metastatic cells must migrate from their primary site of origin to reach the skeleton, MM is characterized by the clonal proliferation of malignant plasma cells within their normal milieu—the bone marrow cavity; accordingly, MM has the greatest incidence of bone involvement among all cancers [1]. For many patients with MM, a pathologic fracture or severe bone pain (frequently within the vertebrae or ribs) due to osteolytic destruction originating from within the marrow cavity is the sentinel event resulting in an MM diagnosis [5]. Patients diagnosed with MM have an approximately 16-fold increased risk of fracture in the year preceding diagnosis [6]. Bone pain, which is usually heightened by movement and improved by rest, is present in approximately 60 % of patients at time of diagnosis [7]. Further, over the course of their disease, approximately 90 % of MM patients will ultimately suffer from osteolytic lesions [1], and approximately 60 % will develop a fracture [6].

The biologic basis for the bone loss and increased fracture risk in multiple myeloma has become increasingly defined over the past several decades, and results from an insidious disruption of the normal bone homeostatic process perpetrated by the myeloma cells themselves.

M.T. Drake, M.D., Ph.D. (✉)
Division of Endocrinology, Mayo Clinic,
200 First Street, Southwest, Rochester, MN 55905, USA
e-mail: drake.matthew@mayo.edu

M.A. Gertz and S.V. Rajkumar (eds.), *Multiple Myeloma: Diagnosis and Treatment*,
DOI 10.1007/978-1-4614-8520-9_17,

Within the normal healthy adult skeleton, a balanced bone remodeling sequence occurs in which fatigued or damaged bone is removed by osteoclast-mediated resorption. This removal is followed both spatially and temporally by replacement of resorbed bone by osteoblast-mediated new bone formation. Any impairment of this normal homeostatic skeletal balance can result in bone loss, disruption in the structural integrity of the affected bone, and an increased risk for potential skeletal complications. It is now clear that bone disease in multiple myeloma is the result of myeloma cell effects on both osteoclasts, leading to increases in osteoclast-mediated bone resorption, and osteoblasts, resulting in a marked decrease in the normal osteoblastic response to bone resorption [8]. Collectively, this unbalanced bone cell activity results in the development of purely osteolytic lesions. This imbalance is also likely a major contributing factor to the generalized systemic bone loss which occurs in MM and leads to the significantly increased risk of osteoporotic-type fractures in MM patients [6, 9].

As a consequence of this marked imbalance in the normal bone remodeling process, patients with MM-associated bone disease suffer from significant morbidity and mortality. Indeed, MM patients who experience a pathologic fracture incur at least a 20 % increased mortality risk [10]. While osteolytic lesions can occur at any skeletal site, the most frequently affected sites are those of the central skeleton [spine (49 %), ribs (33 %), and pelvis (34 %)], skull (35 %), proximal long bones [humeri (22 %) and femora (13 %)], and mandible (10 %) [11]. Frequently occurring skeletal-associated complications [often referred to collectively as skeletal-related events (SREs)] include pathologic fractures (particularly vertebral), intractable bone pain, hypercalcemia, and spinal cord compression [12]. Notably, even patients who achieve at least a very good partial response (VGPR) to chemotherapy may have progression of skeletal disease; likewise, even patients who have sustained complete remission (CR) of their MM generally do not show any radiographic improvement of their skeletal lesions [13].

Molecular Basis for Myeloma Bone Disease

Our understanding of the molecular basis for MM bone disease has increased markedly over the past several decades, primarily due to the identification of factors made by MM cells or within the local bone marrow microenvironment which affect the activity of the primary bone cells—osteoclasts and osteoblasts. The localization of MM cells in close proximity to sites of osteolysis is consistent with a role for locally produced factors in osteolytic lesion development, while the generalized osteoporotic-type bone loss found suggests an important role for circulating factors as well. It is important to recognize that in MM, bone loss is not mediated by the MM cells themselves, but rather results from the ability of MM cells to stimulate osteoclast activity while simultaneously suppressing osteoblast activity. It is also evident that while some MM effects on bone cells are direct, others result from myeloma cells inducing cells normally resident within the bone marrow microenvironment to produce factors which affect bone cell function. In turn, the production of factors both by bone cells and resident cells of the bone marrow microenvironment, in conjunction with the local release of growth factors embedded in the bone matrix during the bone resorption process, leads to further MM cell growth (Fig. 17.1). Accordingly, this process has been appropriately termed the "vicious cycle" [14].

Stimulation of Osteoclast Activity

Studies performed over 3 decades ago demonstrated that human myeloma cells are capable of secreting "osteoclast-activating factors" which support bone resorption in organ culture [15]. Much work since then has characterized many of these factors, while also demonstrating that MM cells can also induce cells within the local marrow microenvironment to produce factors which increase osteoclast production and activity. In a reciprocal relationship as described above,

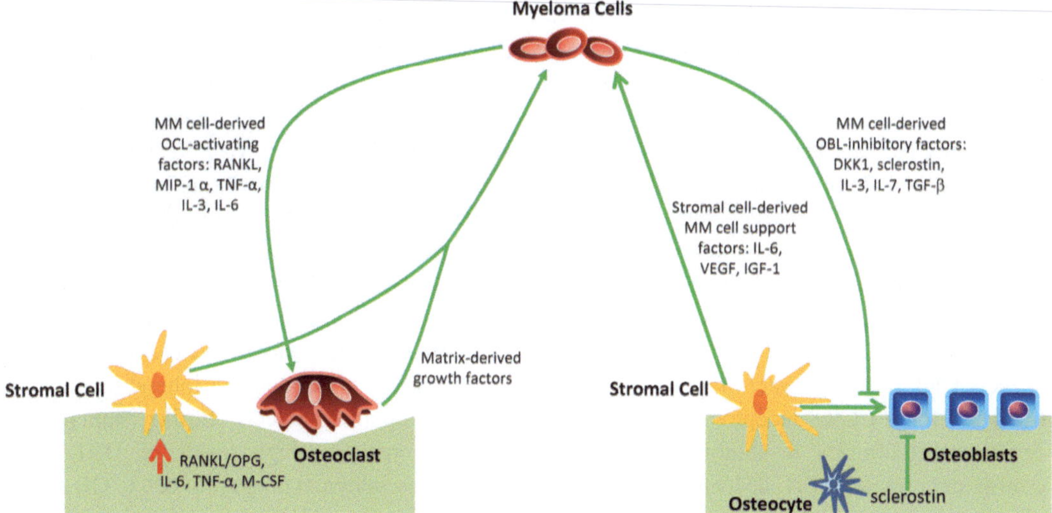

Fig. 17.1 The molecular basis for myeloma bone disease. As described in the text, myeloma cells produce multiple factors which increase osteoclast (*OCL*) activity (*left*) and inhibit osteoblast (*OB*) activity (*right*). Myeloma cells also induce the production of osteoclast activating factors from resident bone marrow stromal cells (*left*), while simultaneously inducing decreased stromal cell production of osteoprotegerin (*OPG*). Osteoclast-mediated digestion of the bone matrix results in local growth factor release to support myeloma cell growth. Further, stromal cell-derived factors produced locally further support myeloma cell growth. The entire process is described as the "vicious cycle" of bone destruction

osteoclast-mediated bone resorption results in the liberation of bone matrix-embedded growth factors which serve to nourish adjacent MM cells. More recently, osteoclasts have also shown to directly release factors which can support myeloma cell growth. Several of these MM cells and osteoclast-produced factors are discussed below (Fig. 17.1).

Receptor Activator of Nuclear Factor Kappa B Ligand

Receptor activator of nuclear factor kappa B ligand (RANKL) binding to its receptor RANK on pre-osteoclasts is critical for osteoclastogenesis. RANKL activity is opposed by osteoprotegerin (OPG), the soluble decoy receptor for RANKL produced by osteoblasts. While myeloma cells can produce low levels of RANKL, whether these low levels are sufficient to promote osteoclastogenesis is unclear [16]. Regardless, MM cells potently induce stromal cell production of RANKL via signaling through interaction of vascular cell adhesion molecule-1 (VCAM-1) on marrow stromal cells and α4β1 integrin on MM cells [17]. Suppression of OPG levels is also important for the establishment of high effective RANKL concentrations, and occurs both through MM cell-mediated suppression of osteoblast differentiation and MM cell-mediated endocytosis of OPG bound to CD138 [18]. Together, these effects create an imbalance in the RANKL/OPG ratio within the marrow cavity, leading to potent stimulation of osteoclast-mediated bone destruction [19]. Recently denosumab, a fully humanized monoclonal antibody against RANKL, has been evaluated in human clinical oncology trials [20]. In a large clinical trial which included a subset of patients with MM, denosumab was found to be non-inferior to zoledronic acid in preventing or delaying first on-study SRE [21]. A large phase III study enrolling only subjects with MM has recently begun, with results anticipated in approximately 2016.

Chemokine (C-C Motif) Ligand 3 (CCL3)/Macrophage Inflammatory Protein-1α (MIP-1α)

CCL3/MIP-1α is another chemokine produced by MM cells which potently increases osteoclastogenesis, particularly when present in conjunction with RANKL. CCLL3/MIP-1α levels are positively correlated with the extent of bone disease in MM, and are negatively correlated with survival [22]. Interestingly, CCL3/MIP-1α levels are also significantly increased in the MM precursor condition monoclonal gammopathy of undetermined significance (MGUS), in which generalized bone loss and increased risk for osteoporotic-type fractures occurs, suggesting that circulating levels of CCL3/MIP-1α can also have systemic skeletal effects [23]. CCL3/MIP-1α functions by binding to the CCR1 receptor. Preclinical studies using small molecule CCR1 receptor inhibitors have demonstrated efficacy in inhibiting both MM growth and osteolysis [24, 25], and CCR1 receptor antagonists are currently in development for future clinical trials in humans [26].

Other Molecules Involved in Osteoclast Activation in Myeloma

A variety of molecules in addition to RANKL and CCL3/MIP-1α with likely roles in increasing osteoclast formation and activity have been described. Among these are tumor necrosis factor-α (TNF-α) [27], interleukin-3 (IL-3) [28], interleukin 6 (IL-6) [29], and ephrinB2/EphB4 [30]. A more complete description of these molecules and their potential roles in the dysregulated osteoclast formation and activity inherent to MM bone disease is beyond the space allowed here.

Suppression of Osteoblast Activity

While the role that increased osteoclast activity plays in the development of osteolytic lesions in MM has long been appreciated, much recent attention has been focused on understanding the molecular basis for osteoblastic suppression in MM bone disease. Intense efforts have now yielded an array of osteoblast inhibitory factors produced either by MM cells or other cells within the bone marrow microenvironment. A description of several of these factors is provided below (Fig. 17.1).

Dickkopf-1 (DKK1)

Activation of the Wnt/β-catenin signaling pathway plays a fundamental role in nearly every aspect of osteoblast development, including the differentiation of osteoblast progenitors into functional osteoblasts, osteoblast proliferation and survival, and ultimately bone formation [31]. DKK1 is a secreted Wnt pathway inhibitor that acts to specifically block Wnt/β-catenin signaling in osteoblasts, thereby inhibiting osteoblast development and activity. Myeloma cells produce high levels of DKK1, and DKK1 also appears to be to be highly expressed by at least some bone marrow stromal cells [32]. Patients whose MM is complicated by osteolytic lesions have elevated levels of DKK1 in BM plasma and peripheral blood compared to control subjects; further, human BM plasma containing high levels of DKK1 can inhibit mesenchymal progenitor cell to OB differentiation in vitro [33]. Serum DKK1 levels correlate with the extent of MM bone disease [34] and decrease in response to anti-myeloma therapy [35]. In murine MM models, antibodies directed against DKK1 increased OB numbers and limited osteolytic disease [36, 37]. Further, pharmacologic stimulation of Wnt signaling in preclinical models also appears to limit myeloma bone disease development [38]. Antibodies directed against DKK1 are now in clinical trials for patients with either smoldering MM or active MM.

Sclerostin

Like DKK1, sclerostin is a secreted inhibitor of the Wnt/β-catenin signaling pathway which is normally expressed by osteocytes, terminally differentiated osteoblasts embedded within the bone matrix. Several recent reports have implicated MM cell sclerostin production as a potential inhibitor of osteoblast activity in MM [39, 40] and demonstrated that circulating sclerostin levels correlate with MM bone disease progression and biochemical markers of bone turnover in humans [41]. Antibodies directed against sclerostin are currently under evaluation for the treatment of human osteoporosis, and encouraging results may stimulate future efforts to assess sclerostin inhibition in other diseases which impact bone including myeloma.

Gfi1

As noted previously, a perplexing aspect of MM bone disease is that even in patients able to achieve a complete remission through chemotherapy, osteolytic lesions do not heal due to continued suppression of osteoblast activity. Insight into this phenomenon has come from the recent discovery that levels of Gfi1, a transcriptional repressor of the *Runx2* master osteoblast gene, are increased in bone marrow stromal cells isolated from patients with MM, and that MM cell induction of Gfi1 in stromal cells potently suppresses osteoblast differentiation [42]. Further studies using a histone deacetylase class I/II inhibitor suggested that Gfi1 may induce epigenetic changes in the *Runx2* gene [42], a result which may explain the irreversible suppression of osteoblast differentiation that occurs in myeloma.

Additional Molecules Involved in Osteoblast Suppression in Myeloma

In addition to DKK1 and the more recently recognized sclerostin, several other molecules with potentially important roles in MM bone disease-associated osteoblast inhibition have been described. These include adiponectin [43], hepatocyte growth factor [44], interleukin-7 (IL-7) [45], activin A [46, 47], and transforming growth factor-β [48]. Again, a more complete discussion of these molecules and their potential roles in the osteoblast suppression seen in MM is beyond the scope of the current chapter; as such, the reader is referred to the referenced publications.

Finally, it is notable that several studies suggest that several agents recently approved for the treatment of MM may also affect bone cell function. Thus, it has been suggested that the immunomodulatory drug lenalidomide may inhibit osteoclast function [49], while members of the proteasome inhibitor class of compounds may both increase osteoblast differentiation [50] and activity and suppress osteoclast function [51–53]. Accordingly, it will be important that future studies that assess therapies for MM bone disease be evaluated in the context of these potentially bone-active molecules now widely used in the treatment of MM.

Skeletal Imaging

Myeloma bone disease reflects both generalized bone loss leading to osteopenia or osteoporosis, and the more well-recognized complication of localized osteolytic destruction. Indeed, the identification of osteolytic lesions serves as one criterion for MM diagnosis. For these reasons, skeletal imaging is an essential component in the evaluation of any patient either suspected or confirmed to have MM.

Since bone scans assess osteoblast-mediated new bone formation by osteoblasts, and osteoblast activity is severely suppressed in MM, standard bone scans often underestimate the extent of bone disease in patients with MM and thus have little clinical utility for either the initial evaluation or the provision of longitudinal care [54]. Thus as detailed in guidelines developed by the International Myeloma Working Group, a metastatic skeletal survey with plain radiographs is recommended as the imaging test of choice at diagnosis; surveys should include all potential areas of myeloma involvement including the entire spine, skull, chest, pelvis, humeri, and femora [55]. However, it should be noted that plain radiographs do have significant limitations. These include the ability to detect osteolytic lesions only following loss of ≥30 % of trabecular bone, and an inability to differentiate between malignant and nonmalignant etiologies (for example, corticosteroid-associated or senile) of generalized bone loss [56]. Despite these limitations, conventional metastatic bone surveys show some form of skeletal involvement (lytic lesions, fractures, or diffuse bone loss) in approximately 80 % of patients. Sites most commonly affected sites are those with active hematopoiesis such as vertebral bodies, ribs, skull, shoulders, pelvis, and proximal humeri and femora. The IMWG guidelines recommend that even in the absence of patient-identified skeletal symptoms, radiographic presence of osteolytic lesions shifts patients to a "symptomatic" categorization and warrants the initiation of MM therapy [55].

Although the majority of skeletal lesions are identifiable by plain radiographs, approximately 10–20 % of patients with complete skeletal surveys do not reveal any evidence of skeletal disease [57]. Thus particularly in patients in whom bone pain is present but corresponding skeletal lesions are not present by standard skeletal survey, the use of alternative imaging methods such as magnetic resonance imaging (MRI) can be very helpful for the detection of bone involvement.

MRI can permit detection of both diffuse and focal bone marrow infiltration prior to the presence of osteolytic lesions found by standard skeletal survey and has been demonstrated to detect focal lesions in the spine, pelvis, and sternum at a higher frequency than that of plain radiographs [58]. Notably, however, the same study also demonstrated that standard metastatic bone surveys could detect some focal lesions (particularly in the ribs and proximal long bones) at a higher frequency than found by MRI. Accordingly, the routine use of MRI to evaluate for skeletal involvement in subjects with myeloma is not justified at present. However, MRI is recommended in patients with apparent solitary plasmacytoma, who should receive an MRI of the entire spine in addition to a standard skeletal survey [55]. In addition, MRI is the recommended method to evaluate suspected spinal cord and/or nerve compression, although computed tomography (CT) can be used for this indication when MRI is unavailable. Positron emission tomography with CT (PET-CT) has also been studied in myeloma. Although PET-CT provides complementary information to MRI, its utility for the evaluation of MM bone disease requires further study prior to its consideration for routine use in myeloma [59].

Treatment of Myeloma Bone Disease

Due to the significant impact of SREs on quality of life and overall survival in patients with MM, careful assessment for bone disease must be continually undertaken in all patients with myeloma. For patients with established skeletal disease, incident or impending fractures, or spinal cord compression, appropriate care is necessary to limit the risk for future complications. While intravenous bisphosphonate therapy remains the cornerstone of current therapies, other approaches including vertebroplasty and kyphoplasty, radiation therapy, or orthopedic or neurosurgical intervention are all important adjuncts which may be necessary to provide optimal patient care.

Vertebroplasty and Kyphoplasty

Both vertebroplasty and balloon kyphoplasty have been evaluated in patients with myeloma. Available data from relatively small, largely retrospective studies suggests that both techniques can provide clinically significant improvements in pain, patient performance status, and mobility [60, 61]. In perhaps the best study available, which involved 134 patients randomized to kyphoplasty or nonsurgical management for the treatment of vertebral compression fractures from solid tumor bone metastases or MM, kyphoplasty was associated with significant improvements in pain, physical function, quality of life, and activities of daily living performance [62]. Although limited safety data exists for the treatment of myeloma-associated vertebral compression fractures, one study did show that when compared to vertebroplasty, kyphoplasty was associated with a slightly reduced risk for cement extravasation [63].

Radiation Therapy

As a primary therapeutic modality, radiation therapy has proven benefit for provision of pain relief and improvement in neurologic symptoms, particularly in the setting of impending spinal cord compression [64]. Dosing should be restricted to the field of therapy in order to spare bone marrow function. In a large retrospective case series, radiation therapy was able to improve motor function in 75 % of subjects with spinal cord compression due to MM, with 1-year control at the site of irradiation of 100 % and survival of 94 % [65].

Surgical Intervention

Surgical intervention is primarily reserved for prevention or repair of proximal appendicular fractures or unstable vertebral fractures. It is also occasionally used in patients with spinal cord compression, in whom radiation therapy is more common as first-line therapy. Surgical treatment is generally palliative and is typically performed in conjunction with other approaches aimed at limiting tumor burden (chemotherapy) and fracture risk (intravenous bisphosphonates) [66].

Bisphosphonate Therapy

The primary clinical approach to limit skeletal-related complications in patients with MM involves the use of bisphosphonates, chemically stable derivatives of inorganic pyrophosphate which due to their affinity for the major constituent of bone (hydroxyapatite), achieve high local concentrations at sites of active osteoclast-mediated bone resorption. Infused bisphosphonate which does not adhere to the skeleton is rapidly cleared from the circulation via renal elimination. Skeletal retention reflects both host factors, including the prevalent rate of bone turnover (which determines binding site availability) and renal function (which determines clearance of unbound bisphosphonate), and bisphosphonate potency for bone matrix [67, 68].

Three bisphosphonates (clodronate, pamidronate, and zoledronic acid) are approved worldwide for the treatment of MM bone disease, although clodronate is not approved in the United States. The oral bisphosphonate clodronate differs from the later-generation intravenous bisphosphonates pamidronate and zoledronate in two important ways. First, oral bisphosphonate absorption is only approximately 1 % compared to 100 % for intravenous bisphosphonate preparations; secondly, clodronate lacks the nitrogen-containing side chain found on both pamidronate and zoledronate, the absence of which significantly limits the ability of clodronate to inhibit osteoclast function [69]. Although the precise biological half-lives of the different nitrogen-containing bisphosphonates in bone remain unknown, they are estimated to be at least several years [70]. Despite bisphosphonate treatment, however, roughly 50 % of myeloma patients experience a skeletal-related complication at disease relapse [71].

Well-performed clinical trials have demonstrated that pamidronate and zoledronate are equally efficacious at limiting SREs and pain in patients with MM [72], and either may be considered as first-line therapy. When compared to placebo, the administration of intravenous pamidronate to patients with myeloma affected by at least one osteolytic lesion significantly diminished SREs (24 % vs. 41 %) and bone pain [73]. A recent double-blind, randomized phase 3 trial assessed reduced monthly pamidronate dosing (30 mg vs. 90 mg) in MM patients initiating treatment, nearly 90 % of whom had skeletal involvement at randomization [74]. Notably, lower dose monthly pamidronate demonstrated comparable time to first SRE, comparable SRE-free survival, comparable overall survival, and comparable progression-free survival. Further, there was a trend in subjects who received the lower pamidronate dose towards reduced risks for developing avascular osteonecrosis of the jaw (ONJ) or renal toxicity.

Recent results from the Medical Research Council Myeloma IX randomized trial, in which patients with newly diagnosed MM were randomized to receive either daily oral clodronate or intravenous zoledronic acid every 3–4 weeks in the setting of additional chemotherapy, have provided additional evidence supporting the role of intravenous bisphosphonates relative to oral bisphosphonate therapy [75]. As expected based on the marked differences in bioavailability and potency for osteoclast inhibition noted above, zoledronic acid treatment reduced the proportion of patients who developed an SRE (27 % vs. 35 %) compared to clodronate, consistent with other work demonstrating the importance of early intravenous bisphosphonate therapy in SRE prevention [76]. Intriguingly, zoledronate also reduced mortality by 16 %, increased overall survival by 5.5 months, and provided slight improvement in median progression-free survival by 2 months. Notably, zoledronate treatment was associated with a higher rate of ONJ (4 %) vs. clodronate (<1 %). Interestingly, most of the survival benefit with zoledronate occurred within the first 4 months of therapy. Although an etiology for this early survival difference is unclear, the substantial differences in bioavailability and potency for osteoclast inhibition are likely significant factors. Importantly, however, the study did not include a pamidronate comparator group; thus whether pamidronate would have provided similar survival benefit is unclear. Notably, secondary trial analyses also demonstrated that compared to clodronate treatment, zoledronate infusion was associated with a lower risk for SRE development in MM patients without bone lesions at baseline [77].

Both the optimal frequency and duration of IV bisphosphonate dosing remain subjects of debate. Based on published trial data, monthly dosing is appropriate for most patients with active myeloma, at least initially, to limit SRE risk. Due to the increased incidence of ONJ which occurs with increased cumulative dose and duration of intravenous bisphosphonate therapy [78], reduced bisphosphonate dosing frequency or discontinuation may be appropriate after 2 years in patients who have achieved a therapeutic CR. Continuation beyond 2 years (at a reduced dose or longer dosing interval) is largely at the discretion of the provider in careful consultation with the patient, but may be appropriate in patients who have achieved less than a CR, and in those patients with myeloma recurrence. Until such data are available to provide guidance, a cautious approach to bisphosphonate therapy beyond 2 years appears prudent.

Complications Associated with Bisphosphonate Use in MM

Bisphosphonate therapy is not without risk, as MM patients treated with intravenous bisphosphonates have the highest incidence of ONJ among all groups of patients with malignancies receiving bisphosphonate therapy [79, 80]. While estimates of ONJ related to oral bisphosphonate therapy for osteoporosis are approximately 1/10,000 to 1/100,000 patient treatment years [80], ONJ incidence in oncology patients (and in particular patients with MM) has approached 10 % in some case series. Identified factors which increase the risk for ONJ development include poor oral hygiene, invasive dental procedures or denture use, and prolonged exposure to high doses of intravenous bisphosphonates [81]. Whether concomitant chemotherapy or glucocorticoid use increases the risk for ONJ is unclear, but has been suggested [82].

Current recommendations for the treatment of ONJ are primarily supportive, and include the use of antiseptic oral rinses, antibiotics, and only occasionally limited surgical debridement in affected patients [83]. The performance of a careful oral examination to detect active or anticipated dental issues, counseling patients on the importance of maintaining good oral hygiene, and continuing with routine dental care after bisphosphonate initiation are also important correlates to limit the risk for ONJ development. Dosing schedule reductions appear to decrease ONJ incidence in MM and may be appropriate for many patients (see previous section on treatment with bisphosphonates) [74, 84]. In addition, a recent retrospective study suggested that antibiotic prophylaxis prior to invasive dental procedures can also limit ONJ incidence in patients with MM receiving intravenous bisphosphonate therapy [85]. Additional prospective studies, however, are required to validate this provocative finding. Finally, a report describing the potential role for biochemical markers of bone formation and resorption has recently been published [86]. Although trials are underway to assess the use of bone turnover markers in guiding bisphosphonate dosing in MM, their routine measurement is not currently recommended outside of clinical trials.

More recently, an association between prolonged bisphosphonate use and increased risk for atypical fractures has been recognized [87]. Although the etiology of these atypical fractures is unclear, currently available data suggests that bisphosphonate-mediated oversuppression of the normal bone remodeling process is a likely contributing factor. Both atypical subtrochanteric femoral fractures [88, 89] and metatarsal stress fractures [90] have been described in patients with MM receiving intravenous bisphosphonate therapy. Though first described in patients receiving prolonged bisphosphonate therapy for osteoporosis [91], clinical features of these fractures appear consistent across disease entities. Salient features for atypical femoral fractures include

(1) fracture location within the subtrochanteric region or femoral shaft; (2) transverse or short oblique orientation; (3) minimal or no associated trauma; (4) presence of a medial spike on fracture completion; and (5) absence of comminution [87]. Importantly, plain radiographic imaging obtained prior to fracture may show thickened cortices and the presence of a localized cortical stress reaction, which may also be present in the contralateral femur. Prodromal thigh pain, discomfort, or subjective weakness at the site of subsequent fracture is also frequently present [92].

Additional potential complications associated with bisphosphonate use which are substantially more common but less widely appreciated are hypocalcemia and acute phase reactions, both of which occur much more commonly following intravenous bisphosphonate infusion [93]. As will be described below, it is important that all patients who receive bisphosphonate therapy have adequate calcium and vitamin D intake to limit their risk for hypocalcemia. Acute phase reactions are idiosyncratic and thought to reflect the activation of $\gamma\delta$T cells; reactions usually last 24–72 h and are characterized by fever, myalgias, and arthralgias. Clinical trials suggest that roughly one in three patients receiving intravenous zoledronic acid experiences such a reaction associated with the first infusion, with the incidence declining progressively with subsequent infusions. Treatment with acetaminophen may ameliorate symptoms, which otherwise resolve spontaneously. Such reactions do not preclude future bisphosphonate therapy.

Supportive Care in Myeloma Bone Disease

As noted previously, in addition to the well-recognized focal osteolytic lesions, patients with myeloma also incur more generalized bone loss due to the significant imbalance which occurs in the normal bone remodeling process. This imbalance leads to significant increases in the risk for osteoporotic-type fractures, risks which are in addition to the already well-recognized pathologic fractures risk.

Thus after treatment of any hypercalcemia initially present, additional efforts to optimize general skeletal health should be undertaken in all patients. These include ensuring adequate intake of both vitamin D (approximately 1,000 IU daily) and calcium (1,200–1,500 mg total daily intake, including all dietary and supplemental sources). Finally, it is important to counsel all patients with MM on the importance of maintaining (as tolerated) an active lifestyle in order to maintain skeletal and muscular strength. Recommend activities should be those which provide skeletal and muscle loading, such as daily walking. Patients should be counseled on the importance of limiting their risks for falls, as well as for limiting activities which require a significant lifting or torsional (twisting) component.

Summary

Symptoms directly related to bone disease frequently precipitate the diagnosis of multiple myeloma. Myeloma bone disease imposes a tremendous burden of morbidity throughout the disease course and increases mortality risk. With continued improvements in chemotherapeutic approaches, life expectancy for many patients following MM diagnosis has significantly increased. As such, efforts to provide optimal skeletal health are paramount to optimizing patient quality of life. Multiple factors dysregulated in MM bone disease have been identified. These include molecules which lead to increases in osteoclast activity such as RANKL and MIP-1α, and others which are involved in suppression of osteoblast activity such as DKK1 and Gfi1. To limit progressive skeletal disability in patients with radiographically evident skeletal disease, treatment with intravenous bisphosphonate therapy remains the current standard of care, although complications such as ONJ and atypical fractures have been observed particularly with prolonged bisphosphonate use. The recent inclusion of novel chemotherapeutic agents including IMiDs and proteasomal inhibitors, which may also affect bone cell function, may lead to improvements in MM bone disease treatments.

Vertebral augmentation, radiotherapy, or surgical interventions are additional potential therapies in appropriately selected patients. Continued efforts to develop novel strategies to improve skeletal-related outcomes are necessary if we are to limit the skeletal morbidity synonymous with myeloma bone disease.

References

1. Roodman GD. Mechanisms of bone metastasis. N Engl J Med. 2004;350:1655–64.
2. Siegel R, Naishadham D, Jemal A. Cancer statistics, 2012. CA Cancer J Clin. 2012;62:10–29.
3. Kumar SK, Lee JH, Lahuerta JJ, Morgan G, Richardson PG, Crowley J, et al. Risk of progression and survival in multiple myeloma relapsing after therapy with imids and bortezomib: a multicenter international myeloma working group study. Leukemia. 2012;26:149–57.
4. Kumar SK, Rajkumar SV, Dispenzieri A, Lacy MQ, Hayman SR, Buadi FK, et al. Improved survival in multiple myeloma and the impact of novel therapies. Blood. 2008;111:2516–20.
5. Kyle RA, Rajkumar SV. Multiple myeloma. N Engl J Med. 2004;351:1860–73.
6. Melton 3rd LJ, Kyle RA, Achenbach SJ, Oberg AL, Rajkumar SV. Fracture risk with multiple myeloma: a population-based study. J Bone Miner Res. 2005; 20:487–93.
7. Kyle RA, Gertz MA, Witzig TE, Lust JA, Lacy MQ, Dispenzieri A, et al. Review of 1027 patients with newly diagnosed multiple myeloma. Mayo Clin Proc. 2003;78:21–33.
8. Roodman GD. Pathogenesis of myeloma bone disease. J Cell Biochem. 2010;109:283–91.
9. Bataille R, Chappard D, Marcelli C, Dessauw P, Baldet P, Sany J, et al. Recruitment of new osteoblasts and osteoclasts is the earliest critical event in the pathogenesis of human multiple myeloma. J Clin Invest. 1991;88:62–6.
10. Saad F, Lipton A, Cook R, Chen YM, Smith M, Coleman R. Pathologic fractures correlate with reduced survival in patients with malignant bone disease. Cancer. 2007;110:1860–7.
11. Kyle RA, Therneau TM, Rajkumar SV, Larson DR, Plevak MF, Melton 3rd LJ. Incidence of multiple myeloma in Olmsted county, Minnesota: trend over 6 decades. Cancer. 2004;101:2667–74.
12. Berenson JR. Myeloma bone disease. Best Pract Res Clin Haematol. 2005;18:653–72.
13. Wahlin A, Holm J, Osterman G, Norberg B. Evaluation of serial bone x-ray examination in multiple myeloma. Acta Med Scand. 1982;212:385–7.
14. Mundy GR. Mechanisms of bone metastasis. Cancer. 1997;80:1546–56.
15. Josse RG, Murray TM, Mundy GR, Jez D, Heersche JN. Observations on the mechanism of bone resorption induced by multiple myeloma marrow culture fluids and partially purified osteoclast-activating factor. J Clin Invest. 1981;67:1472–81.
16. Sezer O, Heider U, Jakob C, Zavrski I, Eucker J, Possinger K, et al. Immunocytochemistry reveals RANKL expression of myeloma cells. Blood. 2002;99:4646–7. author reply 4647.
17. Mori Y, Shimizu N, Dallas M, Niewolna M, Story B, Williams PJ, et al. Anti-alpha4 integrin antibody suppresses the development of multiple myeloma and associated osteoclastic osteolysis. Blood. 2004;104: 2149–54.
18. Tat SK, Padrines M, Theoleyre S, Couillaud-Battaglia S, Heymann D, Redini F, et al. Opg/membranous–rankl complex is internalized via the clathrin pathway before a lysosomal and a proteasomal degradation. Bone. 2006;39:706–15.
19. Giuliani N, Bataille R, Mancini C, Lazzaretti M, Barille S. Myeloma cells induce imbalance in the osteoprotegerin/osteoprotegerin ligand system in the human bone marrow environment. Blood. 2001;98:3527–33.
20. Vij R, Horvath N, Spencer A, Taylor K, Vadhan-Raj S, Vescio R, et al. An open-label, phase 2 trial of denosumab in the treatment of relapsed or plateau-phase multiple myeloma. Am J Hematol. 2009;84:650–6.
21. Henry DH, Costa L, Goldwasser F, Hirsh V, Hungria V, Prausova J, et al. Randomized, double-blind study of denosumab versus zoledronic acid in the treatment of bone metastases in patients with advanced cancer (excluding breast and prostate cancer) or multiple myeloma. J Clin Oncol. 2011;29:1125–32.
22. Terpos E, Politou M, Szydlo R, Goldman JM, Apperley JF, Rahemtulla A. Serum levels of macrophage inflammatory protein-1 alpha (mip-1alpha) correlate with the extent of bone disease and survival in patients with multiple myeloma. Br J Haematol. 2003;123:106–9.
23. Ng AC, Khosla S, Charatcharoenwitthaya N, Kumar SK, Achenbach SJ, Holets MF, et al. Bone microstructural changes revealed by high-resolution peripheral quantitative computed tomography imaging and elevated dkk1 and mip-1alpha levels in patients with mgus. Blood. 2011;118:6529–34.
24. Vallet S, Raje N, Ishitsuka K, Hideshima T, Podar K, Chhetri S, et al. Mln3897, a novel ccr1 inhibitor, impairs osteoclastogenesis and inhibits the interaction of multiple myeloma cells and osteoclasts. Blood. 2007;110:3744–52.
25. Dairaghi DJ, Oyajobi BO, Gupta A, McCluskey B, Miao S, Powers JP, et al. Ccr1 blockade reduces tumor burden and osteolysis in vivo in a mouse model of myeloma bone disease. Blood. 2012;120:1449–57.
26. Sebag M. Ccr1 blockade and myeloma bone disease. Blood. 2012;120:1351–2.
27. Hideshima T, Chauhan D, Schlossman R, Richardson P, Anderson KC. The role of tumor necrosis factor alpha in the pathophysiology of human multiple myeloma: therapeutic applications. Oncogene. 2001;20:4519–27.

28. Lee JW, Chung HY, Ehrlich LA, Jelinek DF, Callander NS, Roodman GD, et al. Il-3 expression by myeloma cells increases both osteoclast formation and growth of myeloma cells. Blood. 2004;103:2308–15.
29. Tamura T, Udagawa N, Takahashi N, Miyaura C, Tanaka S, Yamada Y, et al. Soluble interleukin-6 receptor triggers osteoclast formation by interleukin 6. Proc Natl Acad Sci U S A. 1993;90:11924–8.
30. Pennisi A, Ling W, Li X, Khan S, Shaughnessy Jr JD, Barlogie B, et al. The ephrinb2/ephb4 axis is dysregulated in osteoprogenitors from myeloma patients and its activation affects myeloma bone disease and tumor growth. Blood. 2009;114:1803–12.
31. Day TF, Guo X, Garrett-Beal L, Yang Y. Wnt/beta-catenin signaling in mesenchymal progenitors controls osteoblast and chondrocyte differentiation during vertebrate skeletogenesis. Dev Cell. 2005;8:739–50.
32. Fowler JA, Mundy GR, Lwin ST, Edwards CM. Bone marrow stromal cells create a permissive microenvironment for myeloma development: a new stromal role for wnt inhibitor dkk1. Cancer Res. 2012;72:2183–9.
33. Tian E, Zhan F, Walker R, Rasmussen E, Ma Y, Barlogie B, et al. The role of the wnt-signaling antagonist dkk1 in the development of osteolytic lesions in multiple myeloma. N Engl J Med. 2003;349:2483–94.
34. Kaiser M, Mieth M, Liebisch P, Oberlander R, Rademacher J, Jakob C, et al. Serum concentrations of dkk-1 correlate with the extent of bone disease in patients with multiple myeloma. Eur J Haematol. 2008;80:490–4.
35. Heider U, Kaiser M, Mieth M, Lamottke B, Rademacher J, Jakob C, et al. Serum concentrations of dkk-1 decrease in patients with multiple myeloma responding to anti-myeloma treatment. Eur J Haematol. 2009;82:31–8.
36. Yaccoby S, Ling W, Zhan F, Walker R, Barlogie B, Shaughnessy Jr JD. Antibody-based inhibition of dkk1 suppresses tumor-induced bone resorption and multiple myeloma growth in vivo. Blood. 2007; 109:2106–11.
37. Heath DJ, Chantry AD, Buckle CH, Coulton L, Shaughnessy Jr JD, Evans HR, et al. Inhibiting dickkopf-1 (dkk1) removes suppression of bone formation and prevents the development of osteolytic bone disease in multiple myeloma. J Bone Miner Res. 2009;24:425–36.
38. Edwards CM, Edwards JR, Lwin ST, Esparza J, Oyajobi BO, McCluskey B, et al. Increasing wnt signaling in the bone marrow microenvironment inhibits the development of myeloma bone disease and reduces tumor burden in bone in vivo. Blood. 2008;111:2833–42.
39. Brunetti G, Oranger A, Mori G, Specchia G, Rinaldi E, Curci P, et al. Sclerostin is overexpressed by plasma cells from multiple myeloma patients. Ann N Y Acad Sci. 2011;1237:19–23.
40. Colucci S, Brunetti G, Oranger A, Mori G, Sardone F, Specchia G, et al. Myeloma cells suppress osteoblasts through sclerostin secretion. Blood Cancer J. 2011; 1:e27.
41. Terpos E, Christoulas D, Katodritou E, Bratengeier C, Gkotzamanidou M, Michalis E, et al. Elevated circulating sclerostin correlates with advanced disease features and abnormal bone remodeling in symptomatic myeloma: reduction post-bortezomib monotherapy. Int J Cancer. 2012;131:1466–71.
42. D'Souza S, del Prete D, Jin S, Sun Q, Huston AJ, Kostov FE, et al. Gfi1 expressed in bone marrow stromal cells is a novel osteoblast suppressor in patients with multiple myeloma bone disease. Blood. 2011; 118:6871–80.
43. Fowler JA, Lwin ST, Drake MT, Edwards JR, Kyle RA, Mundy GR, et al. Host-derived adiponectin is tumor-suppressive and a novel therapeutic target for multiple myeloma and the associated bone disease. Blood. 2011;118:5872–82.
44. Standal T, Abildgaard N, Fagerli UM, Stordal B, Hjertner O, Borset M, et al. Hgf inhibits bmp-induced osteoblastogenesis: possible implications for the bone disease of multiple myeloma. Blood. 2007;109:3024–30.
45. Giuliani N, Colla S, Morandi F, Lazzaretti M, Sala R, Bonomini S, et al. Myeloma cells block runx2/cbfa1 activity in human bone marrow osteoblast progenitors and inhibit osteoblast formation and differentiation. Blood. 2005;106:2472–83.
46. Chantry AD, Heath D, Mulivor AW, Pearsall S, Baud'huin M, Coulton L, et al. Inhibiting activin-a signaling stimulates bone formation and prevents cancer-induced bone destruction in vivo. J Bone Miner Res. 2010;25:2633–46.
47. Terpos E, Kastritis E, Christoulas D, Gkotzamanidou M, Eleutherakis-Papaiakovou E, Kanellias N, et al. Circulating activin-a is elevated in patients with advanced multiple myeloma and correlates with extensive bone involvement and inferior survival; no alterations post-lenalidomide and dexamethasone therapy. Ann Oncol. 2012;23:2681–6.
48. Takeuchi K, Abe M, Hiasa M, Oda A, Amou H, Kido S, et al. Tgf-beta inhibition restores terminal osteoblast differentiation to suppress myeloma growth. PLoS One. 2010;5:e9870.
49. Breitkreutz I, Raab MS, Vallet S, Hideshima T, Raje N, Mitsiades C, et al. Lenalidomide inhibits osteoclastogenesis, survival factors and bone-remodeling markers in multiple myeloma. Leukemia. 2008;22: 1925–32.
50. Delforge M, Terpos E, Richardson PG, Shpilberg O, Khuageva NK, Schlag R, et al. Fewer bone disease events, improvement in bone remodeling, and evidence of bone healing with bortezomib plus melphalan-prednisone vs. melphalan-prednisone in the phase iii vista trial in multiple myeloma. Eur J Haematol. 2011;86:372–84.
51. Giuliani N, Morandi F, Tagliaferri S, Lazzaretti M, Bonomini S, Crugnola M, et al. The proteasome inhibitor bortezomib affects osteoblast differentiation in vitro and in vivo in multiple myeloma patients. Blood. 2007;110:334–8.
52. Boissy P, Andersen TL, Lund T, Kupisiewicz K, Plesner T, Delaisse JM. Pulse treatment with the

proteasome inhibitor bortezomib inhibits osteoclast resorptive activity in clinically relevant conditions. Leuk Res. 2008;32:1661–8.
53. Hurchla MA, Garcia-Gomez A, Hornick MC, Ocio EM, Li A, Blanco JF, et al. The epoxyketone-based proteasome inhibitors carfilzomib and orally bioavailable oprozomib have anti-resorptive and bone-anabolic activity in addition to anti-myeloma effects. Leukemia. 2013;27:430–40.
54. Mileshkin L, Blum R, Seymour JF, Patrikeos A, Hicks RJ, Prince HM. A comparison of fluorine-18 fluoro-deoxyglucose pet and technetium-99m sestamibi in assessing patients with multiple myeloma. Eur J Haematol. 2004;72:32–7.
55. Dimopoulos M, Terpos E, Comenzo RL, Tosi P, Beksac M, Sezer O, et al. International myeloma working group consensus statement and guidelines regarding the current role of imaging techniques in the diagnosis and monitoring of multiple myeloma. Leukemia. 2009;23:1545–56.
56. Edelstyn GA, Gillespie PJ, Grebbell FS. The radiological demonstration of osseous metastases. Experimental observations. Clin Radiol. 1967;18:158–62.
57. Collins CD. Multiple myeloma. Cancer Imaging. 2004;4:S47–53.
58. Walker R, Barlogie B, Haessler J, Tricot G, Anaissie E, Shaughnessy Jr JD, et al. Magnetic resonance imaging in multiple myeloma: diagnostic and clinical implications. J Clin Oncol. 2007;25:1121–8.
59. Terpos E, Moulopoulos LA, Dimopoulos MA. Advances in imaging and the management of myeloma bone disease. J Clin Oncol. 2011;29:1907–15.
60. Garland P, Gishen P, Rahemtulla A. Percutaneous vertebroplasty to treat painful myelomatous vertebral deposits-long-term efficacy outcomes. Ann Hematol. 2011;90:95–100.
61. Anselmetti GC, Manca A, Montemurro F, Hirsch J, Chiara G, Grignani G, et al. Percutaneous vertebroplasty in multiple myeloma: Prospective long-term follow-up in 106 consecutive patients. Cardiovasc Intervent Radiol. 2012;35:139–45.
62. Berenson J, Pflugmacher R, Jarzem P, Zonder J, Schechtman K, Tillman JB, et al. Balloon kyphoplasty versus non-surgical fracture management for treatment of painful vertebral body compression fractures in patients with cancer: a multicentre, randomised controlled trial. Lancet Oncol. 2011;12:225–35.
63. La Maida GA, Giarratana LS, Acerbi A, Ferrari V, Mineo GV, Misaggi B. Cement leakage: safety of minimally invasive surgical techniques in the treatment of multiple myeloma vertebral lesions. Eur Spine J. 2012;21 Suppl 1:S61–8.
64. Balducci M, Chiesa S, Manfrida S, Rossi E, Za T, Frascino V, et al. Impact of radiotherapy on pain relief and recalcification in plasma cell neoplasms: long-term experience. Strahlenther Onkol. 2011;187:114–9.
65. Rades D, Veninga T, Stalpers LJ, Basic H, Rudat V, Karstens JH, et al. Outcome after radiotherapy alone for metastatic spinal cord compression in patients with oligometastases. J Clin Oncol. 2007;25:50–6.
66. Utzschneider S, Schmidt H, Weber P, Schmidt GP, Jansson V, Durr HR. Surgical therapy of skeletal complications in multiple myeloma. Int Orthop. 2011;35:1209–13.
67. Cremers SC, Pillai G, Papapoulos SE. Pharmacokinetics/pharmacodynamics of bisphosphonates: use for optimisation of intermittent therapy for osteoporosis. Clin Pharmacokinet. 2005;44:551–70.
68. Drake MT, Clarke BL, Khosla S. Bisphosphonates: mechanism of action and role in clinical practice. Mayo Clin Proc. 2008;83:1032–45.
69. Drake MT, Cremers SC. Bisphosphonate therapeutics in bone disease: the hard and soft data on osteoclast inhibition. Mol Interv. 2010;10:141–52.
70. Khan SA, Kanis JA, Vasikaran S, Kline WF, Matuszewski BK, McCloskey EV, et al. Elimination and biochemical responses to intravenous alendronate in postmenopausal osteoporosis. J Bone Miner Res. 1997;12:1700–7.
71. Lenhoff S, Hjorth M, Turesson I, Westin J, Gimsing P, Wisloff F, et al. Intensive therapy for multiple myeloma in patients younger than 60 years. Long-term results focusing on the effect of the degree of response on survival and relapse pattern after transplantation. Haematologica. 2006;91:1228–33.
72. Rosen LS, Gordon D, Kaminski M, Howell A, Belch A, Mackey J, et al. Long-term efficacy and safety of zoledronic acid compared with pamidronate disodium in the treatment of skeletal complications in patients with advanced multiple myeloma or breast carcinoma: a randomized, double-blind, multicenter, comparative trial. Cancer. 2003;98:1735–44.
73. Berenson JR, Lichtenstein A, Porter L, Dimopoulos MA, Bordoni R, George S, et al. Efficacy of pamidronate in reducing skeletal events in patients with advanced multiple myeloma. Myeloma aredia study group. N Engl J Med. 1996;334:488–93.
74. Gimsing P, Carlson K, Turesson I, Fayers P, Waage A, Vangsted A, et al. Effect of pamidronate 30 mg versus 90 mg on physical function in patients with newly diagnosed multiple myeloma (nordic myeloma study group): a double-blind, randomised controlled trial. Lancet Oncol. 2010;11:973–82.
75. Morgan GJ, Davies FE, Gregory WM, Cocks K, Bell SE, Szubert AJ, et al. First-line treatment with zoledronic acid as compared with clodronic acid in multiple myeloma (mrc myeloma ix): a randomised controlled trial. Lancet. 2010;376:1989–99.
76. Wu EQ, Bensimon AG, Marynchenko M, Namjoshi M, Guo A, Yu AP, et al. Comparison of skeletal complications and treatment patterns associated with early vs. delayed zoledronic acid therapy in multiple myeloma. Clin Lymphoma Myeloma Leuk. 2011;11:326–35.
77. Morgan GJ, Child JA, Gregory WM, Szubert AJ, Cocks K, Bell SE, et al. Effects of zoledronic acid

versus clodronic acid on skeletal morbidity in patients with newly diagnosed multiple myeloma (mrc myeloma ix): secondary outcomes from a randomised controlled trial. Lancet Oncol. 2011;12:743–52.

78. Zervas K, Verrou E, Teleioudis Z, Vahtsevanos K, Banti A, Mihou D, et al. Incidence, risk factors and management of osteonecrosis of the jaw in patients with multiple myeloma: a single-centre experience in 303 patients. Br J Haematol. 2006;134: 620–3.
79. Dimopoulos MA, Kastritis E, Anagnostopoulos A, Melakopoulos I, Gika D, Moulopoulos LA, et al. Osteonecrosis of the jaw in patients with multiple myeloma treated with bisphosphonates: evidence of increased risk after treatment with zoledronic acid. Haematologica. 2006;91:968–71.
80. Khosla S, Burr D, Cauley J, Dempster DW, Ebeling PR, Felsenberg D, et al. Bisphosphonate-associated osteonecrosis of the jaw: report of a task force of the american society for bone and mineral research. J Bone Miner Res. 2007;22:1479–91.
81. Bamias A, Kastritis E, Bamia C, Moulopoulos LA, Melakopoulos I, Bozas G, et al. Osteonecrosis of the jaw in cancer after treatment with bisphosphonates: incidence and risk factors. J Clin Oncol. 2005;23: 8580–7.
82. Tosi P, Zamagni E, Cangini D, Tacchetti P, Di Raimondo F, Catalano L, et al. Osteonecrosis of the jaws in newly diagnosed multiple myeloma patients treated with zoledronic acid and thalidomide-dexamethasone. Blood. 2006;108:3951–2.
83. Snowden JA, Ahmedzai SH, Ashcroft J, D'Sa S, Littlewood T, Low E, et al. Guidelines for supportive care in multiple myeloma 2011. Br J Haematol. 2011;154:76–103.
84. Corso A, Varettoni M, Zappasodi P, Klersy C, Mangiacavalli S, Pica G, et al. A different schedule of zoledronic acid can reduce the risk of the osteonecrosis of the jaw in patients with multiple myeloma. Leukemia. 2007;21:1545–8.
85. Montefusco V, Gay F, Spina F, Miceli R, Maniezzo M, Teresa Ambrosini M, et al. Antibiotic prophylaxis before dental procedures may reduce the incidence of osteonecrosis of the jaw in patients with multiple myeloma treated with bisphosphonates. Leuk Lymphoma. 2008;49:2156–62.
86. Terpos E, Dimopoulos MA, Sezer O, Roodman D, Abildgaard N, Vescio R, et al. The use of biochemical markers of bone remodeling in multiple myeloma: a report of the international myeloma working group. Leukemia. 2010;24:1700–12.
87. Shane E, Burr D, Ebeling PR, Abrahamsen B, Adler RA, Brown TD, et al. Atypical subtrochanteric and diaphyseal femoral fractures: report of a task force of the american society for bone and mineral research. J Bone Miner Res. 2010;25:2267–94.
88. Puhaindran ME, Farooki A, Steensma MR, Hameed M, Healey JH, Boland PJ. Atypical subtrochanteric femoral fractures in patients with skeletal malignant involvement treated with intravenous bisphosphonates. J Bone Joint Surg Am. 2011;93:1235–42.
89. Chang ST, Tenforde AS, Grimsrud CD, O'Ryan FS, Gonzalez JR, Baer DM, et al. Atypical femur fractures among breast cancer and multiple myeloma patients receiving intravenous bisphosphonate therapy. Bone. 2012;51:524–7.
90. Waterman GN, Yellin O, Jamshidinia K, Swift RA, Tamkin JA, Audell RA, et al. Metatarsal stress fractures in patients with multiple myeloma treated with long-term bisphosphonates: a report of six cases. J Bone Joint Surg Am. 2011;93:e106.
91. Odvina CV, Zerwekh JE, Rao DS, Maalouf N, Gottschalk FA, Pak CY. Severely suppressed bone turnover: a potential complication of alendronate therapy. J Clin Endocrinol Metab. 2005;90:1294–301.
92. Drake MT. Bone disease in multiple myeloma. Oncology (Williston Park). 2009;23:28–32.
93. Kennel KA, Drake MT. Adverse effects of bisphosphonates: implications for osteoporosis management. Mayo Clin Proc. 2009;84:632–7. quiz 638.

18 Vertebral Augmentation

Omar Khan and David Kallmes

Introduction

Treatment of painful vertebral compression fractures by spinal augmentation was first introduced in 1987 when Galibert et al. injected acrylic cement percutaneously into the vertebral column of patients with vertebral angiomas [1]. Since that time, it has gained acceptance around the world as a minimally invasive and effective procedure to alleviate painful spinal lesions after more conservative treatment options such as drugs and supportive care prove inadequate. Its use has been expanded, especially in the last decade, to treatment of fractures resulting from osteoporosis, metastatic cancer, and multiple myeloma.

Vertebroplasty Versus Kyphoplasty

Spinal augmentation encompasses both vertebroplasty and kyphoplasty. Vertebroplasty involves the injection of bone cement (polymethylacrylate or PMMA) directly into the vertebral body via a thin needle [2]. In kyphoplasty, the injection occurs after space is created in the vertebra using an inflatable balloon [3–5]. Although the exact mechanism of action is uncertain, it is thought that the infused bone cement stabilizes the vertebral body and thus reduces nerve root compression [6]. In multiple myeloma, the compression results from vertebral lesions caused by the release of osteoclast-activating factors from abnormal plasma cells, which favors bone resorption [7]. These lesions are unique in that they are a result of malignancy, yet express osteoporotic characteristics. They are present in approximately 55–70 % of myeloma patients and are often the first presenting signs of the disease [8]. The ensuing pain can be extremely debilitating, leading to physical and functional disability along with mental distress.

O.Khan • D. Kallmes, M.D. (✉)
Division of Radiology, Mayo Clinic,
200 First Street, Southwest, Rochester, MN 55905, USA
e-mail: Kallmes.david@mayo.edu

Patient Selection

Spinal augmentation, in its present form, should be considered to be a palliative procedure intended to treat painful fractures that are not adequately treated by other means. The use of spinal augmentation for "impending fractures" remains relatively uncommon, and the vast majority of patients undergoing the procedure have already suffered one or more vertebral fractures. Currently, the relative benefit of spinal augmentation to other measures such as medical therapy or radiation treatment remains poorly studied. In any event, consideration for spinal augmentation should be limited to patients who have not responded to various measures of "optimal medical therapy."

M.A. Gertz and S.V. Rajkumar (eds.), *Multiple Myeloma: Diagnosis and Treatment*,
DOI 10.1007/978-1-4614-8520-9_18, © Mayo Foundation for Medical Education and Research 2014

There are numerous factors to consider when working up patients for spinal augmentation. Patients should manifest subjective pain, typically worse with activity, in the region of known fractures. Careful histories should be obtained to discern potential compressive symptoms for cord or nerve root compression. On physical exam, many practitioners strongly rely on the ability to exacerbate pain when pressing gently over the involved vertebral body or bodies.

Imaging workup always included plain radiographs to document the presence of, severity of, and, in the setting of patients with serial radiographs, whether or not the painful fracture is new or old (Fig. 18.1a). In many cases, especially in patients suffering from multiple myeloma, numerous fractures of varying age are present. Current practice in most centers includes, most commonly, spinal MRI or, in patients with contra indications to MRI, bone scan imaging (Fig. 18.1b, c). These tests are used to assess the "activity" of identified fractures. Most practitioners consider that vertebral fractures that manifest edema on MRI or increased activity on bone scan imaging are good targets for spinal augmentation. However, for unknown reasons, vertebral fractures in the setting of multiple myeloma that may respond to spinal augmentation may not show edema on MRI (Fig. 18.1c). CT imaging is used in selected cases where there is concern for involvement of either the fracture line or a plasmacytoma to involve the posterior wall of the vertebral body. In such cases extreme care is used to avoid dorsal deposition of cement that may leak into the spinal canal.

Appropriate lesions for spinal augmentation in patients with multiple myeloma should exist. Patients with multiple myeloma almost universally suffer from systemic osteoporosis. Many or most vertebral fractures in these patients may be the result of this osteoporosis or from osteoporosis resulting from prior spinal irradiation. However, even if local plasmacytoma is present, spinal augmentation may still provide pain relief.

MRI features of benign fractures in the setting of multiple myeloma include the following (Fig. 18.1b, c): (1) areas of "preserved" bone marrow as evidenced by normal T1-weighted imaging hyperintensity; (2) lack of bowing of the posterior wall of the vertebral body; (3) lack of typical plasmacytoma lesions in the vertebral body; (4) lack of involvement of the pedicles with bone edema; and (5) lack of paraspinal mass lesion. If any of these five features causes concern for local myelomatous involvement, then biopsy of the vertebral body at the time of spinal augmentation is readily performed.

Procedure

Preparing for Spinal Augmentation

Once the level or levels for treatment of vertebroplasty have been identified, patients should be appropriately counseled regarding the risk:benefit ratio for spinal augmentation. Acute and subacute risks include infection, fracture, cement pulmonary embolism, allergic reaction, and nerve root or cord compromise from cement leakage. The chronic risk of new onset fractures, as compared to the "natural history" of incident fractures without spinal augmentation, remains unclear.

Procedural Details

In the vast majority of patients, spinal augmentation can be performed on an outpatient basis using conscious sedation rather than general anesthesia. Typical pre-procedural details include fasting after midnight prior to the procedure, reversal or withholding of anticoagulants, if appropriate, exclusion of coexistent infection if any signs or symptoms of such infection are present, and questions about allergies. The safety of spinal augmentation in patients being treated with dual antiplatelet therapy remains poorly studied. Note that iodinated contrast is not given during vertebroplasty.

Patients are typically treated in an angiography suite or operating room with high quality fluoroscopic equipment. After sterile preparation, local anesthesia is given over the skin, soft tissues, and bone. Needles on the order of 11 or

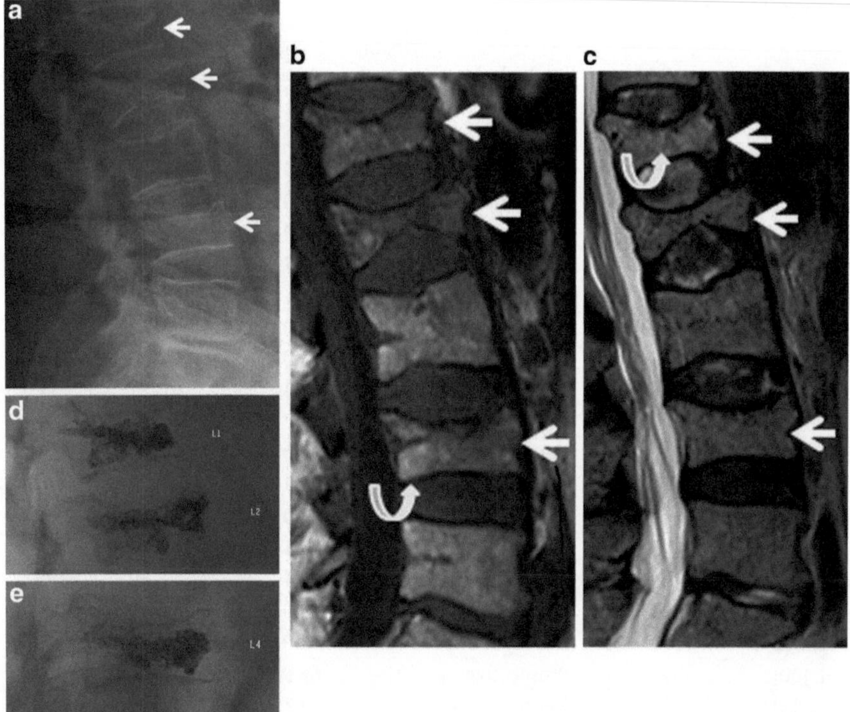

Fig. 18.1 Imaging from a 65-year-old male with multiple myeloma presenting with low back pain. (**a**) Lateral plain radiograph of the lumbar spine. Plain radiograph demonstrates a severe osteopenia. Compression fractures are present at L1, L2, and L4, most severe at L2 (*arrow*). Given plain film findings alone, the chronicity of these fractures is unknown. (**b**) Sagittal T1-weighted MRI image of the lumbar spine. T1-weighted MR demonstrates the fractures noted on the plain radiograph with definite edema in L1, L2, and L4 (*straight arrows*). Notably, there is preserved normal high signal on T1 in the inferoposteral aspect of L4 (*curved arrow*), indicating that this fracture is benign. None of these fractures demonstrate any worrisome features for malignancy, and the T1 findings at L4 are highly suggestive of benignity. (**c**) Sagittal T2 image of lumbar spine. T2-weighted image demonstrates relative lack of T2 hyperintensity, which is typical for myelomatous patients that, for unknown reasons, do not demonstrate substantial edema on T2. There is however some high signal in the L1 vertebral body (*curved arrow*). There is no evidence for epidural extension or for bowing of the posterior wall of vertebral bodies. (**d**) Lateral plain radiograph immediately following L1 and L2 percutaneous vertebroplasty. Note, the barium well-pacified cement filling nearly the entity of both the L1 and L2 vertebral bodies. Note that there is extrusion of cement through the inferior end plate of L2 and partially through the superior end plate of L1. Note also a linear track of cement in L1 that traverses into the L1 pedicle. Each of these findings is typical for successful vertebroplasty and does not indicate adverse event. Indeed, some practitioners believe that cementing the end plate fracture may be a positive prognostic indicator for pain relief. (**e**) Lateral plain radiograph of L4 following percutaneous vertebroplasty demonstrates features similar to that seen above in L1 and L2

13 g are placed into the vertebral body or bodies and barium-opacified cement is infused (Fig. 18.1d, e), either with, in the case of kyphoplasty, or without, in the case of vertebroplasty, the use of cavity creation with a balloon. The infusion needle or needles are removed and band-aids placed over the small incisions. Patients typically are kept on bed rest for 2 h and then discharged.

Current Evidence

Randomized and non-randomized controlled trials in osteoporosis and solid metastatic neoplasms have shown that spinal augmentation consistently reduces pain and improves functional disability [9–12]. Although data from myeloma patients is limited primarily to small

Table 18.1 Study characteristics

#	Authors	SA type	Study design	No. of patients	Average age	Age range	Males	Females
1	Mendoza et al. [13]	Both	Retrospective	79	60.1	30–90	47	32
2	Chen et al. [14]	VP	Retrospective	24	67.0	54–81	4	20
3	Yang et al. [15]	VP	Prospective	38	58.9	54–64	20	18
4	Trumm et al. [16]	VP	Retrospective	39	65.0	58–72	22	17
5	Kasperk et al. [17]	KP	Retrospective	35	58.9	28–90	21	14
6	Basile et al. [18]	VP	Prospective	24	54.7	42–67	11	13
7	Anselmetti et al. [19]	VP	Prospective	106	70.1	35–92	56	50
8	Masala et al. [20]	VP	Retrospective	39	64.0	48–88	17	22
9	Astolfi et al. [21]	KP	Retrospective	30	63.0	54–76	19	11
10	Masala et al. [22]	VP	Retrospective	64	71.4	61–81	34	30
11	McDonald et al. [23]	VP	Retrospective	67	66.2	N/A	N/A	N/A
12	Tran Thang et al. [24]	VP	Retrospective	28	65.0	40–89	17	11
13	Kose et al. [25]	KP	Retrospective	18	63.7	48–82	9	9
13	Kose et al. [25]	VP	Retrospective	16	62.0	65–80	7	9
14	Khanna et al. [26]	KP	Prospective	56	69.4	39–89	N/A	N/A
15	Pflugmacher et al. [27]	KP	Retrospective	20	62.4	52–69	20	0
16	Bosnjakovic et al. [28]	VP	Retrospective	29	68.0	58–79	11	18
17	Huber et al. [29]	KP	Retrospective	76	62.0	28–76	45	31
18	Zou et al. [30]	KP	Prospective	21	65.9	47–81	9	12
19	Julka et al. [31]	KP	Retrospective	32	64.3	44–89	18	14
20	Lane et al. [32]	KP	Prospective	19	60.4	45–74	12	7
21	Garland et al. [33]	VP	Retrospective	26	59.3	42–76	16	10
22	Lim et al. [34]	VP	Retrospective	19	N/A	N/A	N/A	N/A
23	Dudeney et al. [35]	KP	Prospective	18	63.5	48–79	N/A	N/A

SA spinal augmentation, *VP* vertebroplasty, *KP* kyphoplasty, *N/A* not available

experimental case series (Table 18.1), initial studies show similar, promising results in those who have undergone augmentation procedures. One of the largest studies completed to date, performed by Anselmetti et al., included 106 patients who underwent 528 vertebroplasty procedures during a 7-year span. All but five patients had decreased pain and disability. Furthermore, prior to vertebroplasty, 81 patients wore an orthopedic brace and only 11 still needed one after the procedure was administered [19]. Benefits from this study and others are evident both early and late after procedure and appear to be sustained over time (Table 18.2). Vertebroplasty and kyphoplasty show comparable improvement, and there does not appear to be a significant advantage of performing one procedure over the other. Additional favorable outcomes of spinal augmentation presented in the literature include an increase in vertebral height, decrease in patient analgesic use, and a low complication rate due to cement leakage [13–35]. The positive outcomes of vertebroplasty and kyphoplasty have the potential to drastically improve the lives of the myeloma patients. Although there is need for further research, these preliminary studies indicate that spinal augmentation in myeloma patients appears to be palliative and feasible.

Summary

Additional studies are required in order to establish the efficacy of vertebroplasty and kyphoplasty in alleviating pain resulting from myeloma-induced vertebral compression fractures. Specifically, there is a need of larger sample sizes and randomized control trials. Since spinal augmentation with bone cement is a relatively new procedure to treat myeloma patients,

Table 18.2 Pre-procedure and post-procedure data on 10-point pain scales

Authors	Pre-procedure pain	Post-procedure pain (≤1 week)	Post-procedure pain (1 week–1 year)	Post-procedure pain (>1 year)
Mendoza et al. [13]	5.2	3.9	3.9	N/A
Chen et al. [14]	9.0	3.8	3.5	4.7
Yang et al. [15]	9.0	N/A	N/A	3.0
Trumm et al. [16]	6.4	3.9	3.2	N/A
Kasperk et al. [17]	8.1	N/A	3.7	2.3
Basile et al. [18]	N/A	N/A	N/A	N/A
Anselmetti et al. [19]	9.0	1	1.0	1.0
Masala et al. [20]	8.4	2.1	2.4	N/A
Astolfi et al. [21]	8.7	N/A	2.2	3.8
Masala et al. [22]	8.0	N/A	1.9	N/A
McDonald et al. [23]	8.5	3.2	3.2	3.2
Tran Thang et al. [24]	7.5	N/A	N/A	2.1
Kose et al. [25]	3.6	N/A	0.9	1.0
Kose et al. [25]	3.8	N/A	1.2	1.3
Khanna et al. [26]	4.1	N/A	N/A	3.1
Pflugmacher et al. [27]	8.0	2.2	N/A	3.1
Bosnjakovic et al. [28]	7.8	2.3	N/A	N/A
Huber et al. [29]	N/A	N/A	N/A	N/A
Zou et al. [30]	8.1	3.6	3.3	3.4
Julka et al. [31]	N/A	N/A	N/A	N/A
Lane et al. [32]	N/A	N/A	N/A	N/A
Garland et al. [33]	N/A	N/A	N/A	N/A
Lim et al. [34]	8.0	3.23	3.5	5.1
Dudeney et al. [35]	5.5	2.32	2.3	2.3

methodology and technique still need to be refined. There is a need for further investigation to understand the mechanism of action that leads to pain reduction. Additionally, because pain reduction is achieved soon after the procedure and complication rates are low, it may be possible to perform spinal augmentation as a prophylaxis of vertebral bodies that are at risk for fracture [36]. Finally, an effort must be made to increase availability of spinal augmentation to patients with multiple myeloma as a treatment option.

References

1. Galibert P, Deramond H, Rosat P, Le Gars D. Preliminary note on the treatment of vertebral angioma by percutaneous acrylic vertebroplasty. Neurochirurgie. 1987;33(2):166–8. Epub 1987/01/01.
2. Gangi A, Guth S, Imbert JP, Marin H, Dietemann JL. Percutaneous vertebroplasty: indications, technique, and results. Radiographics. 2003;23(2):e10. Epub 2003/08/02.
3. Kasperk C, Hillmeier J, Noldge G, Grafe IA, Dafonseca K, Raupp D, et al. Treatment of painful vertebral fractures by kyphoplasty in patients with primary osteoporosis: a prospective nonrandomized controlled study. J Bone Miner Res. 2005;20(4):604–12. Epub 2005/03/15.
4. Noldge G, DaFonseca K, Grafe I, Libicher M, Hillmeier J, Meeder PJ, et al. Balloon kyphoplasty in the treatment of back pain. Radiologe. 2006; 46(6):506–12. Epub 2006/06/21.
5. Gill JB, Kuper M, Chin PC, Zhang Y, Schutt Jr R. Comparing pain reduction following kyphoplasty and vertebroplasty for osteoporotic vertebral compression fractures. Pain Physician. 2007;10(4):583–90. Epub 2007/07/31.
6. Mathis JM, Barr JD, Belkoff SM, Barr MS, Jensen ME, Deramond H. Percutaneous vertebroplasty: a developing standard of care for vertebral compression fractures. AJNR Am J Neuroradiol. 2001;22(2):373–81. Epub 2001/02/07.
7. Mundy GR, Luben RA, Raisz LG, Oppenheim JJ, Buell DN. Bone-resorbing activity in supernatants from lymphoid cell lines. N Engl J Med. 1974;290(16):867–71. Epub 1974/04/18.
8. Ramos L, de Las Heras JA, Sanchez S, Gonzalez-Porras JR, Gonzalez R, Mateos MV, et al. Medium-term results of percutaneous vertebroplasty in

multiple myeloma. Eur J Haematol. 2006;77(1):7–13. Epub 2006/04/13.
9. Papanastassiou ID, Phillips FM, Van Meirhaeghe J, Berenson JR, Andersson GB, Chung G, et al. Comparing effects of kyphoplasty, vertebroplasty, and non-surgical management in a systematic review of randomized and non-randomized controlled studies. Eur Spine J. 2012;21(9):1826–43. Epub 2012/05/01.
10. Rhyne 3rd A, Banit D, Laxer E, Odum S, Nussman D. Kyphoplasty: report of eighty-two thoracolumbar osteoporotic vertebral fractures. J Orthop Trauma. 2004;18(5):294–9. Epub 2004/04/24.
11. McGirt MJ, Parker SL, Wolinsky JP, Witham TF, Bydon A, Gokaslan ZL. Vertebroplasty and kyphoplasty for the treatment of vertebral compression fractures: an evidenced-based review of the literature. Spine J. 2009;9(6):501–8. Epub 2009/03/03.
12. Han S, Wan S, Ning L, Tong Y, Zhang J, Fan S. Percutaneous vertebroplasty versus balloon kyphoplasty for treatment of osteoporotic vertebral compression fracture: a meta-analysis of randomised and non-randomised controlled trials. Int Orthop. 2011;35(9):1349–58. Epub 2011/06/04.
13. Mendoza TR, Koyyalagunta D, Burton AW, Thomas SK, Phan MH, Giralt SA, et al. Changes in pain and other symptoms in patients with painful multiple myeloma-related vertebral fracture treated with kyphoplasty or vertebroplasty. J Pain. 2012;13(6):564–70. Epub 2012/05/01.
14. Chen LH, Hsieh MK, Niu CC, Fu TS, Lai PL, Chen WJ. Percutaneous vertebroplasty for pathological vertebral compression fractures secondary to multiple myeloma. Arch Orthop Trauma Surg. 2012;132(6):759–64. Epub 2012/02/09.
15. Yang Z, Tan J, Xu Y, Sun H, Xie L, Zhao R, et al. Treatment of MM-associated spinal fracture with percutaneous vertebroplasty (PVP) and chemotherapy. Eur Spine J. 2012;21(5):912–9. Epub 2011/12/17.
16. Trumm C, Jakobs T, Pahl A, Stahl R, Helmberger T, Paprottka P, et al. CT fluoroscopy-guided percutaneous vertebroplasty in patients with multiple myeloma: analysis of technical results from 44 sessions with 67 vertebrae treated. Diagn Interv Radiol. 2012;18(1):111–20. Epub 2011/10/19.
17. Kasperk C, Haas A, Hillengass J, Weiss C, Neben K, Goldschmidt H, et al. Kyphoplasty in patients with multiple myeloma a retrospective comparative pilot study. J Surg Oncol. 2012;105(7):679–86. Epub 2011/10/01.
18. Basile A, Cavalli M, Fiumara P, Di Raimondo F, Mundo E, Caltabiano G, et al. Vertebroplasty in multiple myeloma with osteolysis or fracture of the posterior vertebral wall. Usefulness of a delayed cement injection. Skeletal Radiol. 2011;40(7):913–9. Epub 2011/03/02.
19. Anselmetti GC, Manca A, Montemurro F, Hirsch J, Chiara G, Grignani G, et al. Percutaneous vertebroplasty in multiple myeloma: prospective long-term follow-up in 106 consecutive patients. Cardiovasc Intervent Radiol. 2012;35(1):139–45. Epub 2011/02/10.
20. Masala S, Volpi T, Fucci FP, Cantonetti M, Postorino M, Simonetti G. Percutaneus osteoplasty in the treatment of extraspinal painful multiple myeloma lesions. Support Care Cancer. 2011;19(7):957–62. Epub 2010/05/28.
21. Astolfi S, Scaramuzzo L, Logroscino CA. A minimally invasive surgical treatment possibility of osteolytic vertebral collapse in multiple myeloma. Eur Spine J. 2009;18 Suppl 1:115–21. Epub 2009/05/14.
22. Masala S, Anselmetti GC, Marcia S, Massari F, Manca A, Simonetti G. Percutaneous vertebroplasty in multiple myeloma vertebral involvement. J Spinal Disord Tech. 2008;21(5):344–8. Epub 2008/07/05.
23. McDonald RJ, Trout AT, Gray LA, Dispenzieri A, Thielen KR, Kallmes DF. Vertebroplasty in multiple myeloma: outcomes in a large patient series. AJNR Am J Neuroradiol. 2008;29(4):642–8. Epub 2008/01/19.
24. Tran Thang NN, Abdo G, Martin JB, Seium-Neberay Y, Yilmaz H, Verbist MC, et al. Percutaneous cementoplasty in multiple myeloma: a valuable adjunct for pain control and ambulation maintenance. Support Care Cancer. 2008;16(8):891–6. Epub 2007/10/26.
25. Kose KC, Cebesoy O, Akan B, Altinel L, Dincer D, Yazar T. Functional results of vertebral augmentation techniques in pathological vertebral fractures of myelomatous patients. J Natl Med Assoc. 2006;98(10):1654–8. Epub 2006/10/21.
26. Khanna AJ, Reinhardt MK, Togawa D, Lieberman IH. Functional outcomes of kyphoplasty for the treatment of osteoporotic and osteolytic vertebral compression fractures. Osteoporos Int. 2006;17(6):817–26. Epub 2006/03/07.
27. Pflugmacher R, Kandziora F, Schroeder RJ, Melcher I, Haas NP, Klostermann CK. Percutaneous balloon kyphoplasty in the treatment of pathological vertebral body fracture and deformity in multiple myeloma: a one-year follow-up. Acta Radiol. 2006;47(4):369–76. Epub 2006/06/03.
28. Bosnjakovic P, Ristic S, Mrvic M, Miljkovic AE, Vukicevic T, Marjanovic G, et al. Management of painful spinal lesions caused by multiple myeloma using percutaneous acrylic cement injection. Acta Chir Iugosl. 2009;56(4):153–8. Epub 2009/01/01.
29. Huber FX, McArthur N, Tanner M, Gritzbach B, Schoierer O, Rothfischer W, et al. Kyphoplasty for patients with multiple myeloma is a safe surgical procedure: results from a large patient cohort. Clin Lymphoma Myeloma. 2009;9(5):375–80. Epub 2009/10/28.
30. Zou J, Mei X, Gan M, Yang H. Kyphoplasty for spinal fractures from multiple myeloma. J Surg Oncol. 2010;102(1):43–7. Epub 2010/06/26.
31. Julka A, Tolhurst SR, Srinivasan RC, Graziano GP. Functional outcomes and height restoration for patients with multiple myeloma-related osteolytic vertebral compression fractures treated with kyphoplasty. J Spinal Disord Tech. 2012. Epub 2012/06/01.

32. Lane JM, Hong R, Koob J, Kiechle T, Niesvizky R, Pearse R, et al. Kyphoplasty enhances function and structural alignment in multiple myeloma. Clin Orthop Relat Res. 2004;426:49–53. Epub 2004/09/04.
33. Garland P, Gishen P, Rahemtulla A. Percutaneous vertebroplasty to treat painful myelomatous vertebral deposits-long-term efficacy outcomes. Ann Hematol. 2011;90(1):95–100. Epub 2010/07/08.
34. Lim BS, Chang UK, Youn SM. Clinical outcomes after percutaneous vertebroplasty for pathologic compression fractures in osteolytic metastatic spinal disease. J Korean Neurosurg Soc. 2009;45(6):369–74. Epub 2009/07/18.
35. Dudeney S, Lieberman IH, Reinhardt MK, Hussein M. Kyphoplasty in the treatment of osteolytic vertebral compression fractures as a result of multiple myeloma. J Clin Oncol. 2002;20(9):2382–7. Epub 2002/05/01.
36. Tancioni F, Lorenzetti M, Navarria P, Nozza A, Castagna L, Gaetani P, et al. Vertebroplasty for pain relief and spinal stabilization in multiple myeloma. Neurol Sci. 2010;31(2):151–7. Epub 2010/01/16.

The Role of Radiation Therapy in the Treatment of Multiple Myeloma, Plasmacytoma, and Other Plasma Cell Disorders

19

Prashant Kapoor and James A. Martenson

Introduction

The inherent radioresponsiveness of plasma cell malignancies is well established and radiation therapy has important roles, both adjunctive as well as a primary treatment modality in the management of plasma cell disorders. Nearly 40 % of patients with multiple myeloma require radiotherapy during the course of their disease [1]. Its most common application is in the palliation of symptomatic skeletal and soft tissue lesions in patients with multiple myeloma. Limited field radiation therapy can result in prolonged survival, free of disease, in patients with solitary plasmacytoma. In selected patients with osteosclerotic myeloma, treatment with radiation therapy often results in dramatic relief of debilitating paraneoplastic symptoms. Additionally, it can be used in patients with neurologic compromise due to cord compression or in patients with impending pathologic fractures. Wide-field or total body radiation therapy has been used as part of a pre-transplant conditioning regimen or primary treatment and may occasionally be used in the context of a second stem-cell transplant.

While there are several effective approaches that harness the cell killing potential of radiotherapy in myeloma, including radioimmunotherapy utilizing monoclonal antibodies conjugated with radionuclides [2], radiovirotherapy with recombinant oncolytic viruses [3, 4], and skeletal-targeted radiotherapy involving radiopharmaceuticals [5], this chapter focuses on conventional radiation and chemo-radiation-based management strategies in multiple myeloma and related plasma cell disorders.

P. Kapoor, M.D. (✉)
Division of Hematology, Department of Internal Medicine, Mayo Clinic, 200 First Street, Southwest, Rochester, MN 55905, USA
e-mail: kapoor.prashant@mayo.edu

J.A. Martenson, M.D.
Division of Radiation Oncology, Mayo Clinic, 200 First Street, Southwest, Rochester, MN 55905, USA
e-mail: jmartenson@mayo.edu

Radiation Therapy for Palliation

Bone pain is the most common presenting symptom in multiple myeloma. Bone pain occurred in nearly 60 % of patients in a retrospective analysis of 1,027 myeloma patients from Mayo Clinic [6]. Most bone lesions can be managed effectively with chemotherapy, bisphosphonates, and oral analgesics. However, utilization of radiotherapy to palliate pain that is unresponsive to chemotherapy is not an uncommon clinical practice.

The largest experience with palliative radiation therapy for multiple myeloma evaluated 101 patients treated to 316 sites at the University of Arizona [7]. Patients were generally treated with fractionated radiation therapy. The mean dose was 25 Gy (range 3–60 Gy). Bone pain, present at 94 % of the sites treated, was the most common indication for palliative radiotherapy.

M.A. Gertz and S.V. Rajkumar (eds.), *Multiple Myeloma: Diagnosis and Treatment*,
DOI 10.1007/978-1-4614-8520-9_19, © Mayo Foundation for Medical Education and Research 2014

Neurological impairment (6 %), impending pathologic fracture (3 %), and palpable masses (2 %) were other indications. Symptoms were relieved in 297 of the 306 symptomatic sites (97 %), with complete resolution of symptoms in 26 % and a partial relief rate of 71 %. There was no suggestion of a relationship between the probability of response and the total dose of radiation given to the site. For example, at a total dose of 10.1–15 Gy, 100 % of patients responded with a complete response rate of over 30 %. Response rates for pain, palpable mass, or neurological impairment were 97 %, 100 %, and 90 %, respectively. Lower doses were not associated with a higher risk of relapse over time. Re-treatment at 16 sites resulted in 100 % response rate, a quarter of which were complete responses.

A German study reported on palliative radiation therapy to 67 out of 71 target volumes with a higher dose (median dose 36 Gy, 2–3 Gy 5 times a week) [8]. Pain relief (partial or complete as measured by patients' perception and use of analgesics) was achieved in 85 % of target volumes. Irradiation did not impact the prognosis with respect to overall survival. In a radiosensitive malignancy such as myeloma with limited data on outcomes with radiation therapy, extrapolation of the palliative dose and fractionation of radiation therapy can reasonably be done from randomized controlled trials of radiotherapy for bone metastasis from other cancers. One such meta-analysis of 16 trials for palliation of painful bone metastasis demonstrated no significant difference in attainment of complete or partial pain relief between multi-fractionated and single fraction regimens [9]. Furthermore, no dose–response relationship between single 8 Gy and multi-fractionated higher dose regimens (up to 40 Gy in 15 fractions) was noted [9]. Another group of investigators reported on the suboptimal quality of published randomized studies investigating the role of radiotherapy for painful bone metastases, and as such caution should be exercised in interpretation of the available trials [10].

Another retrospective study from Mallinckrodt Institute of Radiology, St. Louis reported on 128 patients of multiple myeloma, majority of whom were treated for painful bone lesions. The most frequent radiation dose used was 15–20 Gy, and pain relief was obtained in 91 % (21 % complete) [11].

The University of Arizona experience demonstrates that it is not necessary to expose patients to the inconvenience, expense, and toxicity of prolonged courses of treatment. It is important to recognize that the myelotoxicity associated with extensive radiation can impair stem cell collection if future autologous stem cell transplantation is contemplated. Moreover, poor marrow reserves could potentially hinder future administration of chemotherapy. While there is no single optimal dose of radiation therapy for palliation of bone pain in multiple myeloma, it should be possible to effectively palliate nearly all patients with brief courses of therapy, such as 8 Gy in one fraction or 20 Gy in five fractions. A single fraction of 8 Gy has also been recommended by the British Committee for Standards in Hematology and the United Kingdom Myeloma Forum [12]. Such a low dose could potentially permit re-irradiation for local recurrence of symptoms (evident in on 6 % of responding sites in both the Arizona and Mallinckrodt Institute studies) [7, 11]. In most situations, concerns regarding toxicity associated with a single fraction of 8 Gy are misplaced, given results of a large randomized clinical trial in patients with metastatic disease from a variety of primary sites which found 8 Gy in single fraction to be associated with significantly less toxicity when compared to more prolonged courses of therapy [13].

Spinal Cord Compression

During the course of their disease, about 5–15 % of myeloma patients experience spinal cord compression from extramedullary foci, manifesting as sphincter dysfunction, paresthesias, lower extremity weakness, and excruciating back pain [14]. In order to preserve the neurological function and prevent progression of deficits, it is crucial to promptly diagnose the impending nerve root or spinal cord compromise and initiate appropriate treatment emergently.

Although multi-agent combination therapies such as bortezomib, cyclophosphamide, dexamethasone (VCD) or bortezomib, thalidomide, dexamethasone (VTD) can produce rapid responses in patients with mild neurological deficits, radiation therapy with concurrent steroids is recommended for more pronounced symptoms directly attributable to soft tissue disease-related cord compression, provided there is no evidence of spinal instability or retropulsed bone which requires surgical intervention. A recent preclinical study has demonstrated an improvement in the therapeutic efficacy of radiation with incorporation of dexamethasone which selectively augments oxidative stress-induced killing in myeloma cells compared to stromal and stem cells [15].

The absence of level I evidence precludes strong recommendation regarding adequate dose and schedule of radiation therapy. A study from Australia addressing the importance of local control (which in turn favorably influences survival outcomes) in myeloma and lymphoma patients with cord compression demonstrated that local control was better achieved with doses of 40 Gy or higher [16]. However, a more recent retrospective study of patients with myeloma from Mayo Clinic, Arizona and other centers suggested that a regimen involving ten fractions of 3 Gy (total dose 30 Gy) without surgical intervention appears to be appropriate [17]. In this study of 172 patients, a long course of radiation therapy (10×3 Gy, 15×2.5 Gy or 20×2 Gy) demonstrated a better chance of improvement of motor function compared to a single fraction of 8 Gy or 20 Gy in five fractions (76 % vs. 40 % in motor function recovery at 1 year with long and short radiation therapy courses, respectively; $P=0.03$). Similar functional outcomes were noted in a subgroup analysis of patients receiving varying long course RT regimens in this study prompting investigators to recommend the lowest effective dose (30 Gy) [17]. Radiation to the spine may weaken bone, but interestingly, appears to have a protective effect on the development of subsequent new vertebral fractures in myeloma [18, 19]. It is important to avoid extensive radiation as it not only increases toxicity, but can adversely affect bone marrow reserve and compromise subsequent chemotherapeutic strategies. Moreover, extensive radiation may preclude autologous stem cell transplantation-based approaches. Notably, external beam radiation to the affected area without surgical intervention has been found to be an effective approach in selected cases of myeloma involving cervical spine with clinical or radiographic evidence of instability [20].

Pathologic or Impending Pathologic Fracture

A pathologic or impending pathologic fracture of a weight bearing bone in a patient with multiple myeloma or solitary plasmacytoma warrants an orthopedic consultation for stabilization by rod placement, pinning, or arthroplasty. Radiation therapy has been customarily given to the operative field postsurgery in such scenarios. A study involving patients with pathologic fractures owing to bone metastases from a variety of primaries underscored the significance of adjuvant radiation compared to surgery alone. This sequential approach is associated with a reduced incidence of surgical reintervention for local progression or fracture and a higher probability of retaining limb function [21]. The BCSH/UKMF guidelines recommend a single fraction of 8 Gy in the adjuvant setting [12]. We base our approach on the clinical setting. If the disease is chemoresponsive we typically omit adjuvant radiotherapy since comparable results are obtained with systemic therapy alone. On the other hand, adjunctive irradiation or radiation alone can be considered in chemorefractory disease, particularly in patients with short life expectancy. As is the case with other palliative settings in multiple myeloma, short courses of radiation therapy such as 8 Gy in one fraction or 20 Gy in five fractions will be appropriate in most settings.

Radiation Therapy for Solitary Plasmacytoma

Limited field therapy is the primary treatment modality for patients with solitary plasmacytoma. We have discussed our approach to patients with plasmacytomas in a separate chapter in this book. In this section we have focused on the misinformation that exists in regard to the optimal treatment of this disorder.

The 2012 National Comprehensive Cancer Network (NCCN) guidelines recommend that patients with both solitary osseous plasmacytoma and extramedullary plasmacytoma should receive limited field radiation therapy to a dose of at least 45 Gy (http://www.nccn.org/professionals/physician_gls/pdf/myeloma.pdf). Two papers are cited in support of this recommendation. The first is a study of 45 patients treated to a minimum of 30 Gy; 31 received more than 45 Gy. Permanent local control of disease was achieved in the presenting sites of involvement in 43 of 45 patients. Local failure occurred in two patients treated with 40 Gy and 45 Gy, respectively [22]. This study actually suggests that lower doses of radiation therapy may be very effective for the treatment of solitary myeloma. The second citation by the NCCN guidelines is not a reference to a study in support of specific dose, but is instead, a reference to another review article by Hu and Yahalom [23]. The article by Hu and Yahalom, in turn, cites two studies, one by Mendenhall et al. and another by Mill et al. [11]. Mill and colleagues presented a scattergram showing the relationship between total dose and elapsed treatment time for 43 cases from their experience and their review of the literature. They summarized the findings from this data as follows: "A scattergram compiled from the radiation dose, elapsed treatment days, and local control data fails to demonstrate an obvious dose response curve." Mendenhall and colleagues [24] recommended a dose of 40 Gy based on an analysis of 81 patients from their practice and the medical literature. The resulting scattergram (Fig. 19.1) showed that doses associated with local failure are distributed randomly, with no obvious optimal dose. The contention that higher dose treatment results in better local control appears to be derived from a post hoc analysis of the data in which the decision regarding the cut-off between low-dose and high-dose radiation therapy appears to have been made after collection and review of the data, rather than before. In this context it is noteworthy that one report of 45 patients described two cases of local failure, at or above the average dose of 46 Gy [25].

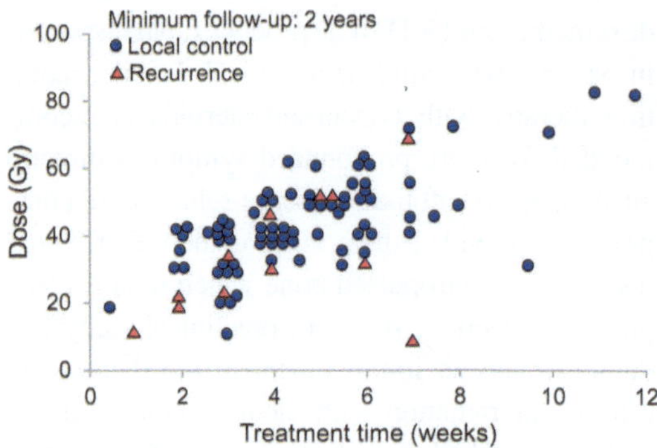

Fig. 19.1 Dose vs. local control in patients with solitary plasmacytoma. Above 20 Gy, there is no obvious relationship between administered dose and local control. Adapted from Mendenhall et al. [24]

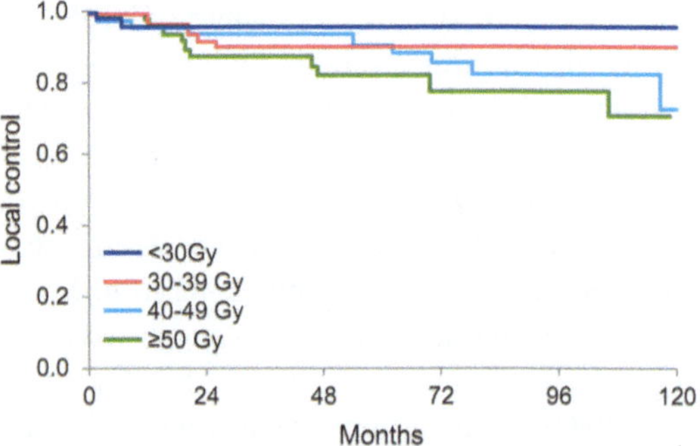

Fig. 19.2 In an analysis of patients treated with radiation therapy from Rare Cancer Network, there was no statistically significant difference in local control according to dose administered. Adapted from Ozsahin et al. [26]

The most definitive study of dose vs. local control in plasmacytoma came from an analysis of 258 patients, published by the Rare Cancer Network [26]. This study is the largest one ever published. The median dose was 40 Gy, with a range of 20–66 Gy. Local control was high in all groups and there was no suggestion that higher doses resulted in better local control; indeed, among patients treated with radiation therapy for plasmacytoma, those who received 50 Gy or more actually have the lowest control (Fig. 19.2). An analysis of local control by dose and tumor bulk did not find improved local control with higher doses of radiation therapy.

Although it has been suggested that extramedullary plasmacytomas are more difficult to con-

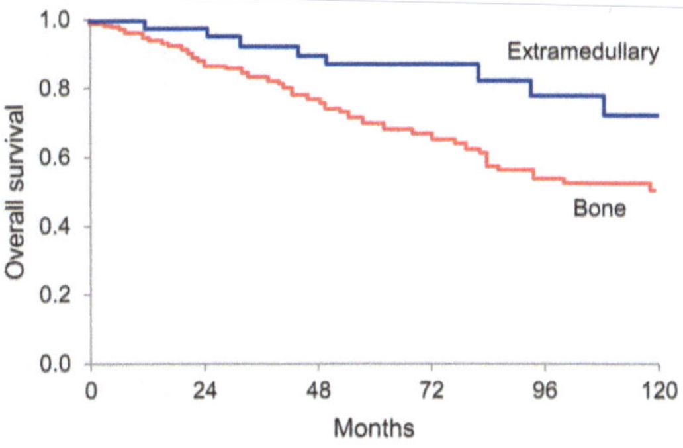

Fig. 19.3 An analysis of Rare Cancer Network Study showed that survival was significantly better among patients with extramedullary plasmacytoma when compared to patients with solitary plasmacytoma of bone ($P=0.04$). Adapted from Ozsahin et al. [26]

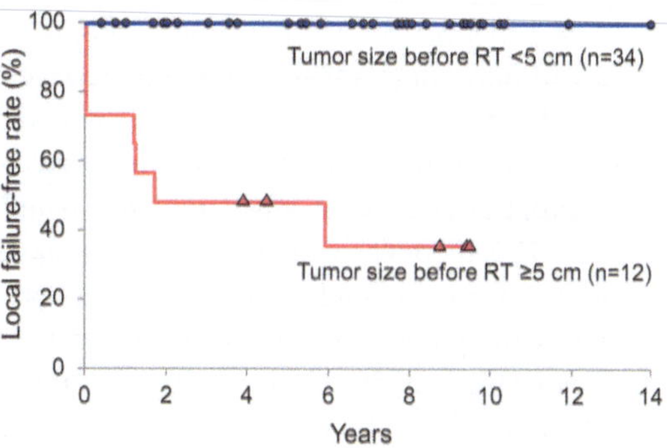

Fig. 19.5 Princess Margaret Hospital experience with solitary plasmacytoma treated with radiation therapy showing higher rate of local control in patients with tumors less than 5 cm, compared to patients with larger tumors. Adapted from Tsang et al. [27]

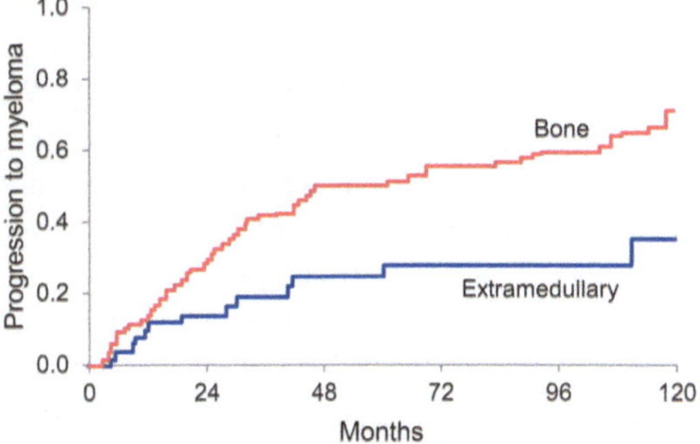

Fig. 19.4 Progression to multiple myeloma in the Rare Cancer Network Study was significantly higher in patients with solitary plasmacytoma of the bone than it was in patients with extramedullary plasmacytoma ($P=0.0009$). Adapted from Ozsahin et al. [26]

trol with radiation therapy [23], this claim was also not supported by this study, which found that the 10-year local control rate was 79 % for osseous plasmacytoma and 74 % for extramedullary plasmacytoma ($P=0.52$). Patients with extramedullary plasmacytomas did have a better prognosis as measured by overall survival (Fig. 19.3) and progression to multiple myeloma (Fig. 19.4).

One of the largest single-institution reports, from Princess Margaret Hospital, provides further support for limiting dose in plasmacytoma [27]. Patients in this study were treated with a range of doses for osseous or soft tissue solitary plasmacytomas; the most common regimen was 35 Gy in 15–20 fractions. The 8-year local disease-free rate was 100 % for patients treated with ≤30 Gy, 81 % for 35 Gy, and 80 % for ≥40 Gy ($P=0.50$). Patient with larger tumors (5 cm or larger) had a much lower rate of local control (Fig. 19.5). Another study from France, however, suggests that the 5-year local control for solitary extramedullary plasmacytoma in the head and neck region was superior when the dose to the clinical target volume is ≥45 Gy (local control 100 % vs. 50 % for those getting a dose less than 45 Gy; $P=0.034$) [28].

As with multiple myeloma, there is no basis for dogmatic assertions that higher doses provide improved local control [29]. Shorter courses of moderate dose treatment, such as 35 Gy in 3 weeks, should be sufficient for most patients with this disease. Given the appreciably worse local control observed in patients with larger tumors, escalation to higher doses (e.g., 45 Gy in 4–4.5 weeks) may be considered, although it must be acknowledged that there are no convincing data with regard to the benefit of this approach. Additionally, we advocate use of adjuvant localized radiation therapy directed at the tumor bed even after complete diagnostic excision of solitary osseous plasmacytoma. The UK Myeloma Forum recommends a dose of 40 Gy in 20 fractions for solitary extramedullary plasmacytomas of 5 cm or less. For larger tumors, it recommends 50 Gy in 25 fractions based on level III evidence from nonexperimental descriptive studies [30].

Most patients with extramedullary plasmacytoma will have tumors that arise in the head and neck [31]. Because of the potential for nodal involvement in these patients, some have advocated prophylactic treatment of regional lymph nodes [23]. Experience with regard to this issue is inconsistent. In one study, 7 of 25 patients presented with lymph node involvement and, in three cases the first site of relapse was in regional lymph nodes [32]. In contrast, a study of 22 patients from MD Anderson hospital found that no patients experienced recurrence in regional lymph nodes [33], while others have reported a regional failure rate of 4–8 % [34–37]. In two reports, patients who experienced progression in regional lymph nodes were effectively salvaged with radiation therapy [37] or surgery [35]. Focal radiation therapy to the primary lesion without extension of fields to cover clinically uninvolved lymph nodes is therefore preferred in patients with extramedullary plasmacytoma, particularly if extension of fields to cover lymph nodes will result in increased morbidity for the patient, such as mucositis or long-term xerostomia.

Osteosclerotic Myeloma

Radiation therapy has a central role in the treatment of selected patients with osteosclerotic myeloma. In this unusual manifestation of multiple myeloma, patients present with one or more sclerotic bone lesions and findings of POEMS syndrome, including polyneuropathy, organomegaly, endocrinopathy, monoclonal plasma proliferative disorder, and skin changes. Additional findings may include edema and effusions, papilledema weight loss [38], and importantly, elevated VEGF levels (a major criterion). Osteosclerotic lesions occur in nearly 95 % of patients with this syndrome and do not usually cause local symptoms such as pain. Radiation therapy, however, is administered to target the underlying plasma cell clone in patients with a single dominant lesion or those with a limited number of lesions (up to three). This approach will usually result in remission of paraneoplastic symptoms and, in some cases, may even be curative. The Mayo Clinic experience suggests that patients who are candidates for radiation therapy have improved survival (Fig. 19.6) [38]. We reserve radiation therapy for patients who have one to three bone lesions who have no evidence of clonality on iliac crest biopsy [39]. A tapering schedule of corticosteroids can be simultaneously given to patients with a rapid decline in clinical condition [40]. The onset of symptom relief can often be delayed by 3–6 months and, in some cases, continued improvement past 2 years has been noted. No reliable information is available with regard to optimal radiotherapy dose in this manifestation.

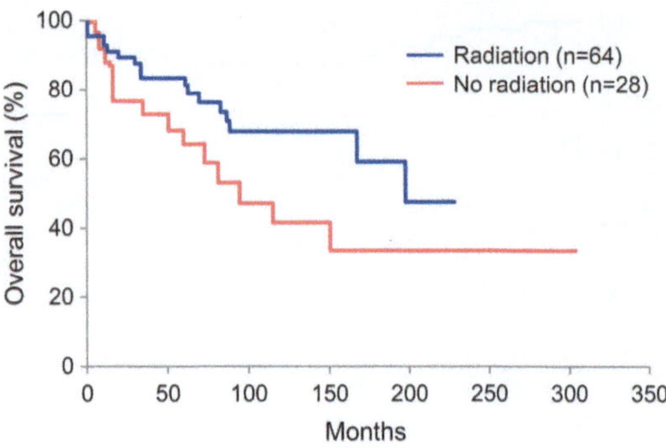

Fig. 19.6 Survival in osteosclerotic myeloma and POEMS syndrome, comparing patients who could be treated with radiation therapy vs. those who were not treated with radiation therapy. The difference is statistically significant ($P=0.04$). Adapted from Dispenzieri et al. [38]

In one study, there was a suggestion of a higher failure rate with radiation doses of less than 40 Gy [38]. In the absence of definitive information regarding optimal dose in this setting, administration of 40–45 Gy to limited fields over the course of 3–4 weeks is appropriate.

Prolonged survival is common in patients with this syndrome; in the Mayo Clinic experience, median survival was 165 months. Patients who have a few persistently FDG-avid osteosclerotic lesions on PET scans without improvement in SUV beyond a year after autologous stem cell transplantation may require adjuvant radiation therapy [39].

In our updated database of 149 patients with established POEMS syndrome seen at Mayo Clinic, Rochester between 1/1999 and 09/2011, 38 (26 %) patients were found to be appropriate candidates for upfront targeted radiation therapy. Median number of lesions was one (range 1–6). In total, 55 lesions of the possible 64 were irradiated, with majority being in the pelvic bones. The median dose was 45 Gy (35–54 Gy). Nearly half of all patients had clinical improvement and hematologic responses. The 4-year overall survival was 95 %. Importantly, the number of bone lesions at baseline did not predict whether subsequent therapies were required by patients [41].

Wide-Field Radiation Therapy

Wide-field radiation therapy has a limited role in the treatment of multiple myeloma. In one study, for example, 3 weeks after completion of 8 cycles of induction therapy with vincristine, melphalan, cyclophosphamide, and prednisone, treatment with sequential hemi-body radiation therapy was initiated. The lower half of the body was first treated to a dose of 3 Gy in a single fraction, followed, 6 weeks later, by upper hemi-body radiation therapy to the same dose. Results of this study were not considered promising [42]. A randomized clinical trial comparing chemotherapy vs. sequential hemi-body radiation therapy for remission consolidation showed that the latter is associated with significantly lower relapse-free survival and overall survival [43]. There is, accordingly, no role for hemi-body radiation therapy in the treatment of multiple myeloma.

The rationale behind using total body irradiation (TBI) for both myeloablative and non-myeloablative conditioning regimens in multiple myeloma takes into account not only the radiosensitivity of myeloma cells but also the cytotoxicity of TBI to lymphocytes which aids in engraftment via immunosuppression. TBI is given in twice daily fractionation with an inter-fraction interval of at least 6 h to potentially spare excessive toxicity to normal tissues and allow time for their repair [44]. The acute side effects of TBI are primarily gastrointestinal (nausea, vomiting, mucositis diarrhea). The incidence of parotitis appears to be reduced with fractionation [45].

Myeloablative chemotherapy and total body radiation therapy were used as part of a preparative regimen prior to autologous stem cell transplant in a phase III clinical trial that used conventional chemotherapy in the control arm [46]. The total dose of radiation therapy was 8 Gy in four fractions. Patients treated with autologous stem cell transplant survived longer. A subsequent clinical trial compared a preparative regimen of melphalan, 140 mg/m^2 and fractionated TBI with melphalan 200 mg/m^2 in patients with newly diagnosed multiple myeloma [47]. Treatment with melphalan alone was associated with significantly faster hematologic recovery, less mucositis, and better survival. Accordingly, there is no role for total body radiation therapy for first autologous transplant in multiple myeloma.

Autologous and myeloablative allogeneic stem cell transplantation have been compared prospectively in two trials. In the US Intergroup trial S9321 of early vs. late autologous stem cell transplantation, a third arm of allogeneic stem cell transplantation for patients younger than 55 years with matched siblings used a myeloablative regimen of TBI and melphalan [48]. Owing to very high transplant-related mortality (53 %), this third arm was prematurely closed. A subsequent analysis, however, at 7 years demonstrated overall survival rates to be equal (39 %) for the recipients of both autologous and allogeneic stem cells. Interestingly, in contrast to the autologous stem cell recipients, survival curve of those patients undergoing allogeneic stem cell transplantation appeared to have plateaued with extended follow-up suggesting a possibility of cure in a subgroup of long term survivors with sustained complete remission. In the other prospective trial by the Haemato Oncology Foundation for Adults in the Netherlands (HOVON-24), overall survival of allogeneic stem cell transplantation recipients after cyclophosphamide/TBI conditioning was lower compared to a matched group receiving autologous stem cell transplantation [49]. Given the excessively high mortality, a full myeloablative transplantation using TBI is not considered a viable option outside of a clinical trial setting [50].

Another approach utilizing TBI in multiple myeloma incorporates a non-myeloablative radiation dose. Bruno and colleagues [51] described the Italian experience in which patients with newly diagnosed myeloma were initially treated with systemic induction therapy. Patients with an HLA compatible sibling were then offered a regimen of an initial autologous stem cell transplant followed by an allogeneic stem cell transplant (biologic randomization). Prior to the allogeneic transplant, a non-myeloablative dose of total body radiation therapy, 2 Gy in a single fraction, was given. Patients who did not have a compatible sibling received two successive autologous stem cell transplants, neither of which used radiation therapy as part of the preparative regimen. Overall survival was superior in patients who completed the allogeneic transplant, when compared to those who received the double autologous transplant protocol. With a median follow-up of 46 months, median survival had not been reached in the patients treated with the autograft-allograft regimen vs. a median survival of 58 months in patients treated with the double autograft regimen ($P=0.03$).

Krishnan and colleagues have recently reported the results of the much awaited Blood and Marrow Transplant Clinical Trials Network (BMT CTN) 0102 phase 3 trial assessing the effectiveness of auto-allo transplantation vs. tandem autologous approach in standard-risk myeloma patients using biological randomization [52]. The former approach incorporated a single fraction 200 cGy of TBI prior to allogeneic peripheral stem cell infusion [52]. In contradistinction to the Italian study, the findings of this largest study to date comparing the two approaches were somewhat similar to most other clinical trials addressing this question [50], suggesting a lack of benefit with the auto-allo approach [52, 53].

Radiation with Novel Agent-Based Therapy

A preclinical study from our institution provided rationale for combining a proteasome inhibitor with radiation therapy. Sensitization of myeloma cells by bortezomib (10 nm) prior to ionizing radiation was shown to result in acute apoptotic response in clonogenic assays [54]. The proposed mechanism for this synergistic activity is abrogation of ionizing radiation-induced activation of NF-KB pathway in myeloma cells. Additionally Fas-mediated cell destruction was observed [54]. In our experience and in a few studies, proteasome inhibitors such as bortezomib and immunomodulators like lenalidomide, but not thalidomide, by themselves have been found to be effective for relapsed/refractory myeloma with extramedullary disease [55–57]. Case reports highlighting successful utilization of concurrent radiation and bortezomib or lenalidomide therapy have been published as well [58, 59]. Although potentially effective and tolerable, clinicians should, in particular, be mindful of gastrointestinal toxicities with concurrent bortezomib use and irradiation [60].

Other Plasma Cell Disorders

Localized Light Chain Amyloidosis (AL)

Radiation therapy has been unsuccessfully used to induce local organ response in systemic AL amyloidosis [61]. In systemic AL amyloidosis, amyloidogenic clonal plasma cells reside within the bone marrow and the amyloid protein infiltrates various organs. Irradiation of the affected enlarged organs does not adversely affect the survival of marrow plasma cells, the potential source of amyloid. Consequently, there is neither any role nor rationale for such an approach in patients with systemic AL amyloidosis. In contrast, radiation therapy has been successfully used in patients with limited AL amyloidosis, including those with tracheobronchial [62–66], nasopharyngeal [67], laryngeal, and orbital or conjunctival amyloidosis [68].

Tracheobronchial amyloidosis, in particular, is a difficult-to-treat, potentially fatal but fortunately a rare variant of localized AL amyloidosis. The characteristic deposition of amyloid, synthesized within the tracheobronchial tree itself by the mucosal plasma cells, results in an obstructive pattern on pulmonary function tests. Tracheobronchial amyloidosis accounts for 25–50 % of all cases of localized pulmonary amyloidosis, and the symptoms are primarily related to airway obstruction. Systemic therapy has been ineffective and is accordingly not indicated in treating this localized phenomenon. Bronchoscopic interventions such as laser resection or balloon dilatation typically result in transient improvement. A small series of seven patients from our institution [65] and a few other case reports from other centers have demonstrated efficacy of external beam radiation therapy, perhaps due to the destruction of local plasma cells and radiation-induced local inflammation. Although optimal dose is unknown, based on the results of our series and other reports, we recommend 20 Gy in ten fractions as a first-line treatment in patients with distal or bulky tracheobronchial amyloidosis not amenable to more invasive approaches. Potential complications of radiation therapy including esophagitis, pericarditis, pneumonitis, pulmonary fibrosis, myelitis, and myocarditis can generally be avoided with this low dose of radiation therapy. This treatment modality is usually well-tolerated, and it can result in durable symptomatic and objective improvement. Moreover, the recommended dose does not preclude re-treatment if necessary [62, 65].

Waldenström's Macroglobulinemia

In this chronic lymphoproliferative disorder, there are specific clinical scenarios where radiation therapy may have a role. These include management of the Bing–Neel syndrome which results from infiltration of the central nervous system by malignant plasmacytoid lymphocytes in Waldenström's macroglobulinemia. This rare complication appears to respond to various approaches, including focal or whole brain radiation therapy (20–40 Gy), chemotherapy or a combination of both [69, 70].

Rarely, splenic radiation and splenectomy have successfully controlled advanced disease in patients of Waldenström's macroglobulinemia with marked splenomegaly [71, 72].

Future Directions

The use of fractionated TBI has declined as a result of unacceptable toxicities. The role of low-dose TBI for non-myeloablative regimens in myeloma has still not been completely defined. The concept, efficacy, and feasibility of total marrow irradiation (TMI) with helical tomotherapy, a technique utilized to preferentially deliver more targeted dose of TBI to marrow and reduced doses to adjacent organs, is being investigated in multiple myeloma and other radiosensitive hematologic malignancies [73, 74]. This approach has the potential to permit dose escalation to sites of tumor burden and simultaneously reduce delivery, and therefore, associated toxicities to the uninvolved organs. A recent phase I study incorporating TMI as sole ablative modality prior to second tandem autologous stem cell transplantation in patients with myeloma has demonstrated feasibility and tolerability of this modality at maximal tolerated dose of 1,600 cGy [75]. Further evaluation of this approach in phase 2 trials is required.

Intensity modulated radiation therapy (IMRT) is being used with increasing frequency in patients receiving radiotherapy for malignant disease. The advantage of IMRT is that it can deliver high doses of radiation therapy that conform closely to a tumor, thus providing greater sparing of normal organs. In plasma cell disorders, however, IMRT is generally not needed because relatively low doses of radiation therapy are able to provide good tumor control without exceeding normal tissue tolerance. In rare circumstances, IMRT may be beneficial in plasma cell disorders. In some patients with head and neck plasmacytoma, for example, IMRT may be indicated if it is able to provide greater sparing of upper aerodigestive mucosa or salivary glands in comparison to conventional three-dimensional radiation therapy [76]. IMRT is extraordinarily expensive and labor-intensive. It also gives a higher integral dose to normal structures, even while minimizing the volume of normal organs exposed to high-dose radiation therapy. The vast majority of patients with plasma cell disorders should be treated with conventional radiation therapy rather than IMRT.

Proton therapy shares with IMRT the ability to deliver highly conformal doses of radiation therapy. Radiation dose delivered by protons can be concentrated over a modulated Bragg Peak. As a result, protons can deliver a low entrance dose, and deep to the Bragg Peak, minimal exit dose. These characteristics can result in delivery of highly conformal radiation doses to malignant tumors without the increased integral dose associated with IMRT. Proton therapy is similar to IMRT in that it is extraordinarily expensive and labor-intensive. Because relatively low-dose radiation therapy is sufficient for the vast majority of patients with plasma cell disorders, protons should not be used except under very rare circumstances where a clear and clinically meaningful dosimetric advantage is possible with this modality.

The vast majority of patients with plasma cell disorders can be treated with relatively low dose, carefully planned conventional radiation therapy.

References

1. Featherstone C, et al. Estimating the optimal utilization rates of radiotherapy for hematologic malignancies from a review of the evidence: part II-leukemia and myeloma. Cancer. 2005;103(2):393–401.
2. Kapoor P, et al. Anti-CD20 monoclonal antibody therapy in multiple myeloma. Br J Haematol. 2008;141(2): 135–48.
3. Dingli D, et al. Image-guided radiovirotherapy for multiple myeloma using a recombinant measles virus expressing the thyroidal sodium iodide symporter. Blood. 2004;103(5):1641–6.
4. Goel A, et al. Radioiodide imaging and radiovirotherapy of multiple myeloma using VSV(Delta51)-NIS, an attenuated vesicular stomatitis virus encoding the sodium iodide symporter gene. Blood. 2007;110(7): 2342–50.
5. Dispenzieri A, et al. A phase II study of (153) Sm-EDTMP and high-dose melphalan as a peripheral blood stem cell conditioning regimen in patients with multiple myeloma. Am J Hematol. 2010;85(6):409–13.
6. Kyle RA, et al. Review of 1027 patients with newly diagnosed multiple myeloma. Mayo Clin Proc. 2003;78(1):21–33.
7. Leigh BR, et al. Radiation therapy for the palliation of multiple myeloma. Int J Radiat Oncol Biol Phys. 1993;25(5):801–4.
8. Mose S, et al. Role of radiotherapy in the treatment of multiple myeloma. Strahlenther Onkol. 2000;176(11): 506–12.
9. Wu JS, et al. Meta-analysis of dose-fractionation radiotherapy trials for the palliation of painful bone metastases. Int J Radiat Oncol Biol Phys. 2003; 55(3):594–605.
10. Shakespeare TP, Thiagarajan A, Gebski V. Evaluation of the quality of radiotherapy randomized trials for painful bone metastases. Cancer. 2005;103(9):1976–81.
11. Mill WB, Griffith R. The role of radiation therapy in the management of plasma cell tumors. Cancer. 1980; 45(4):647–52.
12. Bird JM, et al. Guidelines for the diagnosis and management of multiple myeloma 2011. Br J Haematol. 2011;154(1):32–75.
13. Hartsell WF, et al. Randomized trial of short- versus long-course radiotherapy for palliation of painful bone metastases. J Natl Cancer Inst. 2005;97(11):798–804.
14. Rades D, et al. Prognostic factors for local control and survival in patients with spinal cord compression from myeloma. Strahlenther Onkol. 2012;188(7):628–31.
15. Bera S, et al. Dexamethasone-induced oxidative stress enhances myeloma cell radiosensitization while sparing normal bone marrow hematopoiesis. Neoplasia. 2010;12(12):980–92.
16. Wallington M, et al. Local control and survival in spinal cord compression from lymphoma and myeloma. Radiother Oncol. 1997;42(1):43–7.
17. Rades D, et al. Short-course radiotherapy is not optimal for spinal cord compression due to myeloma. Int J Radiat Oncol Biol Phys. 2006;64(5):1452–7.
18. Lecouvet F, et al. Long-term effects of localized spinal radiation therapy on vertebral fractures and focal lesions appearance in patients with multiple myeloma. Br J Haematol. 1997;96(4):743–5.
19. Yeh HS, Berenson JR. Treatment for myeloma bone disease. Clin Cancer Res. 2006;12(20 Pt 2): 6279s–84.
20. Rao G, et al. Multiple myeloma of the cervical spine: treatment strategies for pain and spinal instability. J Neurosurg Spine. 2006;5(2):140–5.
21. Townsend PW, et al. Role of postoperative radiation therapy after stabilization of fractures caused by metastatic disease. Int J Radiat Oncol Biol Phys. 1995; 31(1):43–9.
22. Dimopoulos MA, et al. Curability of solitary bone plasmacytoma. J Clin Oncol. 1992;10(4):587–90.
23. Hu K, Yahalom J. Radiotherapy in the management of plasma cell tumors. Oncology. 2000;14(1):101–8, 111; discussion 111–2, 115.

24. Mendenhall CM, Thar TL, Million RR. Solitary plasmacytoma of bone and soft tissue. Int J Radiat Oncol Biol Phys. 1980;6(11):1497–501.
25. Galieni P, et al. Clinical outcome of extramedullary plasmacytoma. Haematologica. 2000;85(1):47–51.
26. Ozsahin M, et al. Outcomes and patterns of failure in solitary plasmacytoma: a multicenter Rare Cancer Network study of 258 patients. Int J Radiat Oncol Biol Phys. 2006;64(1):210–7.
27. Tsang RW, et al. Solitary plasmacytoma treated with radiotherapy: impact of tumor size on outcome. Int J Radiat Oncol Biol Phys. 2001;50(1):113–20.
28. Tournier-Rangeard L, et al. Radiotherapy for solitary extramedullary plasmacytoma in the head-and-neck region: a dose greater than 45 Gy to the target volume improves the local control. Int J Radiat Oncol Biol Phys. 2006;64(4):1013–7.
29. Koh H, Kim I, Kim C, Kim H, Yoon S, Heo D. Clinical and prognostic features of plasmacytoma: outcome analysis of 29 cases in SNUH. Int J Radiat Oncol Biol Phys. 2010;78:S557.
30. Soutar R, et al. Guidelines on the diagnosis and management of solitary plasmacytoma of bone and solitary extramedullary plasmacytoma. Clin Oncol. 2004;16(6):405–13.
31. Dolin S, Dewar JP. Extramedullary plasmacytoma. Am J Pathol. 1956;32(1):83–103.
32. Knowling MA, Harwood AR, Bergsagel DE. Comparison of extramedullary plasmacytomas with solitary and multiple plasma cell tumors of bone. J Clin Oncol. 1983;1(4):255–62.
33. Liebross RH, et al. Clinical course of solitary extramedullary plasmacytoma. Radiother Oncol. 1999; 52(3):245–9.
34. Bachar G, et al. Solitary extramedullary plasmacytoma of the head and neck—long-term outcome analysis of 68 cases. Head Neck. 2008;30(8):1012–9.
35. Chao MW, et al. Radiotherapy in the management of solitary extramedullary plasmacytoma. Intern Med J. 2005;35(4):211–5.
36. Mayr NA, et al. The role of radiation therapy in the treatment of solitary plasmacytomas. Radiother Oncol. 1990;17(4):293–303.
37. Susnerwala SS, et al. Extramedullary plasmacytoma of the head and neck region: clinicopathological correlation in 25 cases. Br J Cancer. 1997;75(6):921–7.
38. Dispenzieri A, et al. POEMS syndrome: definitions and long-term outcome. Blood. 2003;101(7): 2496–506.
39. Dispenzieri A. How I treat POEMS syndrome. Blood. 2012;119(24):5650–8.
40. Dispenzieri A. POEMS syndrome: update on diagnosis, risk-stratification, and management. Am J Hematol. 2012;87(8):804–14.
41. Humeniuk MS, Gertz MA, Lacy MQ, Kyle RA, Hayman SR, Kumar SK, et al. Outcomes of patients with POEMS syndrome treated initially with radiation. Blood. 2013;122(1):68–73.
42. MacKenzie MR, et al. Consolidation hemibody radiotherapy following induction combination chemotherapy in high-tumor-burden multiple myeloma. J Clin Oncol. 1992;10(11):1769–74.
43. Salmon SE, et al. Chemotherapy is superior to sequential hemibody irradiation for remission consolidation in multiple myeloma: a Southwest Oncology Group study. J Clin Oncol. 1990;8(9):1575–84.
44. Shrieve D. The role of radiotherapy. In: Mehta J, Singhal S, editors. Myeloma. London: Martin Dunitz; 2002.
45. Ozsahin M, et al. Total-body irradiation before bone marrow transplantation. Results of two randomized instantaneous dose rates in 157 patients. Cancer. 1992;69(11):2853–65.
46. Attal M, et al. A prospective, randomized trial of autologous bone marrow transplantation and chemotherapy in multiple myeloma. Intergroupe Francais du Myelome. N Engl J Med. 1996;335(2):91–7.
47. Moreau P, et al. Comparison of 200 mg/m(2) melphalan and 8 Gy total body irradiation plus 140 mg/m(2) melphalan as conditioning regimens for peripheral blood stem cell transplantation in patients with newly diagnosed multiple myeloma: final analysis of the Intergroupe Francophone du Myelome 9502 randomized trial. Blood. 2002;99(3):731–5.
48. Barlogie B, et al. Standard chemotherapy compared with high-dose chemoradiotherapy for multiple myeloma: final results of phase III US Intergroup Trial S9321. J Clin Oncol. 2006;24(6):929–36.
49. Lokhorst HM, et al. Partially T-cell-depleted allogeneic stem-cell transplantation for first-line treatment of multiple myeloma: a prospective evaluation of patients treated in the phase III study HOVON 24 MM. J Clin Oncol. 2003;21(9):1728–33.
50. Lokhorst H, et al. International Myeloma Working Group consensus statement regarding the current status of allogeneic stem-cell transplantation for multiple myeloma. J Clin Oncol. 2010;28(29):4521–30.
51. Bruno B, et al. A comparison of allografting with autografting for newly diagnosed myeloma. N Engl J Med. 2007;356(11):1110–20.
52. Krishnan A, et al. Autologous haemopoietic stem-cell transplantation followed by allogeneic or autologous haemopoietic stem-cell transplantation in patients with multiple myeloma (BMT CTN 0102): a phase 3 biological assignment trial. Lancet Oncol. 2011; 12(13):1195–203.
53. Dispenzieri A. Is there a future for auto-allo HSCT in multiple myeloma? Lancet Oncol. 2011;12(13): 1176–7.
54. Goel A, et al. PS-341-mediated selective targeting of multiple myeloma cells by synergistic increase in ionizing radiation-induced apoptosis. Exp Hematol. 2005;33(7):784–95.
55. Blade J, et al. Soft-tissue plasmacytomas in multiple myeloma: incidence, mechanisms of extramedullary spread, and treatment approach. J Clin Oncol. 2011;29(28):3805–12.
56. Rosinol L, et al. Extramedullary multiple myeloma escapes the effect of thalidomide. Haematologica. 2004;89(7):832–6.

57. Laura R, et al. Bortezomib: an effective agent in extramedullary disease in multiple myeloma. Eur J Haematol. 2006;76(5):405–8.
58. Berges O, et al. Concurrent radiation therapy and bortezomib in myeloma patient. Radiother Oncol. 2008;86(2):290–2.
59. Marchand V, et al. Concurrent radiation therapy and lenalidomide in myeloma patient. Radiother Oncol. 2008;87(1):152–3.
60. Mohiuddin MM, Harmon DC, Delaney TF. Severe acute enteritis in a multiple myeloma patient receiving bortezomib and spinal radiotherapy: case report. J Chemother. 2005;17(3):343–6.
61. Thibault I, Vallieres I. Macroglossia due to systemic amyloidosis: is there a role for radiotherapy? Case Rep Oncol. 2011;4(2):392–9.
62. Gallivan GJ, Gallivan HK. Laryngeal amyloidosis causing hoarseness and airway obstruction. J Voice. 2010;24(2):235–9.
63. Kalra S, et al. External-beam radiation therapy in the treatment of diffuse tracheobronchial amyloidosis. Mayo Clin Proc. 2001;76(8):853–6.
64. Monroe AT, et al. Tracheobronchial amyloidosis: a case report of successful treatment with external beam radiation therapy. Chest. 2004;125(2):784–9.
65. Neben-Wittich MA, Foote RL, Kalra S. External beam radiation therapy for tracheobronchial amyloidosis. Chest. 2007;132(1):262–7.
66. O'Regan A, et al. Tracheobronchial amyloidosis. The Boston University experience from 1984 to 1999. Medicine. 2000;79(2):69–79.
67. Tesei F, et al. Extramedullary plasmocytoma (EMP) of the head and neck: a series of 22 cases. Acta Otorhinolaryngol Ital. 1995;15(6):437–42.
68. Pecora JL, Sambursky JS, Vargha Z. Radiation therapy in amyloidosis of the eyelid and conjunctiva: a case report. Ann Ophthalmol. 1982;14(2):194–6.
69. Grewal JS, et al. Bing-Neel syndrome: a case report and systematic review of clinical manifestations, diagnosis, and treatment options. Clin Lymphoma Myeloma. 2009;9(6):462–6.
70. Malkani RG, et al. Bing-Neel syndrome: an illustrative case and a comprehensive review of the published literature. J Neurooncol. 2010;96(3): 301–12.
71. Kapoor P, et al. Splenectomy in plasma cell dyscrasias: a review of the clinical practice. Am J Hematol. 2006;81(12):946–54.
72. Takemori N, et al. Durable remission after splenectomy for Waldenstrom's macroglobulinemia with massive splenomegaly in leukemic phase. Leuk Lymphoma. 1997;26(3–4):387–93.
73. Shueng PW, et al. Total marrow irradiation with helical tomotherapy for bone marrow transplantation of multiple myeloma: first experience in Asia. Technol Cancer Res Treat. 2009;8(1):29–38.
74. Wong JY, et al. Image-guided total-marrow irradiation using helical tomotherapy in patients with multiple myeloma and acute leukemia undergoing hematopoietic cell transplantation. Int J Radiat Oncol Biol Phys. 2009;73(1):273–9.
75. Somlo G, et al. Total marrow irradiation: a new ablative regimen as part of tandem autologous stem cell transplantation for patients with multiple myeloma. Clin Cancer Res. 2011;17(1):174–82.
76. Vosmik M, et al. Solitary extramedullary plasmacytoma in the oropharynx: advantages of intensity-modulated radiation therapy. Clin Lymphoma Myeloma. 2007;7(6):434–7.

Neurologic Complications of Myeloma

20

Chafic Y. Karam and Michelle L. Mauermann

Introduction

Patients with multiple myeloma (MM) frequently develop neurological complications related to the disease or its treatment [1–3]. These neurological complications may affect the central nervous system (CNS) [4] or more commonly the peripheral nervous system (PNS) [1, 5]. Neurological complications can result from:

(a) Direct infiltration of the nervous system by neoplastic cells [4]
(b) Indirect effect such as paraneoplastic syndrome or amyloid deposition [5]
(c) Iatrogenic effect during multiple myeloma treatment [1]
(d) Toxic-metabolic syndrome related to systemic complications of multiple myeloma [6]
(e) A combination of the above

Furthermore, a neurological syndrome can be the presenting sign of multiple myeloma [7]. In this chapter we will discuss these different neurological complications of myeloma by system (CNS vs. PNS) and the management of these complications (Table 20.1).

C.Y. Karam, M.D. • M.L. Mauermann, M.D. (✉)
Department of Neurology, Mayo Clinic,
200 1st St. SW, Rochester, MN 55905, USA
e-mail: Chafickaram@gmail.com;
Mauermann.Michelle@mayo.edu

Central Nervous System

Toxic-Metabolic Encephalopathy

Patients with multiple myeloma that present with altered mental status (confusion, agitation), persistent headache, lethargy, or hypersomnolence should be screened for metabolic and electrolyte disturbances. For instance, high blood levels of ammonia, even in the absence of liver involvement, may be observed in certain patients with multiple myeloma. One explanation of this syndrome is the possible secondary elevation of ammonia by myeloma cell lines [8–11]. Advanced renal failure in patients with multiple myeloma can result in uremia and metabolic acidosis leading to altered mental status [12]. While the CNS dysfunction in patients with a metabolic condition usually presents with global symptoms, occasionally patients may present with seizures or focal neurological deficits in the setting of hypercalcemia [12].

Cord Compression

Spinal cord compression in patients with multiple myeloma is common and may be caused by either an extramedullary plasmacytoma or a bone

M.A. Gertz and S.V. Rajkumar (eds.), *Multiple Myeloma: Diagnosis and Treatment*,
DOI 10.1007/978-1-4614-8520-9_20,

Table 20.1 Neurological complications of multiple myeloma

Central nervous system	Peripheral nervous system
Toxic-metabolic encephalopathy	MM-associated PN without amyloidosis
Cord compression	MM-associated PN with amyloidosis
CNS myelomatosis	Treatment-emergent PN
Intracranial plasmacytomas	Radiculopathy
Acute disseminated encephalomyelitis	Myopathy
Stiff-person syndrome	
Hyperviscosity	
Hypoperfusion	

fragment due to vertebral body fracture [13–16]. Patients with cord compression present with severe back pain associated with weakness or numbness in lower limbs (+/−upper limbs depending on level of compression) with or without difficulty initiating urination or incontinence. Some patients, however, may present with an indolent syndrome of dull pain and chronic progressive weakness and urinary incontinence. A high level of suspicion is required in patients with multiple myeloma and leg weakness and an urgent MRI of the spine should be obtained along with a neurological and a neurosurgical consultation. If there is contraindication to MRI (e.g., pacemaker), CT myelography can be obtained in lieu of an MRI. Treatment usually consists of high-dose steroids with radiation therapy, or decompressive surgery to avoid permanent paraplegia.

CNS Myelomatosis

CNS invasion by plasma cells is an unusual complication of MM and results from metastases to leptomeninges, brain parenchyma, choroid plexus, and cranial nerves. Patients may present with extremity weakness, changes of mental status, speech and gait disturbance, cranial nerve palsies, and symptoms of increased intracranial pressure (headaches, nausea, vomiting) [4, 17]. Pituitary failure (hypopituitarism) can occur if the lesion interferes with the pituitary gland. CSF will generally reveal increased protein levels and cytology may show the neoplastic cells. CSF opening pressure may be elevated [4].

Intracranial Plasmacytomas

Intracranial plasmacytomas are rare depositions of malignant plasma cells and almost always represent extensions of myelomatous lesions of the skull or plasmacytomas involving the clivus or base of the skull [18].

Acute Disseminated Encephalomyelitis

Rare cases of acute disseminated encephalomyelitis (ADEM) occur in MM. ADEM is a condition presenting with multifocal neurological symptoms with or without alteration of mental status due to multiple inflammatory lesions in the brain and spinal cord that result from autoimmune demyelination. Whether truly caused by an MM-induced paraneoplastic syndrome, chemotherapy, or simply due to chance association is not clear [19, 20].

Stiff-Person Syndrome

Stiff-person syndrome presents with progressive stiffness and rigidity of the axial or limb musculature with bouts of spasms in the back or limbs. It is thought to be an autoimmune process. Rare cases of MM with stiff-person syndrome have been reported [21, 22]. This may be either the result of a paraneoplastic syndrome or due to chance association.

Hyperviscosity

Hyperviscosity in MM usually results from an increase in the protein fraction of the circulating blood as well as abnormal polymerization and abnormal shape of immunoglobulin molecules. Symptoms of hyperviscosity usually appear when the serum viscosity reaches 4–5 cp which corresponds to a serum immunoglobulin M (IgM) level of at least 3 g/dL, an IgG level of 4 g/dL, and an IgA level of 6 g/dL. Patients with hyperviscosity may present with focal neurological signs, visual disturbance, and gum bleeding [23, 24].

Hypoperfusion

Brain hypoperfusion syndrome manifested by dizziness, syncope, or focal neurological symptoms with or without stroke can occur in the setting of heart failure caused by bortezomib treatment [25] or from amyloidosis complicating MM.

Peripheral Neuropathies

Peripheral neuropathies in patients with MM can be divided into those caused by the disease itself (MM-associated PN) and the others caused by the treatment of MM (treatment-emergent PN).

MM-Associated PN

Clinically, peripheral neuropathy can be found in about 5–20 % [1, 2, 26–29] of patients with untreated myeloma. Furthermore, nerve conduction studies (NCS) may demonstrate neuropathy in patients without clinical symptoms, increasing the incidence to up to 39 % of patients with untreated MM [27]. The mechanism of peripheral neuropathy in patients with untreated MM is not very well elucidated [26–28, 30]. Several studies have demonstrated amyloid deposition in some but not all neuropathy cases [26–28]. However, it remains difficult to interpret these findings in cases with only positive fat aspirates as these can be false positives, especially in laboratories that are not highly specialized in this test [30].

MM-associated PN without amyloidosis: The peripheral neuropathy of patients without amyloidosis is usually one of three types: sensorimotor, sensory, or motor [1, 2, 26–29]. In these patients the neuropathy is considered secondary to a paraneoplastic syndrome and not due to amyloid deposition inside the nerve or nerve invasion by neoplastic cells. Nerve biopsy shows both axonal degeneration and demyelination [26].

Sensorimotor

Patients with a sensorimotor peripheral neuropathy demonstrate slow progression of distal sensory (numbness, tingling) and motor symptoms. Examination shows involvement of all sensory modalities and mild distal weakness in a length-dependent, symmetric pattern. Ankle reflexes may be reduced or absent. These patients do not have prominent autonomic involvement. NCS show mild slowing of motor conduction velocities and low-to-absent compound muscle action potentials. Sensory nerve action potentials are usually low to absent [1, 2, 26–29].

Sensory

Patients with a sensory neuropathy or ganglionopathy may present with a progressive history of bilateral leg numbness without pain, autonomic features, or complaints of muscle weakness [26]. Examination of these patients usually reveals a moderately severe loss of vibration and proprioception in the legs and hands, with relative preservation of touch-pressure, pain, and thermal discrimination. Motor function is usually normal but can be challenging to assess due to severe proprioceptive loss. Deep tendon reflexes are usually absent. Sensory ataxia and Rombergism may be present. NCS demonstrate reduced or absent sensory nerve action potentials in both the upper and lower limbs. Motor nerve conduction studies and needle electromyography are usually normal or relatively preserved compared to the extent of sensory abnormalities. In these patients, somatosensory-evoked potentials (SSEPs) may help discriminate a ganglionopathy vs. a polyneuropathy.

Motor

Patients with a motor-predominant peripheral neuropathy may present with slowly progressive symptoms that can be distal or proximal and involve both upper and lower limbs. They may even have facial, bulbar, or respiratory weakness. Patients may complain of sensory symptoms (acral paresthesia) but these do not dominate the clinical picture [2, 26, 29]. They may exhibit muscle atrophy and fasciculations upon examination.

Deep tendon reflexes are reduced or absent. NCS may show moderate slowing of motor conduction velocities and abnormal sensory nerve action potentials. Needle electromyography reveals fibrillation potentials in proximal and distal muscles with neurogenic motor unit potential changes.

MM-associated PN with amyloidosis: The neuropathy of patients with amyloidosis can present initially with carpal tunnel syndrome [31]. Later patients may complain of prominent dysesthesias, dissociated sensory loss with predominant involvement of nociception (pain) and thermal (temperature) discrimination, autonomic insufficiency (i.e., postural lightheadedness, constipation, urinary retention, early satiety, dry eyes/mouth, erectile dysfunction, or sweating abnormalities), or rarely painless weakness without autonomic dysfunction [26]. NCS frequently show carpal tunnel syndrome. Motor conduction studies show mixed axonal and demyelinating features including low-amplitude compound muscle action potentials, slight slowing of conduction velocities, and slight prolongation of distal latencies. Sensory nerve action potentials tend to be markedly reduced or unobtainable. Needle electromyography demonstrates fibrillation potentials and neurogenic motor unit potentials which tend to be more prominent distally [26].

Treatment-Emergent PN

Treatment-emergent peripheral neuropathy is the most frequent neurological complication in patients with MM. It can affect up to 65 % of patients receiving chemotherapy [2]. In addition, patients with severe iatrogenic neuropathy may discontinue the treatment which can result in reduced rates of treatment responsiveness [32]. The type of neuropathy and the extent of its reversibility depend on the agent used. Since peripheral neuropathy may be present in up to 39 % of patients with MM prior to treatment [27] it is helpful to evaluate patients with MM for neuropathy prior to treatment. Screening questions such as the presence of numbness, tingling, pain, weakness, postural lightheadedness, urinary retention, or constipation are essential. Furthermore, since the neuropathy may not be symptomatic, careful neurological examination including supine and erect blood pressure measurements as well as NCS should be performed in patients with MM prior to treatment. If patients have a neuropathy prior to treatment, care should be given in choosing the least neurotoxic agent if possible. During the course of their treatment, patients with MM should be carefully monitored for new signs and symptoms suggestive of neuropathy. The definition and grading of peripheral neuropathy according to National Cancer Institute are summarized in Table 20.2. The most common offending medications include bortezomib and thalidomide.

Table 20.2 Definition of peripheral neuropathy according to National Cancer Institute

Grade 1	Asymptomatic
Grade 2	Loss of deep tendon reflexes or paraesthesia (including tingling), not interfering with function; weakness on examination or testing only
Grade 3	Sensory alteration or paraesthesia (including tingling), interfering with function but not with activities of daily living (ADL); symptomatic weakness, interfering with function but not with ADL
Grade 4	Sensory alteration or paraesthesia interfering with ADL; weakness interfering with ADL; bracing or assistance to walk (i.e., cane- or walker-indicated), life-threatening, disabling (i.e., paralysis)

Bortezomib: Bortezomib is the first member of a new class of chemotherapeutic agents that inhibit the proteasome-ubiquitination pathway. The primary target may be the dorsal root ganglia [33]. Bortezomib-induced peripheral neuropathy is one of the most common and important drug-related adverse events and occurs in up to 70 % of multiple myeloma patients [34], and severe neuropathy affecting activities of daily living occurs in approximately 13 % of patients [35–38]. The incidence of neuropathy increases with cumulative dose and plateaus at the fifth treatment cycle [39]. Dose reduction is required in up to 30 % of patients due to [40] peripheral neuropathy and

Table 20.3 Proposed dose-modification guidelines for bortezomib-related neuropathic pain and/or peripheral sensory or motor neuropathy [34]

Grade 1 (paresthesias, weakness, and/or loss of reflexes) without pain or loss of function	Reduce current bortezomib dose by one level (1.3 → 1.0 → 0.7 mg/m^3) or, for patients receiving a twice-weekly schedule, change to a once-per-week schedule using the same dose Consider starting with 1.3 mg/m^2 once per week in patients with history of prior peripheral neuropathy	Prior peripheral neuropathy was the only risk factor associated with bortezomib-related peripheral neuropath in newly diagnosed patients treated with VMP [81] Baseline peripheral neuropathy was a risk factor for development bortezomib-related peripheral neuropathy of Grade ≥3 in relapsed/refractory MM patients treated with single-agent bortezomib [39] A VMP regimen using bortezomib 1.3 mg/m^2 once weekly from the start of therapy showed reduced neurotoxicity and delivered a similar cumulative dose of bortezomib to that in VISTA, and resulted in similar efficacy [82]
Grade 1 with pain or Grade 2 (with no pain, but limiting instrumental activities of daily living)	For patients receiving twice-weekly bortezomib, reduce current dose by one level, or change to a once-per-week schedule using the same dose For patients receiving bortezomib on a once-per-week schedule: reduce current dose by one level, or consider temporary discontinuation; upon resolution (Grade ≤1), restart once-per-week dosing at lower dose level in cases of favorable benefit-to-risk ratio	Early reduction of bortezomib from 1.3 mg/m^2 twice weekly to once weekly in patients receiving VMP showed reduced neurotoxicity, delivered similar cumulative dose of bortezomib to that in VISTA, and resulted in similar efficacy [41] Dose-reduction strategies including dose reduction from 1.3 to 1.0 mg/m^2, changing from twice-weekly to once-weekly dosing, and withholding of bortezomib resulted in improvement or resolution of peripheral neuropathy in most patients with bortezomib-related peripheral neuropathy [81, 40]
Grade 2 with pain, Grade 3 (limiting self care and activities of daily living), or Grade 4	Discontinue bortezomib	Discontinuation as part of a peripheral neuropathy management strategy resulted in improvement or resolution of clinically significant neuropathy in 71 % of patients in an analysis of two phase 2 studies of bortezomib [39]

Source: Leukemia (2012) 26, 595–608. © 2012 Macmillan Publishers Limited All rights reserved 0887-6924/12. www.nature.com/leu

In part A, grading for this currently recommended dose-modification guideline is based on National Cancer Institute Common Terminology Criteria for Adverse Events (NCI CTCAE) version 3.0. In APEX, the dose-modification guideline used was the same, but based on NCI CTC version 2.0 grading; in addition, patients experiencing Grade 3 peripheral neuropathy with pain were to discontinue bortezomib. In part B, as for part A, grading is based on NCI CTCAE v3.0
MM multiple myeloma, *VMP* bortezomib, melphalan–prednisone

5 % require discontinuation of treatment [2, 39] (Table 20.3). The use of once-weekly dosing [41] or twice weekly, but via subcutaneous administration [42], can reduce rates of neuropathy. The neuropathy is of mild (Grade 1) to moderate (Grade 2) severity in 22 % [43]. Severe weakness (Grade 3 or 4) occurs in 14 % and interferes with ability to perform daily activities [43]. Grade 3 or Grade 4 peripheral neuropathy is more frequent in patients with preexisting neuropathy [2, 39].

The typical bortezomib-induced neuropathy is often a painful sensory predominant and length-dependent neuropathy [43]. Several types of neuropathic pain symptoms are described including allodynia, paresthesia, burning, electrical shocks, and lightning-like pain. Quantitative sensory testing (QST) shows that there is dysfunction in all fiber types in sensory nerves. Impaired Aβ and C sensory function also extends into areas of skin that are not perceived as affected by pain [44].

On QST, patients have significantly elevated touch-detection threshold and slotted peg board time (assess dexterity), impaired pinprick detection, and elevated thresholds for the detection of skin warming and heat pain [44]. NCS most often demonstrate low-amplitude sensory nerve action potentials consistent with axonal injury [39]. The neuropathy often improves or resolves within weeks when a dose-modification algorithm is used (64–71 %) [39, 40]. The median time to improvement of resolution is 110 days [40].

In addition to the common painful neuropathy in patients receiving bortezomib, there is a small subgroup of patients that develop a severe neuropathy soon after commencing bortezomib [40, 45, 46]. These patients present with a severe, motor-predominant polyradiculoneuropathy with less prominent pain, areflexia, electrophysiological features of conduction block, elevated CSF protein, and mild nerve T2 hyperintensity [46, 47]. Nerve biopsy has demonstrated inflammatory collections [45] which in one case had diagnostic evidence of microvasculitis [47].

Lenalidomide: Neuropathy in patients with MM treated with lenalidomide appears to be much less common than bortezomib. It may affect up to 25 % of patients treated with lenalidomide but it does not usually cause a greater than a Grade 2 neuropathy [48–51]. The neuropathy in these patients was not as well defined as in the bortezomib studies.

Thalidomide: The incidence of thalidomide-induced neuropathy depends on the dosage and treatment duration. Up to 50 % of patients taking thalidomide for conditions other than MM may develop a neuropathy [52]. In MM patients, the neuropathy might occur more frequently, because of either the higher dosage or underlying neuropathy associated with myeloma. Thus, neuropathy may occur in 58–81 % of patients with underlying myeloma [53, 54]. The symptoms of thalidomide neuropathy can present after treatment has stopped [34]. Patients usually present with sensory more than motor complaints. Sensory complaints may be in the form of either painful paresthesias or numbness. These symptoms typically begin in the feet and progress to involve the hands in a stocking-glove fashion. If weakness is present, it is usually mild and can present as tremor. Neurological examination demonstrates reduced light touch, vibration, and pinprick in the feet. There may be mild distal weakness and reduced ankle reflexes [55, 56]. Symptoms may progress for several months after stopping thalidomide and then stabilize or improve. NCS demonstrate reduced sensory nerve action potentials and may show reduced compound muscle action potentials as well [55, 57–61].

Some authors demonstrated there may be additional dorsal root ganglia involvement [59]. Patients with sensory ganglionopathy have a different clinical presentation than the length-dependent sensorimotor polyneuropathy. There is gait ataxia that worsens with eye closure, loss of large fiber sensation (vibration and proprioception) which can cause pseudoathetosis. Pain and temperature sensation and muscle strength are preserved. Reflexes are usually diffusely absent. NCS demonstrate absent sensory nerve action potentials. SSEPs usually show absent spinal and cortical potentials which are very suggestive of ganglionopathy [59]. Peripheral nerve biopsies show loss of predominantly large myelinated fibers, myelin ovoids, lack of inflammation, and a few regenerative clusters [55].

The severity and reversibility of the neuropathy depend on the length of the treatment and the cumulative dose [55, 56] and nerve damage may not be reversible. Care should be taken when patients are on this drug for a long duration (e.g., more than 200 mg/day for more than a year) [61]. As with bortezomib, genetic factors and underlying neuropathy may play an important role in determining the risk for developing a neuropathy in patients receiving thalidomide [62].

Vincristine: The incidence of vincristine-induced neuropathy in MM is 10–15 % [63–65] but as high as 34 % in one study possibly due to bolus administration [66]. Vincristine neuropathy is typically a distal symmetric sensorimotor peripheral neuropathy [67]. Frequently, paresthesias are the first symptom and begin in the fingers before the feet. With further exposure patients develop loss of pinprick and touch sensation and progress to distal sensory loss in the hands and feet. Weakness and autonomic dysfunction can be prominent features. NCS demonstrate reduced sensory nerve action potentials and compound muscle action potentials consistent with axonal neuropathy [68]. Peripheral nerve biopsies demonstrate axonal degeneration [69]. Most patients improve with withdrawal of the drug; however, mild distal sensory loss often persists [68].

POEMS Syndrome

The polyneuropathy in POEMS syndrome (polyneuropathy, organomegaly, endocrinopathy, M protein, and skin changes) is more studied than MM-associated polyneuropathies but it is unclear whether the pathophysiology is different. Peripheral neuropathy is a major criteria required for the diagnosis of POEMS syndrome. In addition, whereas MM-related neuropathy appears to be axonal or at least mixed axonal and demyelinating, the neuropathy in POEMS syndrome is predominantly demyelinating. Patients with POEMS syndrome usually present with distal, symmetric, progressive weakness and sensory changes in the legs more than the arms [26]. Patients have positive sensory symptoms in their legs and hands, and less frequently pain. Pain can be prominent in some patients but autonomic symptoms are infrequent. Complaints of weakness are more prominent than sensory complaints in these patients, and many are severely incapacitated [26]. Patients with POEMS should be distinguished from patients with chronic inflammatory demyelinating polyneuropathy (CIDP) [70, 71]. NCS are helpful in distinguishing POEMS patients from CIDP as there is greater reduction of motor amplitudes, greater slowing of motor and sensory conduction velocities, less prolonged motor distal latencies, less frequent temporal dispersion and conduction block, no sural sparing, greater number of fibrillation potentials in a length-dependent pattern, and higher terminal latency indices [71]. Levels of vascular endothelial growth factor and interleukin 12 are increased in POEMS syndrome and may be useful for diagnosis and as a measure of disease activity [72, 73].

Management of the Polyneuropathy in Patients with MM

Management of polyneuropathies in general focuses on several approaches: (1) identifying the cause of the neuropathy, (2) treating of the cause of the neuropathy, (3) removing offending agents, (4) treating neuropathy symptoms, and (5) attending to rehabilitation needs.

As discussed throughout this chapter, the neuropathy in patients with MM may be due to the disease itself or to the treatment. When it is related to the disease itself, prior to initiation of any therapy, it should be determined whether there is systemic amyloidosis (uncommon) or there is a paraneoplastic syndrome causing the neuropathy (more common but mechanism unknown). Melphalan, which is commonly used in patients with MM in combination with other chemotherapeutic agents, may have a modest effect on the amyloid itself [74]. However, the combination of melphalan with stem-cell transplantation may benefit the patients more, although it is unclear if it also affects the neuropathy [74]. For the treatment-related peripheral neuropathies, dose reduction or even stopping the treatment may be needed as outlined earlier in this chapter. For the positive sensory symptoms such as painful burning or tingling sensation, symptomatic management may be needed. These can include local treatments such as cold soaks of the feet, topical patches, or gels/creams. If the symptoms are not limited to the feet or the prior approach is not sufficient, systemic medications including calcium channel α_2-δ ligands, tricyclic antidepressants, or selective serotonin norepinephrine reuptake inhibitors can be used. Rarely opioids can be tried if patient has acute neuropathic pain or while titrating another agent. Autonomic involvement in patients with amyloidosis may be severe and the symptoms should be managed accordingly and may need a multisystemic approach with a urologist, cardiologist, and gastroenterologist. Physical and occupational therapy is often beneficial when there is muscle weakness or gait imbalance. Many patients with foot drop benefit from ankle foot orthoses. POEMS syndrome and other severe neuropathies can have prominent contractures and require vigilance in management.

Radiculopathy

Radiculopathy in patients with multiple myeloma is common. It may occur with or without a compressive myelopathy as described above. It usually occurs in the thoracic or lumbosacral area. The radiculopathy results from compression of the nerve by direct extension of the vertebral plasmacytoma lesion, foraminal stenosis secondary to the collapsed bone itself or, least commonly, leptomeningeal disease [75]. Patients with radiculopathy complain of pain radiating along the root dermatome. For instance if root compression is in the neck, the patient may complain of pain radiating from the neck down to the upper extremity sometimes to the fingertips. They may also have weakness in the limbs and signs of cord compression (see above). If the compression occurs in the thoracic region, patients may complain of band-like pain across the chest or abdomen in addition to cord compression symptoms. Depending on the rapidity and severity of the compression these symptoms may be indolent or acute. Urgent MRI or, if there is a contraindication to the MRI, CT scan of the spine is needed to confirm the diagnosis. Steroids and systemic chemotherapy may provide rapid relief of pain. If there is soft tissue component causing the stenosis, radiation may be of benefit.

Myopathy

Patient with multiple myeloma may have a myopathy that is either secondary to the disease itself or secondary to its treatment. When it is due to the disease, it is likely secondary to amyloid myopathy [76, 77]. Myopathy related to the treatment of MM can be seen in patients treated with (1) bortezomib which may cause rhabdomyolysis [78] or (2) more commonly secondary to steroid treatment [79]. Furthermore, patients may develop pyomyositis which if not recognized early can lead to septicemia and death [80]. The myopathy may be difficult to suspect and may be underdiagnosed because of the absence of sensory complaints and because weakness is usually multifactorial and attributed to the chronic systemic disease and treatment. A myopathy is suspected when the patient reports trouble getting out of a chair without using the arms, trouble climbing stairs, or trouble raising the arms above the head such us when reaching for items on a shelf or washing or combing the hair. Needle electromyography may help with confirming the diagnosis of myopathy. Rarely a muscle biopsy may be needed. The treatment of the myopathy depends on the cause. If the myopathy is due to high-dose steroids, reducing or stopping steroids is beneficial. Physical therapy is also helpful in patients with myopathies.

Summary

In the last few years, there has been many advances and improved survival in patients with multiple myeloma. However, patients with multiple myeloma frequently develop neurological complications secondary to the disease or its treatment and the incidence of these complications may rise because of improved life expectancy. The neurological complications may affect the CNS or PNS. Physicians treating patients with myeloma need to be aware and have a high suspicion of these complications. Prevention and/or prompt treatment may prevent permanent neurological damage. Initial and subsequent examinations and documentation of baseline and new neurological findings are essential, especially when trying to differentiate complications caused by the disease vs. its treatment. Imaging and nerve biopsy may aid in diagnosis and may direct the physician to the correct treatment. Genetic studies may help prevent treatment-emergent peripheral neuropathies in the future.

References

1. Plasmati R, Pastorelli F, Cavo M, Petracci E, Zamagni E, Tosi P, et al. Neuropathy in multiple myeloma treated with thalidomide: a prospective study. Neurology. 2007;69(6):573–81.
2. Richardson PG, Xie W, Mitsiades C, Chanan-Khan AA, Lonial S, Hassoun H, et al. Single-agent bortezomib in previously untreated multiple myeloma: efficacy, characterization of peripheral neuropathy, and molecular correlations with response and neuropathy. J Clin Oncol. 2009;27(21):3518–25.
3. Dispenzieri A, Kyle RA. Neurological aspects of multiple myeloma and related disorders. Best Pract Res Clin Haematol. 2005;18(4):673–88.
4. Fassas AB, Ward S, Muwalla F, Van Hemert R, Schluterman K, Harik S, et al. Myeloma of the central nervous system: strong association with unfavorable chromosomal abnormalities and other high-risk disease features. Leuk Lymphoma. 2004;45(2):291–300.
5. Smestad C, Monstad P, Lindboe CF, Mygland A. Amyloid myopathy presenting with distal atrophic weakness. Muscle Nerve. 2004;29(4):605–9.
6. Camacho J, Arnalich F, Anciones B, Pena JM, Gil A, Barbado FJ, et al. The spectrum of neurological manifestations in myeloma. J Med. 1985;16(5–6):597–611.
7. Hogan MC, Lee A, Solberg LA, Thome SD. Unusual presentation of multiple myeloma with unilateral visual loss and numb chin syndrome in a young adult. Am J Hematol. 2002;70(1):55–9.
8. Matsuzaki H, Hata H, Sonoki T, Matsuno F, Kuribayashi N, Yoshida M, et al. Serum amino acid disturbance in multiple myeloma with hyperammonemia. Int J Hematol. 1995;61(3):131–7.
9. Talamo G, Cavallo F, Zangari M, Barlogie B, Lee CK, Pineda-Roman M, et al. Hyperammonemia and encephalopathy in patients with multiple myeloma. Am J Hematol. 2007;82(5):414–5.
10. Otsuki T, Yamada O, Sakaguchi H, Ichiki T, Kouguchi K, Wada H, et al. In vitro excess ammonia production in human myeloma cell lines. Leukemia. 1998;12(7): 1149–58.
11. Kwan L, Wang C, Levitt L. Hyperammonemic encephalopathy in multiple myeloma. N Engl J Med. 2002;346(21):1674–5.
12. Swash M, Rowan AJ. Electroencephalographic criteria of hypocalcemia and hypercalcemia. Arch Neurol. 1972;26(3):218–28.
13. Lourbopoulos A, Ioannidis P, Balogiannis I, Stavrinou P, Koletsa T, Karacostas D. Cervical epidural plasmacytoma presenting as ascending paraparesis. Spine J. 2011;11(5):e1–4.
14. Okacha N, Chrif E, Brahim E, Ali A, Abderrahman E, Gazzaz M, et al. Extraosseous epidural multiple myeloma presenting with thoracic spine compression. Joint Bone Spine. 2008;75(1):70–2.
15. Zeng Z, Zheng L, Lin J, Chen J. Successful bortezomib treatment in combination with dexamethasone and thalidomide for previously untreated epidural plasmacytoma. Oncol Lett. 2012;3(3):557–9.
16. Svien HJ, Price RD, Bayrd ED. Neurosurgical treatment of compression of the spinal cord caused by myeloma. J Am Med Assoc. 1953;153(9):784–6.
17. Lupu VD, Saini N, Balish M. CNS myelomatosis. Neurology. 2005;64(6):1007.
18. Yaman E, Benekli M, Coskun U, Sezer K, Ozturk B, Kaya AO, et al. Intrasellar plasmacytoma: an unusual presentation of multiple myeloma. Acta Neurochir. 2008;150(9):921–4; discussion 4.
19. Sheng B, Mak VW, Lee HK, Li HL, Lee IP, Wong S. Multiple myeloma presenting with acute disseminated encephalomyelitis: causal or chance link? Neurology. 2006;67(10):1893–4.
20. Vokaer M, de Zegers Beyl D, Bier JC. Multiple myeloma presenting with acute disseminated encephalomyelitis: causal or chance link? Neurology. 2007; 68(21):1873–4; author reply 4.
21. Clow EC, Couban S, Grant IA. Stiff-person syndrome associated with multiple myeloma following autologous bone marrow transplantation. Muscle Nerve. 2008;38(6):1649–52.
22. Schiff D, Dalmau J, Myers DJ. Anti-GAD antibody positive stiff-limb syndrome in multiple myeloma. J Neurooncol. 2003;65(2):173–5.
23. Adams BD, Baker R, Lopez JA, Spencer S. Myeloproliferative disorders and the hyperviscosity syndrome. Emerg Med Clin North Am. 2009;27(3) :459–76.
24. Mehta J, Singhal S. Hyperviscosity syndrome in plasma cell dyscrasias. Semin Thromb Hemost. 2003; 29(5):467–71.
25. Gupta A, Pandey A, Sethi S. Bortezomib-induced congestive cardiac failure in a patient with multiple myeloma. Cardiovasc Toxicol. 2012;12(2):184–7.
26. Kelly Jr JJ, Kyle RA, Miles JM, O'Brien PC, Dyck PJ. The spectrum of peripheral neuropathy in myeloma. Neurology. 1981;31(1):24–31.
27. Walsh JC. The neuropathy of multiple myeloma. An electrophysiological and histological study. Arch Neurol. 1971;25(5):404–14.
28. Malhotra P, Choudhary PP, Lal V, Varma N, Suri V, Varma S. Prevalence of peripheral neuropathy in multiple myeloma at initial diagnosis. Leuk Lymphoma. 2011;52(11):2135–8.
29. Stork AC, van der Pol WL, van Kessel D, Lokhorst HM, Notermans NC. Effect of stem cell transplantation for B-cell malignancies on disease course of associated polyneuropathy. J Neurol. 2012;259(10): 2100–4.
30. Ansari-Lari MA, Ali SZ. Fine-needle aspiration of abdominal fat pad for amyloid detection: a clinically useful test? Diagn Cytopathol. 2004;30(3):178–81.
31. Murakami T, Tachibana S, Endo Y, Kawai R, Hara M, Tanase S, et al. Familial carpal tunnel syndrome due to amyloidogenic transthyretin His 114 variant. Neurology. 1994;44(2):315–8.
32. Jagannath S, Durie BG, Wolf JL, Camacho ES, Irwin D, Lutzky J, et al. Extended follow-up of a phase 2 trial of bortezomib alone and in combination with dexamethasone for the frontline treatment of multiple myeloma. Br J Haematol. 2009;146(6):619–26.

33. Cavaletti G, Gilardini A, Canta A, Rigamonti L, Rodriguez-Menendez V, Ceresa C, et al. Bortezomib-induced peripheral neurotoxicity: a neurophysiological and pathological study in the rat. Exp Neurol. 2007;204(1):317–25.
34. Richardson PG, Delforge M, Beksac M, Wen P, Jongen JL, Sezer O, et al. Management of treatment-emergent peripheral neuropathy in multiple myeloma. Leukemia. 2012;26(4):595–608.
35. Jagannath S, Barlogie B, Berenson J, Siegel D, Irwin D, Richardson PG, et al. A phase 2 study of two doses of bortezomib in relapsed or refractory myeloma. Br J Haematol. 2004;127(2):165–72.
36. Richardson PG, Barlogie B, Berenson J, Singhal S, Jagannath S, Irwin D, et al. A phase 2 study of bortezomib in relapsed, refractory myeloma. N Engl J Med. 2003;348(26):2609–17.
37. Richardson PG, Sonneveld P, Schuster MW, Irwin D, Stadtmauer EA, Facon T, et al. Bortezomib or high-dose dexamethasone for relapsed multiple myeloma. N Engl J Med. 2005;352(24):2487–98.
38. San Miguel JF, Schlag R, Khuageva NK, Dimopoulos MA, Shpilberg O, Kropff M, et al. Bortezomib plus melphalan and prednisone for initial treatment of multiple myeloma. N Engl J Med. 2008;359(9):906–17.
39. Richardson PG, Briemberg H, Jagannath S, Wen PY, Barlogie B, Berenson J, et al. Frequency, characteristics, and reversibility of peripheral neuropathy during treatment of advanced multiple myeloma with bortezomib. J Clin Oncol. 2006;24(19):3113–20.
40. Richardson PG, Sonneveld P, Schuster MW, Stadtmauer EA, Facon T, Harousseau JL, et al. Reversibility of symptomatic peripheral neuropathy with bortezomib in the phase III APEX trial in relapsed multiple myeloma: impact of a dose-modification guideline. Br J Haematol. 2009;144(6):895–903.
41. Mateos MV, Oriol A, Martinez-Lopez J, Gutierrez N, Teruel AI, de Paz R, et al. Bortezomib, melphalan, and prednisone versus bortezomib, thalidomide, and prednisone as induction therapy followed by maintenance treatment with bortezomib and thalidomide versus bortezomib and prednisone in elderly patients with untreated multiple myeloma: a randomised trial. Lancet Oncol. 2010;11(10):934–41.
42. Moreau P, Pylypenko H, Grosicki S, Karamanesht I, Leleu X, Grishunina M, et al. Subcutaneous versus intravenous administration of bortezomib in patients with relapsed multiple myeloma: a randomised, phase 3, non-inferiority study. Lancet Oncol. 2011;12(5):431–40.
43. Argyriou AA, Iconomou G, Kalofonos HP. Bortezomib-induced peripheral neuropathy in multiple myeloma: a comprehensive review of the literature. Blood. 2008;112(5):1593–9.
44. Cata JP, Weng HR, Burton AW, Villareal H, Giralt S, Dougherty PM. Quantitative sensory findings in patients with bortezomib-induced pain. J Pain. 2007;8(4):296–306.
45. Saifee TA, Elliott KJ, Lunn MP, Blake J, Reilly MM, Rabin N, et al. Bortezomib-induced inflammatory neuropathy. J Peripher Nerv Syst. 2010;15(4):366–8.
46. Ravaglia S, Corso A, Piccolo G, Lozza A, Alfonsi E, Mangiacavalli S, et al. Immune-mediated neuropathies in myeloma patients treated with bortezomib. Clin Neurophysiol. 2008;119(11):2507–12.
47. Mauermann ML, Blumenreich MS, Dispenzieri A, Staff NP. A case of peripheral nerve microvasculitis associated with multiple myeloma and bortezomib treatment. Muscle Nerve. 2012;46(6):970–7.
48. Chanan-Khan AA, Lonial S, Weber D, Borrello I, Foa R, Hellmann A, et al. Lenalidomide in combination with dexamethasone improves survival and time-to-progression in patients ≥65 years old with relapsed or refractory multiple myeloma. Int J Hematol. 2012; 96(2):254–62.
49. Kroger N, Zabelina T, Klyuchnikov E, Kropff M, Pfluger KH, Burchert A, et al. Toxicity-reduced, myeloablative allograft followed by lenalidomide maintenance as salvage therapy for refractory/relapsed myeloma patients. Bone Marrow Transplant. 2012; 48(3):403–7.
50. Jakubowiak AJ, Dytfeld D, Griffith KA, Lebovic D, Vesole DH, Jagannath S, et al. A phase 1/2 study of carfilzomib in combination with lenalidomide and low-dose dexamethasone as a frontline treatment for multiple myeloma. Blood. 2012;120(9):1801–9.
51. Berenson JR, Yellin O, Kazamel T, Hilger JD, Chen CS, Cartmell A, et al. A phase 2 study of pegylated liposomal doxorubicin, bortezomib, dexamethasone and lenalidomide for patients with relapsed/refractory multiple myeloma. Leukemia. 2012;26(7):1675–80.
52. Bastuji-Garin S, Ochonisky S, Bouche P, Gherardi RK, Duguet C, Djerradine Z, et al. Incidence and risk factors for thalidomide neuropathy: a prospective study of 135 dermatologic patients. J Invest Dermatol. 2002;119(5):1020–6.
53. Rajkumar SV, Hayman S, Gertz MA, Dispenzieri A, Lacy MQ, Greipp PR, et al. Combination therapy with thalidomide plus dexamethasone for newly diagnosed myeloma. J Clin Oncol. 2002;20(21):4319–23.
54. Rajkumar SV, Dispenzieri A, Fonseca R, Lacy MQ, Geyer S, Lust JA, et al. Thalidomide for previously untreated indolent or smoldering multiple myeloma. Leukemia. 2001;15(8):1274–6.
55. Chaudhry V, Cornblath DR, Corse A, Freimer M, Simmons-O'Brien E, Vogelsang G. Thalidomide-induced neuropathy. Neurology. 2002;59(12):1872–5.
56. Fullerton PM, Kremer M. Neuropathy after intake of thalidomide (distaval). Br Med J. 1961;2(5256): 855–8.
57. Lagueny A, Rommel A, Vignolly B, Taieb A, Vendeaud-Busquet M, Doutre MS, et al. Thalidomide neuropathy: an electrophysiologic study. Muscle Nerve. 1986;9(9):837–44.
58. Molloy FM, Floeter MK, Syed NA, Sandbrink F, Culcea E, Steinberg SM, et al. Thalidomide neuropathy in patients treated for metastatic prostate cancer. Muscle Nerve. 2001;24(8):1050–7.
59. Giannini F, Volpi N, Rossi S, Passero S, Fimiani M, Cerase A. Thalidomide-induced neuropathy: a ganglionopathy? Neurology. 2003;60(5):877–8.

60. Mileshkin L, Stark R, Day B, Seymour JF, Zeldis JB, Prince HM. Development of neuropathy in patients with myeloma treated with thalidomide: patterns of occurrence and the role of electrophysiologic monitoring. J Clin Oncol. 2006;24(27):4507–14.
61. Richardson P, Schlossman R, Jagannath S, Alsina M, Desikan R, Blood E, et al. Thalidomide for patients with relapsed multiple myeloma after high-dose chemotherapy and stem cell transplantation: results of an open-label multicenter phase 2 study of efficacy, toxicity, and biological activity. Mayo Clin Proc. 2004; 79(7):875–82.
62. Johnson DC, Corthals SL, Walker BA, Ross FM, Gregory WM, Dickens NJ, et al. Genetic factors underlying the risk of thalidomide-related neuropathy in patients with multiple myeloma. J Clin Oncol. 2011;29(7):797–804.
63. Harousseau JL, Attal M, Avet-Loiseau H, Marit G, Caillot D, Mohty M, et al. Bortezomib plus dexamethasone is superior to vincristine plus doxorubicin plus dexamethasone as induction treatment prior to autologous stem-cell transplantation in newly diagnosed multiple myeloma: results of the IFM 2005–01 phase III trial. J Clin Oncol. 2010; 28(30):4621–9.
64. Dimopoulos MA, Pouli A, Zervas K, Grigoraki V, Symeonidis A, Repoussis P, et al. Prospective randomized comparison of vincristine, doxorubicin and dexamethasone (VAD) administered as intravenous bolus injection and VAD with liposomal doxorubicin as first-line treatment in multiple myeloma. Ann Oncol. 2003;14(7):1039–44.
65. Sonneveld P, Suciu S, Weijermans P, Beksac M, Neuwirtova R, Solbu G, et al. Cyclosporin A combined with vincristine, doxorubicin and dexamethasone (VAD) compared with VAD alone in patients with advanced refractory multiple myeloma: an EORTC-HOVON randomized phase III study (06914). Br J Haematol. 2001;115(4): 895–902.
66. Oken MM, Harrington DP, Abramson N, Kyle RA, Knospe W, Glick JH. Comparison of melphalan and prednisone with vincristine, carmustine, melphalan, cyclophosphamide, and prednisone in the treatment of multiple myeloma: results of Eastern Cooperative Oncology Group Study E2479. Cancer. 1997;79(8): 1561–7.
67. Pal PK. Clinical and electrophysiological studies in vincristine induced neuropathy. Electromyogr Clin Neurophysiol. 1999;39(6):323–30.
68. Casey EB, Jellife AM, Le Quesne PM, Millett YL. Vincristine neuropathy. Clinical and electrophysiological observations. Brain. 1973;96(1):69–86.
69. McLeod JG, Penny R. Vincristine neuropathy: an electrophysiological and histological study. J Neurol Neurosurg Psychiatry. 1969;32(4):297–304.
70. Nasu S, Misawa S, Sekiguchi Y, Shibuya K, Kanai K, Fujimaki Y, et al. Different neurological and physiological profiles in POEMS syndrome and chronic inflammatory demyelinating polyneuropathy. J Neurol Neurosurg Psychiatry. 2012;83(5):476–9.
71. Mauermann ML, Sorenson EJ, Dispenzieri A, Mandrekar J, Suarez GA, Dyck PJ. Uniform demyelination and more severe axonal loss distinguish POEMS syndrome from CIDP. J Neurol Neurosurg Psychiatry. 2012;83(5):480–6.
72. Kanai K, Sawai S, Sogawa K, Mori M, Misawa S, Shibuya K, et al. Markedly upregulated serum interleukin-12 as a novel biomarker in POEMS syndrome. Neurology. 2012;79(6):575–82.
73. D'Souza A, Hayman SR, Buadi F, Mauermann M, Lacy MQ, Gertz MA, et al. The utility of plasma vascular endothelial growth factor levels in the diagnosis and follow-up of patients with POEMS syndrome. Blood. 2011;118(17):4663–5.
74. Skinner M, Sanchorawala V, Seldin DC, Dember LM, Falk RH, Berk JL, et al. High-dose melphalan and autologous stem-cell transplantation in patients with AL amyloidosis: an 8-year study. Ann Intern Med. 2004;140(2):85–93.
75. Brenner B, Carter A, Freidin N, Malberger E, Tatarsky I. Pancoast's syndrome in multiple myeloma. Acta Haematol. 1984;71(5):353–5.
76. Prayson RA. Amyloid myopathy: clinicopathologic study of 16 cases. Hum Pathol. 1998;29(5):463–8.
77. Lawson TM, Bevan MA, Williams BD. Clinical images: skeletal muscle pseudo-hypertrophy in myeloma-associated amyloidosis. Arthritis Rheum. 2002;46(8):2251.
78. Cibeira MT, Mercadal S, Arenillas L, Muntanola A, Salamero O, Blade J. Bortezomib-induced rhabdomyolysis in multiple myeloma. Acta Haematol. 2006;116(3):203–6.
79. Perrot S, Le Jeunne C. Steroid-induced myopathy. Presse Med. 2012;41(4):422–6.
80. Kalambokis G, Theodorou A, Kosta P, Tsianos EV. Multiple myeloma presenting with pyomyositis caused by community-acquired methicillin-resistant Staphylococcus aureus: report of a case and literature review. Int J Hematol. 2008;87(5):516–9.
81. Dimopoulos MA, Mateos MV, Richardson PG, Schlag R, Khuageva NK, Shpilberg O et al. Risk factors for, and reversibility of, peripheral neuropathy associated with bortezomib-melphalan-prednisone in newly diagnosed patients with multiple myeloma: subanalysis of the phase 3 VISTA study. Eur J Haematol. 2011;86:23–31.
82. Bringhen S, Larocca A, Rossi D, Cavalli M, Genuardi M, Ria R et al. Efficacy and safety of once weekly bortezomib in multiple myeloma patients. Blood 2010;116:4745–4753.

21 Myeloma Cast Nephropathy

Nelson Leung

Introduction

Myeloma cast nephropathy (MCN) is the sine qua non renal lesion of multiple myeloma (MM). It was first reported in 1909, some 60 years after the description of Bence Jones protein [1]. Studies have now confirmed Bence Jones protein to be the same as monoclonal immunoglobulin free light chain (FLC) [2]. The term "cast nephropathy" was first used by Oliver in 1945 to describe the intraluminal obstruction of renal tubules by monoclonal FLC casts and the resulting inflammatory reaction around these tubules. Other than rare incidences where MCN can be the result of a lymphoplasmacytic lymphoma, it is always associated with MM [3]. While other renal lesions can be seen with low-grade plasma cell dyscrasias, lymphoproliferative disorders, and MM, the development of MCN signifies the progression of monoclonal gammopathy of undetermined significance (MGUS) or smoldering multiple myeloma (SMM) to symptomatic multiple myeloma (MM) [4].

Even though cast nephropathy is the signature lesion of MM, it is not defined in the CRAB (hyper*C*alcemia, *R*enal impairment, *A*nemia and *B*one lesions) criteria. Renal involvement is defined as a serum creatinine (Scr) of >2 mg/dL attributable to the plasma cell dyscrasia [5]. Because several other lesions may be responsible for the renal impairment in MM, the criterion is made general to encompass all causes [6]. Unfortunately, this has also made it more difficult to study cast nephropathy as patients enrolled in some trials had only acute renal failure with MM but not necessarily MCN. Currently, the only method capable of accurately diagnosing MCN is a kidney biopsy. In practice, this is not always feasible as patients may be anticoagulated or have coagulopathy. It is therefore important to keep this in mind when interpreting studies that involve MM patients with renal impairment as a percentage of these patients may not have MCN which may impact the results.

Incidence

The true incidence of cast nephropathy is unknown. Acute renal impairment as defined by an Scr of 2 mg/dL or more is present in approximately 20 % of the newly diagnosed patients with MM [7]. The incidence is higher with more advanced disease. For example, Durie-Salmon stage III disease is diagnosed in 44 % of patients with normal Scr vs. 87 % of patients with Scr > 2 mg/dL. Unfortunately, this does not indicate the prevalence of MCN since several renal lesions are associated with MM. MCN was found in 32 % of patients in one autopsy study making

N. Leung, M.D. (✉)
Division of Hematology, Mayo Clinic, 200 First Street, Southwest, Rochester, MN 55905, USA
e-mail: leung.nelson@mayo.edu

M.A. Gertz and S.V. Rajkumar (eds.), *Multiple Myeloma: Diagnosis and Treatment*,
DOI 10.1007/978-1-4614-8520-9_21, © Mayo Foundation for Medical Education and Research 2014

it the most common renal lesion in that study [8]. In this series, immunoglobulin light chain (AL) amyloidosis was found in 11 % and light chain deposition disease was found in 5 %. In another autopsy study, MCN was noted in up to 48–62 % of patients [9]. Five percent of the patients from this study had AL amyloidosis. Interestingly, nephrocalcinosis was seen in 42 % of patients and 10 % had plasma cell infiltrates. Pyelonephritis was also seen in 20 % of the patients from this study. In a renal biopsy study of 190 patients with MM from the Mayo Clinic, 33 % had MCN, 22 % had monoclonal immunoglobulin deposition disease (MIDD), and 21 % had AL amyloidosis [6]. In addition, acute tubular necrosis (ATN) was noted in 9 %, acute interstitial nephritis in 2 %, and up to 25 % of the patient had a non-paraprotein-related kidney injury. It is important to point out that since the indication for the renal biopsy is not the same for all diseases, the incidences are not likely to reflect the true values. On the other hand, these studies all indicate that MCN is not the only renal disease that can affect these patients.

Clinical Manifestations

MCN can be the first manifestation of MM or may occur during relapse disease [10]. MCN usually presents as acute renal failure resulting in an acute rise in Scr over a period of days. The severity of renal impairment is variable and can range from modest to severe requiring dialysis. Unfortunately, MCN is often asymptomatic until uremic symptoms appear. Symptoms such as lower extremity edema and severe hypertension are usually absent as they are more typical of glomerular diseases while damage from MCN is purely confined to the tubulointerstitial compartment.

Several risk factors have been identified to be associated with MCN. One of the most important is the presence of urinary FLC. The risk of renal impairment is up to 25-folds higher in patients with high urinary FLC excretion vs. those without [11]. In patients with >12 g/g (FLC/creatinine) the risk of renal impairment is approximately 50 %. Other risk factors include nonsteroidal anti-inflammatory drugs (NSAIDs), dehydration (vomiting and diarrhea), infection, and intravenous contrast [12]. NSAIDs are sometimes taken or prescribed as a result of back pain due to boney lesions or compression fracture. Vomiting and diarrhea can precipitate MCN through dehydration. Whether intravenous contrast is truly a risk factor of MCN is debatable but one study found the incidence of acute renal failure in increasing approximately fivefolds in patients with multiple myeloma. The commonality of these risk factors is an alteration in the intrarenal hemodynamics. This may also explain why the use of angiotensin converting enzyme (ACE) inhibitors has been reported to precipitate MCN [13].

One of the most striking features of MCN is the inferior survival reported in patients who develop acute renal failure. In one study, the median survival was 36 months for patients with normal renal function vs. 18 and 13 months for those who had moderate and severe renal failure, respectively [14]. Results were similar in another study where the median survival of patients with normal renal function was 34.5 months and 8.6 months in patients with renal failure [7]. Even more important is the fact that both studies found recovery of renal function was associated with improved survival. In fact, patients who recovered their renal function had similar survival to those who never developed renal failure. On the other hand, patients with irreversible renal failure had a median survival as short as 3.8 months [7]. Recently, the impact of renal impairment on survival has been called into question. A retrospective study evaluating 203 patients treated with novel agents (thalidomide, lenalidomide, and bortezomib) found that while an estimate glomerular filtration rate (eGFR) of <60 mL/min/1.73 m^2 was associated with poorer survival in the univariate analysis, it was not significant in the multivariate analysis [15]. The factors associated with survival from this study were age ≤75 years, platelet ≤ 130 × 10^9/L, international staging system (ISS) stage, LDH ≥ 300 IU/L. The benefits of bortezomib were also demonstrated in a recent phase III trial comparing vincristine doxorubicin dexamethasone (VAD) to bortezomib doxorubicin dexamethasone (PAD) for induction therapy followed by autologous stem cell transplantation and maintenance therapy with thalidomide in the

VAD-treated group and bortezomib in the PAD group [16]. Significant improvement in both progression-free survival (PFS) and overall survival (OS) was seen in the patients with renal impairment treated with PAD as compared to ones treated with VAD. The biggest effect was in the first 12 months of therapy. It was unclear if bortezomib maintenance had an advantage over thalidomide.

Diagnosis of Cast Nephropathy

Currently, MCN can only be diagnosed via a kidney biopsy. On light microscopy, intraluminal casts are seen in the distal tubule of the nephron [17]. The appearance of these casts can be waxy to crystalline in nature. Shape edges can sometime be seen as a result of "fracture" during the slide preparation which is quite characteristic of light chain casts. The number of casts can vary and may have prognostic significance in regard to recovery of kidney function in some studies. Another characteristic feature is the presence of macrophage-derived giant cell reaction around the casts. Tubular rupture may occur as a result of the obstruction. Where this occurs, an intense inflammatory infiltrate can be seen resulting in an interstitial nephritis. On immunofluorescence study, only a single light chain corresponding to the circulating monoclonal immunoglobulin should stain in the casts.

While no other method can accurately distinguish among the different renal lesions, a recent study found urinary albumin excretion can be quite useful [18]. In a study of patients with biopsy-proven MCN, AL amyloidosis, MIDD, and ATN, urinary albumin excretion was the only parameter that can separate MCN from the other three lesions in the multivariate analysis. Patients with MCN have much lower albuminuria than patients with AL amyloidosis and MIDD. The median percentage of urine albumin in patients with MCN was 7 % vs. 70 % for AL amyloidosis and 55 % for MIDD. Patient with ATN had a median of 25 % albumin in the urine resulting in some overlap between MCN and ATN. Although it is not perfect, a low urinary albumin excretion strongly suggests the acute kidney injury is due to MCN.

Pathogenesis

The discovery of the urinary protein Tamm-Horsfall glycoprotein in light chain casts was a major advance in the understanding of the pathogenesis of MCN [19]. The binding and aggregation of FLC to THP is now recognized to be the essential step in formation of cast and development of MCN [20]. Normally, a small amount of polyclonal FLCs are present in the blood and are cleared by the kidney. They are freely filtered by the glomerulus and reabsorbed in the proximal tubule. Up to 30 g of FLC can be removed by the proximal tubule each day [21]. The small amount that is left is excreted in the urine without any problem. In patients with MM, the overproduction of FLC overwhelms the proximal tubules' ability to reabsorb all of the FLC. In addition, some monoclonal FLC are toxic to the proximal tubular cells further reducing the FLC reabsorption capability [10]. The result is a higher than usual concentration of FLC in the distal tubule. This by itself however is not enough for cast formation. Reports of patients excreting 10–20 g/day of Bence Jones protein without renal impairment are well recognized. In fact, the famous patient Thomas McBean whose urine was responsible for the discovery of Bence Jones protein was estimated to have excreted 67 g/day without any impairment to his kidney function and had no evidence of kidney disease on autopsy [22]. The most important aspect is the affinity of the FLC toward THP.

Studies have found that not all FLCs bind THP. Even among the ones that do, there is a wide range of affinity. A single binding site has been identified on THP that interacts with both κ and λ FLC. The binding site on FLC has been localized to complementarity determining region (CDR) specifically CDR3 [23]. Small changes in the amino acid sequence can have large effects on the affinity of an FLC toward THP. Therefore, in order for MCN to occur, there must be sufficient concentration of monoclonal FLC and significant affinity of the FLC toward THP. Studies have found that MCN is rare in patients without urinary FLC, yet high serum or urine FLC levels do not guarantee MCN. In a study of MM patients with renal biopsy, the patient with the highest serum FLC level (>8,000 mg/dL) did not have MCN but rather MIDD [24]. On the other hand, there appears to be a minimum concentration that is required for the cast formation. The lowest level of serum FLC reported to be associated with MCN was 85 mg/dL.

Treatment

Initially treatment of cast nephropathy is similar to other types of kidney injury. Effort should be made to reverse dehydration and discontinue all potential nephrotoxins. Studies have found increased cast formation with sodium chloride concentrations >80 mmol/L [25]. Therefore, in this setting half normal saline may be more advantageous than the isotonic normal saline. In addition, although a high urine output is usually desired, furosemide should be avoided unless it is necessary for volume overload because furosemide has been found to increase cast formation. It does this by increasing the sodium chloride concentration in the distal tubule, but furosemide has also been found to be capable of increasing co-aggregation of light chain to THP.

Rapid reduction of the serum FLC concentration is of the utmost importance with regard to recovery of renal function. In a study of patients treated with plasma exchange (PLEX), no patient with biopsy-proven cast nephropathy recovered renal function with less than a 50 % reduction in the serum FLC [24]. Similarly, a minimum of 50 % reduction was also noted in a pilot study using the high cutoff dialyzer to remove serum FLC [26]. Using the data from these studies, a mathematical model predicts that a 60 % reduction in serum FLC by day 14 is associated with an 80 % chance of recovery of renal function [27]. This was irrespective of the baseline FLC at the time of kidney injury.

Chemotherapy

Chemotherapy is essential for sustained reduction of serum FLC. One of the most effective agents in this setting is bortezomib. Bortezomib is a reversible proteasome inhibitor that has high activity against myeloma cells [28]. Because it is non-nephrotoxic and not renally metabolized or cleared, it can be used without dosage adjustment making it an excellent choice in patients with renal failure. In the VISTA trial, previously untreated patients were randomized to melphalan and prednisone (MP) vs. bortezomib melphalan and prednisone (VMP) [29]. The addition of bortezomib significantly increased the overall hematologic response rate from 47 % in the MP group to 71 % in the VMP group. In a subgroup analysis of patients with creatinine clearance (CrCl) of ≤30 mL/min, the addition of bortezomib to MP increased the hematologic complete response (CR) rate from 13 % (MP) to 37 % (VMP). The time to response was reduced from 3.4 months (MP) to 1.0 month (VMP) in the renally impaired patients. Reversal of renal impairment as defined by raising a baseline CrCl of <50 to >60 mL/min was experienced by more patients in the VMP group (44 %) than MP-treated patients (34 %). The biggest difference was in the patients whose baseline CrCl was <30 mL/min. In these patients, 37 % of the VMP-treated patients recovered to a CrCl of >60 mL/min vs. 7 % of the MP-treated patients.

A phase II study using PAD was performed on patients with acute renal failure (within 4 weeks of study) with eGFR of <50 mL/min/1.73 m^2 [30]. The study found PAD was able to achieve a hematologic response rate of 72 %. Median renal function improved from 20.5 to 48.4 mL/min. The improvement in renal function correlated with hematologic response. Patients who achieved a very good partial response (VGPR) or better had a median renal function of 59.6 mL/min compared with 38.9 mL/min in those with partial (PR) or minimal response (MR) and 16.8 mL/min in those who were only able to achieve stable disease (SD) or progressed.

A phase III trial was performed that compared VAD with PAD in patients from the Dutch-Belgium HOVON-65 trial and the German multicenter GMMG trial [16]. As a part of the trial, patients either received a single or double autologous stem cell transplantation depending on the original trial (HOVON-65 = single,

GMMG = double) the patient had been enrolled. Patients assigned to PAD were then given bortezomib as maintenance; VAD-treated patients were given thalidomide for 2 years as maintenance after ASCT. Eleven percent of the VAD-treated patients had a baseline Scr of >2 mg/dL as compared to 9 % in the PAD-treated group. Overall response (>partial response (PR)) rates were 83 % in the VAD group vs. 90 % in the PAD group, $p = 0.002$. CR rate was also superior in the PAD group with 36 % vs. 24 %, $p < 0.001$. In the subgroup analysis, PAD was found to be superior to VAD in patients with renal impairment in terms of both progression-free survival (PFS: 30 vs. 13 months) and overall survival (OS: 54 vs. 21 months), respectively. Renal impairment was found to be associated with inferior PFS and OS only in the VAD-treated patients but had no effect on the PAD-treated patients.

Extracorporeal Therapies

To date, three randomized trials had been performed to evaluate the benefit of extracorporeal removal of FLC. These trials all involve the use of PLEX. The first is the Zucchelli study involving 29 patients with severe acute renal failure with 83 % of the patients requiring dialysis at the time of study [31]. Renal biopsy was obtained on 17 patients. Patients were randomized to hemodialysis and PLEX ($n = 15$) while the control group ($n = 14$) received peritoneal dialysis. This study found 11 of the 13 patients who required dialysis in the PLEX group recovered renal function while only two in the control group recovered enough renal function to be dialysis-independent. The authors observed that patients who had significant reduction in the Bence Jones proteinuria were more likely to recover than those who did not. Not only was the study criticized for the difference in dialysis modalities, but also the higher early mortality in the control group. The Johnson study involved 21 patients again with severe acute renal failure [32]. Seven (64 %) of 11 patients in the PLEX group and 5 (50 %) of 10 patients in the control group required dialysis. This time, both groups received hemodialysis. Renal biopsy was obtained on 76 % of patients. This study found no difference in the recovery of renal function. Seven of the 11 patients randomized to receive PLEX recovered while 5 of 10 control patients also had improvement in renal function. In this study, of the patients who were dialysis-dependent, only those who received PLEX recovered renal function.

The largest study of PLEX was the Clark study where 104 patients were randomized to PLEX or control arm [33]. Seven patients either withdrew or were lost to follow-up thus the analysis was performed on 97 patients (58 in the PLEX arm and 39 in the control arm). The degree of renal impairment was less severe in this study as 35 % of the control group and 26 % of the PLEX group were dialysis-dependent at the time of the study. This study also used a composite end point which consisted of death, dialysis dependence, and eGFR of <30 mL/min/1.73 m^2. The results of this study found composite end point was reached in 57.9 % of the PLEX group and 69.2 % of the control group, $p = 0.36$. Excluding death, 36.8 % became dialysis-independent in the control group vs. 41.6 % in the PLEX-treated group. Morality at 6 months was similar (33.3 % control vs. 32.8 % PLEX) between the two groups. The authors concluded that PLEX was not superior. However, while the conclusion is applicable to patients with undifferentiated acute renal failure, it may not be applicable to MCN since few patients from the study had a renal biopsy. In addition, serum FLC was not measured as part of the study so it was unclear whether sufficient PLEX was performed. In a retrospective study evaluating factors that influence response to PLEX, the two most important factors that determined the renal outcome were diagnosis of MCN and >50 % reduction in serum FLC [24]. Thus, both of these factors need to be incorporated into future trials.

In addition to PLEX, the use of large pore dialyzers has been reported to be beneficial in the recovery of renal function. Using a dialyzer with a molecular weight cutoff of 50 kDa, 19 patients with biopsy-proven MCN were treated [26]. Dialysis independence was achieved for 14 patients (13 who completed chemotherapy and

1 of 6 who had chemotherapy withheld). Once again, no one with less than 50 % reduction of serum FLC recovered renal function. The promising results have inspired two randomized trials that are currently ongoing to evaluate the effectiveness of large pore dialyzers.

Non-chemotherapeutic Agents

Currently, treatments of MCN have focused on the reduction in FLC concentration either by killing of the plasma cells or removal as in PLEX and large pore dialyzers. However, two compounds have been reported to help recovery of renal function without treating the underlying MM. The first compound is pituitary adenylate cyclase-activating polypeptide (PACAP38) [34]. In addition to tubular obstruction, monoclonal FLCs have also been shown to produce intense inflammatory reaction via mitogen-activating protein kinases (MAPKs), extracellular signal-regulated kinases (ERKs), C-jun N-terminal kinases (JNK), p38 and most importantly nuclear factor kappa-light-chain-enhancer of activated B cells (NFκB). PACAP38 was able to inhibit the activation of ERK1/2, JNK, and p38 MAPKs in renal tubule cell culture. PACAP38 and dexamethasone completely suppressed the activation of NFκB by monoclonal FLC. In vivo study with PACAP38 shows near-complete suppression of TNFα where animals treated with sham and monoclonal FLC had a six-fold increase. PACAP38 were also found to suppress myeloma growth and IL-6 production by stromal cells especially when dexamethasone was added. However, therapeutic benefits in MCN remain undetermined for PACP38.

The first inhibitor of binding and cast formation was recently described. An inhibitor was created to block binding site between the CDR3 region of FLC and THP [35]. This oligopeptide inhibitor was fashioned after amino acid sequences known to have strong affinity toward THP. The inhibitory effect was further enhanced by cyclizing the synthetic peptide. Coadministration of this cyclized peptide with monoclonal FLC reduced cast formation and prevented acute kidney injury. Even more exciting was benefits demonstrated in a rescue experiment. The cyclized peptide was capable of reducing the rise in Scr and number of cast formed (6.2 ± 0.64 (vehicle) vs. 0.38 ± 0.16 (cyclized peptide)) 4 h after injection of monoclonal FLC. The cyclized peptide represents the first treatment of MCN not dependent on the response of the myeloma. Despite the optimism, the results are still preliminary and more study is needed to discover its full potential.

Summary

Although monoclonal gammopathy is associated with many kidney diseases, MCN is the one that is intimately linked to multiple myeloma. Its presence indicates the myeloma has become symptomatic and treatment is required. The pathogenesis of cast formation is promoted by high concentration of FLC in the distal tubule allowing the binding and coprecipitation with THP. Reversal of the renal injury requires rapid reduction of serum FLC levels by at least 60 %. In the past, acute renal failure in MM denotes a poor prognosis. However, this may have changed with the use of novel agents especially bortezomib which can be used without dosage adjustment in renal failure. Its rapid action may help recovery of renal function and reverse the adverse effect of renal failure. Recently, a molecule that blocks the binding of FLC to THP has been discovered and that is capable of reversing the renal failure without any effect on the FLC level. This opens the possibility of treating MCN without relying on response of the tumor to chemotherapy. Not only is this a huge advance in terms of treatment, but it also allows better understanding of the impact of renal failure in these patients by decoupling the recovery of renal function from response of the myeloma.

References

1. Leung N. Treating myeloma cast nephropathy without treating myeloma. J Clin Invest. 2012;122(5):1605–8.
2. Edelman GM, Gally JA. The nature of Bence-Jones proteins. Chemical similarities to polypetide chains of myeloma globulins and normal gamma-globulins. J Exp Med. 1962;116:207–27.

3. Perez NS, et al. Lymphoplasmacytic lymphoma causing light chain cast nephropathy. Nephrol Dial Transplant. 2012;27(1):450–3.
4. Leung N, Rajkumar SV. Renal manifestations of plasma cell disorders. Am J Kidney Dis. 2007;50(1):155–65.
5. Dimopoulos MA, et al. Renal impairment in patients with multiple myeloma: a consensus statement on behalf of the International Myeloma Working Group. J Clin Oncol. 2010;28(33):4976–84.
6. Nasr SH, et al. Clinicopathologic correlations in multiple myeloma: a case series of 190 patients with kidney biopsies. Am J Kidney Dis. 2012;59(6):786–94.
7. Blade J, et al. Renal failure in multiple myeloma: presenting features and predictors of outcome in 94 patients from a single institution. Arch Intern Med. 1998;158(17):1889–93.
8. Ivanyi B. Frequency of light chain deposition nephropathy relative to renal amyloidosis and Bence Jones cast nephropathy in a necropsy study of patients with myeloma. Arch Pathol Lab Med. 1990;114(9):986–7.
9. Kapadia SB. Multiple myeloma: a clinicopathologic study of 62 consecutively autopsied cases. Medicine. 1980;59(5):380–92.
10. Winearls CG. Acute myeloma kidney. Kidney Int. 1995;48(4):1347–61.
11. Drayson M, et al. Effects of paraprotein heavy and light chain types and free light chain load on survival in myeloma: an analysis of patients receiving conventional-dose chemotherapy in Medical Research Council UK multiple myeloma trials. Blood. 2006;108(6):2013–9.
12. Sanders PW, Booker BB. Pathobiology of cast nephropathy from human Bence Jones proteins. J Clin Invest. 1992;89(2):630–9.
13. Rabb H, et al. Acute renal failure from multiple myeloma precipitated by ACE inhibitors. Am J Kidney Dis. 1999;33(2):E5.
14. Knudsen LM, Hjorth M, Hippe E. Renal failure in multiple myeloma: reversibility and impact on the prognosis. Nordic Myeloma Study Group. Eur J Haematol. 2000;65(3):175–81.
15. Eleftherakis-Papapiakovou E, et al. Renal impairment is not an independent adverse prognostic factor in patients with multiple myeloma treated upfront with novel agent-based regimens. Leuk Lymphoma. 2011;52(12):2299–303.
16. Sonneveld P, et al. Bortezomib induction and maintenance treatment in patients with newly diagnosed multiple myeloma: results of the randomized phase III HOVON-65/GMMG-HD4 trial. J Clin Oncol. 2012;30(24):2946–55.
17. Markowitz GS. Dysproteinemia and the kidney. Adv Anat Pathol. 2004;11(1):49–63.
18. Leung N, et al. Urinary albumin excretion patterns of patients with cast nephropathy and other monoclonal gammopathy-related kidney diseases. Clin J Am Soc Nephrol. 2012;7(12):1964–8.
19. Start DA, et al. Myeloma cast nephropathy: immunohistochemical and lectin studies. Mod Pathol. 1988;1(5):336–47.
20. Sanders PW, et al. Mechanisms of intranephronal proteinaceous cast formation by low molecular weight proteins. J Clin Invest. 1990;85(2):570–6.
21. Hutchison CA, et al. Efficient removal of immunoglobulin free light chains by hemodialysis for multiple myeloma: in vitro and in vivo studies. J Am Soc Nephrol. 2007;18(3):886–95.
22. Bence Jones H. On a new substance occurring in the urine of a patient with mollities ossium. Philos Trans R Soc Lond B Biol Sci. 1848;138:55–62.
23. Ying WZ, Sanders PW. Mapping the binding domain of immunoglobulin light chains for Tamm-Horsfall protein. Am J Pathol. 2001;158(5):1859–66.
24. Leung N, et al. Improvement of cast nephropathy with plasma exchange depends on the diagnosis and on reduction of serum free light chains. Kidney Int. 2008;73(11):1282–8.
25. Sanders PW. Pathogenesis and treatment of myeloma kidney. J Lab Clin Med. 1994;124(4):484–8.
26. Hutchison CA, et al. Treatment of acute renal failure secondary to multiple myeloma with chemotherapy and extended high cut-off hemodialysis. Clin J Am Soc Nephrol. 2009;4(4):745–54.
27. Hutchison CA, et al. Early reduction of serum-free light chains associates with renal recovery in myeloma kidney. J Am Soc Nephrol. 2011;22(6):1129–36.
28. Mateos MV, San Miguel JF. Bortezomib in multiple myeloma. Best Pract Res Clin Haematol. 2007;20(4):701–15.
29. Dimopoulos MA, et al. VMP (bortezomib, melphalan, and prednisone) is active and well tolerated in newly diagnosed patients with multiple myeloma with moderately impaired renal function, and results in reversal of renal impairment: cohort analysis of the phase III VISTA study. J Clin Oncol. 2009;27(36):6086–93.
30. Ludwig H, et al. Light chain-induced acute renal failure can be reversed by bortezomib-doxorubicin-dexamethasone in multiple myeloma: results of a phase II study. J Clin Oncol. 2010;28(30):4635–41.
31. Zucchelli P, et al. Controlled plasma exchange trial in acute renal failure due to multiple myeloma. Kidney Int. 1988;33(6):1175–80.
32. Johnson WJ, et al. Treatment of renal failure associated with multiple myeloma. Plasmapheresis, hemodialysis, and chemotherapy. Arch Intern Med. 1990;150(4):863–9.
33. Clark WF, et al. Plasma exchange when myeloma presents as acute renal failure: a randomized, controlled trial [see comment] [summary for patients in Ann Intern Med. 2005 Dec 6;143(11):120; PMID: 16330784]. Ann Intern Med. 2005;143(11):777–84.
34. Arimura A, Li M, Batuman V. Potential protective action of pituitary adenylate cyclase-activating polypeptide (PACAP38) on in vitro and in vivo models of myeloma kidney injury. Blood. 2006;107(2):661–8.
35. Ying WZ, et al. Mechanism and prevention of acute kidney injury from cast nephropathy in a rodent model. J Clin Invest. 2012;122(5):1777–85.

Amyloidosis

22

Morie A. Gertz and Steven R. Zeldenrust

Introduction

Amyloidosis is defined by its tinctorial properties. Deposits seen in tissues that bind Congo red and demonstrate green birefringence when viewed under polarized light is the *sine qua non*. Amyloid deposits are extracellular and amorphous when seen with a light microscope. They are pinkish-appearing when stained with hematoxylin and eosin. By electron microscopy, amyloid deposits are rigid, nonbranching fibrils of indefinite length and a width of approximately 9.5 nm [1]. Amyloid deposits can be purified because they are insoluble in saline and represent the residue after repeated homogenizations in water [2]. Historically, amyloidosis was classified as familial when seen with an autosomal dominant inheritance pattern [3]. Amyloidosis was defined as secondary when it occurred in the presence of a longstanding inflammatory process bronchiectasis, osteomyelitis, tuberculosis, leprosy, inflammatory bowel disease, or abscess. All unknown forms of amyloidosis were referred to as primary amyloidosis. With the advent of modern biochemical techniques, amyloidosis can be classified based on the subunit protein comprising the amyloid fibril. An abbreviated nomenclature for amyloidosis is given in Table 22.1 [4]. Forms other than immunoglobulin light chain amyloidosis are unlikely to be encountered by a practicing oncologist. All forms of AL are composed of immunoglobulin light chains or heavy chains or fragments thereof.

Experimentally, it is possible to digest immunoglobulin light chains in vitro and have them form amyloid fibrils [5]. Most light chain amyloid fibrils are composed of a fragment of the immunoglobulin light or heavy chain and have a molecular weight of approximately 12 kDa. The clinical characteristics of light and heavy chain amyloidosis are not distinct, and the determination can be made by mass spectroscopy. Light chains from the urine of patients with amyloidosis can produce amyloid deposits in mice when injected [6]. It is, therefore, assumed that certain Bence Jones proteins have an amyloidogenic predisposition. This suggests they are more prone to misfolding into the beta-pleated sheet configuration. Additional evidence of the amyloidogenicity of light chains is derived from the fact that in multiple myeloma and MGUS, κ light chains account for two-thirds of the immunoglobulin proteins; but in light chain amyloidosis, λ light chains represent three-quarters of the deposits seen [7] (Fig. 22.1). Moreover, the λ_{VI} subclass of light chain amyloidosis is virtually always associated with AL [8]. Patients with amyloidosis may be classified into those with and those without multiple myeloma. It appears that the percentage of plasma cells has an impact on outcome [9].

M.A. Gertz, M.D., M.A.C.P. (✉)
S.R. Zeldenrust, M.D., Ph.D.
Division of Hematology, Mayo Clinic, 200 First Street, Southwest, Rochester, MN 55905, USA
e-mail: gertz.morie@mayo.edu; zeldenrust.steven@mayo.edu

M.A. Gertz and S.V. Rajkumar (eds.), *Multiple Myeloma: Diagnosis and Treatment*,
DOI 10.1007/978-1-4614-8520-9_22, © Mayo Foundation for Medical Education and Research 2014

Table 22.1 Amyloid nomenclature

Protein	Subclinical	Clinical
AL or AH (primary)	Immunoglobulin	Cardiomyopathy Nephrotic syndrome Peripheral neuropathy Hepatomegaly
AA (secondary)	SAA	Goiter Diarrhea Nephrotic syndrome
ATTR (familial)	Transthyretin	Neuropathy Cardiomyopathy Senile systemic amyloidosis
Aβ	ABPP	Alzheimer's
Aβ_2M (dialysis)	Beta 2 microglobulin	Carpal tunnel Arthropathy
A LECT2 (familial)	Leukocyte chemotactic factor	Kidney disease
A fib (familial)	Fibrinogen A α	Kidney disease

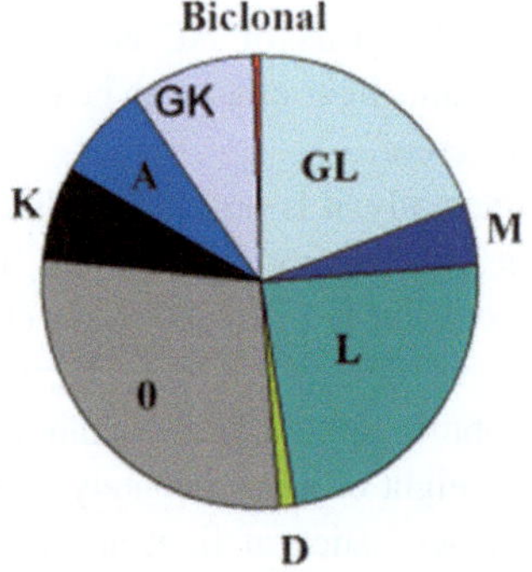

Fig. 22.1 Distribution of serum monoclonal protein found by immunofixation in amyloidosis

However, only the rare patient actually develops lytic bone disease, cast nephropathy, or cytopenias related to marrow infiltration. If a patient does not present with multiple myeloma at the time of diagnosis, the likelihood of overt myeloma developing during the course of the disease is <1 % [10]. Amyloidosis has an incidence of 8 per million per year with a median age of approximately 67. The ratio of patients seen with multiple myeloma to amyloidosis is approximately 5:1. The median number of plasma cells seen at the time of diagnosis ranges from 5 to 7 % [11]. Generally, in amyloidosis, the cells are nonproliferative, fail to carry the genetic abnormalities typically seen in multiple myeloma, and have a very small percent in S phase.

Diagnosis

The symptoms and physical findings in light chain amyloidosis are nonspecific, and physical findings that are diagnostic are seen only in a small percentage of patients. The question of when a clinician should consider amyloidosis in the differential diagnosis is, therefore, important.

Age is a major part of the differential. Only 1 % of patients with light chain amyloidosis present under the age of 40. Males represent 65 % of patients compared with multiple myeloma where 52 % are male [12]. The most common symptoms seen in light chain amyloidosis are fatigue and weight loss, which are nonspecific and are not helpful in determining whether a patient should be screened. Fatigue is seen most often in the presence of cardiac amyloidosis in which the objective evidence can be very subtle. Lightheadedness frequently accompanies the fatigue but is also nonspecific. The etiology of lightheadedness in amyloidosis can be either plasma volume contraction in patients with nephrotic syndrome or the low stroke volume seen in patients who have a poorly filling left ventricle during diastole [13]. Orthostatic hypotension can be seen in renal, cardiac, or autonomic amyloidosis [14].

The physical findings of amyloidosis are seen in only 15 % of patients. Periorbital purpura is

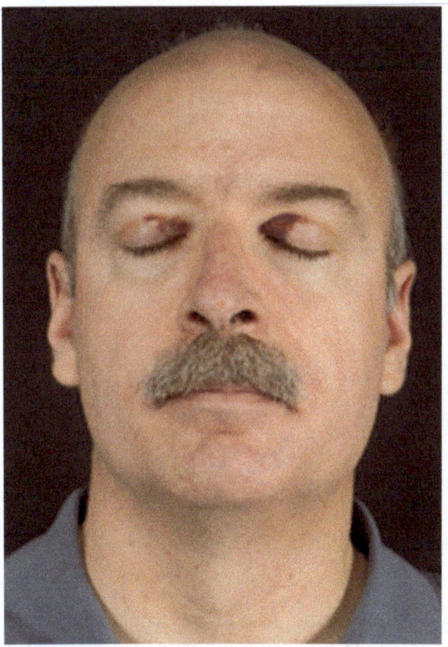

Fig. 22.2 Eyelid purpura only visible with eyes closed

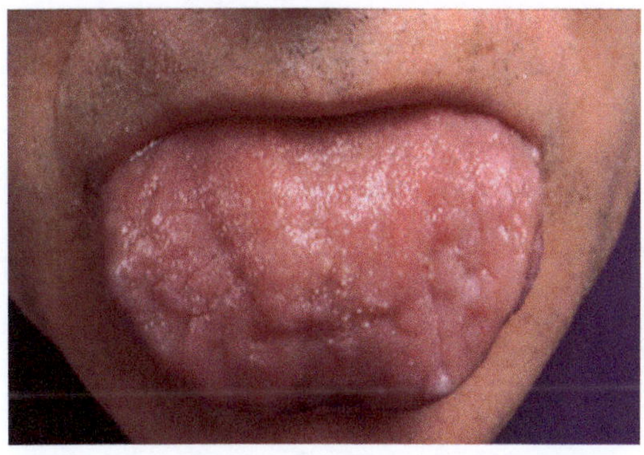

Fig. 22.3 Enlarged tongue in a patient with light chain amyloidosis

diagnostic when recognized but is only seen in 15 % of patients and has been misdiagnosed as "autoimmune ophthalmopathy" or "coagulation disorder." The purpura is seen in the webbing of the neck, eyelids, and face (Fig. 22.2) [15]. Hepatomegaly is seen in 25 % of patients but is palpable >5 cm below the right costal margin in 10 %. Macroglossia is highly specific but can be misdiagnosed as carcinoma of the tongue or as a sign of acromegaly (Fig. 22.3). Macroglossia is seen in <10 % of patients and is easily overlooked since the most common finding is dental indentations on the underside of the tongue [16].

Table 22.2 Dominant amyloid syndrome

	%
Nephrotic syndrome	45
Hepatomegaly	20
Cardiomyopathy	43
Carpal tunnel	18
Peripheral neuropathy	15
Autonomic neuropathy	8
Atypical myeloma	17

Submandibular lymph gland enlargement is common and can be misinterpreted as submandibular lymphadenopathy.

Patients with amyloidosis have been misdiagnosed as having temporal arteritis [17]. Amyloid occlusion of small vessels can lead to jaw, calf, and buttock claudication. The sedimentation rate is often elevated due to the monoclonal protein. Skeletal muscle, pseudohypertrophy, and periarticular infiltration causing shoulder-pad sign occurs but is rare [18]. Most patients have some degree of xerostomia due to infiltration of the minor salivary glands. Sjögren's syndrome can be incorrectly diagnosed.

Amyloid Syndromes

In view of the fact that the symptoms of amyloid (fatigue, weight loss, and edema) are very nonspecific and the diagnostic findings (purpura, arthropathy, and tongue enlargement) are seen only in a minority of patients, clinicians need to be alert to the five common syndromes associated with light chain amyloidosis and screen when these are found [19].

- Nephrotic range proteinuria with or without renal insufficiency
- Hepatomegaly without imaging abnormalities
- Heart failure with normal systolic function; usually restrictive cardiomyopathy
- Peripheral neuropathy, particularly associated with a monoclonal gammopathy
- Atypical multiple myeloma

Any time an adult is seen with one of these syndromes, amyloid should be included in the differential diagnosis [20]. Table 22.2 shows the frequency with which amyloidosis syndromes are seen.

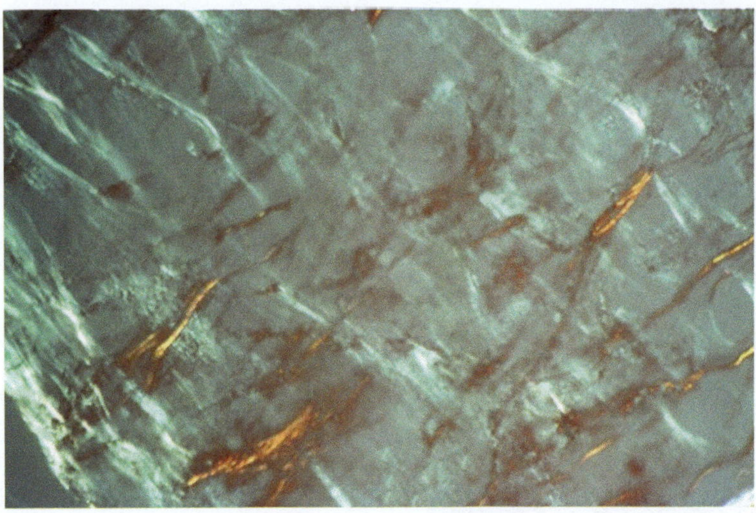

Fig. 22.4 Subcutaneous fat stained with Congo red viewed under polarized light ×1,000

When seeing a patient with one of these five syndromes, the most appropriate screening test is immunoelectrophoresis and immunofixation of the serum and urine as well as an immunoglobulin free light chain assay. Virtually all patients with light chain amyloidosis by definition have a clonal plasma cell producing a light chain or heavy chain fragment. Detection of a monoclonal immunoglobulin, particularly light chain proteinuria or proteinemia, is highly suspicious of amyloidosis with an appropriate clinical syndrome. The immunoglobulin free light chain assay is an important component of the diagnostic evaluation since a high proportion of patients will only have a free light chain in the serum and will have a negative immunofixation test [21]. A screening serum protein electrophoresis is inadequate for screening of patients with a compatible clinical syndrome. An M-spike is visible in only 40 % of patients. Thirty-five percent of M-spikes seen in amyloidosis are <0.5 g/dL.

Half of patients with light chain amyloidosis excrete >1 g of albumin in the urine. The presence of proteinuria should trigger immunofixation since the presence of a light chain suggests a diagnosis must be one of the following three [22].

1. Myeloma cast nephropathy
2. Light chain amyloidosis
3. K immunoglobulin deposition disease

If the serum and urine and the free light chain assay are performed in a patient with a compatible clinical syndrome, one of the three will be abnormal in 99 % of patients. These screening blood and urine tests represent the best noninvasive studies when a clinician is seeing a patient with any of the five syndromes. In the 1 % of patients in which an M component is not seen, alternate possibilities need to be considered including localized amyloidosis or non-light chain amyloidosis. In these situations, mass spectroscopic analysis of a known amyloid deposit is the best next step.

Confirming a Diagnosis of Amyloidosis

In patients that have a compatible clinical syndrome and are found to have a light chain in the serum or urine or an abnormal free light chain ratio, biopsy confirmation of the diagnosis is required before proceeding with any form of further assessment. The most sensitive imaging technique for recognizing light chain amyloidosis is radio-iodine amyloid P component scanning [23]. Unfortunately, this test is not available in the United States and, although highly sensitive, still requires biopsy confirmation to demonstrate Congo red-positive deposits in the tissue. It is always possible to directly biopsy the kidney, heart, liver, or peripheral nerve to confirm the diagnosis, but this is rarely necessary. By performing a subcutaneous fat aspiration [24] (Fig. 22.4) and a

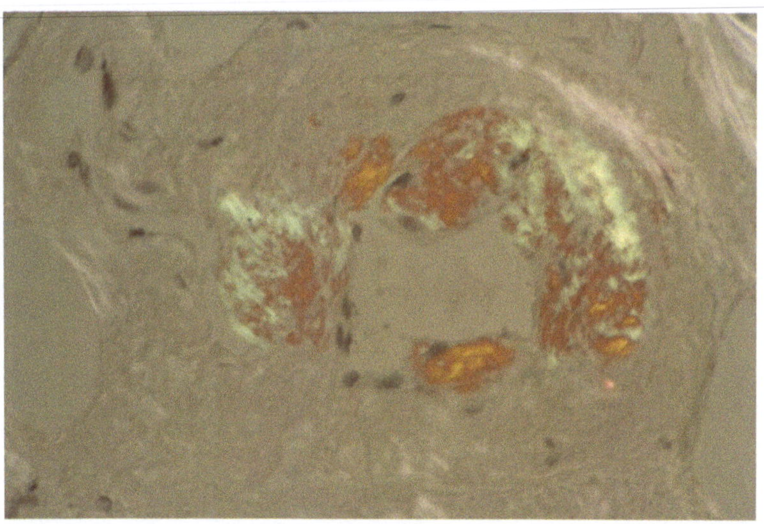

Fig. 22.5 Bone marrow arteriole stained with Congo red and viewed under polarized light ×1,000

bone marrow biopsy (required in any case to exclude myeloma), 85 % of patients with amyloid will have one of these tissues positive (Fig. 22.5). An algorithm is provided in Fig. 22.6 to follow for the diagnosis of amyloid.

At the time of diagnosis, amyloid is widely deposited in the vascular system. Biopsy of tissues that contain blood vessels will frequently demonstrate amyloid deposits even when there is no clinical involvement at those sites. Endoscopic biopsies of the stomach [25], the rectum, and the salivary gland have been reported to show amyloid in patients without symptoms in 60–90 % [26]. Biopsy of uninvolved skin is frequently positive. These techniques are acceptable, although occasionally rectal bleeding is seen from endoscopic biopsy, and superficial biopsy that failed to include submucosa can result in false negatives.

The current practice at Mayo is to obtain a simultaneous bone marrow and subcutaneous fat aspirate. Neither of these tests is performed by a physician. Turnaround time is 48 h. The risk to the patient is minimal. If the subcutaneous fat and marrow biopsy are negative, direct biopsy of the affected organ yields the diagnosis. Caution in interpreting Congo red stains is warranted [27]. False positives can occur due to precipitation of the dye. Moreover, in some circumstances, collagen and elastin fibrils will pick up Congo red, making it difficult to distinguish from amyloid deposits.

Once amyloid deposits are detected in tissue, it is imperative that the correct type of amyloidosis be diagnosed. Previously, this was done by a combination of clinical criteria and immunohistochemistry. However, this has repeatedly been shown to be unreliable; and today, the standard of care is mass spectroscopic analysis of the amyloid deposit [28]. Using laser capture microdissection, amyloid deposits can be removed from a glass slide and undergo mass spectroscopic sequencing [29]. In this way, the subunit protein can be identified, making it relatively easy to distinguish light chain amyloidosis from secondary amyloidosis as well as the multiple forms of familial amyloidosis, including those associated with transthyretin, LECT2 [30], fibrinogen A α, apolipoprotein, and lysozyme. In most instances, patients who have TTR-amyloidosis detected by mass spectroscopic sequencing are able to distinguish inherited mutations from native transthyretin deposition based on the molecular weight of the TTR protein as determined by mass spectroscopic analysis [31]. There have been instances where patients who have clinical syndromes that are consistent with amyloid but have Congo red negative fat aspirates have undergone mass

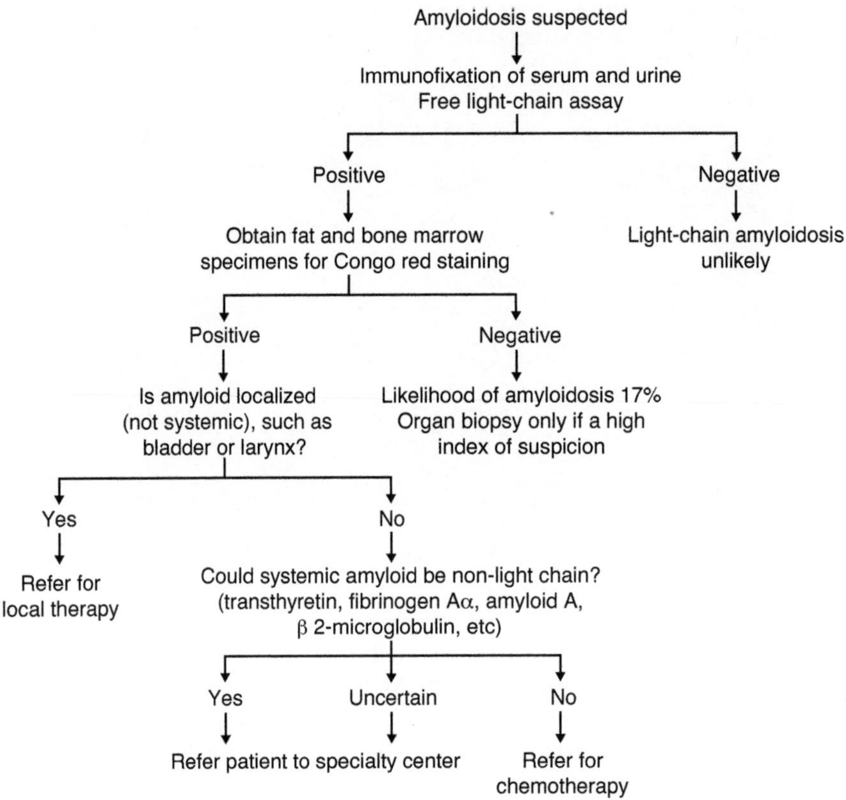

Fig. 22.6 Algorithm designed to evaluate a newly diagnosed patient with amyloidosis

spectroscopic analysis, and amyloid-related peptides have been found, including apolipoprotein-E, serum amyloid P component, and immunoglobulin light chain fragments in the absence of a Congo red-positive deposit. Whenever a pathologist makes a diagnosis of amyloid in tissue sections, the automatic next question should be—What type? Mass spectroscopic analysis represents the most sensitive and specific technique for making this determination [32].

Organ-Specific Syndromes

Kidney

Renal involvement is seen in light chain amyloidosis in 45 % of patients. Amyloid is seen in 2.5 % of renal biopsy specimens. In nondiabetic nephrotic syndrome over the age of 50, amyloid is seen in 10 % of renal biopsy specimens [33] (Fig. 22.7). The serum creatinine has been shown to predict survival in patients with amyloidosis where the 24-h urine total protein excretion has no impact on survival [34]. In renal amyloid, λ light chains far exceed κ light chains. Clinically, nephrotic range protein results in hypoalbuminemia. This lowers the plasma oncotic pressure and results in a leakage of plasma into the extravascular space. The most common presentation of this leak is lower extremity edema [35]. Diuretics remain the mainstay of edema therapy. However, excessive diuretic use can aggravate intravascular volume, compromise renal blood flow, and aggravate orthostatic hypotension. Both midodrine [36] and fludrocortisone have been used to manage orthostatic hypotension but can cause supine hypertension and aggravate edema. The greatest threat from the loss of urinary protein is the continuous albuminuria damaging the tubulointerstitial system, resulting in the development of end-stage renal disease. One-third of patients with renal amyloidosis will ultimately require dialysis. The serum creatinine at presentation is a major

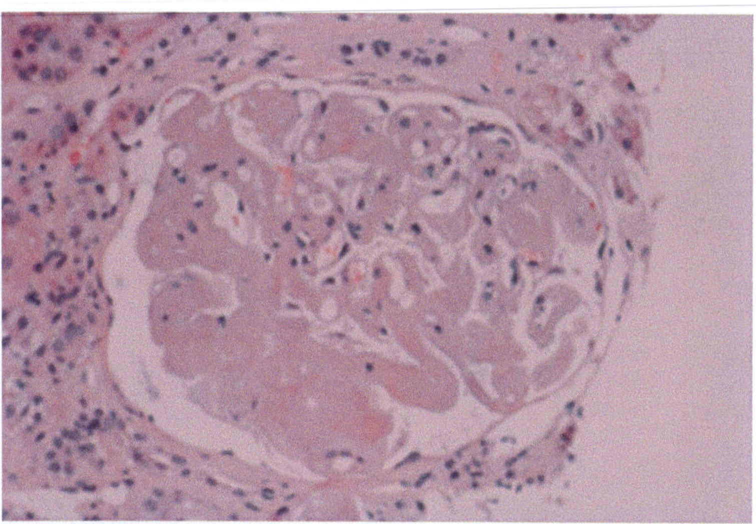

Fig. 22.7 Renal glomerulus showing the amorphous eosinophilic deposit of amyloid. Note the amyloid deposit is acellular

factor in determining which patients will ultimately require dialysis support. No survival differences have been reported between hemodialysis and peritoneal dialysis.

Patients with high levels of proteinuria, usually in excess of 10 g/day, can have serum albumin levels fall below 1 g/dL. These patients can develop anasarca and are disabled due to the fluid leak [37]. In these situations, percutaneous ligation of the renal artery and/or percutaneous clips on the ureter to result in anuria has been performed to stop the urinary protein leak and normalize the plasma oncotic pressure. Early initiation of dialysis may have a similar effect when it results in anuria [38].

There is no correlation between the extent of amyloid deposits seen on renal biopsy and the extent of proteinuria. The urinalysis in patients with AL is not specific, showing an inactive urinary sediment containing protein and fat [39]. Most patients with renal amyloid die due to the subsequent development or concordant presence of cardiac amyloidosis with congestive heart failure.

Heart

Heart failure with normal systolic function, a consequence of restrictive cardiomyopathy, is the next most common clinical presentation of light chain amyloidosis and is the most challenging to diagnose [40]. Patients present with fatigue and dyspnea on exertion. However, because this is not a consequence of systolic failure, the cardiac silhouette is often normal [41]. Echocardiography will show a preserved ejection fraction, and the coronary anatomy will be normal, often leading to a misdiagnosis of noncardiac dyspnea [42]. Low voltage and pseudoinfarction patterns are regularly seen on EKG but are often overlooked when this rare diagnosis is not considered in the differential diagnosis of a patient [43]. In our anecdotal experience, the use of beta adrenergic blockers and angiotensin receptor blockers can often aggravate the symptoms of fatigue and dyspnea on exertion. Echocardiography typically demonstrates infiltration of the cardiac wall resulting in thickening. This is often misinterpreted as hypertrophy if not accompanied by echocardiographic Doppler and strain studies to look at cardiac relaxation [44, 45] (Fig. 22.8). When a patient presents with fatigue that is unexplained, dyspnea on exertion, and no history of ischemic heart disease, immunofixation of the serum and urine and an immunoglobulin free light chain analysis becomes an important screening test.

The underlying physiology of cardiac amyloidosis is the so-called stiff heart [46]. Filling of the left ventricular chamber during diastole is impaired. The rapid rise in left ventricular

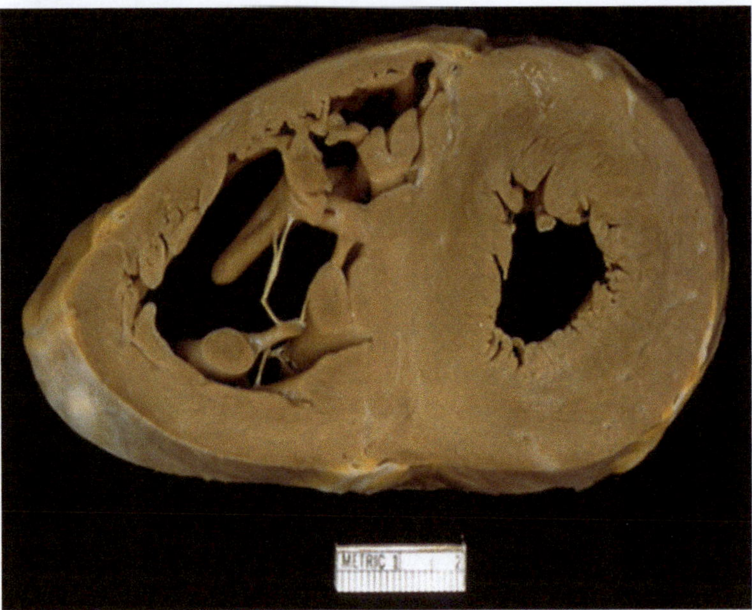

Fig. 22.8 Heart from a patient with light chain amyloid with massive infiltration of the ventricle causing thickening of the heart walls

end-diastolic pressure leads to reduced diastolic filling and, therefore, reduced stroke volume. Even in the presence of a normal ejection fraction, reduced stroke volume will result in a reduced cardiac output. Most patients with amyloidosis early in the course have a hyperdynamic myocardium with a resting pulse of 100. An elevation of ejection fraction to 70–75 % is not rare. Doppler echocardiography is useful in recognizing the rapid decline in filling velocity during diastole. Echocardiography remains the most useful test for imaging amyloid. It shows a median septal wall thickness of 15 mm with normal being 12 or less. Hypertension can cause hypertrophy of the ventricle. It would be rare for patients with hypertension in the modern era to have a wall thickness >15 mm related to poor blood pressure control. Other characteristic features of amyloid include thickening of the right ventricle and reduction in left ventricular chamber size. Using echocardiography alone, amyloid can be diagnosed in 40 % of patients; frank heart failure is seen in only 15 %. The presence of cardiac amyloid has a profound impact on survival, and cardiac amyloid is the most common cause of death from amyloid, even in those patients presenting with hepatomegaly, peripheral neuropathy, and nephrotic syndrome [47]. A reduction in the ejection fraction of amyloid is a late sign and is associated with survival measured in months. Magnetic resonance imaging has been introduced for the diagnosis of cardiac amyloidosis [48]. It shows thickening of the myocardium as does echocardiography. However, a characteristic finding after the injection of gadolinium is subendocardial enhancement, which is considered diagnostic of amyloidosis [49]. Gadolinium is contraindicated in patients who have renal insufficiency [50].

Because of the high prevalence of ischemia and coronary artery disease in the United States, amyloid should not be considered in patients who have obvious risk factors for coronary artery disease. However, a patient who presents with cardiomyopathy without a history of ischemia or risk factors for ischemia, such as smoking and diabetes, or evidence of valvular heart disease should be screened with immunofixation of the serum and urine and an immunoglobulin free light chain ratio. Low voltage electrocardiography can be seen in upwards of two-thirds of patients with cardiac amyloidosis [51].

Late consequences of advanced cardiac involvement include valvular thickening and valvular regurgitation [52]. It is important not to confuse the restrictive cardiomyopathy of amyloid with restrictive pericardial disease. Case reports in the literature of patients with cardiac amyloid who underwent unnecessary pericardial stripping procedures with poor outcomes exist [53]. Endomyocardial biopsy will reveal the correct diagnosis in all patients if five specimens are obtained [54]. The poor ventricular inflow and the high incidence of atrial fibrillation have been recognized to be associated with a significant incidence of thrombi in the left atrial appendage [55]. These are potential sources of cardiac embolism [56]. Some have proposed routine anticoagulation in patients with cardiac amyloidosis, but this has not been adopted in the Mayo practice. Occasionally, amyloid can deposit through the coronary microcirculation and produce ischemic symptoms of exertional angina as well as infarction with a normal cardiac catheterization since the large vessels are not involved [57].

Sudden cardiac death occurs in approximately 10 % of patients with amyloidosis [58]. Whether afterload reduction plays any role in the treatment of cardiac amyloid has not been the subject of randomized trials. Diuretics remain the mainstay of management of fluid retention, but these patients require a very high filling pressure in order to fill the ventricular chamber, and diuretic therapy can result in hypotension and syncope.

Cardiac amyloidosis can occur as an inherited disorder of late onset [59]. The most common mutation in the United States represents a mutation in transthyretin at position 122, which is most commonly associated with African-Americans and causes late-onset heart failure [60]. The presence of cardiac amyloid in the absence of an immunoglobulin light chain abnormality should prompt genetic study and mass spectroscopic analysis of the amyloid tissue to confirm that it is of light chain origin.

Cardiac biomarkers play an important role in assessing function in cardiac amyloidosis [61]. The B-natriuretic peptide and the serum troponin levels have repeatedly been shown to predict outcomes in patients with amyloidosis and form, with the immunoglobulin free light chain assay, the staging system for amyloidosis. All patients with amyloidosis are assigned a point: 1—if the difference between the involved and uninvolved free light chain is ≥18 mg/dL, 1—if the cardiac troponin-T level is >0.025 ng/mL, and 1—patients who have an NT-proBNP >1,800 pg/mL, creating four stages with scores of 0–3 points. In an analysis of 583 patients using the staging system, median survivals range from 60 months for stage I to 6 months for stage IV [62].

Elderly patients with congestive heart failure can have amyloid cardiomyopathy due to senile systemic amyloidosis [63]. These patients have native transthyretin deposits in the myocardium, do not have light chain amyloidosis, and have a much improved median survival when compared with light chain amyloidosis. Senile systemic amyloid (formerly known as senile cardiac amyloid) often requires an endomyocardial biopsy to establish the diagnosis [64]. Echocardiographically, the two disorders are indistinguishable. Chemotherapy is contraindicated in familial and senile cardiac amyloidosis.

Liver

Hepatomegaly is seen in up to a quarter of patients with light chain amyloidosis. Most commonly, these patients present with hepatomegaly and an increased serum alkaline phosphatase level. Half of these patients will have proteinuria related to renal amyloidosis [65]. Suspicion of amyloidosis involving the liver should occur whenever hepatomegaly is seen with:

1. Proteinuria
2. Presence of a monoclonal protein in the serum or urine
3. Peripheral blood smear that shows evidence of hyposplenism
4. Hepatomegaly out of proportion to the degree of alkaline phosphatase elevation

Rarely, patients with amyloidosis will present with hepatic or splenic rupture [66]. Jaundice, when seen in light chain amyloidosis, is a preterminal finding. Portal hypertension is rare and esophageal varices are reported in <1 % of all patients. Ascites is regularly seen, in part, related to the associated nephrotic range proteinuria and low albumin, not due to portal hypertension. Liver biopsy is a safe technique that will demonstrate perisinusoidal and portal amyloid deposition [67]. In our experience, the median survival of patients who have liver biopsy proof of amyloidosis is 1 year.

Gastrointestinal Tract

If the rectum or stomach is biopsied in patients with light chain amyloidosis, vascular deposits are invariably seen but are not reflective of intestinal involvement with amyloid. Weight loss is common but does not correlate well with intestinal involvement. Steatorrhea is seen in fewer than 5 % of patients with amyloidosis. Advanced amyloid in the gastrointestinal tract can cause intestinal pseudo-obstruction, and a rare patient requires long-term parenteral nutrition because all attempts at enteral feeding fail [68]. Abdominal distention and pain are common. Pharmacologic therapy of intestinal amyloidosis is frustrating. Diarrhea often with fecal incontinence can be seen in patients with amyloidosis [69]. Often loperamide and diphenoxylate are ineffective. We have used Paregoric and tincture of opium in an attempt to manage the diarrhea. We have experience in the placement of diverting colostomies as the only way to manage the diarrhea.

Rarely, amyloid presents with ischemic colitis due to microvascular obstruction [70]. Radiographic studies in amyloidosis are rarely of value and are generally nonspecific. In a series of 769 patients with amyloidosis, only eight had symptomatic gastric amyloid. The symptoms were nonspecific: prolonged nausea, vomiting, and weight loss. Gastroparesis was found in three. Six of the eight had concomitant small bowel amyloid. Recovery of motility with systemic therapy is not to be expected.

Nervous System

The most common nervous system manifestation of amyloid is mixed axonal and demyelinating peripheral neuropathy [71]. This tends to be a symmetric ascending neuropathy preferentially involving the lower extremities. Sensory symptoms precede motor symptoms. Lower extremity dysesthesias precede upper extremity dysesthesias. The progression of amyloid neuropathy is slow; and oftentimes, years can elapse between the first development of paresthesias and the histologic diagnosis. Muscle weakness can be seen in up to two-thirds [72]. Autonomic symptoms are seen in approximately one in six. Carpal tunnel syndrome is associated with peripheral neuropathy in half of patients. Electromyography is often not helpful since the amyloid deposits preferentially are found in small fibers, and nerve conduction studies preferentially measure large myelinated fibers [73]. In these instances, the patient's symptoms can be more severe than the EMG/NCV findings. All patients with an unexplained peripheral neuropathy (nondiabetic) should have immunofixation of serum and urine and an immunoglobulin free light chain assay performed. Cranial neuropathy has been reported but is rare [74]. Sural nerve biopsy is the most sensitive technique for the diagnosis of amyloidosis. Reports exist where sural nerve biopsies missed the diagnosis of amyloidosis; and by mass spectroscopic analysis, light chain deposits can be detected in the sural nerve specimen without Congo red-positive deposits [75]. Multiple sections of a sural nerve biopsy must be examined to exclude the diagnosis.

Respiratory Tract

Anatomic involvement with the pulmonary arteriolar blood vessels is commonly seen, but clinical symptoms of pulmonary amyloidosis are rare and are overshadowed by the high frequency of cardiac involvement. Gas exchange is preserved until late into the disease. Pulmonary function testing shows restrictive pulmonary function. The most common finding is radiographic evidence of an interstitial or reticulonodular infiltrate [76]. The finding of an amyloid nodule is usually a localized form of amyloidosis and not associated with systemic disease or a plasma cell dyscrasia [77]. The chest radiograph is not specific and is often misdiagnosed as interstitial pulmonary fibrosis or usual interstitial pneumonia. To distinguish a patient with interstitial disease from pulmonary amyloidosis requires finding a monoclonal protein in the serum or urine or a free light chain abnormality.

Coagulation System

Bleeding is seen in light chain amyloidosis. Factor X deficiency is well recognized and is seen in approximately 5 % of patients [78]. Fragile blood vessels can lead to periorbital and skin purpura. The most common abnormal coagulation test is the thrombin time due to the development of a dysfibrinogenemia [79]. Abnormal platelet aggregation has been reported. Therapy of factor X deficiency has been reported to be successful with melphalan and prednisone, autologous stem cell transplantation, splenectomy, and the infusion of activated clotting factor concentrate VII [80].

Response Assessment

It is very difficult to assess organ responses in amyloidosis, and these responses are often delayed. Therefore, assessment of hematologic response is the first step in assessing response to therapy. Current response criteria for amyloidosis divide responses into four categories. The first is a complete response, which requires negative immunofixation of the serum and urine as well as a normal κ to λ immunoglobulin free light chain ratio. A very good partial response requires that the difference between the involved and uninvolved free light chain absolute values are <4 mg/dL. A partial response is defined as a difference in the free light chain, involved and uninvolved, fall by >50 %. All other patients are considered nonresponders to therapy [81]. Light chain responses can be rapid and typically can be seen as early as 6 weeks after the initiation of chemotherapy, which would allow for change in a therapeutic regimen if an inadequate decline in the light chain values is seen.

Although the light chains are the first measures of response, the intent of therapy in amyloidosis is to improve organ function so criteria exist for the assessment of organ function in amyloidosis [82]. A response in renal amyloidosis required a 50 % decrease in 24-h urine protein loss and this decrease must be at least 0.5 g/day without a change in the serum creatinine or creatinine clearance. Conversely, a 50 % increase in urinary protein loss of at least 1 g/day or a 25 % worsening of serum creatinine or creatinine clearance is indicative of renal progression. Historically, assessment of cardiac response was with echocardiography, but this has been supplanted due to interobserver variability as well as the inability to validate outcomes using serial echocardiography. Currently, response and progression in cardiac amyloidosis is measured by the NT-proBNP (the same test used in the staging system as outlined above). A cardiac response is defined as a 30 % reduction in the NT-proBNP, at least 300 ng/L, in patients whose baseline NT-proBNP was >650 ng/L [83]. Alternatively, an improvement in New York Heart Association class from class IV to class II or class III to class I is considered a response. Progression of cardiac amyloidosis is defined as an NT-proBNP rise of >30 % and >300 ng/dL, or a 33 % increase in cardiac troponin T, or a fall in ejection fraction by >10 % that is not attributable to variability in technique.

Liver response is defined as a 50 % decrease in the abnormal alkaline phosphatase value. Progression is defined as a 50 % increase of alkaline phosphatase above the lowest value. Criteria to define response and progression of soft tissue, gastrointestinal tract, or lung amyloidosis do not currently exist.

Treatment

The treatment of amyloidosis is advancing rapidly with the refinement in novel agent-based chemotherapy and autologous stem cell transplantation. Melphalan and prednisone, for many years, was considered the standard of therapy for the treatment of amyloidosis. However, the response rate was never >20–30 %, and the overall impact on survival was considered minimal [84]. Despite the introduction of new drugs, 30 % of patients with amyloidosis die of the disease in the first year after diagnosis [85]. Given the fact that most patients with cardiac amyloidosis are often diagnosed at an advanced stage, no therapy is likely to improve outcomes until the diagnosis is made at an earlier stage. Moreover, the resolution of amyloid from an organ is often slow even when the production of precursor light chain is eliminated. Patients who have a hematologic response often die of end organ damage before sufficient time elapses for a response to occur.

Conventional Chemotherapy

The combination of melphalan and high-dose dexamethasone has been reported to produce hematologic complete responses in up to 33 % of patients with a day-100 mortality of only 4 %. Resolution of cardiac failure was seen in 6 of 32 patients with a median time to response of 4.5 months. A 5-year actuarial survival in patients treated with melphalan and dexamethasone is 50 %. Melphalan and dexamethasone could be used successfully a second time after relapse [86]. Success with melphalan and dexamethasone is often dependent upon the fraction of patients with cardiac amyloidosis. In a study of parenteral melphalan with dexamethasone, the median survival was only 17.5 months [87]; and in a second study, a median survival of only 10.5 months has been reported [88]. Therefore, the range of reported survivals are anywhere from 10.5 to 61 months, reflecting heterogeneity of patient populations enrolled into various trials. For future trials, stratification of stage based on light chain, BNP, and troponin is essential to understand the fraction of patients being treated based on severity of cardiac function. Melphalan and dexamethasone has replaced melphalan and prednisone as the new standard of care in patients who are not eligible for stem cell transplant.

Autologous Stem Cell Transplantation

At Mayo Clinic, we are very enthusiastic about the use of stem cell transplantation for the treatment of light chain amyloidosis. However, patients need to be carefully selected and in our experience, approximately 20–25 % of patients are actually eligible for this technique. However, in properly selected patients, the treatment-related mortality can be lowered below 5 % [89], and the 10-year overall survival is as high as 43 % [90]. Validation of organ responses following stem cell transplantation using amyloid P component scanning has been performed. Significant organ regression and improved quality of life has also been reported. The best outcomes following stem cell transplant are achieved in those patients who have a complete hematologic response or VGPR [91]. Careful patient selection, avoiding patients above the age of 65–70, patients who have a serum creatinine >1.8 mg/dL, a serum troponin T >0.06 [92], or an NT-proBNP >5,000, is important for a successful outcome with low treatment-related mortality. Because patients with advanced cardiac involvement are excluded, patients who receive stem cell transplant are disproportionately renal, with 70 % of patients showing evidence of renal involvement. Half show evidence of cardiac involvement by echo, but these tend to be milder than other patients seen with cardiac amyloidosis. Peripheral nerve involvement is seen in 12 % and hepatic involvement in 14 %. The median urinary protein excretion for patients who receive stem cell transplant is 3.8 g/24-h period with 7 % plasma cells in the bone marrow [93]. The median age of a transplanted patient is 57 years.

In our program, stem cell mobilization is done without cytotoxic chemotherapy. It usually requires two aphereses to collect an adequate number of stem cells. Melphalan-200 is our standard conditioning regimen; however, new conditioning regimens are being explored. Median length of hospital stay is 8 days. Nineteen percent of patients never require hospitalization. We do not use GCSF post-transplantation because of fluid retention. A hematologic response is seen in three-quarters of patients, with complete hematologic responses in 40 % of patients. We do not use induction chemotherapy if the patients do not have multiple myeloma at the time of diagnosis [94]. Organ responses are seen in nearly half. At the beginning of our program, treatment-related mortality was as high as 10 %. In the last 3.5 years, it has fallen to 1 %. After the first 100 days, hematologic response is the strongest predictor of long-term survival. The median survival for complete responders has not been reached and is 107 months for partial responders. The most important predictors of outcome following stem cell transplant are NT-proBNP and troponin levels [95]. There is only one prospective randomized study comparing conventional chemotherapy with stem cell transplant. It did not show an advantage for stem cell transplantation, but the study has been criticized for its high treatment-related mortality [96].

Immunomodulatory Agents

Melphalan, dexamethasone, and lenalidomide have been reported for the treatment of light chain amyloidosis. In a phase I dose-escalation study, the lenalidomide dose was increased from 5 to 20 mg on days 1–21 of a 28-day cycle. The melphalan dose was lower than that used in patients with multiple myeloma at 0.17 mg/kg per day for 4 days instead of the standard 0.25 mg/kg per day. This was given for 4 days every 28 days. Deep vein thrombosis prophylaxis is required for patients receiving an immunomodulatory drug. The maximum tolerated dose of lenalidomide was 15 mg/day. The reported complete response rate was 42 % with partial responses seen in 9 of 26, giving an overall response rate of 58 % and a 2-year overall survival of 81 % [97].

A combination of cyclophosphamide, thalidomide, and dexamethasone has been shown to be safe and effective in the treatment of amyloidosis. In a risk-adapted oral regimen of cyclophosphamide, thalidomide, and dexamethasone, 75 patients with advanced amyloidosis were treated. Hematologic response was seen in 74 % of patients treated with this all-oral regimen, including 21 % complete responses. Median overall survival from initiation of therapy was 41 months with a 3-year estimated overall survival of 82 %. Grade II toxicity was seen in 52 % [98].

Lenalidomide and dexamethasone has been used in the treatment of amyloidosis. Lenalidomide can increase the NT-proBNP level [99]. Lenalidomide, 25 mg, as is used in myeloma, is not tolerated by the majority, and 15 mg should be considered the starting dose. A Mayo Clinic study enrolled 23 patients; 10 patients discontinued within the first three cycles. There were ten responses to treatment. Common adverse events were neutropenia, thrombocytopenia, rash, and fatigue [100]. A recent study of lenalidomide and dexamethasone in amyloid patients refractory to both melphalan- and bortezomib-based therapy has been reported. Twenty-four patients were enrolled, and 19 were also refractory to thalidomide. Two died before evaluation of response, and 50 % had severe adverse effects. Survival was significantly shorter in patients with a troponin I >0.1 ng/mL and in patients diagnosed <18 months before treatment initiation. The hematologic response rate was 41 %. The median overall survival was 14 months [101]. Lenalidomide has been combined with dexamethasone and cyclophosphamide. In a cohort of patients treated with 12 cycles, two-thirds of whom had no prior therapy, the maximum tolerated dose of lenalidomide was 15 mg/day and that of cyclophosphamide was 100 mg/day. A greater than partial response was seen in 55 % and a complete response was seen in 8 % [102]. Four out of the five patients who received prior bortezomib responded, and organ response was seen in 40 % of the patients who survived 6 months. The 2-year overall survival was 41 %.

The investigational immunomodulatory agent, pomalidomide, has been used with dexamethasone in patients with relapsed amyloidosis. In a cohort of patients in whom 33 were evaluable for organ response, the response rate was 48 % with a median time to response of 1.9 months. Organ improvement was documented in 5 of 33 patients. The overall and progression-free survival median times were 28 and 14 months, respectively. The 1-year overall survival and progression-free survival rates were 76 and 59 %, respectively [103].

Bortezomib

Bortezomib is a highly active agent in the treatment of light chain amyloidosis. The combination of bortezomib and dexamethasone has been reported in untreated patients to have a 47 % complete response rate with higher responses in patients treated with twice-weekly bortezomib.

The cardiac response rate is 29 %. Hematologic responses were associated with cardiac organ responses with reduction in the NT-proBNP. A 1-year survival rate of 76 % has been reported [104]. The NT-proBNP is independently associated with survival. Bortezomib has been combined with melphalan and dexamethasone as well as cyclophosphamide and dexamethasone. The so-called CyBorD regimen has been reported using bortezomib 1.5 mg/m^2 weekly, cyclophosphamide 300 mg/m^2 once weekly, and dexamethasone 40 mg weekly. In a phase II study of 17 patients that received 2–6 cycles of therapy, 10 (58 %) had symptomatic cardiac involvement and 14 (82 %) had >1 organ involved. Responses were seen in 16 (94 %) patients with 71 % complete response and 24 % partial response. The time to response was 2 months median. Some patients not previously eligible for stem cell transplant became eligible [105].

Summary

For patients who can be transplanted safely, stem cell transplantation is a preferred option for the treatment of amyloid. For non-transplant candidates, melphalan and dexamethasone remains the default standard. Bortezomib and lenalidomide have clear activity, but integrating it into practice is not fully defined. Combinations including cyclophosphamide, thalidomide, dexamethasone, melphalan, lenalidomide, and dexamethasone currently are being actively explored.

- Amyloidosis should be considered in all patients with nephrotic syndrome, unexplained cardiomyopathy, peripheral neuropathy, hepatomegaly, and atypical myeloma.
- When a patient with any of those syndromes is seen, immunofixation of serum and urine and a free light chain assay is mandatory.
- If a light chain is detected, a bone marrow and a fat stained with Congo red and subjected to mass spectroscopy is mandatory.
- The prognosis is determined by the serum troponin level, the brain natriuretic peptide level, and the immunoglobulin free light chain level.
- Systemic chemotherapy is warranted and can include chemotherapy without novel agents, with novel agents, and high-dose therapy with stem cell transplantation.

References

1. Gertz MA, Comenzo R, Falk RH, et al. Definition of organ involvement and treatment response in immunoglobulin light chain amyloidosis (AL): a consensus opinion from the 10th International Symposium on amyloid and amyloidosis, Tours, France, 18–22 April 2004. Am J Hematol. 2005;79(4):319–28. Prepublished on 2005/07/27 as doi:10.1002/ajh.20381.
2. Vilhjalmsson DT, Ingolfsdottir IE, Thormodsson FR. Isolation of amyloid by solubilization in water. Methods Mol Biol. 2012;849:403–10. Prepublished on 2012/04/25 as doi:10.1007/978-1-61779-551-0_27.
3. Koike H, Hashimoto R, Tomita M, et al. Diagnosis of sporadic transthyretin Val30Met familial amyloid polyneuropathy: a practical analysis. Amyloid. 2011;18(2):53–62. Prepublished on 2011/04/06 as doi:10.3109/13506129.2011.565524.
4. Sipe JD, Benson MD, Buxbaum JN, et al. Amyloid fibril protein nomenclature: 2012 recommendations from the nomenclature committee of the International Society of Amyloidosis. Amyloid. 2012;19(4):167–70. Prepublished on 2012/11/02 as doi:10.3109/13506129.2012.734345.
5. Buxbaum J. Aberrant immunoglobulin synthesis in light chain amyloidosis. Free light chain and light chain fragment production by human bone marrow cells in short-term tissue culture. J Clin Invest. 1986;78(3):798–806. Prepublished on 1986/09/01 as doi:10.1172/JCI112643.
6. Solomon A, Weiss DT, Kattine AA. Nephrotoxic potential of Bence Jones proteins. N Engl J Med. 1991;324(26):1845–51. Prepublished on 1991/06/27 as doi:10.1056/NEJM199106273242603.
7. Palladini G, Russo P, Bosoni T, et al. Identification of amyloidogenic light chains requires the combination of serum-free light chain assay with immunofixation of serum and urine. Clin Chem. 2009;55(3):499–504. Prepublished on 2009/01/10 as doi:10.1373/clinchem.2008.117143.
8. del Pozo Yauner L, Ortiz E, Sanchez R, et al. Influence of the germline sequence on the thermodynamic stability and fibrillogenicity of human lambda 6 light chains. Proteins. 2008;72(2):684–92. Prepublished on 2008/02/09 as doi:10.1002/prot.21934.
9. Merlini G, Seldin DC, Gertz MA. Amyloidosis: pathogenesis and new therapeutic options. J Clin Oncol. 2011;29(14):1924–33. Prepublished on 2011/04/13 as doi:10.1200/JCO.2010.32.2271.
10. Rajkumar SV, Gertz MA, Kyle RA. Primary systemic amyloidosis with delayed progression to

multiple myeloma. Cancer. 1998;82(8):1501–5. Prepublished on 1998/04/29 as doi.

11. Katoh N, Poshusta TL, Manske MK, et al. A reappraisal of immunoglobulin variable gene primers and its impact on assessing clonal relationships between PB B cells and BM plasma cells in AL amyloidosis. J Clin Immunol. 2011;31(6):1029–37. Prepublished on 2011/09/13 as doi:10.1007/s10875-011-9582-y.
12. Sirohi B, Powles R. Epidemiology and outcomes research for MGUS, myeloma and amyloidosis. Eur J Cancer. 2006;42(11):1671–83. Prepublished on 2006/07/28 as doi:10.1016/j.ejca.2006.01.065.
13. Phelan D, Collier P, Thavendiranathan P, et al. Relative apical sparing of longitudinal strain using two-dimensional speckle-tracking echocardiography is both sensitive and specific for the diagnosis of cardiac amyloidosis. Heart. 2012;98(19):1442–8. Prepublished on 2012/08/07 as doi:10.1136/heartjnl-2012-302353.
14. Pandit A, Gangurde S, Gupta SB. Autonomic failure in primary amyloidosis. J Assoc Physicians India. 2008;56:995–6. Prepublished on 2009/03/28 as doi.
15. Riazance-Lawrence JH, Toumadje A, Johnson Jr WC. The circular dichroism of tumor necrosis factor-alpha: measurement into the vacuum UV and analysis for secondary structure. Chirality. 1991;3(4):254–6. Prepublished on 1991/01/11 as doi:10.1002/chir.530030407.
16. Pau M, Reinbacher KE, Feichtinger M, Karcher H. Surgical treatment of macroglossia caused by systemic primary amyloidosis. Int J Oral Maxillofac Surg. 2013;42(2):294–7. Prepublished on 2012/06/26 as doi:10.1016/j.ijom.2012.05.015.
17. Legault K, Shroff A, Crowther M, Khalidi N. Amyloidosis and giant cell arteritis/polymyalgia rheumatica. J Rheumatol. 2012;39(4):878–80. Prepublished on 2012/04/03 as doi:10.3899/jrheum.111013.
18. Guerreiro de Moura CG, Pinto de Souza S. Images in clinical medicine. “Shoulder pad” sign. N Engl J Med. 2004;351(25):e23. Prepublished on 2004/12/17 as doi:10.1056/ENEJMicm040061.
19. Gertz MA, Dispenzieri A. Immunoglobulin light-chain amyloidosis: growing recognition, new approaches to therapy, active clinical trials. Oncology. 2012;26(2):152–61. Prepublished on 2012/04/12 as doi.
20. Gertz MA. Immunoglobulin light chain amyloidosis: 2011 update on diagnosis, risk-stratification, and management. Am J Hematol. 2011;86(2):180–6. Prepublished on 2011/01/26 as doi:10.1002/ajh.21934.
21. Rao M, Yu WW, Chan J, et al. Serum free light chain analysis for the diagnosis, management, and prognosis of plasma cell dyscrasias. Rockville, MD: Agency for Healthcare Research and Quality; 2012.
22. Herrera GA, Turbat-Herrera EA. Ultrastructural immunolabeling in the diagnosis of monoclonal light-and heavy-chain-related renal diseases. Ultrastruct Pathol. 2010;34(3):161–73. Prepublished on 2010/05/12 as doi:10.3109/01913121003672873.
23. Hawkins PN, Pepys MB. Imaging amyloidosis with radiolabelled SAP. Eur J Nucl Med. 1995;22(7):595–9. Prepublished on 1995/07/01 as doi.
24. Kettwich LG, Sibbitt Jr WL, Emil NS, et al. New device technologies for subcutaneous fat biopsy. Amyloid. 2012;19(2):66–73. Prepublished on 2012/03/29 as doi:10.3109/13506129.2012.666508.
25. Sawada T, Adachi Y, Akino K, et al. Endoscopic features of primary amyloidosis of the stomach. Endoscopy. 2012;44 Suppl 2 UCTN:E275-6. Prepublished on 2012/07/21 as doi:10.1055/s-0032-1309750.
26. Foli A, Palladini G, Caporali R, et al. The role of minor salivary gland biopsy in the diagnosis of systemic amyloidosis: results of a prospective study in 62 patients. Amyloid. 2011;18 Suppl 1:75–7. Prepublished on 2011/08/16 as doi:10.3109/13506129.2011.574354029.
27. Leung N, Nasr SH, Sethi S. How I treat amyloidosis: the importance of accurate diagnosis and amyloid typing. Blood. 2012;120(16):3206–13. Prepublished on 2012/09/06 as doi:10.1182/blood-2012-03-413682.
28. Brambilla F, Lavatelli F, Merlini G, Mauri P. Clinical proteomics for diagnosis and typing of systemic amyloidoses. Proteomics Clin Appl. 2013;7(1–2):136–43. Prepublished on 2012/11/28 as doi:10.1002/prca.201200097.
29. Sethi S, Vrana JA, Theis JD, et al. Laser microdissection and mass spectrometry-based proteomics aids the diagnosis and typing of renal amyloidosis. Kidney Int. 2012;82(2):226–34. Prepublished on 2012/04/13 as doi:10.1038/ki.2012.108.
30. Murphy C, Wang S, Kestler D, et al. Leukocyte chemotactic factor 2 (LECT2)-associated renal amyloidosis. Amyloid. 2011;18 Suppl 1:218–20. Prepublished on 2011/08/16 as doi:10.3109/13506129.2011.574354084.
31. Roden AC, Aubry MC, Zhang K, et al. Nodular senile pulmonary amyloidosis: a unique case confirmed by immunohistochemistry, mass spectrometry, and genetic study. Hum Pathol. 2010;41(7):1040–5. Prepublished on 2010/04/13 as doi:10.1016/j.humpath.2009.11.019.
32. Lavatelli F, Vrana JA. Proteomic typing of amyloid deposits in systemic amyloidoses. Amyloid. 2011;18(4):177–82. Prepublished on 2011/11/15 as doi:10.3109/13506129.2011.630762.
33. Yao Y, Wang SX, Zhang YK, Qu Z, Liu G, Zou WZ. The clinicopathological analysis in a large cohort of Chinese patients with renal AL amyloidosis. Nephrol Dial Transplant. 2013;28(3):689–97. Prepublished on 2012/11/28 as doi:10.1093/ndt/gfs501.
34. Suzuki K. Diagnosis and treatment of multiple myeloma and AL amyloidosis with focus on improvement of renal lesion. Clin Exp Nephrol. 2012;16(5):659–71. Prepublished on 2012/09/13 as doi:10.1007/s10157-012-0684-5.

35. Pinney JH, Hawkins PN. Amyloidosis. Ann Clin Biochem. 2012;49(Pt 3):229–41. Prepublished on 2012/03/10 as doi:10.1258/acb.2011.011225.
36. Gupta V, Lipsitz LA. Orthostatic hypotension in the elderly: diagnosis and treatment. Am J Med. 2007;120(10):841–7. Prepublished on 2007/10/02 as doi:10.1016/j.amjmed.2007.02.023.
37. Gertz MA, Leung N, Lacy MQ, et al. Clinical outcome of immunoglobulin light chain amyloidosis affecting the kidney. Nephrol Dial Transplant. 2009;24(10):3132–7. Prepublished on 2009/05/01 as doi:10.1093/ndt/gfp201.
38. Montseny JJ, Kleinknecht D, Meyrier A, et al. Long-term outcome according to renal histological lesions in 118 patients with monoclonal gammopathies. Nephrol Dial Transplant. 1998;13(6):1438–45. Prepublished on 1998/06/26 as doi.
39. Herrera GA. Renal manifestations of plasma cell dyscrasias: an appraisal from the patients' bedside to the research laboratory. Ann Diagn Pathol. 2000;4(3): 174–200. Prepublished on 2000/08/05 as doi.
40. Dubrey SW. Amyloid heart disease: a brief review of treatment options. Postgrad Med J. 2012;88(1046):700–5. Prepublished on 2012/06/30 as doi:10.1136/postgradmedj-2012-130854.
41. Dubrey SW, Comenzo RL. Amyloid diseases of the heart: current and future therapies. QJM. 2012;105(7):617–31. Prepublished on 2012/01/10 as doi:10.1093/qjmed/hcr259.
42. Kapoor P, Thenappan T, Singh E, Kumar S, Greipp PR. Cardiac amyloidosis: a practical approach to diagnosis and management. Am J Med. 2011;124(11):1006–15. Prepublished on 2011/10/25 as doi:10.1016/j.amjmed.2011.04.013.
43. Marcu CB, Niessen HW, Beek AM, Brouwer WP, Robbers LF, Van Rossum AC. Cardiac involvement with amyloidosis: mechanisms of disease, diagnosis and management. Conn Med. 2011;75(10):581–90. Prepublished on 2012/01/06 as doi.
44. Bellavia D, Pellikka PA, Dispenzieri A, et al. Comparison of right ventricular longitudinal strain imaging, tricuspid annular plane systolic excursion, and cardiac biomarkers for early diagnosis of cardiac involvement and risk stratification in primary systematic (AL) amyloidosis: a 5-year cohort study. Eur Heart J Cardiovasc Imaging. 2012;13(8):680–9. Prepublished on 2012/02/07 as doi:10.1093/ehjci/jes009.
45. Liu D, Niemann M, Hu K, et al. Echocardiographic evaluation of systolic and diastolic function in patients with cardiac amyloidosis. Am J Cardiol. 2011;108(4):591–8. Prepublished on 2011/08/03 as doi:10.1016/j.amjcard.2011.03.092.
46. Bhupathi SS, Chalasani S, Rokey R. Stiff heart syndrome. Clin Med Res. 2011;9(2):92–9. Prepublished on 2010/09/21 as doi:10.3121/cmr.2010.899.
47. Sanchorawala V. Role of high-dose melphalan and autologous peripheral blood stem cell transplantation in AL amyloidosis. Am J Blood Res. 2012;2(1):9–17. Prepublished on 2012/03/21 as doi.
48. Robbers LF, Baars EN, Brouwer WP, et al. T1 mapping shows increased extracellular matrix size in the myocardium due to amyloid depositions. Circ Cardiovasc Imaging. 2012;5(3):423–6. Prepublished on 2012/05/18 as doi:10.1161/CIRCIMAGING.112.973438.
49. Syed IS, Glockner JF, Feng D, et al. Role of cardiac magnetic resonance imaging in the detection of cardiac amyloidosis. JACC Cardiovasc Imaging. 2010;3(2):155–64. Prepublished on 2010/02/18 as doi:10.1016/j.jcmg.2009.09.023.
50. Romero JR, Preis SR, Beiser AS, et al. Lipoprotein phospholipase A2 and cerebral microbleeds in the Framingham Heart Study. Stroke. 2012;43(11):3091–4. Prepublished on 2012/09/11 as doi:10.1161/STROKEAHA.112.656744.
51. Piper C, Butz T, Farr M, Faber L, Oldenburg O, Horstkotte D. How to diagnose cardiac amyloidosis early: impact of ECG, tissue Doppler echocardiography, and myocardial biopsy. Amyloid. 2010;17(1):1–9. Prepublished on 2010/02/12 as doi:10.3109/13506121003619310.
52. Cacoub P, Axler O, De Zuttere D, et al. Amyloidosis and cardiac involvement. Ann Med Interne. 2000; 151(8):611–7. Prepublished on 2001/02/15 as doi.
53. Singh V, Fishman JE, Alfonso CE. Primary systemic amyloidosis presenting as constrictive pericarditis. Cardiology. 2011;118(4):251–5. Prepublished on 2011/07/16 as doi:10.1159/000329062.
54. Kieninger B, Eriksson M, Kandolf R, et al. Amyloid in endomyocardial biopsies. Virchows Arch. 2010;456(5):523–32. Prepublished on 2010/04/09 as doi:10.1007/s00428-010-0909-5.
55. Feng D, Edwards WD, Oh JK, et al. Intracardiac thrombosis and embolism in patients with cardiac amyloidosis. Circulation. 2007;116(21):2420–6. Prepublished on 2007/11/07 as doi:10.1161/CIRCULATIONAHA.107.697763.
56. Nakagawa M, Tojo K, Sekijima Y, Yamazaki KH, Ikeda S. Arterial thromboembolism in senile systemic amyloidosis: report of two cases. Amyloid. 2012;19(2):118–21. Prepublished on 2012/05/16 as doi:10.3109/13506129.2012.685131.
57. Tsai SB, Seldin DC, Wu H, O'Hara C, Ruberg FL, Sanchorawala V. Myocardial infarction with "clean coronaries" caused by amyloid light-chain AL amyloidosis: a case report and literature review. Amyloid. 2011;18(3):160–4. Prepublished on 2011/04/21 as doi:10.3109/13506129.2011.571319.
58. Morin J, Schreiber WE, Lee C. Sudden death due to undiagnosed primary amyloidosis. J Forensic Sci. 2013;58 Suppl 1:S250–2. Prepublished on 2012/11/28 as doi:10.1111/1556-4029.12029.
59. Benson MD. Ostertag revisited: the inherited systemic amyloidoses without neuropathy. Amyloid. 2005;12(2):75–87. Prepublished on 2005/07/14 as doi:10.1080/13506120500106925.
60. Yamashita T, Hamidi Asl K, Yazaki M, Benson MD. A prospective evaluation of the transthyretin Ile122 allele frequency in an African-American population.

Amyloid. 2005;12(2):127–30. Prepublished on 2005/07/14 as doi:10.1080/13506120500107162.
61. Dispenzieri A, Lacy MQ, Katzmann JA, et al. Absolute values of immunoglobulin free light chains are prognostic in patients with primary systemic amyloidosis undergoing peripheral blood stem cell transplantation. Blood. 2006;107(8):3378–83. Prepublished on 2006/01/07 as doi:10.1182/blood-2005-07-2922.
62. Kumar S, Dispenzieri A, Lacy MQ, et al. Revised prognostic staging system for light chain amyloidosis incorporating cardiac biomarkers and serum free light chain measurements. J Clin Oncol. 2012;30(9):989–95. Prepublished on 2012/02/15 as doi:10.1200/JCO.2011.38.5724.
63. Dungu JN, Anderson LJ, Whelan CJ, Hawkins PN. Cardiac transthyretin amyloidosis. Heart. 2012;98(21):1546–54. Prepublished on 2012/08/14 as doi:10.1136/heartjnl-2012-301924.
64. Falk RH. Senile systemic amyloidosis: are regional differences real or do they reflect different diagnostic suspicion and use of techniques? Amyloid. 2012;19 Suppl 1:68–70. Prepublished on 2012/06/01 as doi:10.3109/13506129.2012.674074.
65. Gertz MA, Kyle RA. Amyloidosis: prognosis and treatment. Semin Arthritis Rheum. 1994;24(2):124–38. Prepublished on 1994/10/01 as doi.
66. Skok P, Knehtl M, Ceranic D, Glumbic I. Splenic rupture in systemic amyloidosis—case presentation and review of the literature. Z Gastroenterol. 2009;47(3):292–5. Prepublished on 2009/03/13 as doi:10.1055/s-2008-1027628.
67. Park MA, Mueller PS, Kyle RA, Larson DR, Plevak MF, Gertz MA. Primary (AL) hepatic amyloidosis: clinical features and natural history in 98 patients. Medicine. 2003;82(5):291–8. Prepublished on 2003/10/08 as doi:10.1097/01.md.0000091183.93122.c7.
68. Cowan AJ, Skinner M, Seldin DC, et al. Amyloidosis of the gastrointestinal tract: a 13-year single center referral experience. Haematologica. 2013;98(1):141–6. Prepublished on 2012/06/27 as doi:10.3324/haematol.2012.068155.
69. Sattianayagam P, Hawkins P, Gillmore J. Amyloid and the GI tract. Expert Rev Gastroenterol Hepatol. 2009;3(6):615–30. Prepublished on 2009/11/26 as doi:10.1586/egh.09.59.
70. Maza I, Vlodavsky E, Eliakim RA. Rectal bleeding as a presenting symptom of AL amyloidosis and multiple myeloma. World J Gastrointest Endosc. 2010;2(1):44–6. Prepublished on 2010/12/17 as doi:10.4253/wjge.v2.i1.44.
71. Adams D, Lozeron P, Lacroix C. Amyloid neuropathies. Curr Opin Neurol. 2012;25(5):564–72. Prepublished on 2012/09/04 as doi:10.1097/WCO.0b013e328357bdf6.
72. Matsuda M, Gono T, Morita H, Katoh N, Kodaira M, Ikeda S. Peripheral nerve involvement in primary systemic AL amyloidosis: a clinical and electrophysiological study. Eur J Neurol. 2011;18(4):604–10. Prepublished on 2010/09/24 as doi:10.1111/j.1468-1331.2010.03215.x.
73. Montel S, Albertini L, Spitz E. Coping strategies in relation to quality of life in amyotrophic lateral sclerosis. Muscle Nerve. 2012;45(1):131–4. Prepublished on 2011/12/23 as doi:10.1002/mus.22270.
74. Adams D. Hereditary and acquired amyloid neuropathies. J Neurol. 2001;248(8):647–57. Prepublished on 2001/09/25 as doi.
75. Rajkumar SV, Gertz MA, Kyle RA. Prognosis of patients with primary systemic amyloidosis who present with dominant neuropathy. Am J Med. 1998;104(3):232–7. Prepublished on 1998/04/29 as doi.
76. Wallaert B, Renard B, Ars C, Copin MC, Remy J. CT features of primary systemic pulmonary amyloidosis mimicking pulmonary sarcoidosis. Presse Med. 2012;41(1):82–4. Prepublished on 2011/07/29 as doi:10.1016/j.lpm.2011.05.015.
77. Eguchi T, Yoshida K, Kobayashi N, et al. Localized nodular amyloidosis of the lung. Gen Thorac Cardiovasc Surg. 2011;59(10):715–7. Prepublished on 2011/10/11 as doi:10.1007/s11748-010-0748-y.
78. Manikkan AT. Factor X, deficiency: an uncommon presentation of AL amyloidosis. Ups J Med Sci. 2012;117(4):457–9. Prepublished on 2012/06/02 as doi:10.3109/03009734.2012.690457.
79. Suga N, Miura N, Kitagawa W, Morita H, Banno S, Imai H. Differential diagnosis of localized and systemic amyloidosis based on coagulation and fibrinolysis parameters. Amyloid. 2012;19(2):61–5. Prepublished on 2012/03/16 as doi:10.3109/13506129.2012.663425.
80. Ma Y, Kwon EH, Lee JE, Kim K, Kim HJ, Kim SH. Acquired factor X deficiency in light chain amyloidosis: a report of 2 Korean cases. Korean J Lab Med. 2011;31(3):154–6. Prepublished on 2011/07/23 as doi:10.3343/kjlm.2011.31.3.154.
81. Palladini G, Dispenzieri A, Gertz MA, et al. New criteria for response to treatment in immunoglobulin light chain amyloidosis based on free light chain measurement and cardiac biomarkers: impact on survival outcomes. J Clin Oncol. 2012;30(36):4541–9. Prepublished on 2012/10/24 as doi:10.1200/JCO.2011.37.7614.
82. Palladini G, Merlini G. Uniform risk-stratification and response criteria are paving the way to evidence-based treatment of AL amyloidosis. Oncology. 2011;25(7):633, 637–8. Prepublished on 2011/09/06 as doi.
83. Perlini S, Musca F, Salinaro F, et al. Functional correlates of N-terminal natriuretic peptide type B (NT-proBNP) response to therapy in cardiac light chain (AL) amyloidosis. Amyloid. 2011;18 Suppl 1:91–2. Prepublished on 2011/08/16 as doi:10.3109/13506129.2011.574354035.
84. Gertz MA, Lacy MQ, Dispenzieri A. Therapy for immunoglobulin light chain amyloidosis: the new and the old. Blood Rev. 2004;18(1):17–37. Prepublished on 2003/12/20 as doi.
85. Kumar SK, Gertz MA, Lacy MQ, et al. Recent improvements in survival in primary systemic amyloidosis and the importance of an early mortality risk

score. Mayo Clin Proc. 2011;86(1):12–8. Prepublished on 2011/01/05 as doi:10.4065/mcp.2010.0480.
86. Palladini G, Russo P, Nuvolone M, et al. Treatment with oral melphalan plus dexamethasone produces long-term remissions in AL amyloidosis. Blood. 2007;110(2):787–8. Prepublished on 2007/07/04 as doi:10.1182/blood-2007-02-076034.
87. Dietrich S, Schonland SO, Benner A, et al. Treatment with intravenous melphalan and dexamethasone is not able to overcome the poor prognosis of patients with newly diagnosed systemic light chain amyloidosis and severe cardiac involvement. Blood. 2010;116(4):522–8. Prepublished on 2010/04/09 as doi:10.1182/blood-2009-11-253237.
88. Lebovic D, Hoffman J, Levine BM, et al. Predictors of survival in patients with systemic light-chain amyloidosis and cardiac involvement initially ineligible for stem cell transplantation and treated with oral melphalan and dexamethasone. Br J Haematol. 2008;143(3):369–73. Prepublished on 2008/08/12 as doi:10.1111/j.1365-2141.2008.07327.x.
89. Gertz MA, Lacy MQ, Dispenzieri A, et al. Refinement in patient selection to reduce treatment-related mortality from SCT in amyloidosis. Bone Marrow Transplant. 2013;48(4):557–61. Prepublished on 2012/09/12 as doi:10.1038/bmt.2012.170.
90. Cordes S, Dispenzieri A, Lacy MQ, et al. Ten-year survival after autologous stem cell transplantation for immunoglobulin light chain amyloidosis. Cancer. 2012;118(24):6105–9. Prepublished on 2012/06/19 as doi:10.1002/cncr.27660.
91. Sher T, Hayman SR, Gertz MA. Treatment of primary systemic amyloidosis (AL): role of intensive and standard therapy. Clin Adv Hematol Oncol. 2012;10(10):644–51. Prepublished on 2012/11/29 as doi.
92. Gertz M, Lacy M, Dispenzieri A, et al. Troponin T level as an exclusion criterion for stem cell transplantation in light-chain amyloidosis. Leuk Lymphoma. 2008;49(1):36–41. Prepublished on 2008/01/19 as doi:10.1080/10428190701684518.
93. Gertz MA, Buadi FK, Hayman SR. Treatment of immunoglobulin light chain (primary or AL) amyloidosis. Oncology. 2011;25(7):620–6. Prepublished on 2011/09/06 as doi.
94. Gertz MA, Lacy MQ, Dispenzieri A, et al. Autologous stem cell transplant for immunoglobulin light chain amyloidosis: a status report. Leuk Lymphoma. 2010;51(12):2181–7. Prepublished on 2010/10/21 as doi:10.3109/10428194.2010.524329.
95. Kumar SK, Dispenzieri A, Lacy MQ, et al. Changes in serum-free light chain rather than intact monoclonal immunoglobulin levels predicts outcome following therapy in primary amyloidosis. Am J Hematol. 2011;86(3):251–5. Prepublished on 2011/02/18 as doi:10.1002/ajh.21948.
96. Jaccard A, Moreau P, Leblond V, et al. High-dose melphalan versus melphalan plus dexamethasone for AL amyloidosis. N Engl J Med. 2007;357(11):1083–93. Prepublished on 2007/09/15 as doi:10.1056/NEJMoa070484.
97. Moreau P, Jaccard A, Benboubker L, et al. Lenalidomide in combination with melphalan and dexamethasone in patients with newly diagnosed AL amyloidosis: a multicenter phase 1/2 dose-escalation study. Blood. 2010;116(23):4777–82. Prepublished on 2010/08/21 as doi:10.1182/blood-2010-07-294405.
98. Wechalekar AD, Goodman HJ, Lachmann HJ, Offer M, Hawkins PN, Gillmore JD. Safety and efficacy of risk-adapted cyclophosphamide, thalidomide, and dexamethasone in systemic AL amyloidosis. Blood. 2007;109(2):457–64. Prepublished on 2006/09/23 as doi:10.1182/blood-2006-07-035352.
99. Dispenzieri A, Dingli D, Kumar SK, et al. Discordance between serum cardiac biomarker and immunoglobulin-free light-chain response in patients with immunoglobulin light-chain amyloidosis treated with immune modulatory drugs. Am J Hematol. 2010;85(10):757–9. Prepublished on 2010/09/28 as doi:10.1002/ajh.21822.
100. Dispenzieri A, Lacy MQ, Zeldenrust SR, et al. The activity of lenalidomide with or without dexamethasone in patients with primary systemic amyloidosis. Blood. 2007;109(2):465–70. Prepublished on 2006/09/30 as doi:10.1182/blood-2006-07-032987.
101. Palladini G, Russo P, Foli A, et al. Salvage therapy with lenalidomide and dexamethasone in patients with advanced AL amyloidosis refractory to melphalan, bortezomib, and thalidomide. Ann Hematol. 2012;91(1):89–92. Prepublished on 2011/05/03 as doi:10.1007/s00277-011-1244-x.
102. Kastritis E, Terpos E, Roussou M, et al. A phase 1/2 study of lenalidomide with low-dose oral cyclophosphamide and low-dose dexamethasone (RdC) in AL amyloidosis. Blood. 2012;119(23):5384–90. Prepublished on 2012/04/21 as doi:10.1182/blood-2011-12-396903.
103. Dispenzieri A, Buadi F, Laumann K, et al. Activity of pomalidomide in patients with immunoglobulin light-chain amyloidosis. Blood. 2012;119(23):5397–404. Prepublished on 2012/04/12 as doi:10.1182/blood-2012-02-413161.
104. Reece DE, Hegenbart U, Sanchorawala V, et al. Efficacy and safety of once-weekly and twice-weekly bortezomib in patients with relapsed systemic AL amyloidosis: results of a phase 1/2 study. Blood. 2011;118(4):865–73. Prepublished on 2011/05/13 as doi:10.1182/blood-2011-02-334227.
105. Mikhael JR, Schuster SR, Jimenez-Zepeda VH, et al. Cyclophosphamide-bortezomib-dexamethasone (CyBorD) produces rapid and complete hematologic response in patients with AL amyloidosis. Blood. 2012;119(19):4391–4. Prepublished on 2012/02/15 as doi:10.1182/blood-2011-11-390930.

IgM Multiple Myeloma

23

Steven R. Schuster and Joseph Mikhael

Introduction

IgM myeloma (IgM MM) is a unique, rare subtype of multiple myeloma (MM) comprising just 0.5 % of all cases of MM. Like other types of myeloma with monoclonal gammopathies of other immunoglobulins (e.g., IgG, IgA), patients with IgM MM often have classic symptoms including hypercalcemia, anemia, renal failure, and lytic bone lesions ("CRAB" symptoms). However, unlike the other types of MM, IgM MM shares the finding of an IgM monoclonal gammopathy with another hematologic process, Waldenstrom's macroglobulinemia (WM). Clinicians are presented with a diagnostic dilemma when a patient presents with a variety of concerning symptoms and an IgM monoclonal gammopathy. Distinguishing these two diagnoses is critical as the approach to therapy and prognosis greatly differ [1, 2].

This chapter intends to summarize recent literature that help define IgM MM, highlight clinical features of this rare subtype, and review treatment considerations for this rare disease.

S.R. Schuster, M.D. • J. Mikhael, M.D. (✉)
Division of Hematology and Medical Oncology, Mayo Clinic Arizona, 13400 East Shea Boulevard, Scottsdale, AZ 85259-5494, USA
e-mail: schuster.steven1@mayo.edu; mikhael.joseph@mayo.edu

Disease Definition

Findings of IgM monoclonal gammopathy, plasma cell proliferation on bone marrow biopsy, and "CRAB" symptoms (hypercalcemia, renal impairment, anemia, and lytic bone lesions) classically distinguished the rare diagnosis of IgM MM from the more common WM. Of these symptoms, lytic bone lesions are common in MM and exceedingly rare in WM. However, some patients may not have all of these findings and symptoms can overlap between the two diagnoses, making the diagnosis difficult. Cytogenetics can help further define the differences between IgM MM and WM. Initial studies of patients with IgM MM demonstrated the presence of t(11;14), leading to cyclin D1 dysregulation, in seven of eight patients with IgM MM, but it was absent in all 17 cases of WM [3, 4]. Another group demonstrated the association of 6q-deletion with WM, and proposed it to be able to distinguish WM from IgM MGUS [5]. More importantly, whole genome sequencing of 30 patients with WM revealed an oncogenic mutation of MYD88 on chromosome 3p22 in 26 of these 30 patients (86.6 %) [6]. These studies suggested that cytogenetic findings, in conjunction with clinical features, may be utilized to define IgM MM.

Based on these observations, IgM MM is now defined as a symptomatic clonal plasma cell proliferative disorder characterized by an IgM monoclonal protein (regardless of size), 10 % or more plasma cells on bone marrow biopsy, plus

M.A. Gertz and S.V. Rajkumar (eds.), *Multiple Myeloma: Diagnosis and Treatment*,
DOI 10.1007/978-1-4614-8520-9_23, © Mayo Foundation for Medical Education and Research 2014

the presence of lytic bone lesions and/or cytogenetic abnormalities involving chromosome 14 (e.g., the translocation t(11;14)) [7].

Indeed, with so many therapeutic options available, the clinician must have a rational, risk stratified and feasible approach to patients in relapse [8]. Lytic bone lesions are objective evidence of end organ damage, and can be considered specific to MM and are not a feature of WM. High expression of IL-1β, a potent osteoclast activating factor that also upregulates IL-6, is seen in MM with no increased expression in WM [9]. Based on review of these data, cytogenetic findings of translocations involving chromosome 14 affecting cyclin D1 and lytic bone lesions are a critical component of the disease definition of IgM MM [7].

After making this definition a priori, 23 patients diagnosed with IgM MM at any of the three Mayo Clinic sites (Rochester, Arizona, Jacksonville) were reviewed. Twenty-one of these 23 patients were defined as having IgM MM based on the above definition. The remaining two patients were diagnosed based on immunophenotype analysis and may have had either WM or IgM MM early in its disease course. All 21 patients that fit the definition of IgM MM had lytic bone lesions. Of the 16 patients evaluated with FISH, six (38 %) demonstrated the t(11;14) abnormality.

The principles used to define this entity are similar to those that have been used in the past to define monoclonal gammopathy of undetermined significance (MGUS), light chain MGUS, and smoldering multiple myeloma [10]. When defining a disease entity, it is critical that the disease definition be highly specific, such that the definition can reliably differentiate it from closely related disorders. More importantly, the definition should be consistent with the expected natural history of the disease defined as such. Figure 23.1 shows the Kaplan–Meier curve for overall survival of 21 patients with IgM MM and reveals an overall survival of 30 months, more consistent with the diagnosis of MM than WM [7].

Importantly, other clinical features, such as immunophenotype analysis and the presence of anemia, hypercalcemia, and renal failure, are not specific enough to MM to be included as clinical diagnostic criteria. It would be ideal to define IgM MM in an identical way to non-IgM MM. However, IgM MM is a rare subset of MM, and it is frequently misdiagnosed and treated as WM. The definition of IgM MM must be strict and specific to allow for a clear separation from WM.

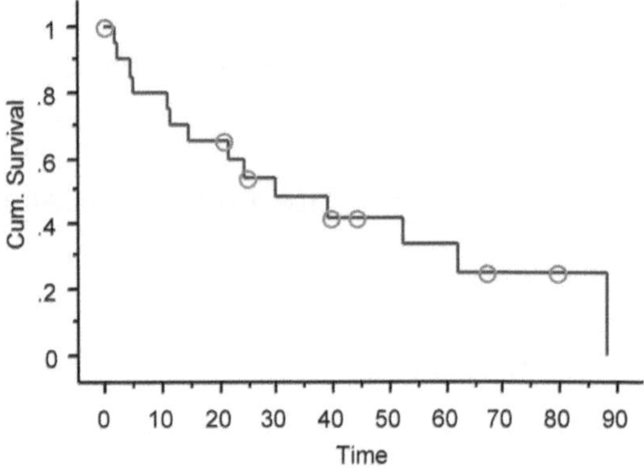

Fig. 23.1 Kaplan–Meier survival curve for 21 patients with IgM MM diagnosed at the Mayo Clinic

Previous studies show that 17.2 % of cases of MGUS have the IgM isotype [11]. IgM MGUS can be a precursor condition to IgM MM, similar to the well-documented progression seen in non-IgM MM. One of the limitations in establishing a strict disease definition is that it may miss patients who have less advanced stages of the disease.

Of the 15 cases in the Mayo Clinic series with known immunophenotype analysis, ten demonstrated the usual immunophenotype for MM (CD138+, CD20). Three cases were considered "CD20 partial," one case exhibited an unusual CD138+ CD20+ immunophenotype, and one case was CD20 positive. IgM MM is most often CD20 negative, but we do not believe it can be a stringent requirement for diagnosis based on this study.

Clinical Characteristics

In the largest review of patients with IgM Myeloma, the baseline characteristics at the time of diagnosis are typical of non-IgM MM and are shown in Table 23.1 [7]. Interestingly, 85 % of patients with IgM MM had abnormal serum

Table 23.1 Clinical characteristics of patients with IgM myeloma at time of diagnosis

Clinical characteristics	Median value (range)	Percentage of patients with abnormal level
Age, years	66 (51–77)	
Hemoglobin, g/dL	10.2 (6.1–13.3)	95.2 % (Hgb < 13.2)
Creatinine, mg/dL	1.4 (0.7–3.6)	47.6 % (Cr > 1.3)
Corrected calcium, mg/dL	10.4 (8.5–14.4)	61.9 % (Ca > 10.1)
IgM, quantitative, mg/dL	4,660 (160–11,400)	90.5 % (IgM > 300)
M-spike, mg/dL	3.1 (0.001–6.2)	47.6 % (M-spike ≥ 3)
β2-Macroglobulin, μg/mL	3.61 (1.7–8.51)	92.3 % (level > 1.8)
Viscosity, centipoise	4.0 (0.9–12.7)	85.0 % (level ≥ 1.5)
Bone marrow plasma cell, %	50 (20–100)	100 % (>10 %)

viscosity. Hyperviscosity can be an emergent situation requiring immediate plasmapheresis and can occur in both IgM MM and WM.

Treatment

WM is a disorder of B-lymphocytes with plasmacytic differentiation, and first-line therapy includes rituximab, a monoclonal antibody directed against the B-lymphocyte antigen CD20, with or without additional agents [12]. In contrast, anti-CD20 immunotherapy has not shown benefit in MM, which is consistent with the infrequent expression of this antigen by mature plasma cells [13]. Further, first-line therapy in appropriate candidates with MM should include consideration of an early autologous stem cell transplant [2, 14]. Cytogenetic analysis can risk stratify patients with MM and guidelines are available regarding consolidation with autologous stem cell transplant after initial therapy [14]. In WM, stem cell transplant may have a potential role, but it is currently reserved for refractory or relapsed disease with no first-line indication. This critical difference in first-line therapy contributes to the paramount importance of distinguishing these two entities at diagnosis. Differences in treatment of patients with newly diagnosed disease are summarized in Table 23.2.

In general, the clinical course and prognosis of WM tends to be more indolent than MM. These disparities in treatment and prognosis create the need for an accurate diagnostic approach for these two disease processes. Without it, clinicians are at risk of treating patients suboptimally. Of the 16 patients with known treatment plans in the retrospective Mayo Clinic series, six patients (37.5 %) received autologous bone marrow transplant for MM [7]. Eight patients (50 %) received initial therapy for MM, and eight patients (50 %) received initial treatment with conventional chemotherapy regimens appropriate for WM. These findings affirm the importance of a specific disease definition.

Summary

IgM MM is a rare subtype of MM with clinical features and prognosis consistent with non-IgM MM. As the finding of an IgM monoclonal gammopathy occurs in both IgM MM and WM, a specific disease definition is required to create a distinct separation between these two disease entities.

Diagnosis of IgM MM requires: (1) a symptomatic clonal plasma cell proliferative disorder, (2) an IgM monoclonal protein (regardless of size), (3) 10 % or more plasma cells on bone marrow biopsy, and (4) the presence of lytic bone lesions and/or cytogenetic abnormalities involving chromosome 14 (e.g., the translocation t(11;14)) [7].

The key studies that led to the definition of IgM MM are retrospective, and additional data would be useful to support the diagnostic criteria. The recent finding of a mutation that acts as an

Table 23.2 Recommended treatment regimens for multiple myeloma and Waldenstrom's Macroglobulinemia for newly diagnosed disease

	Waldenstrom's macroglobulinemia [1, 12]	Multiple myeloma [14–16]
Asymptomatic (e.g., SMM or SWM)[a]	Observation	Observation
Transplant candidate	Rituximab, cyclophosphamide, dexamethasone (RCD); or rituximab alone[b]	Induction followed by autologous stem cell transplantation and lenalidomide maintenance therapy[c, d]
Non-transplant candidate with good performance status	Rituximab, cyclophosphamide, dexamethasone (RCD); purine nucleoside analogs with or without rituximab; or rituximab alone	Several options: (e.g., melphalan, prednisone, thalidomide (MPT) or melphalan, prednisone, bortezomib (MPV))
Non-transplant candidate with poor performance status	Rituximab alone or Chlorambucil alone	Melphalan and prednisone (MP) or lenalidomide and dexamethasone [17]

[a] *SMM* smoldering multiple myeloma or *SWM* smoldering Waldenstrom's macroglobulinemia
[b] Avoid use of alkylating agents and nucleoside analogs in transplant candidates due to possibility of compromising future stem cell collection
[c] Induction with one of several appropriate non-alkylator-based regimens such as lenalidomide plus dexamethasone or cyclophosphamide and bortezomib plus dexamethasone
[d] Benefits of lenalidomide maintenance should be weighed against the risks in the individual patient

oncogene in WM, MYD88 L265P, can further help distinguish IgM MM from WM. Perhaps whole genome sequencing or other similar method in IgM MM will reveal additional information that alters the disease definition in the future.

As treatment differs significantly between these two diagnoses (e.g., role of stem cell transplant) and will continue to diverge with the further drug development and discovery, IgM MM is a rare subtype of MM with a unique disease definition.

References

1. Dimopoulos MA et al. Update on treatment recommendations from the Fourth International Workshop on Waldenstrom's macroglobulinemia. J Clin Oncol. 2009;27(1):120–6.
2. Harousseau J-L, Moreau P. Autologous hematopoietic stem-cell transplantation for multiple myeloma. N Eng J Med. 2009;360(25):2645–54.
3. Avet-Loiseau H et al. Translocation t(11;14)(q13;q32) is the hallmark of IgM, IgE, and nonsecretory multiple myeloma variants. Blood. 2003;101(4):1570–1.
4. Feyler S et al. IgM myeloma: a rare entity characterized by a CD20-CD56-CD117- immunophenotype and the t(11;14). Br J Haematol. 2008;140(5): 547–51.
5. Schop RFJ et al. 6q deletion discriminates Waldenstrom macroglobulinemia from IgM monoclonal gammopathy of undetermined significance. Cancer Genet Cytogenet. 2006;169(2):150–3.
6. Treon SP et al. MYD88 L265P somatic mutation in Waldenström's macroglobulinemia. N Eng J Med. 2012;367(9):826–33.
7. Schuster SR et al. IgM multiple myeloma: disease definition, prognosis, and differentiation from Waldenstrom's macroglobulinemia. Am J Hematol. 2010;85(11):853–5.
8. Avet-Loiseau H et al. 14q32 translocations discriminate IgM multiple myeloma from Waldenstrom's macroglobulinemia. Semin Oncol. 2003;30(2):153–5.
9. Donovan KA et al. IL-1beta expression in IgM monoclonal gammopathy and its relationship to multiple myeloma. Leukemia. 2002;16(3):382–5.
10. Rajkumar SV, Kyle RA, Buadi FK. Advances in the diagnosis, classification, risk stratification, and management of monoclonal gammopathy of undetermined significance: implications for recategorizing disease entities in the presence of evolving scientific evidence. Mayo Clin Proc. 2010;85(10):945–8.
11. Kyle RA et al. Prevalence of monoclonal gammopathy of undetermined significance. N Eng J Med. 2006;354(13):1362–9.
12. Ansell SM et al. Diagnosis and management of Waldenstrom macroglobulinemia: Mayo stratification of macroglobulinemia and risk-adapted therapy (mSMART) guidelines. Mayo Clin Proc. 2010;85(9): 824–33.
13. Baz R et al. Combination of rituximab and oral melphalan and prednisone in newly diagnosed multiple myeloma. Leuk Lymphoma. 2007;48(12):2338–44.

14. Kumar SK et al. Management of newly diagnosed symptomatic multiple myeloma: updated Mayo Stratification of Myeloma and Risk-Adapted Therapy (mSMART) consensus guidelines. Mayo Clin Proc. 2009;84(12):1095–110.
15. Attal M et al. Lenalidomide maintenance after stem-cell transplantation for multiple myeloma. N Eng J Med. 2012;366(19):1782–91.
16. McCarthy PL et al. Lenalidomide after stem-cell transplantation for multiple myeloma. N Eng J Med. 2012;366(19):1770–81.
17. Chanan-Khan AA et al. Lenalidomide in combination with dexamethasone improves survival and time-to-progression in patients >/=65 years old with relapsed or refractory multiple myeloma. Int J Hematol. 2012;96(2):254–62.

24 Waldenström's Macroglobulinemia

Stephen M. Ansell, Lucy S. Hodge, and Suzanne R. Hayman

Introduction

Waldenström's macroglobulinemia (WM) is a B-cell lymphoproliferative disorder defined by a lymphoplasmacytic infiltration in the bone marrow or lymphatic tissue and a monoclonal immunoglobulin M (IgM) protein in the serum [1, 2]. The infiltration of the bone marrow and extramedullary sites by malignant B-cells, as well as elevated IgM levels, accounts for the symptoms associated with this disease. This may result in patients developing constitutional symptoms, pancytopenia, organomegaly, neuropathy, symptoms associated with immunoglobulin deposition, or hyperviscosity [3, 4]. There is significant heterogeneity, however, in the symptoms with which patients present. While some patients present with the symptoms listed above, many are asymptomatic at the time of diagnosis.

Waldenström's macroglobulinemia remains incurable with current therapy with a median survival for symptomatic patients of approximately 8 years [5]. However, because many patients are diagnosed with this disease at an advanced age, approximately half of the patients die from causes unrelated to Waldenström's macroglobulinemia. Due to the incurable nature of the disease, the heterogeneity of clinical presentation, as well as the comorbid conditions and competing causes of death, the decision to treat patients and the choice of treatment can be rather complex. A number of consensus meetings have listed reasonable treatment options [6–8], but the treating physician is still faced with a difficult treatment decision in a patient with an uncommon disease.

Epidemiology

The overall incidence of Waldenström's macroglobulinemia is approximately 5 per million persons per year accounting for approximately 1–2 % of hematological cancers [9, 10]. The incidence of this disease is highest among Caucasians and is rare in other population groups [11]. The median age at diagnosis varies between 63 and 68 years, and the majority of new patients (55–70 %) are male [3].

Patients with monoclonal gammopathy of undetermined significance (MGUS) are at increased risk for progression to Waldenström's macroglobulinemia [12]. In a population-based study of 1,384 individuals with MGUS, researchers showed an increased risk factor of 46 for developing Waldenström's macroglobulinemia [12]. The rate of progression from IgM MGUS to Waldenström's macroglobulinemia was further noted to be 1.5–2 % a year [13–15].

S.M. Ansell, M.D., Ph.D. (✉) • L.S. Hodge
S.R. Hayman
Division of Hematology, Mayo Clinic,
200 First Street, South West, Rochester,
MN 55905, USA
e-mail: ansell.stephen@mayo.edu; Hodge.lucy@mayo.edu; Hayman.suzanne@mayo.edu

M.A. Gertz and S.V. Rajkumar (eds.), *Multiple Myeloma: Diagnosis and Treatment*,
DOI 10.1007/978-1-4614-8520-9_24, © Mayo Foundation for Medical Education and Research 2014

While the development of Waldenström's macroglobulinemia is thought to be sporadic, there are a few studies demonstrating familial linkage and predisposition to the disease [16–18]. Both familial clustering of Waldenström's macroglobulinemia and a notable increase (~10-fold) in the frequency of IgM MGUS in first-degree relatives of Waldenström's patients are suggestive of familial risk [17]. Under the assumption that Waldenström's macroglobulinemia and IgM MGUS share common susceptibility genes, strong linkages involving chromosomes 1q, 3q, and 4q have been identified [13]. Additionally, several studies have indicated a causal relationship between MGUS/Waldenström's macroglobulinemia and chronic antigenic stimulation [18–21]. Recently, it was shown that 11 % of patients with IgM MGUS/Waldenström's macroglobulinemia reacted with paratarg-7 (P-7), a protein of unknown function [22]. Analyses of relatives of patients with IgM MGUS/Waldenström's macroglobulinemia with an anti-P-7-paraprotein showed that the hyperphosphorylated state of this protein (pP7) is inherited as a dominant trait, and carriers of pP7 have more than a sixfold increased risk of developing IgM MGUS/Waldenström's macroglobulinemia ($p=0.001$) [22]. Thus, pP-7 is the first biological entity that provides a plausible explanation for the familial clustering of cases of IgM MGUS/Waldenström's macroglobulinemia.

Diagnosis

Attempts to better define Waldenström's macroglobulinemia have been made in recent years by the World Health Organization (WHO) Lymphoma Classification [23], the consensus group formed at the Second International Workshop on Waldenström's Macroglobulinemia [1], and the Mayo Clinic [24]. However, the respective definitions of the diagnostic criteria for Waldenström's macroglobulinemia by these groups are not identical. All groups recognize Waldenström's macroglobulinemia as a lymphoplasmacytic lymphoma associated with an IgM monoclonal protein in the serum. The WHO definition includes lymphomas other than lymphoplasmacytic lymphoma and also allows the monoclonal protein to be IgG or IgA. In contrast, the Second International Workshop on Waldenström's Macroglobulinemia restricts the diagnosis exclusively to cases with lymphoplasmacytic lymphoma and an IgM monoclonal protein. The Second International Workshop on Waldenström's Macroglobulinemia also eliminated the requirement for either a minimum amount of bone marrow involvement or a threshold concentration of IgM in the serum to fulfill the diagnosis, allowing for any detectable amount of either. In contrast, Mayo Clinic criteria require at least 10 % marrow involvement by lymphoplasmacytic lymphoma in asymptomatic patients. Furthermore, in regard to pathologic features, the WHO criteria focus predominantly on nodal involvement, whereas studies at Mayo Clinic indicate that most cases of Waldenström's macroglobulinemia are bone marrow-based.

Lymphoplasmacytic lymphoma involving either the bone marrow or the extramedullary sites typically exhibits a cytologic spectrum ranging from small lymphocytes with clumped chromatin, inconspicuous nucleoli, and sparse cytoplasm to well-formed plasma cells [1, 25]. Frequently present are "plasmacytoid lymphocytes," which have cytologic features of both lymphocytes and plasma cells, although the cytologic composition and the degree of plasmacytic differentiation vary from case to case. Nodal involvement is typically characterized by paracortical and hilar infiltration with frequent sparing of the subscapular and marginal sinuses. The bone marrow usually has some combination of nodular, paratrabecular, and interstitial infiltration; in approximately one-half of cases, plasma cells that contain Dutcher bodies are present.

The broad cytologic spectrum of the malignant cells composing Waldenström's macroglobulinemia tumors is reflected in their immunophenotypic attributes. A monotypic lymphocytic component is almost always detected, typically with high levels of surface CD19, CD20, and immunoglobulin light chain expression [25]. The lymphoid component typically lacks CD10. In approximately 40 % of cases, the lymphocytes show some degree of CD5 expression; however, these cases usually do not express this antigen as strongly as tumor cells derived from patients with chronic lymphocytic leukemia (CLL)/small lymphocytic lymphoma or mantle cell lymphoma. By comparison, the plasmacytic component expresses the same immunoglobulin light chain as the lymphocytic component, is positive for CD138 (particularly when assessed by immunohistochemistry), and shows diminished expression of B-cell-associated antigens such as CD19, CD20, and PAX5. Typically, the lymphoplasmacytic lymphoma cells are positive for surface IgM, but on the basis of the WHO criteria, they may express any immunoglobulin isotype. In cases with isotype switch, the phenotype of the plasma cells closely resembles that of myelomatous plasma cells with strong CD38 and CD138 co-expression and complete lack of CD19. Waldenström's macroglobulinemia tumor cells have also been shown to be $CD25^+$, $CD27^+$, $CD75^-$, $FMC7^+$, $Bcl2^+$, and $Bcl6^-$.

Conventional cytogenetic analyses initially determined the deletion of 6q to be the most common recurrent chromosomal abnormality in Waldenström's macroglobulinemia, identified in approximately 50 % of patients [26]. Schop et al. observed 23 % of patients with an abnormal karyotype to have a 6q deletion, while FISH analysis confirmed deletion of 6q in 42 % of patients [27]. Further studies to assess minimal areas of deletion used multiple FISH probes on the 6q arm, and a minimal deleted region at 6q23–24.3 was suggested [28]. Although the deletion of 6q is present in around 50 % of WM patients, its presence cannot be used for diagnosis as it is widely observed in several B-cell malignancies, such as marginal zone lymphomas, multiple myeloma, and chronic lymphocytic leukemias [29–32].

Preliminary data obtained from whole genome sequencing of 30 Waldenström's macroglobulinemia cases have recently been reported [33]. Strikingly, a mutation in *MYD88* leading to a leucine to proline substitution in codon 265 (L265P) was found in 90 % of the cases (46/51). The *MYD88* mutation provides a potential biomarker for differentiating Waldenström's macroglobulinemia from other related entities such as marginal zone lymphoma, where *MYD88* L265P was detected in less than 10 % of cases. Furthermore, the low prevalence of *MYD88* mutations in IgM MGUS suggests either that the abnormality is associated with disease progression or that there is more than one type of IgM MGUS, with only some types progressing to Waldenström's macroglobulinemia.

Gene expression profile (GEP) analysis of Waldenström's macroglobulinemia also provides valuable information regarding the transcriptional signature of the disease. Data gathered from two independent studies highlight the similarities and differences in GEP between Waldenström's macroglobulinemia, CLL, multiple myeloma, normal B-cells, and normal plasma cells [34, 35]. These studies specifically highlight similarities between GEP in malignant Waldenström's macroglobulinemia cells and CLL. When analyzed in unsupervised clusters, Waldenström's macroglobulinemia clustered far more with CLL expressions than with multiple myeloma [34]. Both Waldenström's macroglobulinemia and CLL have strong B-cell signatures, characterized by the common marker CD20, and are defined by low proliferation rates and a lack of IgH translocations [35]. The GEP of both Waldenström's macroglobulinemia and CLL shared similar profiles, particularly with regard to cell markers and IL-10 [34, 35].

One of the most significant findings in both studies was the high level of IL-6 transcript expression in Waldenström's macroglobulinemia compared to multiple myeloma, CLL, and normal B-cells [34, 35]. IL-6 is a potent inflammatory cytokine that stimulates both local and systemic activating physiological functions in a multitude of cells [36]. Locally, it acts to increase lymphocyte activity, including antibody production. Additionally, IL-6 plays a key role by activating the MAPK pathway. While there were no specific mutations found in *MAPK*, its activity was notably increased, likely correlating with the upregulation of IL-6 [34]. The increase in IL-6 expression in Waldenström's macroglobulinemia cells, more so than in normal B-cells, is suggestive of its autocrine activity.

Interestingly, IL-6 binds to the tyrosine kinase receptor Janus kinases (JAK) 1 and 2, which activate the downstream transcription factor Stat3, leading to increases in gene transcription, IgM production, and the activation of other signaling pathways [37]. Recently, a functional relationship between IL-6, Rantes (CCL5), and IgM secretion was observed and appears to be mediated through the JAK/STAT and PI3K pathways [38]. For the moment, the specific mechanisms of hyperimmunoglobulin secretion in Waldenström's macroglobulinemia are still not known. GEP data combined with studies of the JAK/STAT pathway could be useful in future investigations into the pathogenic role of IL-6 and the JAK/STAT pathway in Waldenström's macroglobulinemia.

Clinical Presentation

The infiltration of the bone marrow with malignant cells and the high levels of serum IgM protein circulating in patients with Waldenström's macroglobulinemia are responsible for the majority of the morbidity associated with this malignancy. While some patients with Waldenström's macroglobulinemia have no symptoms at diagnosis, others present with anemia, bleeding, or neurological complaints [39]. Additionally, as IgM protein is capable of forming large pentameric molecules in the circulation, many patients present with symptoms associated with immunoglobulin deposition and hyperviscosity syndrome [3]. Symptoms due to hyperviscosity syndrome have been reported in around 30 % of Waldenström's macroglobulinemia patients and include skin and mucosal bleeding, retinopathy and visual disturbances, and cold sensitivity [39, 40].

Due to a shortage of effective therapies and a wide variability in clinical presentation and comorbidities, the process involved in deciding when and how to treat patients diagnosed with Waldenström's macroglobulinemia can be a challenging one. However, before treatment can even be considered, an appropriate differential diagnosis between Waldenström's macroglobulinemia, IgM MGUS, and smoldering Waldenström's macroglobulinemia must be made as the appropriate treatment strategy may vary depending on the diagnosis. To this end, Mayo Clinic has created diagnostic criteria to differentiate between these IgM gammopathies based on the extent of bone marrow involvement and the presence or absence of symptomatic disease (see Table 24.1) [24].

Prognostic Factors

Following a diagnosis of Waldenström's macroglobulinemia, the next step is to determine how best to manage the disease using a risk-adapted approach. Criteria commonly used for risk stratification are shown in Table 24.2. A multicenter collaborative project known as the International Prognostic Staging System for Waldenstrom's Macroglobulinemia (IPSSWM) has incorporated five adverse prognostic factors to define three different risk groups for patients with Waldenström's

Table 24.1 Diagnostic criteria for Waldenström's macroglobulinemia [24]

Waldenström's macroglobulinemia	IgM monoclonal gammopathy (regardless of the size of the M protein) with >10 % bone marrow lymphoplasmacytic infiltration (usually intertrabecular) by small lymphocytes that exhibit plasmacytoid or plasma cell differentiation and a typical immunophenotype (surface IgM^+, $CD5^-$, $CD10^-$, $CD19^+$, $CD20^+$, $CD23^-$) that satisfactorily excludes other lymphoproliferative disorders including chronic lymphocytic leukemia and mantle cell lymphoma
IgM MGUS	Serum IgM monoclonal protein level <3 g/dL, bone marrow lymphoplasmacytic infiltration <10 %, and no evidence of anemia, constitutional symptoms, hyperviscosity, lymphadenopathy, or hepatosplenomegaly
Smoldering Waldenström's macroglobulinemia (also referred to as indolent or asymptomatic Waldenström's macroglobulinemia)	Serum IgM monoclonal protein level ≥3 g/dL and/or bone marrow lymphoplasmacytic infiltration ≥10 % and no evidence of end-organ damage, such as anemia, constitutional symptoms, hyperviscosity, lymphadenopathy, or hepatosplenomegaly, that can be attributed to a lymphoplasmacytic disorder

Table 24.2 Criteria used for risk stratification in Waldenström's macroglobulinemia

Clinical parameters
Hyperviscosity symptoms
Constitutional symptoms
Bulky lymphadenopathy/splenomegaly
Presence of symptomatic or unresponsive neuropathy
Hemolytic anemia
Laboratory parameters
Hemoglobin
Platelet count
Bone marrow infiltration

macroglobulinemia [3]. These factors include age >65 years, hemoglobin <11.5 g/dL, platelet count <100,000/μL, β_2-microglobulin >3 mg/L, and monoclonal IgM protein >7 g/dL. Patients with 0–1, 2, or >2 of these factors are considered to be at low-, intermediate-, or high-risk, respectively, with corresponding 5-year survival rates of 87, 68, and 37 % [41]. While not currently used to determine the most appropriate treatment regimen, understanding a patient's level of risk may be taken into account in deciding if and when treatment is necessary. Conversely, many asymptomatic patients may not require any therapy at all. For example, in a study by Garcia-Sanz et al., 50 % of patients who were asymptomatic at diagnosis did not require therapy for almost 3 years [39]. Similarly, one in ten patients who were managed with a watch-and-wait approach did not require therapy for 10 years. Taken together, these data underscore the need to carefully consider a patient's prognostic risk prior to the initiation of any treatment to limit therapy to only those patients in whom it is required.

Indications for Treatment

To better determine which patients with Waldenström's macroglobulinemia should receive treatment, a consensus panel at the Second International Workshop on Waldenström's Macroglobulinemia agreed that therapy should be initiated in patients with a defined set of clinical findings and/or laboratory values [42]. Specifically, treatment was deemed appropriate in patients presenting with any of the following: constitutional symptoms including fever, night sweats, or weight loss; lymphadenopathy or splenomegaly; hemoglobin <10 g/dL or a platelet count lower than 100×10^9/L due to bone marrow infiltration; complications of the disease including symptomatic sensorimotor peripheral neuropathy, systemic amyloidosis, renal insufficiency, or symptomatic cryoglobulinemia. It was also recommended that patients with IgM MGUS and smoldering (asymptomatic) Waldenström's macroglobulinemia with preserved hematologic function should be managed with a watch-and-wait approach. Additionally, all patients should be evaluated for symptoms of hyperviscosity syndrome (rarely observed with IgM levels <4 g/dL) such as visual deterioration, neurological symptoms, or unexplained bleeding, and should undergo plasmapheresis if necessary prior to receiving chemotherapy or immunotherapy [43].

Initial Therapy

Initial therapy for previously untreated patients with symptomatic Waldenström's macroglobulinemia may involve various chemotherapeutic combinations with or without the addition of the CD20$^+$-targeted antibody rituximab [44]. Rituximab is also used successfully as a single agent as first-line treatment in low-risk patients with symptomatic Waldenström's macroglobulinemia. Treatment regimens containing nucleoside analogs (NA) such as fludarabine, with combinations including fludarabine/cyclophosphamide/rituximab (FCR) and fludarabine/rituximab (FR), have demonstrated good efficacy in symptomatic Waldenström's macroglobulinemia patients. In a multicenter prospective study of 43 previously untreated patients with symptomatic disease, the FCR regimen was associated with an overall response rate of 79 %, including 11.6 % complete remission and 20.9 % very good partial remissions [45]. However, significant myelosuppression may limit the utility of this combination, as grade 3–4 neutropenia was reported in 45 % of courses and was the main reason for treatment discontinuation. Similarly, a separate study examined the combination of six cycles of fludarabine and eight infusions of rituximab (FR) [7].

Of the 43 patients enrolled, complete responses were achieved in two patients, with 81 % of patients achieving either a very good partial response or partial response. Neutropenia, thrombocytopenia, and pneumonia of grade 3 or higher were reported in 63 % of patients receiving the FR combination.

While NA-based therapies have demonstrated activity in the treatment of Waldenström's macroglobulinemia, an increased incidence of transformation to non-Hodgkin's lymphoma and the development of myelodysplasia have been associated with the use of these agents. A recent study followed 439 patients with Waldenström's macroglobulinemia, of which 193 were previously treated with NA, 136 were treated without an NA, and 110 of whom had follow-up without treatment, for a median of 5 years [46, 47]. Overall, 5 % of patients transformed and 2 % developed myelodysplasia among the NA-treated cohort whereas only one patient transformed within the other groups. These data suggest that while NA-based therapeutic regimens are effective, the additional long-term risks associated with these therapies must be taken into account by clinicians when deciding upon an initial treatment strategy for patients with Waldenström's macroglobulinemia.

Initially considered to be the standard of care, alkylating agents have also been used successfully in the treatment of Waldenström's macroglobulinemia. Over time, combinations of alkylating agents, including chlorambucil and cyclophosphamide, with vinca alkaloids, nucleoside analogs, and/or anthracyclines have been studied and deemed effective [48–51]. The addition of rituximab to alkylating agent-based combinations has further increased patient response rates. In a prospective, randomized trial including 34 Waldenström's macroglobulinemia patients treated with R-CHOP and 30 patients treated with CHOP but no rituximab, a significantly higher overall response rate was achieved in the patient group receiving chemoimmunotherapy (94 % vs. 67 %, $p=0.0085$) as compared to chemotherapy alone, with no major differences noted in toxicity [52]. Furthermore, patients in the R-CHOP group experienced a significantly longer time to treatment failure (median of 63 months) as compared to patients in the CHOP arm (22 months $p=0.0033$).

Significant activity coinciding with improved toxicity profiles has been achieved in Waldenström's macroglobulinemia with other alkylating agents administered in combination with rituximab, suggesting that such regimens may be preferable as initial therapy for this disease [43]. For example, a regimen including dexamethasone, rituximab, and cyclophosphamide (DRC) yielded an overall response rate of 83 % in previously untreated Waldenström's macroglobulinemia patients, of which 7 % were complete responders [53]. Furthermore, only 9 % of patients experienced grade 3 or 4 neutropenia. Alkylating agents combined with rituximab are also useful in treating relapsed or refractory patients. Treon et al. reported an overall response rate of 83.3 % in 30 such WM patients treated with bendamustine in combination with rituximab (BR) [54]. While the therapy was well tolerated, there was an increased incidence of myelosuppression in patients who had previously been treated with nucleoside analogs, as has been reported previously [47]. Further support for the use of BR as initial therapy comes from a comparison with R-CHOP in 41 Waldenström's macroglobulinemia patients [55]. When compared with R-CHOP, treatment with BR resulted in fewer relapses, was better tolerated, and was associated with a longer progression-free survival, despite identical response rates for both regimens.

Rapid and durable patient responses have also been achieved with the proteasome inhibitor bortezomib when used in combination with rituximab in Waldenström's macroglobulinemia. When bortezomib, dexamethasone, and rituximab (BDR) were administered to 23 previously untreated, but symptomatic Waldenström's macroglobulinemia patients, overall response rates neared 96 % with responses occurring at a median of 1.4 months [56]. However, a high incidence of peripheral neuropathy led to the discontinuation of bortezomib in 61 % of patients. A separate study by Ghobrial et al. reported overall response rates of 88 % when bortezomib and rituximab were administered concurrently in patients with symptomatic Waldenström's macroglobulinemia

[57]. However, in this study, no grade 3 or 4 neuropathies were documented, with the most significant adverse event being neutropenia, which occurred in 12 % of patients.

The therapeutic benefit of adding rituximab to chemotherapeutic regimens for the treatment of Waldenström's macroglobulinemia has been well documented. However, when used as a single agent, rituximab has been associated with response rates ranging from 29 to 65 %, making single agent rituximab a viable option in the treatment of Waldenström's macroglobulinemia, specifically in low-risk patients with symptomatic disease and modest hematologic compromise and in patients with IgM-related neuropathy requiring treatment [43]. In a study of 69 symptomatic patients, 35 of whom had received treatment previously, overall response rates of 52 % were reported following administration of rituximab as a single agent [58]. Yet, when using rituximab as a single agent, clinicians must be made aware of the paradoxical rituximab-associated increase in IgM protein levels occurring in some patients, known as the rituximab "flare" [43, 59]. While IgM levels may remain elevated out to 4 months following treatment with rituximab, this does not necessarily indicate a treatment failure, although additional plasmapheresis may be necessary to alleviate symptoms of hyperviscosity.

Based on the array of agents that are clinically active in this disease, a risk-adapted approach to the management of Waldenström's macroglobulinemia is recommended. Three groups of patients can be identified [43]. Patients with IgM MGUS or smoldering (asymptomatic) Waldenström's macroglobulinemia and preserved hematological function constitute a low-risk group. Symptomatic Waldenström's macroglobulinemia patients with modest hematological compromise, IgM-related neuropathy, or hemolytic anemia have an intermediate risk of disease progression and subsequent morbidity or mortality. Waldenström's macroglobulinemia patients who have significant constitutional symptoms, profound hematological compromise, bulky disease, or hyperviscosity have a high-risk of disease progression and early mortality.

Utilizing the risk groups outlined above, we recommend the following: (1) Patients with IgM MGUS or smoldering (asymptomatic) Waldenström's macroglobulinemia and preserved hematological function should be observed without initial pharmacotherapy. (2) Symptomatic Waldenström's macroglobulinemia patients with modest hematological compromise, IgM-related neuropathy requiring treatment, or hemolytic anemia unresponsive to corticosteroids should receive standard doses of rituximab alone without maintenance therapy. (3) Waldenström's macroglobulinemia patients who have significant constitutional symptoms, profound hematological compromise, bulky disease, or hyperviscosity should be treated with the DRC regimen (dexamethasone, rituximab, cyclophosphamide). Any patient with symptoms of hyperviscosity should first be started on plasmapheresis (see mSMART algorithm in Fig. 24.1) [43].

Management of Relapsed Disease

Despite the high overall response rates associated with the aforementioned treatment regimens and the introduction of new therapeutic agents in the past few decades, studies have not demonstrated a significant improvement in the outcome of patients with Waldenström's macroglobulinemia treated over the last 25 years [60]. These data underscore the need for more effective agents to further improve patient survival, especially in those who have failed previous treatment regimens. Fortunately, new therapies and treatment combinations are currently in clinical testing in patients with refractory and relapsed disease. For example, drugs classified as immunomodulators (IMiDs), including thalidomide and lenalidomide, have been studied in Waldenström's macroglobulinemia in combination with rituximab as these agents enhance rituximab-mediated, antibody-dependent, cell-mediated cytotoxicity [61]. However, despite relatively high overall response rates, the use of both thalidomide and lenalidomide has been associated with substantial toxicity [62]. In the case of lenalidomide and rituximab, the clinical trial was closed early due

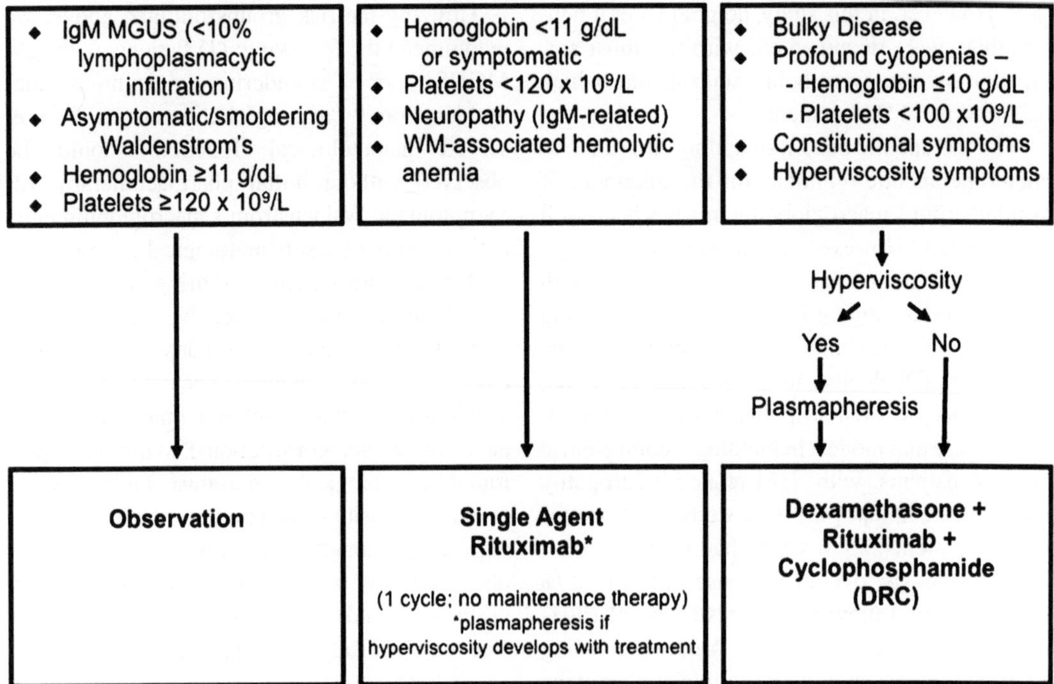

Fig. 24.1 Mayo Clinic (Mayo stratification of macroglobulinemia and risk-adapted therapy [mSMART]) consensus for management of newly diagnosed Waldenström's macroglobulinemia (WM) [43]. MGUS = monoclonal gammopathy of undetermined significance. SI conversion factor: To convert hemoglobin values to g/L, multiply by 10

to reports of significant anemia, which occurred in 13 of 16 enrolled patients [63]. Thus, while these agents have demonstrated significant activity and durable responses, further studies are necessary to identify the optimal dose of drug required to achieve maximal activity with minimal toxicity.

The mammalian target of rapamycin (mTOR) inhibitor everolimus has also been studied in Waldenström's macroglobulinemia, due to the known role of the PI3K/Akt/mTOR signal transduction pathway as a driver of tumor survival in various hematologic malignancies, including Waldenström's macroglobulinemia [64]. When used as a single agent in 50 patients with symptomatic, relapsed, or refractory Waldenström's macroglobulinemia, overall response rates reached 70 % with a 12-month progression-free survival of 62 % [65]. However, significant toxicities occurred with the use of everolimus, with 56 % of patients developing grade 3 or higher toxicities requiring dose reductions in 52 % of patients. Yet while bearing in mind its toxicity profile, single agent everolimus appears to be a potential new therapeutic option for the treatment of Waldenström's macroglobulinemia.

As preclinical studies indicated activity of the nonselective histone deacetylase inhibitor panobinostat in Waldenström's macroglobulinemia cell lines, this agent has also been studied in a phase II trial of 27 patients with refractory or relapsed/refractory disease [66]. Panobinostat was observed to be an active therapeutic agent in this patient population with an overall response rate of 60 %. Due to a high incidence of hematological toxicities, the initial protocol required modifications to decrease the panobinostat dose from 30 mg 3 times per week to 25 mg 3 times per week; the lower dosing schedule was better tolerated.

In addition to chemotherapeutics, novel immunotherapies targeting CD20 are currently in development in an effort to try and improve upon the response rates achieved with single agent

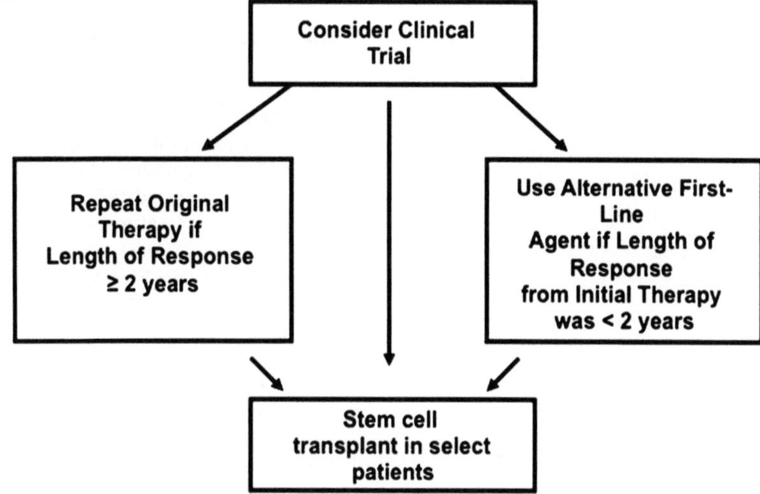

Fig. 24.2 Mayo Clinic (Mayo stratification of macroglobulinemia and risk-adapted therapy [mSMART]) consensus for management of relapsed Waldenström's macroglobulinemia [43]

rituximab while limiting the rituximab "flare" in IgM. One such monoclonal antibody is ofatumumab (OFA), which targets an epitope encompassing both the large and small extracellular loops of CD20, whereas rituximab targets only the large loop alone [67]. OFA has been studied as a single agent in a cohort of 37 patients with Waldenström's macroglobulinemia, 28 of whom had received a median of three prior therapies [68]. An overall response rate of 59 % was reported along with a lower incidence of IgM "flare" as compared to rituximab. The toxicity profile, which included the development of infection in 15 patients, was deemed to be acceptable, making OFA another potential therapeutic option in Waldenström's macroglobulinemia, especially in patients with refractory disease.

Lastly, stem cell transplantation is another potential option for the treatment of patients with advanced Waldenström's macroglobulinemia. Autologous stem cell transplants are relatively well tolerated and long-lasting complete responses have been reported [43]. In a retrospective analysis of 158 young, but heavily pretreated, patients with Waldenström's macroglobulinemia who underwent autologous stem cell transplantation (ASCT), nearly half of the patients remained in remission at 5 years, with a non-relapse mortality rate of only 3.8 %. Five-year progression-free survival and overall survival rates were 40 % and 68.5 %, respectively [69]. While additional prospective studies are warranted, these initial data suggest that ASCT may have a place in the treatment of Waldenström's macroglobulinemia, especially in younger, heavily pretreated, or relapsed patients. A similar retrospective study has also been performed to assess the role of allogeneic stem cell transplantation (alloSCT) in the treatment of Waldenström's macroglobulinemia. Kyriakou et al. assessed 86 patients with Waldenström's macroglobulinemia who received an allograft after either myeloablative (MAC) or reduced-intensity conditioning (RIC) regimens [69]. However, both the MAC and RIC regimens were associated with significantly higher risks of non-relapse mortality at 3 years (33 % and 23 %, respectively) as compared with ASCT, and therefore alloSCT is not considered an appropriate therapeutic option for patients with Waldenström's macroglobulinemia outside of a clinical trial.

As there is currently no standard approach to the management of patients with relapsed Waldenström's macroglobulinemia, our approach (Fig. 24.2) is to consider all patients for participation in a clinical trial either as definitive therapy for their disease or as preparative therapy prior to transplant [43]. For patients who are ineligible or unwilling to go on a clinical trial, the choice of therapy is determined by their response to frontline treatment. Because responses to initial therapies are often delayed and can occur 12 months or more after initiating treatment, we recommend using a 2-year cutoff to determine treatment. For patients with a durable response that lasted >2 years, the original therapy can be repeated. For patients who have an inadequate response to initial therapy or a response lasting <2 years, an alternative agent or combination should be used. An autologous stem cell transplant should be considered in all eligible patients with relapsed disease.

Summary

Waldenström's macroglobulinemia is a rare disease, and practicing hematologists and oncologists may infrequently treat these patients. Patients may present with a spectrum of clinical findings, and many patients do not require treatment initially. When patients do require therapy, it is important to select therapies that do not negatively impact future treatment options. To provide a simple risk-adapted approach to managing patients with Waldenström's macroglobulinemia, we have outlined a rational approach to this disease [43]. These recommendations are regularly modified as new data become available and the most current guidelines are available at www.mSMART.org.

References

1. Owen RG, Treon SP, Al-Katib A, et al. Clinicopathological definition of Waldenstrom's macroglobulinemia: consensus panel recommendations from the Second International Workshop on Waldenstrom's macroglobulinemia. Semin Oncol. 2003;30:110–5.
2. Dimopoulos MA, Kyle RA, Anagnostopoulos A, Treon SP. Diagnosis and management of Waldenstrom's macroglobulinemia. J Clin Oncol. 2005; 23:1564–77.
3. Dimopoulos MA, Panayiotidis P, Moulopoulos LA, Sfikakis P, Dalakas M. Waldenstrom's macroglobulinemia: clinical features, complications, and management. J Clin Oncol. 2000;18:214–26.
4. Vijay A, Gertz MA. Waldenstrom macroglobulinemia. Blood. 2007;109:5096–103.
5. Kastritis E, Kyrtsonis MC, Hatjiharissi E, et al. No significant improvement in the outcome of patients with Waldenström's macroglobulinemia treated over the last 25 years. Am J Hematol. 2011;86(6):479–83.
6. Gertz MA, Anagnostopoulos A, Anderson K, et al. Treatment recommendations in Waldenstrom's macroglobulinemia: consensus panel recommendations from the second international workshop on Waldenstrom's macroglobulinemia. Semin Oncol. 2003;30:121–6.
7. Treon SP, Gertz MA, Dimopoulos M, et al. Update on treatment recommendations from the third international workshop on Waldenstrom's macroglobulinemia. Blood. 2006;107:3442–6.
8. Dimopoulos MA, Gertz MA, Kastritis E, et al. Update on treatment recommendations from the fourth international workshop on Waldenstrom's macroglobulinemia. J Clin Oncol. 2009;27:120–6.
9. Herrinton LJ, Weiss NS. Incidence of Waldenstrom's macroglobulinemia. Blood. 1993;82:3148–50.
10. Groves FD, Travis LB, Devesa SS, Ries LA, Fraumeni Jr JF. Waldenstrom's macroglobulinemia: incidence patterns in the United States, 1988–1994. Cancer. 1998;82:1078–81.
11. Benjamin M, Reddy S, Brawley OW. Myeloma and race: a review of the literature. Cancer Metastasis Rev. 2003;22:87–93.
12. Kyle RA, Therneau TM, Rajkumar SV, et al. A long-term study of prognosis in monoclonal gammopathy of undetermined significance. N Engl J Med. 2002;346(8):564–9.
13. McMaster ML, Goldin LR, Bai Y, et al. Genome wide linkage screen for Waldenstrom macroglobulinemia susceptibility loci in high-risk families. Am J Hum Genet. 2006;79(4):695–701.
14. Kyle RA, Therneau TM, Rajkumar SV, et al. Long-term follow-up of IgM monoclonal gammopathy of undetermined significance. Blood. 2003;102(10): 3759–64.
15. Kyle RA, Therneau TM, Rajkumar SV, et al. Long-term follow-up of IgM monoclonal gammopathy of undetermined significance. Semin Oncol. 2003;30(2): 169–71.
16. Treon SP, Hunter ZR, Aggarwal A, et al. Characterization of familial Waldenstrom's macroglobulinemia. Ann Oncol. 2006;17(3):488–94.
17. McMaster ML. Familial Waldenstrom's macroglobulinemia. Semin Oncol. 2003;30(2):146–52.
18. Royer RH, Koshiol J, Giambarresi TR, et al. Differential characteristics of Waldenstrom macroglobulinemia according to patterns of familial aggregation. Blood. 2010;115(22):4464–71.
19. Aoki H, Takishita M, Kosaka M, Saito S. Frequent somatic mutations in D and/or JH segments of Ig gene in Waldenstrom's macroglobulinemia and chronic lymphocytic leukemia (CLL) with Richter's syndrome but not in common CLL. Blood. 1995;85(7): 1913–9.

20. Wagner SD, Martinelli V, Luzzatto L. Similar patterns of V kappa gene usage but different degrees of somatic mutation in hairy cell leukemia, prolymphocytic leukemia, Waldenstrom's macroglobulinemia, and myeloma. Blood. 1994;83(12):3647–53.
21. Martin-Jimenez P, Garcia-Sanz R, Balanzategui A, et al. Molecular characterization of heavy chain immunoglobulin gene rearrangements in Waldenstrom's macroglobulinemia and IgM monoclonal gammopathy of undetermined significance. Haematologica. 2007;92(5):635–42.
22. Grass S, Preuss KD, Wikowicz A, et al. Hyperphosphorylated paratarg-7: a new molecularly defined risk factor for monoclonal gammopathy of undetermined significance of the IgM type and Waldenstrom macroglobulinemia. Blood. 2011; 117(10):2918–23.
23. Swerdlow SH, Campo E, Harris NL, et al. WHO classification of tumours of haematopoietic and lymphoid tissues, vol. 2. 4th ed. Geneva, Switzerland: International Agency for Research on Cancer (IARC); 2008. p. 441.
24. Kyle RA, Rajkumar SV. Criteria for diagnosis, staging, risk stratification and response assessment of multiple myeloma. Leukemia. 2009;23:3–9.
25. Morice WG, Chen D, Kurtin PJ, Hanson CA, McPhail ED. Novel immunophenotypic features of marrow lymphoplasmacytic lymphoma and correlation with Waldenstrom's macroglobulinemia. Mod Pathol. 2009;22:807–16.
26. Mansoor A, Medeiros LJ, Weber DM, et al. Cytogenetic findings in lymphoplasmacytic lymphoma/ Waldenstrom macroglobulinemia. Chromosomal abnormalities are associated with the polymorphous subtype and an aggressive clinical course. Am J Clin Pathol. 2001;116(4):543–9.
27. Schop RF, Kuehl WM, Van Wier SA, et al. Waldenstrom macroglobulinemia neoplastic cells lack immunoglobulin heavy chain locus translocations but have frequent 6q deletions. Blood. 2002; 100(8):2996–3001.
28. Schop RF, Van Wier SA, Xu R, et al. 6q deletion discriminates Waldenstrom macroglobulinemia from IgM monoclonal gammopathy of undetermined significance. Cancer Genet Cytogenet. 2006;169(2): 150–3.
29. Braggio E, Dogan A, Keats JJ, et al. Genomic analysis of marginal zone and lymphoplasmacytic lymphomas identified common and disease-specific abnormalities. Mod Pathol. 2012;25(5):651–60.
30. Ferreira BI, Garcia JF, Suela J, et al. Comparative genome profiling across subtypes of lowgrade B-cell lymphoma identifies type-specific and common aberrations that target genes with a role in B-cell neoplasia. Haematologica. 2008;93(5):670–9.
31. Rinaldi A, Mian M, Chigrinova E, et al. Genome-wide DNA profiling of marginal zone lymphomas identifies subtype-specific lesions with an impact on the clinical outcome. Blood. 2011;117(5):1595–604.
32. Dohner H, Stilgenbauer S, Benner A, et al. Genomic aberrations and survival in chronic lymphocytic leukemia. N Engl J Med. 2000;343(26):1910–6.
33. Treon SP, Xu L, Yang G, et al. MYD88 L265P somatic mutation in Waldenström's macroglobulinemia. N Engl J Med. 2012;367(9):826–33.
34. Chng WJ, Schop RF, Price-Troska T, et al. Gene expression profiling of Waldenstrom macroglobulinemia reveals a phenotype more similar to chronic lymphocytic leukemia than multiple myeloma. Blood. 2006;108(8):2755–63.
35. Gutierrez NC, Ocio EM, de Las Rivas J, et al. Gene expression profiling of B lymphocytes and plasma cells from Waldenstrom's macroglobulinemia: comparison with expression patterns of the same cell counterparts from chronic lymphocytic leukemia, multiple myeloma and normal individuals. Leukemia. 2007;21(3):541–9.
36. Hodge DR, Hurt EM, Farrar WL. The role of IL-6 and STAT3 in inflammation and cancer. Eur J Cancer. 2005;41(16):2502–12.
37. Hodge LS, Ansell SM. Jak/stat pathway in Waldenstrom's macroglobulinemia. Clin Lymphoma Myeloma Leuk. 2011;11(1):112–4.
38. Elsawa SF, Novak AJ, Ziesmer SC, et al. Comprehensive analysis of tumor microenvironment cytokines in waldenstrom macroglobulinemia identifies CCL5 as a novel modulator of IL-6 activity. Blood. 2011;118(20):5540–9.
39. Garcia-Sanz R, Montoto S, Torrequebrada A, et al. Waldenstrom macroglobulinemia: presenting features and outcome in a series with 217 cases. Br J Haematol. 2001;115:575–82.
40. Stone MJ, Pascual V. Pathophysiology of Waldenstrom's macroglobulinemia. Haematologica. 2010;95:359–64.
41. Morel P, Duhamel A, Gobbi P, et al. International prognostic scoring system for Waldenstrom macroglobulinemia. Blood. 2009;113:4163–70.
42. Kyle RA, Treon SP, Alexanian R, et al. Prognostic markers and criteria to initiate therapy in Waldenstrom's macroglobulinemia: consensus panel recommendations from the second international workshop on Waldenstrom's macroglobulinemia. Semin Oncol. 2003;30:116–20.
43. Ansell SM, Kyle RA, Reeder CB, et al. Diagnosis and management of Waldenstrom macroglobulinemia: mayo stratification of macroglobulinemia and risk-adapted therapy (mSMART) guidelines. Mayo Clin Proc. 2010;85:824–33.
44. Tedeschi A, Benevolo G, Varettoni M, et al. Fludarabine plus cyclophosphamide and rituximab in Waldenstrom macroglobulinemia: an effective but myelosuppressive regimen to be offered to patients with advanced disease. Cancer. 2012;118:434–43.
45. Treon SP, Branagan AR, Ioakimidis L, et al. Long-term outcomes to fludarabine and rituximab in Waldenstrom macroglobulinemia. Blood. 2009;113: 3673–8.

46. Leleu X, Soumerai J, Roccaro A, et al. Increased incidence of transformation and myelodysplasia/acute leukemia in patients with Waldenstrom macroglobulinemia treated with nucleoside analogs. J Clin Oncol. 2009;27:250–5.
47. Annibali O, Petrucci MT, Martini V, et al. Treatment of 72 newly diagnosed Waldenstrom macroglobulinemia cases with oral melphalan, cyclophosphamide, and prednisone: results and cost analysis. Cancer. 2005;103:582–7.
48. Petrucci MT, Avvisati G, Tribalto M, Giovangrossi P, Mandelli F. Waldenstrom's Macroglobulinaemia: results of a combined oral treatment in 34 newly diagnosed patients. J Intern Med. 1989;226:443–7.
49. Leblond V, Levy V, Maloisel F, et al. Multicenter, randomized comparative trial of fludarabine and the combination of cyclophosphamide-doxorubicin-prednisone in 92 patients with Waldenstrom macroglobulinemia in first relapse or with primary refractory disease. Blood. 2001;98:2640–4.
50. Tamburini J, Levy V, Chaleteix C, Fermand JP, Delmer A, Stalniewicz L, et al. Fludarabine plus cyclophosphamide in Waldenstrom's macroglobulinemia: results in 49 patients. Leukemia. 2005;19: 1831–4.
51. Buske C, Hoster E, Dreyling M, et al. The addition of rituximab to front-line therapy with CHOP (R-CHOP) results in a higher response rate and longer time to treatment failure in patients with lymphoplasmacytic lymphoma: results of a randomized trial of the German Low-Grade Lymphoma Study Group (GLSG). Leukemia. 2009;23:153–61.
52. Dimopoulos MA, Anagnostopoulos A, Kyrtsonis MC, et al. Primary treatment of Waldenstrom macroglobulinemia with dexamethasone, rituximab, and cyclophosphamide. J Clin Oncol. 2007;25:3344–9.
53. Treon SP, Hanzis C, Tripsas C, et al. Bendamustine therapy in patients with relapsed or refractory Waldenstrom's macroglobulinemia. Clin Lymphoma Myeloma Leuk. 2011;11:133–5.
54. Rummel MJ, Niederle N, von Grunhagen U, et al. Bendamustine plus rituximab versus CHOP plus rituximab as first-line treatment in patients with indolent lymphomas and Waldenstrom's macroglobulinemia. In: Sixth International Workshop on Waldenstrom's Macroglobulinemia. Venice, Italy 2010.
55. Treon SP, Ioakimidis L, Soumerai JD, et al. Primary therapy of Waldenstrom macroglobulinemia with bortezomib, dexamethasone, and rituximab: WMCTG clinical trial 05–180. J Clin Oncol. 2009;27:3830–5.
56. Ghobrial IM, Xie W, Padmanabhan S, et al. Phase II trial of weekly bortezomib in combination with rituximab in untreated patients with Waldenstrom macroglobulinemia. Am J Hematol. 2010;85:670–4.
57. Gertz MA, Rue M, Blood E, Kaminer LS, Vesole DH, Greipp PR. Multicenter phase 2 trial of rituximab for Waldenstrom macroglobulinemia (WM): an Eastern Cooperative Oncology Group Study (E3A98). Leuk Lymphoma. 2004;45:2047–55.
58. Ghobrial IM, Fonseca R, Greipp PR, et al. Initial immunoglobulin M 'flare' after rituximab therapy in patients diagnosed with Waldenstrom macroglobulinemia. Cancer. 2004;101:2593–8.
59. Kastritis E, Kyrtsonis M-C, Hatjiharissi E, et al. No significant improvement in the outcome of patients with Waldenström's macroglobulinemia treated over the last 25 years. Am J Hematol. 2011;86:479–83.
60. Davies FE, Raje N, Hideshima T, et al. Thalidomide and immunomodulatory derivatives augment natural killer cell cytotoxicity in multiple myeloma. Blood. 2001;98:210–6.
61. Treon SP, Soumerai JD, Branagan AR, et al. Thalidomide and rituximab in Waldenstrom macroglobulinemia. Blood. 2008;112:4452–7.
62. Treon SP, Soumerai JD, Branagan AR, et al. Lenalidomide and rituximab in Waldenstrom's macroglobulinemia. Clin Cancer Res. 2009;15:355–60.
63. Leleu X, Jia X, Runnels J, et al. The Akt pathway regulates survival and homing in Waldenstrom macroglobulinemia. Blood. 2007;110:4417–26.
64. Ghobrial IM, Gertz M, Laplant B, et al. Phase II trial of the oral mammalian target of rapamycin inhibitor everolimus in relapsed or refractory Waldenstrom macroglobulinemia. J Clin Oncol. 2010;28:1408–14.
65. Ghobrial IM, Poon T, Rourke M, et al. Phase II trial of single agent pabinostat (LBH589) in relapsed or relapsed/refractory Waldenstrom macroglobulinemia. San Diego, CA: American Society of Hematology; 2010.
66. Cheson BD. Ofatumumab, a novel anti-CD20 monoclonal antibody for the treatment of B-cell malignancies. J Clin Oncol. 2010;28:3525–30.
67. Furman RR, Eradat H, DiRienzo CG, et al. A phase II trial of ofatumumab in subjects with Waldenstroms macroglobulinemia. San Diego, CA: American Society for Hematology; 2011.
68. Kyriakou C, Canals C, Sibon D, et al. High-dose therapy and autologous stem-cell transplantation in Waldenstrom macroglobulinemia: the Lymphoma Working Party of the European Group for Blood and Marrow Transplantation. J Clin Oncol. 2010;28: 2227–32.
69. Kyriakou C, Canals C, Cornelissen JJ, et al. Allogeneic stem-cell transplantation in patients with Waldenstrom macroglobulinemia: report from the Lymphoma Working Party of the European Group for Blood and Marrow Transplantation. J Clin Oncol. 2010;28: 4926–34.

Index

M.A. Gertz and S.V. Rajkumar (eds.), *Multiple Myeloma: Diagnosis and Treatment*,
DOI 10.1007/978-1-4614-8520-9, © Mayo Foundation for Medical Education and Research 2014

MIX
Papier aus verantwortungsvollen Quellen
Paper from responsible sources
FSC® C105338

If you have any concerns about our products,
you can contact us on
ProductSafety@springernature.com

In case Publisher is established outside the EU,
the EU authorized representative is:
Springer Nature Customer Service Center GmbH
Europaplatz 3, 69115 Heidelberg, Germany

Printed by Libri Plureos GmbH
in Hamburg, Germany